Atlas of orthotics

BIOMECHANICAL PRINCIPLES AND APPLICATION

Atlas of orthotics

BIOMECHANICAL PRINCIPLES AND APPLICATION

American Academy of Orthopaedic Surgeons

with 836 illustrations

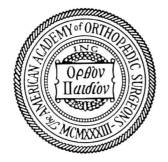

Saint Louis

The C. V. Mosby Company

1975

Library of Congress Cataloging in Publication Data

American Academy of Orthopaedic Surgeons.
　　Atlas of orthotics.

　　Bibliography: p.
　　Includes index.
　　1. Orthopedic apparatus.　I. Title.　[DNLM:
1. Biomechanics.　2. Orthopedic equipment. WE172
A512a]
RD755.A43 1975　　　　617'.307　　　　75-22185
ISBN 0-8016-0021-9

TS/NK/B　9　8　7　6　5　4　3　2　1

Contributors

ANNE G. ALEXANDER, R.P.T.

Chief of Rehabilitation, Prosthetic Research Study, Seattle, Washington.

NORMAN BERGER, M.S.

Associate Co-ordinator, Prosthetics and Orthotics, New York University Post-Graduate Medical School, New York, New York.

THOMAS R. BIDWELL, C.P.O.

Attending Orthotist, Northwestern University Prosthetic and Orthotic Education, Chicago, Illinois.

WALTER P. BLOUNT, M.D.

Clinical Professor of Orthopaedic Surgery, Emeritus, Medical College of Wisconsin, Orthopaedic Surgery, Milwaukee, Wisconsin.

JOHN H. BOWKER, M.D.

Professor, Department of Orthopaedic Surgery, University of Arkansas College of Medicine, Little Rock, Arkansas.

WILTON H. BUNCH, M.D., Ph.D.

Professor and Chairman of the Department of Orthopaedic Surgery, Loyola University, Maywood, Illinois.

ERNEST M. BURGESS, M.D.

Clinical Professor in Orthopaedic Surgery, University of Washington, School of Medicine, Seattle; Principal Investigator, Prosthetics Research Study, Seattle, Washington.

ALBERT H. BURSTEIN, B.M.E., M.M.E., Ph.D.

Associate Professor, Department of Mechanical Design, School of Engineering; Associate Professor, Department of Surgery, The School of Medicine, Case Western Reserve University, Cleveland, Ohio.

JAMES M. CARY, M.D.

Assistant Clinical Professor of Orthopaedic Surgery, Yale University School of Medicine, New Haven; Assistant Medical Director, Newington Children's Hospital, Newington, Connecticut.

MARIA T. COTCH, M.D.

Resident, Los Angeles County Medical Center, Los Angeles, California.

RONALD L. DeWALD, M.D.

Professor, Orthopaedic Surgery, Rush Medical College, Chicago, Illinois.

ARTHUR GUILFORD, C.P.O.

Rancho Los Amigos Hospital, Downey, California.

†CAMERON B. HALL, M.D.

Formerly Associate Clinical Professor of Surgery (Orthopaedics), School of Medicine, University of California at Los Angeles, Los Angeles, California.

————————

†Deceased.

MELVIN H. JAHSS, M.D.

Associate Professor of Orthopaedic Surgery, Mount Sinai School of Medicine; Chief, Foot Services, Hospital for Joint Disease, New York; Chief, Foot Services, Mount Sinai Hospital, New York, New York.

RICHARD H. JONES, M.D.

Clinical Assistant Professor, Orthopaedic Surgery, University of Minnesota, Minneapolis, Minnesota.

HENRY LaROCCA, M.D.

Associate Professor, Section of Orthopaedic Surgery, Tulane University School of Medicine, New Orleans, Louisiana.

MAURICE LeBLANC, M.S.M.E., C.P.

Chief, Department of Rehabilitation Engineering, Children's Hospital at Stanford, Palo Alto, California; Formerly Staff Engineer, Committee on Prosthetics Research and Development, National Academy of Sciences–National Research Council, Washington, D.C.

RALPH LUSSKIN, M.D.

Professor of Clinical Orthopaedic Surgery, Department of Orthopaedic Surgery, New York University School of Medicine, New York, New York.

NEWTON C. McCOLLOUGH, III, M.D.

Associate Professor, Department of Orthopaedics and Rehabilitation, Director of Rehabilitation, University of Miami School of Medicine, Miami, Florida.

COLIN A. McLAURIN, Sc.D.

Director, Rehabilitation Engineering, Ontario Crippled Children's Centre, Toronto, Ontario, Canada.

ROGER A. MANN, M.D.

Assistant Clinical Professor, Department of Orthopaedic Surgery, California Medical School, San Francisco; Director, Gait Analysis Laboratory, Shriners' Hospital, San Francisco, California.

KEITH L. MARKOLF, Ph.D.

Assistant Professor of Bioengineering, Department of Surgery, Division of Orthopaedic Surgery, University of California, Los Angeles, California.

JOHN H. MOE, M.D.

Director, Twin City Scoliosis Center, Professor Emeritus, University of Minnesota, Minneapolis, Minnesota.

JAMES M. MORRIS, M.D.

Associate Professor of Orthopaedic Surgery, Department of Orthopaedic Surgery, University of California, School of Medicine, San Francisco, California.

EUGENE F. MURPHY, Ph.D.

Director, Research Center for Prosthetics, Veterans Administration, New York, New York.

PAUL H. NEWELL, Jr., P.E., Ph.D.

President, New Jersey Institute of Technology, Newark, New Jersey.

TIMOTHY J. NUGENT, Ph.D.

Professor and Director, Rehabilitation-Education Services and Rehabilitation-Education Center, University of Illinois, Urbana, Illinois.

EDWARD PEIZER, Ph.D.

Assistant Director, Research Center for Prosthetics, Veterans Administration, New York, New York.

JACQUELIN PERRY, M.D.

Chief, Kinesiology Service, Rancho Los Amigos Hospital, Downey, California; Professor of Surgery (Orthopedic), University of Southern California School of Medicine, Los Angeles, California.

ANTON J. REICHENBERGER

Project Manager, Component Development, Bioengineering Research Service, Prosthetics Center, Veterans Administration, New York, New York.

JOHN ROGERS, M.D.

Director of Tissue Trauma Study Group, Rehabilitation Engineering Center of Rancho Los Amigos Hospital, University of Southern California, Los Angeles, California.

AUGUSTO SARMIENTO, M.D.

Professor and Chairman, Department of Orthopaedics and Rehabilitation, University of Miami School of Medicine, Miami, Florida.

SHAHAN K. SARRAFIAN, M.D., F.A.C.S.

Assistant Professor, Orthopaedic Surgery, Northwestern University Medical School, Chicago, Illinois.

WILLIAM F. SINCLAIR, C.P.O.

Adjunct Instructor, Department of Orthopaedics and Rehabilitation, University of Miami School of Medicine, Miami, Florida.

ANTHONY STAROS, M.S.M.E., P.E.

Director, Prosthetics Center, Veterans Administration, New York, New York.

ROBERT G. THOMPSON, M.D.

Associate Professor, Department of Orthopaedic Surgery, Northwestern University Medical School, Chicago, Illinois.

DONALD W. WRIGHT, M.Ed.

Projects Manager of Physiology and Human Factors Laboratory, Veterans Administration Prosthetics Center, New York, New York.

Preface

The *Atlas of Orthotics* is designed to provide information in, and an understanding of, the fields of orthotics and human disability. Material presented in this volume is directed to orthotists, residents in orthopaedic surgery and physical medicine, orthopaedic surgeons, physiatrists, physical therapists, occupational therapists, biomedical engineers, and other individuals who require specialized orthotic knowledge to assist in the treatment of the handicapped.

The *Orthopaedic Appliances Atlas,* published in 1952, is a collection of diverse material pertaining to the field of orthotics, gathered for the first time in one text. Perusal of that edition reveals a wealth of information covering orthotic materials, components, and appliances for the spine and the upper and lower limbs. Careful appraisal of the contents of that volume reveals the emphasis on the application of orthoses (braces) believed to be specific for a particular disease or disease process. The individual's biomechanical deficiencies, independent of etiology, were less thoroughly appreciated at that time.

Since the publication of that volume, close cooperation between the fields of medicine and engineering has established that, regardless of the type or origin of a disease process, attention should be focused on the biomechanical deficit of the patient, with less emphasis on the specific disease process. The growth of applied biomechanics has provided the practicing orthopaedic surgeon and others treating the handicapped with a rational and generic basis for prescription of an orthosis best suited for a particular patient's needs.

As new bioengineering knowledge burgeoned, the Board of Directors of the American Academy of Orthopaedic Surgeons authorized revision of the *Orthopaedic Appliances Atlas,* volume 1, to provide a necessary reference. The Committee on Prosthetics and Orthotics undertook a critical review of the material in volume 1 in light of new knowledge of biomechanics and materials. They agreed that the new volume must emphasize a biomechanical approach to orthotic prescription and design.

To provide for intelligent assessment of biomechanical deficits in any patient, some form of biomechanical physical examination was sought. An *ad hoc* committee[1] developed and field tested a system-and-record form that permits a reasonable biomechanical analysis of lower-limb dysfunction. Although this type of analysis probably will not be required routinely by the knowledgeable practitioner, it will be helpful in teaching the neophyte physician how to develop an appropriate orthotic prescription. It also serves as a basis of communication between the physician and the orthotist who is required to fill the physician's sometimes complex orthotic prescription.

After successful completion of the lower-limb biomechanical-analysis form, an upper-limb

---

[1]McCollough, N. C., III, Fryer, C. M., and Glancy, J.: A new approach to patient analysis for orthotic prescription. Part 1. The lower extremity, Artif. Limbs 14(2):68-80, 1970.

ix

analysis system was developed and tested. Dysfunctions of the lower and upper limbs lent themselves more easily to this type of evaluation than did the spine. It was possible, nonetheless, to develop a form useful in evaluation of spine deficits that could serve as a rational basis for prescription of a spinal orthosis.

At about the same time, a task force appointed by The National Academy of Sciences began deliberations on a new orthotics terminology that could more accurately describe an orthosis.[2] After several deliberations, the task force recommended that orthoses could be best described by enumeration of the joints they encompass and also by their effect on the control of anatomic joint motions. This new nomenclature is used throughout the present volume.

Once the committee dedicated itself to the concept of biomechanical analysis of the handicapped individual as the basis for orthotic prescription

[2]Harris, E. E.: A new orthotics terminology, Orthot. Prosthet. 27(2):6-10, June 1973.

and application, material for the remainder of the atlas was gathered and its biomechanical aspects were identified. Each member of the committee was assigned a section or sections of the table of contents for which he assumed direct supervision.

The committee extends its thanks to Dr. Robert Stewart, former Director of the Prosthetic and Sensory Aids Division of the Veterans Administration, Washington, D.C., for his support of the Committee on Prosthetics and Orthotics in its efforts to revise the previous volume. The Veterans Administration provided moral and financial support for the first volume and has continued its similar support for this volume. We greatly appreciate this support.

The Committee on Prosthetics and Orthotics also wishes to thank the Board of Directors of the American Academy of Orthopaedic Surgeons for its support of the effort to provide this volume of useful information on orthotics.

The Committee on Prosthetics and Orthotics, American Academy of Orthopaedic Surgeons

Robert G. Thompson, M.D., *Chairman*
John H. Bowker, M.D.
Ernest Burgess, M.D.
James M. Cary, M.D.
†Cameron B. Hall, M.D.
Richard Jones, M.D.
Claude N. Lambert, M.D.
Ralph Lusskin, M.D.
Newton C. McCollough, III, M.D.
Raymond Pellicore, M.D.
Jacquelin Perry, M.D.

Contents

Atlas of orthotics

BIOMECHANICAL PRINCIPLES AND APPLICATION

PART ONE

Introduction

CHAPTER 1

Physical properties of materials including solid mechanics

EUGENE F. MURPHY, Ph.D.
ALBERT H. BURSTEIN, Ph.D.

Availability of materials

The increasing availability of a wide variety of materials for orthotic appliances—some with centuries of use, others with the background of decades, and a growing number from the space age —imposes greater responsibility for wise selection. In addition, new materials open possibilities for novel designs and offer opportunities for solutions to perennial problems such as breakage, bulkiness, clothing damage, poor hygiene, or inadequate support.

Selection of the correct material in the right place for each specific appliance depends partially on understanding the elementary principles of mechanics of materials, concepts of forces, deformations and failure of structures under load, improvements in mechanical properties by heat treatments or other means, and design of structures. The choice, today, among materials is already extensive. Metals used for structures include several types of steels, numerous alloys of aluminum, and (to a limited extent) titanium and its alloys. Copper or brass rivets and successive platings of copper, nickel, and chromium illustrate important but minor uses of other metals. Plastics, fabrics, rubbers, and leathers have wide indications and composite structures (of epoxy or plastic matrix plus reinforcing metal "whiskers" or boron or graphite fibers) are being studied. In the field of plastics the laminates are in competition with thermoplastics such as polyethylene and polypropylene.

Despite publicity for exotic new materials, and remarkably accelerating progress, there is no single magic material that will serve as a panacea for all orthotic problems. One reason is that different and even diametrically opposite properties are needed for special clinical situations or even parts of the same device. Elastic properties offer one example. Stiffness of the structure may be desirable for a knee-ankle orthosis (KAO) intended to support body weight. In contrast considerable flexibility and range of motion are necessary if an ankle orthosis is to allow plantar flexion in response to heel strike.

Static strength and resistance to deformation are needed to support heavy patients. At the same time ductility is essential during the process of fitting a metal bar to the contours of the individual patient. These rigid members are permanently deformed by the very high local stresses the orthotist deliberately applies with his bending irons. Despite that need for a permanent set, the orthotist dislikes excessive elasticity, which would require overbending to allow for springback, and he certainly hopes the patient's weight will not cause further plastic deformation or breakage.

Combinations of material are commonly used

to construct an orthosis so that widely divergent mechanical demands can be met. The cuffs generally are made of steel or aluminum. These are then fitted with felt pads and leather covers held in place with rivets of copper or a softer grade of cuff metal.

Bearings often are combinations of materials. A low-friction washer or bushing of nylon, graphite-impregnated nylon, bronze, or oil-impregnated porous bronze may be placed between structural parts of steel or aluminum. If ball, roller, or needle bearings are used—such as in a balanced forearm orthosis or "feeder" for upper-limb weakness—the rolling parts and races are of hardened high-carbon steel, there may be plastic or felt seals, and the entire assembly is then mounted on a structure of other materials.

Springs, dampers, or locks also often involve combinations of materials. A spring, typically formed from a strip of high-strength wire, is often inserted in a structure of another material. In recent years, flexible plastics such as polypropylene, capable of indefinitely large numbers of repeated bends, have been used as hinges with or without significant spring-return effect. Sometimes these hinges are attached to plastic laminates or other structures (such as body jackets). In some cases, they serve as an integral joint (such as an ankle joint) in an orthotic structure that is stiffened in other portions by inherent shape or by deliberate addition of corrugations.

Another example of combinations of materials occurs in many efforts to protect against corrosion. A steel frame, if not made of stainless steel, may be coated with plastisol and heated or cured, or it may be plated with a combination of materials, such as copper first, then nickel, and perhaps chromium. Aluminum orthoses may be given an electrochemical anodizing treatment to form a tough, relatively thick film of aluminum oxide on the surface, a special case of combination of materials.

Plastic laminates form an increasingly important category of combination of materials. Though celluloid jackets (fabric impregnated with that pioneer plastic) were used for spinal orthoses many decades ago, plastic laminates of polyester resins and stockinet fabric were only introduced into orthotics after World War II, partly as a carry-over from training in the later prosthetic schools. The ability to make closely fitting flesh-colored orthoses instead of more bulky and conspicuous metal-bar appliances has increasingly attracted attention, despite the greater labor involved in fabrication.

Composite materials are still not widely used though availability is improving, working techniques are better understood, and costs are decreasing as uses are found for these materials. Most composites were developed for extremely demanding applications in aerospace or in high-performance aircraft. Boron-coated tungsten filaments laminated with epoxy resin have been used experimentally in orthotics although brittle failure with low energy absorption is a severe limitation. They may be useful in orthotics in special cases where very great stiffness is needed. Graphite fibers laminated with epoxy also have extreme stiffness and they are becoming less expensive than the boron composites.

Some metals, particularly aluminum, can be greatly strengthened by incorporation of tiny needle-like crystals or "whiskers" of various materials like synthetic sapphire (a far cry from the ancient use of chopped straw to reinforce bricks!). The engineering literature increasingly carries both theoretical analyses and test data on various composites. Some composites may prove feasible for critical parts like orthoses joints or locks. Conversely, incorporation of lubricants within a material, though often weakening the structure, may be useful in a joint.

The unit cost of material used in orthotic devices is relatively insignificant in the total cost of the finished orthosis. The requirement may be just a few ounces, a few pounds, or even fewer kilograms. A far greater investment has been made to assure adequate skill in fabrication and assembly and professional services in fitting and aligning to the individual. Hence even large variations in unit prices of competitive materials are of minor significance.

More important than unit price of materials are factors like physical properties, stability during use over a substantial range of temperatures, endurance under repeated loading, resistance to wear and corrosion, and ease of working in the shop and adjusting in the fitting room. The economic choice among suitable materials may also depend on the number of steps and time required for initial processing, for adjustments, and for maintenance.

The direct use of expensive stainless steel is often economically justified in comparison with the additional steps and delays in delivery involved in plating of the ordinary steels. Similarly the speed and simplicity of molding thermoplastic synthetic balata directly on the body without discomfort is very attractive, particularly for temporary orthoses, in comparison with the additional cost and delays involved in preparing a plaster cast, and then a plaster model before one uses other thermoplastics with higher softening points or preparing a thermosetting plastic laminate. Nevertheless, vacuum forming of a hot sheet of thermoplastic material against a plaster model appears to have advantages.

Now at least 20 and perhaps 30 elements from the periodic table have some application in prosthetics or orthotics for either shop processes or final products. In addition new materials are continually being developed at great expense for a wide variety of aerospace or industrial uses. A small specialty like orthotics can profit from this progress by directing its more limited resources to testing the promising materials and to designing appropriate fabrication methods for efficient use.

To test materials and to specify reproducible recipes once proved successful in clinical application, we need detailed standards and specifications for raw materials, treatments, and methods of construction. Fortunately many exist already and more are being developed by professional societies, trade associations, and commercial companies.

Both individual laboratories and the postgraduate prosthetics-orthotics education schools are writing manuals detailing step by step those construction methods proved most successful.[4,18,37] The federal, state, and local governments have a variety of procurement specifications. The American Society for Testing and Materials, in its 32-volume *Annual Book of ASTM Standards*,[2] includes a number of specifications, test methods, and recommended practices applicable to orthotics and to surgical implants.[3] The American Iron and Steel Institute has specifications for numerous types of steel alloys, of which some are appropriate for orthotics. Individual companies have standards for steel, aluminum, and titanium alloys. Major chemical companies maintain specific stock numbers for different grades of resin to make, for instance, rigid or flexible plastic laminate.

Occasionally a company makes a subtle change in its product to improve a particular property, a change that may lead to unexpected problems in a different direction, but ordinarily a quality-control program assures that successive batches of a given product will behave alike.

Perhaps 90% of all breakage of orthotic devices are caused by the large number of repeated loadings at seemingly moderate levels. These repeated load levels are well below the load needed to break a fresh appliance with a single application of load. This *fatigue failure* process[7] is *not* prevented by periods of rest between loads, in contrast to self-healing biologic systems.[34] Parts broken by mechanical fatigue failure typically show successive parallel markings resembling oyster shells, where an initially tiny crack has successively opened slightly farther at later application of loads, thus propagating itself across the structure until the remaining area is so small that further repetition of the seemingly safe load causes sudden rupture leaving an irregular crystalline surface. (Decades ago, the metal was believed to have "crystallized" mysteriously initiating the failure. More recently the nature of fatigue failure became better understood.)

When a newly designed appliance withstands daily stress for weeks or months, the designer naturally becomes optimistic. Yet there still may be danger of a fatigue failure within a normal period of usefulness. Thus laboratory fatigue tests of initial models should be routine. Also there should be systematic inspection of appliances undergoing early clinical trials. During such inspections, any cracks indicating impending fatigue failure may be detected.

In a structure under load, any notch, crack, or geometric discontinuity is particularly serious because it tends to increase the local risk of failure above that which would otherwise be present. The sharp bottom of the notch concentrates the forces; so the load per unit area (stress) may be doubled or trebled. This may initiate a crack, which raises the stress even further and creates a self-propagating situation until the entire structure is fatally weakened and fails under an ordinary load. Obviously, the goal must be to avoid the "sharp-blade" effect of a narrow crack and to blunt the "cutting edge" of any notch or reentrant corner by making it as shallow and rounded as feasible.[35] In this direction, paradoxically, a part may be strengthened very greatly by having a hole drilled to blunt the leading edge of a crack, or by the *removal* of material on either side of a V-shaped notch to create a smoother, broader U-shaped trough.

Electrolytic corrosion can occur when there is

electrical contact between dissimilar metals or even between similar metals in fluids with differing concentrations of oxygen at two separated points. The latter situation may occur, for example, if there is a little circulation deep within a crevice between two contacting metal pieces of an implant, so that oxygen is quickly depleted but not replaced. Greater awareness of stress-raising factors and alertness to avoid them may be far more valuable in preventing failures of devices in clinical usage than a change to a novel, highly publicized, but largely unproved material.

Most metals are mined as ores in oxide form. The various smelting and refining processes used to win the desired metal from its ore primarily involve reducing processes. In service, though, these metals tend to oxidize again. If the surface coating of oxide readily flakes, peels, or wears away, bare metal is exposed to further oxidations. If this new layer in turn peels off and leaves fresh metal exposed, progressive destructive corrosion ultimately ruins the structure. One answer is protective coating.

Painting or plating will protect the base metal, but scratches may expose the base metal and thus allow corrosion. The reactive metallic oxide typically occupies more volume, leading to a wedgelike expansion near the edge of the scratch, which tends to crack and peel off more of the protective coating.

Fortunately many materials like stainless steels or aluminum tend to form tough, thin, highly adherent oxide films. Under most circumstances, these films protect the great bulk of metal against further attack. Special processes such as passivating steel or anodizing aluminum deliberately create tougher films. Care must be taken though to avoid repeated abrasion capable of breaking off the oxide film as rapidly as it reforms.

Reasons for engineering mechanics and solid mechanics

For a number of reasons, a general, even if intuitive, understanding of engineering mechanics, solid mechanics, and strength of materials is important to the members of the orthotics clinic team and especially to the orthotist. A general understanding of stresses arising from loading of structures, particularly from the bending of beams, is needed. The physician and the orthotist can then appreciate the importance of simple methods to allow controlled deformation during fitting, to provide stiffness or resiliency as prescribed, and to reduce breakage whether from impact or from repeated loading.

Certain problems can be solved by a branch of study called "engineering mechanics," usually subdivided into statics (analysis of forces on an orthosis when it is stationary) and dynamics (analysis of a moving force). From knowledge of *external* gross forces on a structure, whether animate or inanimate, it is often possible to calculate the major *internal* forces at joints, pins, or other connections or within major beams, bones, and so forth. The basic concepts of solid mechanics applicable to orthotics will be presented in a relatively nonmathematical fashion.

Much also can be learned from kinematics, "the mathematics of motion," the science that describes motion without immediate regard to the forces involved. The complex motions of the human knee, for example, have been described by use of kinematic techniques.

This chapter does not attempt to cover the engineering mechanics of structure or the kinematics of the body or the experimental and analytical methods of analysis. Some sources, however, are suggested in the reading list.[8, 19, 20, 24, 36, 45]

SOLID MECHANICS

When a force is applied to an object, either some type of motion is created or, when this cannot occur, the energy is absorbed within the structure to cause a change in shape. This static situation is significant to decisions relating to orthotic design. *Stress* and *strain* are the terms employed to define the acting forces and their effects.

Definitions

Strain. The term *strain* refers to the change in shape within a material whether it is visible or microscopic. There are two basic types of change—length and angle.

Length change or normal strain. When an external load is applied to the ends of a bar, a change in length occurs. This deformation is called *normal strain* because the force is perpendicular or normal to the displaced force. Normal strain is designated by the Greek letter ϵ (epsilon). It is defined as the change in length as a proportion of the original length. With change being designated by the Greek letter Δ (capital delta), this relationship is expressed as $\Delta L/L$ (Fig. 1-1).

Normal strain is therefore a dimensionless

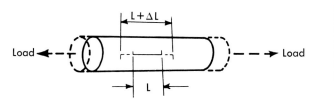

Fig. 1-1. Normal strain.

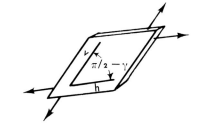

Fig. 1-3. Shear strain.

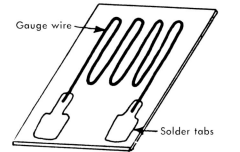

Fig. 1-2. Instrument for measuring strain.

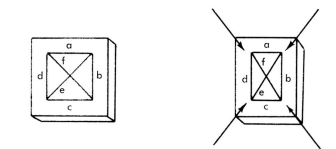

Fig. 1-4. Compressive and shear strain.

quantity (such as cm/cm, in./in.). Since most of the normal strains with which we deal in using metals are very small, on the order of several millionths or 10^{-6}, we often talk in terms of "microstrain." One microstrain (10^{-6}) represents a change in length of one part in one million (such as 0.000,001 cm/cm or inch/inch).

Two types of normal strain can occur—lengthening and shortening. When the length of the structure increases, it is called a *tensile strain* and recorded as a positive number. Shortening is a *compressive strain* and is expressed as a negative number.

Normal strain is easily measured by a variety of techniques. One common strain-measuring device is a *strain gauge,* which translates the length change into an electrical signal. Constructed of a small coil of wire (Fig. 1-2), it is glued onto the surface of the object to be measured. The electrical resistance of the wire alters as the material to which it is fastened is strained. The change in electrical resistance is proportional to the normal strain. Such instrumentation is capable of measuring strains as small as one one-hundredth of a microstrain.

The distribution of strains on the surface of an object can be described by applying a brittle coating and then studying the pattern of the cracks that result from loading. Mechanical devices that magnify small motions and display the results optically are also used.

Angular change of shear strain. When the external load is applied obliquely, the change in the object is an angular deformity. This is called a *shear strain.* One may most readily demonstrate the event by drawing on the object's surface two lines at right angles to each other and noting their change (Fig. 1-3). After the material on which the lines are scribed is subjected to an external load, they are no longer perpendicular. Now the lines have deformed by an angle that is expressed by the Greek letter γ (gamma). Hence shear is an angular deformity from the original normal (perpendicular) state. Shear strain is defined as the tangent of the angle γ. For most materials, the magnitude of shear is sufficiently small to allow the approximation $\gamma \cong \tan \gamma$, where γ is measured in radians. (A complete circle of 360 degrees equals 2π radians; so 1 radian is approximately 57.3 degrees, and 90 degrees equals $\pi/2$ radians.)

Combined normal and shear strain. The existence of strain in a material is not a simple one-dimensional condition. Tension and compression strains are always associated with shear strains. This is demonstrated by drawing a square and its diagonals on the object's surface (Fig. 1-4). An

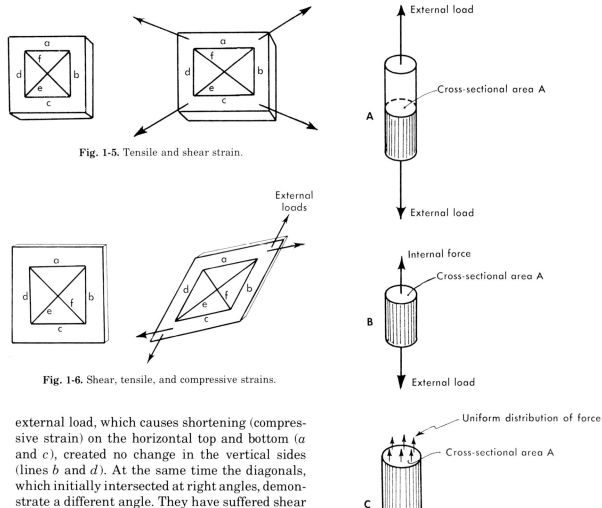

Fig. 1-5. Tensile and shear strain.

Fig. 1-6. Shear, tensile, and compressive strains.

Fig. 1-7. Stress forces in equilibrium.

external load, which causes shortening (compressive strain) on the horizontal top and bottom (*a* and *c*), created no change in the vertical sides (lines *b* and *d*). At the same time the diagonals, which initially intersected at right angles, demonstrate a different angle. They have suffered shear strain. A similar pattern of deformity occurs with a tensile strain (Fig. 1-5). We have chosen to examine only a limited number of lines of the infinite number that could have been drawn on the square. It is easily demonstrated that only lines parallel to lines *b* and *d* remain strain-free. All others undergo either tension or compression, while all line pairs not parallel to the edges strain in shear as well.

The reciprocal behavior occurs if the sample of material is deformed by an oblique load (Fig. 1-6). In this case, the square deforms into a parallelogram. Line pairs *a-b, b-c, c-d,* and *d-a* undergo shear strain but not normal strain. The diagonal lines *e* and *f,* however, do undergo tension strain, *E,* and compressive strain, *F,* but *do not* suffer shear strain; the diagonals remain perpendicular to each other.

This inherent interaction between induced strains is vital to an understanding of material behavior. These general principles are valid for all solid materials.[24]

Stress. When an object is stationary, it is said to be in equilibrium. This is the case when the net force acting on the object is zero. At the same time each portion of the structure also is in equilibrium and all the forces acting on any portion should sum to zero. In response to externally applied loads new internal forces (intermolecular) are generated. These forces may be imagined as "glue" holding the structure together. They may also be consid-

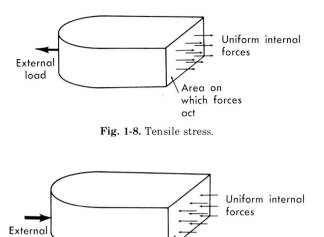

Fig. 1-8. Tensile stress.

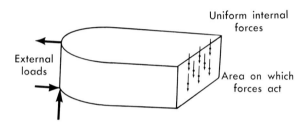

Fig. 1-9. Compression stress.

Fig. 1-10. Shear stress on internal surface area.

ered as small forces at every point on any cross section. The distribution of these forces over the particular areas of concern is described as *stress*.

Stress is generally defined as the load per unit cross-sectional area of a material. Because the concern usually relates to internal changes, stress may also be defined as the ratio of the force applied on an internal surface to the area of this surface (Fig. 1-7). For analysis one imagines the original body being separated at a designated plane; the internal forces on this area are now "external." The area represents an internal surface with a uniform distribution of forces acting on it exactly equal and opposite to the forces on the formerly contiguous wall of the other portion, which has been removed.

When the internal force distribution is not of uniform intensity, the determination of the magnitude of the stress on any portion of the surface requires that the total area be subdivided into sufficiently small portions so as to allow the force to be considered uniformly distributed over each small region.

Normal stress. When the forces are perpendicular to the surface upon which they act, the ratio of force to area is called *normal stress*. This is designated by the Greek letter σ (sigma).

If the force acting on a particular area is directed outward from the surface, it is said to be *tensile stress* (Fig. 1-8). Conversely, a *compressive stress* exists when the perpendicular force is directed into the surface in question (Fig. 1-9). The distribution of normal stress acting on a plane may include both tensile and compressive stresses.[24,45]

Shear stress. When, instead of acting perpendicularly to the internal surface, a distributed force is parallel to the surface, the ratio of the force to the surface area upon which it is acting is called *shear stress* (Fig. 1-10).

Combined normal and shear stresses. It is important to note that shear stress and normal tensile or compressive stress may simultaneously exist on any internal surface. Actually, coexistence is the far more usual situation. The analysis of a section from the bar of an orthosis subjected to a compressive load would be an example (Fig. 1-11). It is reasonable to expect that the small element selected for analysis will also be subjected to compressive forces on its transverse planes (planes a and b). One can demonstrate the combined stresses by slicing the cube on a diagonal and examining the lower portion (Fig. 1-11).

A force F is required on diagonal plane c to keep the small element from moving upward in response to the force on the lower face. It is the stresses acting on surface c that produce this net downward force, thus maintaining equilibrium. Such a force F can be considered to have two components F_n perpendicular (normal) to plane c and F_t parallel. Each of these components of force F is related to a stress on surface c. The condition of stress on surface c is thus composed of compression stress attributable to F_n and shear stress attributable to F_t. In an analogous manner, if the strut were subjected to a pulling or tensile load, the diagonal plane would have tension and shear stresses imposed on it. In general, when a member has normal stresses on transverse planes, all other internal planes except longitudinal planes have stresses on them. Each plane has normal and shear stresses in a proportion dependent on its angle relative to the longitudinal axis. On those planes located at 45 degrees there is a tension (compression) stress equal to one half the tension (compression) stress on the transverse planes.

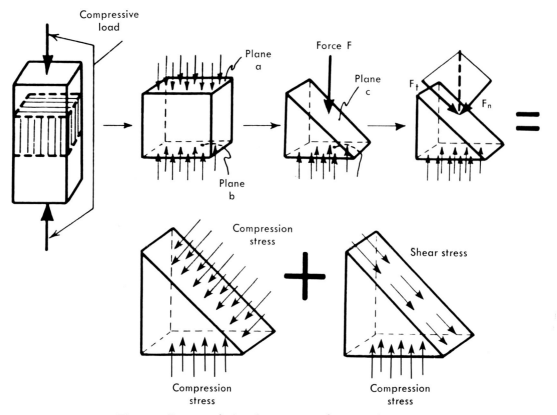

Fig. 1-11. Forces producing shear stress and compressive stresses.

Twisting or loading a structure in *torsion* induces shear stress. Fig. 1-12 shows a small piece of material in a tubular strut that is being twisted. The shear stress that is created on each longitudinal *(a)* and transverse *(b)* face is the same as the other shear stresses. The small cube is in equilibrium, since the forces and moments produced by the shear stresses sum to zero. If we examine one half of the cube after slicing along one 45-degree diagonal (Fig. 1-12), we see that with forces produced by the shear stresses on only two surfaces (*a* and *b*), the piece of material would not be in equilibrium. What is needed for equilibrium is a force acting on surface *d*. This required force $\overline{D}$ on surface *d* is perpendicular to the surface and therefore produces a tension stress. A similar argument would show that the other 45-degree diagonal plane *e* would be subject to a compressive stress (Fig. 1-12). In general, then, if a material is directly subjected to shear stress (such as caused by torsional loading), there are shear stresses of equal intensity on the transverse and longitudinal planes. On the 45-degree diagonal planes there are only tension or compression stresses. The magni-

tude of these stresses on the 45-degree planes is equal to the magnitude of the shear stress on the transverse and longitudinal planes. However on diagonal planes not at 45 degrees to the axis there are both normal (tension or compression) stresses and shear stresses.

Note that the concept of stress involves a force distributed over an internal surface in a material. Because this internal force distribution is inaccessible, it is not possible to measure stresses directly in solids. We can only calculate stresses by knowing the shape of the structure, the nature of loading, and the properties of the material.

Experimental relationship between stress and strain. Many times it is desirable to know the ultimate loading condition that a material can tolerate in terms of stress. For instance, aluminum 2024-T81, e.g., Duralumin, is classed as capable of resisting in tension 414 MN/m² (meganewtons per square meter, or 60,000 psi [lb/inch²]) before deforming permanently. Although stress is not directly measurable, the stress levels in a complex shape can be determined by measuring the strain exhibited in response to controlled loading

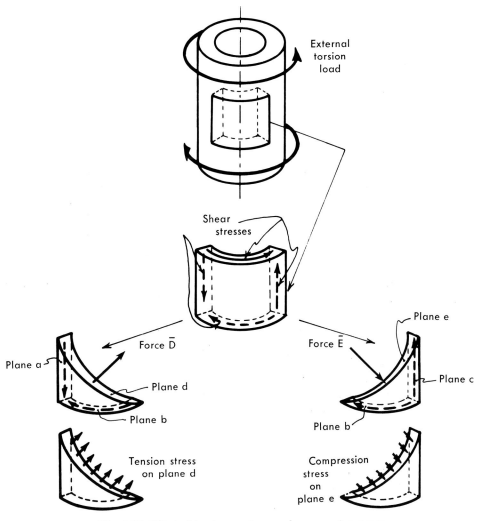

Fig. 1-12. Effect of torsion on shear and compressive stress.

and applying known stress-strain relationships.

To determine the relationship between stress and strain for a particular material, several standard tests have been established. The most common of these is the tension test. This procedure requires the gradual elongation of a carefully prepared sample of material along with simultaneous measurement of the induced load and the elongation of a gauge section of uniform cross-sectional area. One may calculate the tensile stress by dividing the load by this area. The specimen is designed to provide uniform stress distribution across the area of the gauge section. The strain is calculated as the ratio of the change in length of the gauge section to its original length. Stress is then plotted against strain (Fig. 1-13).

A stress-strain curve for a mild steel depicts

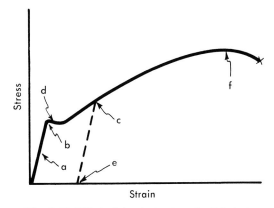

Fig. 1-13. Effect of simple tension of mild steel.

the most important parameters of the usual structural materials: elastic range, yield point, plastic range, and fracture point. The initial portion of the curve is virtually linear. If the material is loaded up to point *a* within this linear region and then unloaded, both stress and strain will return to zero. This type of behavior is termed "elastic" and the linear portion of the curve *(0-b)* is called the elastic region. Springs, for instance, are designed to operate within this region. Any elastic deformation is reversible upon removal of the stress. The slope of this region is known as the *modulus of elasticity,* elastic modulus, or Young's modulus *(E),* and is a measure of the stiffness of the material.

If the stress is increased significantly beyond the linear region, say, to point *c,* then permanent strain is produced. If the induced load is allowed to return to zero, the decreasing curve will be parallel to the elastic region, but will intersect the horizontal axis with a residual strain *e.* There will remain a *plastic deformation* equal to *0-e.* This concept is deliberately used in forming orthotic components with bending irons. Though the "snapback" strain that occurs elastically is reversible, that which occurs plastically is permanent.

To distinguish more clearly between these two behavioral regions, one must define a measurable point *d.* A sample loaded to this value and then unloaded will retain a deformation of 0.2%. The stress at condition *d* is called the *yield stress.* The highest point on the stress-strain curve *f* represents maximum nominal stress calculated from the original cross-sectional area of the test specimen. The stress at this condition is called the *ultimate stress.* Further loading at this point

causes the material to reduce its cross-sectional area at some point. This necking is caused by shear strain on the 45-degree planes and can be easily seen in a steel or aluminum tensile specimen.

The amount of permanent or plastic deformation that a material will undergo before failure is called its *ductility.* Most steels and surgical metals are ductile materials to varying degrees.

Materials that do not plastically deform before fracture are called *brittle* materials. Glass is an example of a brittle material. The stress-strain curve for such a material shows no flattening to the right of the elastic curve (Fig. 1-14), that is, no plastic deformation before fracture. The strain is completely reversible in this material for any loading cycle before failure.

For many materials, on release of the load, the curve does not retrace itself as the specimen regains its original shape. The closed loop formed by the loading and unloading cycle is called the *hysteresis* curve. It is a measure of the amount of energy the material absorbs each loading cycle.

Brittle materials, though sometimes attractive because of high ultimate strength, may be unsuitable for shock loading under impact because they cannot absorb much energy before fracturing. For example, a hard brittle steel with an ultimate stress of 650 MN/m² (94,000 psi) and a 5% ultimate strain (Fig. 1-15) can absorb, before breaking, only one half the energy of a mild steel with a yield stress of 325 MN/m² (47,000 psi) and a 20% ultimate strain. One may best visualize this behavior by observing the area under the stress-strain curve, a direct measure of energy required for failure. This comparison, however, is based on the total energy required for *failure, not* the amount of energy required to deform permanently

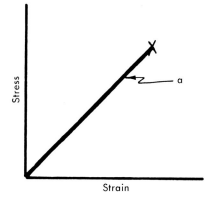

Fig. 1-14. Stress-strain curve for glass.

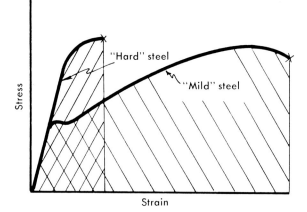

Fig. 1-15. Stress-strain curve for steel.

the material. In certain cases, permanent deformation is tantamount to failure. For an elastic material, the amount of energy required to deform it permanently is dependent on the yield stress and the elastic modulus. Actually, the energy required to deform permanently a volume of metal is given by the equation

$$\frac{\sigma_y^2 \cdot Volume}{2 \cdot E}$$

where E is the elastic modulus and σ_y is the yield stress. The higher the yield stress for a given modulus (Fig. 1-16, A) or the lower the elastic modulus for a given yield stress (Fig. 1-16, B), the greater the energy required before plastic deformation occurs. Under shock loading then a material of high yield stress but relatively low modulus—a "resilient" material—may be desirable.

Failure of materials. There are two general types of elastic materials—*brittle* and *ductile*. These terms actually describe failure modes under customary loading conditions. Unusual conditions such as sharp notches, extreme stiffening, or other unusual configurations may alter the customary behavior of many ductile materials so as to cause brittle fracture. For most applications, though,

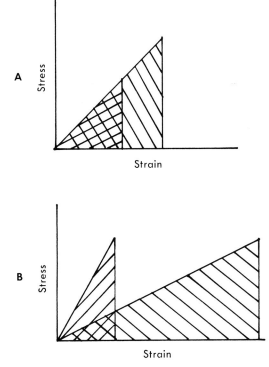

Fig. 1-16. Comparison of **A**, yield stress, **B**, moduli.

the ductility of a material, expressed as a percent elongation to failure, will indicate the mechanism of probable failure under a single overload. Most engineering metals have a ductility falling between 10% and 40%. The general tendency within a family of materials is for increasing yield strength to correspond to decreasing ductility. Thus structural steel has lower yield stress but much greater ductility than the hardened tool steel in a chisel; a softer Duralumin alloy, such as 2024, likewise has lower yield stress but higher ductility than hardened 7075 T6 aluminum alloy.

A ductile failure is indicative of simple one-cycle overload generally arising from an emergency. In an orthotic device, permanent deformation—or even rupture after extensive distortion—may indicate desirable energy absorption protecting the patient during an accidental fall. Such failures are identified by distortion of the structure in the region of the fracture. The pieces when reassembled do not reproduce the shape of the original structure. The fracture area will usually be reduced in cross section. Such failures suggest reevaluation of the design because of functional overload even if this is under emergency conditions. Decisions must be made as to the probability of future similar loads as well as on the safest course of events. There is little value in protecting an external orthotic device against failure but ensuring that the patient will fracture a bone!

Brittle fractures can be caused by discontinuities in structural members. A discontinuity such as a hole or especially a sharp notch—"an invisible knife"—will cause a significant local buildup of stress. This phenomenon is called *stress concentration*. The metal may actually yield in the immediate vicinity of the hole, but overall failure will resemble a brittle fracture if caused by a single, suddenly applied load. The stress near a small cylindrical hole may be three times higher in tension or four times higher in shear than the stresses in the more remote material; the stress at the root of a sharp notch may be even more exaggerated.

Fatigue fracture. Multiple loadings producing stresses of insufficient intensity to cause yielding may cause a structure to fail by a process known as *metal fatigue*. This rather complex process entails the initiation and slow propagation of cracks through the material. These cracks, which usually start at the surface or at an internal flaw, effectively reduce the cross-sectional area. One final load, nominally as safe as similar earlier loads, causes a stress at the ultimate strength and a brittle-like failure results.[7,39]

Fatigue failure depends on the establishment and growth of crack planes through the material. Anything that aids either the initiation or propagation of these crack planes enhances fatigue. Factors that stimulate the formation of surface cracks are stress concentrations, surface imperfections attributable to material or finish, corrosion, and gross intensity of stress. The growth rate of a crack is a function of both the number and the intensity of the loading cycles in a given time period. It is important to note that the effect of loading is cumulative. Resting periods do not allow the metal to regain strength or repair cracks. Mechanical structures, unlike bones, lack physiologic systems, which respond to stress levels; so there is no remodeling or hypertrophy to meet the new demands. Nor is there a means to conserve and reform available raw materials by selective atrophy of structures when they are no longer needed.

The ability of a material to resist fatigue failure is demonstrated by the relation of allowable stress to the number of cycles that stress can be tolerated (Fig. 1-17). Curves for a particular steel and a particular aluminum are shown. Although these curves represent the most likely lifetime of a material, usually a considerable scatter of actual data is found.

Endurance limit. Ferrous alloys typically can withstand some level of stress for an unlimited number of cycles. The greatest repetitive stress for which the material does not fail is called the *endurance limit.* The limit is reached where the curve of stress versus cycles becomes horizontal. If a ferrous alloy can withstand 10^6 (1 million) cycles, it will probably withstand an indefinitely larger number of similar cycles.

This indefinite "life" is not true for other metals, especially aluminum alloys. In this case, the nominal tensile endurance limit is defined as the greatest tensile stress that would allow 5×10^8 (or 500 million) cycles. Actually, it is possible to cause fatigue failure in aluminum alloys at the nominal endurance limit simply by increasing the number of cycles. Because the curve of tolerable stress versus the number of cycles is so nearly horizontal at a large number of cycles, only a small reduction in stress will prolong the probable useful life before failure by 10, 100, or 1000 times.

Generally, the endurance limit of a metal is between 30% and 50% of its yield stress. Any tensile stress of higher value repeatedly applied will induce fatigue failure. Because notches, roughness, or corrosion are such serious sources of increased stress-accelerated fatigue failure, much attention should be given to their prevention in orthoses and other structures that experience critical loading under constraints of weight and bulk; such attention is more effective than searching for nominally stronger materials.

Stress in complex loading situations

Bending. The most common and crucial complex stress condition existing in orthotic devices is

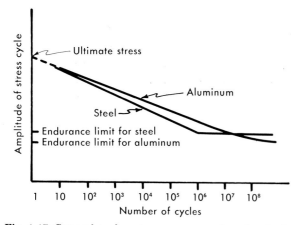

Fig. 1-17. Curves based on stress versus number of cycles before failure for steel and aluminum.

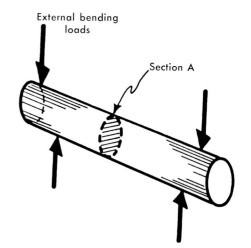

Fig. 1-18. Effect of external bending loads on body.

bending. The stresses associated with bending loads are combinations of shear, compression, and tension. To understand the stress condition caused by bending, one can examine a beam of uniform cross section subjected to a bending force on each end (Fig. 1-18). By isolating a portion of the structure (a "free body" in engineering terms) and analyzing the external forces and moments acting upon one surface, A, we can discern the resultant internal reaction on it. If a condition of equilibrium exists, the resultant of the internal reaction must be equal to the moment applied to the beam. If this were not true, the body would not be in equilibrium and it would tend to spin. This internal reaction moment is achieved by a stress distribution consisting of both tension and compression (Fig. 1-19). The greater the internal reaction moment (bending moment) the greater these stresses. Maximum compression occurs on the cross section near the surface on the inside of the curve. Maximum tension occurs opposite this at the convex surface.

The normal stress distribution in bending of any beam varies evenly from maximum tension at one surface to maximum compression at the opposite surface. The stresses are zero (changing from tension to compression) at the *neutral axis*. The amount of stress in a beam depends on the amount and distribution of material in the cross-sectional area. The parameter that measures this is called the *section modulus, z*. For instance, a three-flanged nail has a much lower section modulus than does an I beam of similar size (Fig. 1-20).

The I shape places more material farther from the neutral axis and as a result can sustain a higher bending moment perpendicular to that plane. The I beam has a lower modulus, however, for bending across its face than does the nail. The use of such special shapes requires knowledge as to the direction of the load as well as the magnitude.

The greater the section modulus, the lower the stress. The stress for a bending load is always maximum at the outermost point on the cross section. Usually a beam breaks because of failure of this outermost fiber with subsequent rupture of the succeeding fiber. For an asymmetric cross section like the tibia, the maximum compressive stress may be less than the maximum tensile stress because the distance to the outermost fiber in compression is less (Fig. 1-21). Since a knowledge of bending stresses is useful in the understanding of the mechanics of orthoses, this concept will be further examined by separate study of the variables of bending moment and section modulus.

The value of the internal bending moment, *M*, in any section of a cantilever beam or a simply loaded beam supported at the ends is the product of a force and a distance. This means that given the same transverse force acting on one end of the beam, the internal moment and thus the stress at any section distal to the force will vary with the

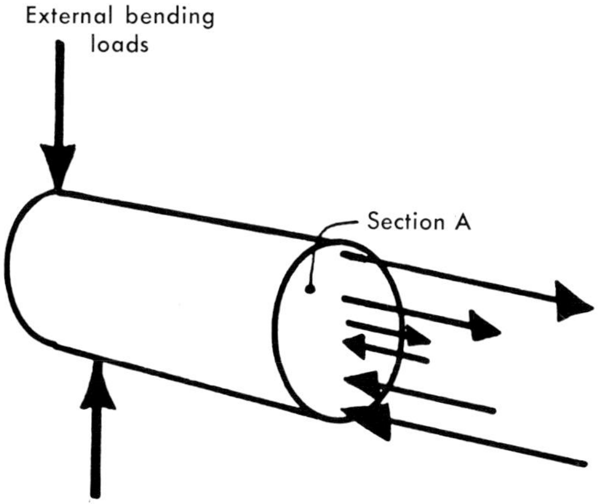

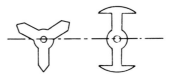

Fig. 1-20. Effect of cross-sectional shape on section modulus.

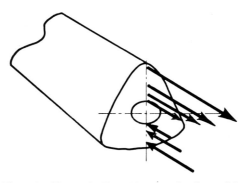

Fig. 1-21. Unequal effect of bending loads on tibia.

External bending loads

Section A

Fig. 1-19. Effect of external bending forces on internal forces within beam.

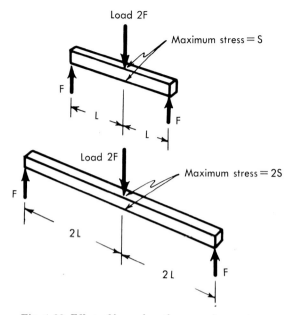

Fig. 1-22. Effect of beam length on maximum stress.

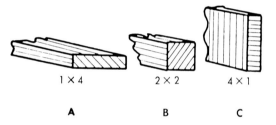

Fig. 1-23. Effect of distribution of material on section moduli.

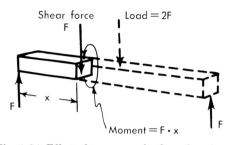

Fig. 1-24. Effect of transverse loads on long beam.

length of the beam. For equal sections, a simple beam that is twice as long will have twice the maximum resulting stress since its maximum moment at its center is twice the value of the shorter beam (Fig. 1-22).

The section modulus is an important parameter in consideration of the strength of beams. The section modulus is a property of the cross-sectional area that takes into account not only the total amount of area but also the disposition of the area with respect to the neutral axis.

Beams may possess the same area but have widely differing section moduli. Three beams with the same area, 4 square centimeters, but with various distributions of material, demonstrate different section moduli. For a beam positioned as a plank (Fig. 1-23, *A*) the section modulus is $2/3$ cm³. When the same area is formed into a square

shape (Fig. 1-23, *B*), the section modulus will be $1^{1}/_{3}$ cm³. If the beam is turned up on edge as a joist (Fig. 1-23, *C*) the section modulus increases to $2^{2}/_{3}$ cm³. There is a factor of 4 between the first and last illustration. The value of the section modulus (calculated as the base multiplied by the square of the height divided by 6 for rectangular cross sections) is a measure of the strength of the beam. That is, for a given bending moment the beam that has a maximum value of section modulus will have the minimum bending stress and will thus have the least tendency to fail. Thus, a beam on edge will support a larger bending moment than can be supported by the same beam when oriented flat.

Normal stress is not the only type of stress produced in a beam under bending. Consider a section of a centrally loaded beam near the center force (Fig. 1-24). Not only is there a moment at this section, but also there must be a shear force in order for the beam to be in equilibrium. This shear force produces shear stresses whose distribution depends on the shape of the cross section. They are zero at the top and bottom and rise to a maximum at the center of the cross section.

For most applications, the bending shear stress is not critical; for its magnitude is usually much lower than that of the bending tension and the bending compression stresses. Nevertheless the compromises between tension, compression, and shear illustrate the problems facing a designer. For a given weight of beam, the designer—if he is confident of the direction of loading—may attempt to move material outward from the neutral axis, like a joist or an I beam to minimize tension and compression stresses. If he goes too far, though, he will have a deep narrow joist, likely to buckle or wrinkle in the center; or two planks, flanges of an exaggerated I beam, connected by a thin membrane-like web, so overstressed in shear that the web is nearly useless in connecting the two flanges for mutual support. A real orthosis may

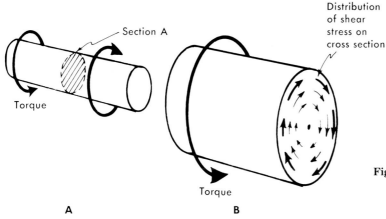

Fig. 1-25. Effect of torsion on cylinder.

well have practical limitations of cosmesis, clothing damage, or difficulties of fitting to the particular patient. Thus, there are realistic limits to changes in cross section in efforts to reduce stress.

Torsional loading. When a body is subjected to a moment or torque tending to twist about its axis, it is said to be subjected to *torsion.* As a result of this applied load, the body undergoes a complex state of deformation and stress. Consider the simple case of a solid cylinder subjected to a torque (Fig. 1-25). For the portion of the cylinder to the left of section *A* (isolated as a free body), the stress distribution on the section must produce a resultant moment equal and opposite to the net torque imposed on the left end of the cylinder. This must be true if this element of the body is to remain in equilibrium. In addition, there can be no resulting axial or radial force, as there are no comparable applied loads. The stress distribution that satisfies these criteria is shown in Fig. 1-25, *B.* Note that all of the stresses on the cross section are shear stresses. The shear stress is distributed over the entire cross section *A.* The magnitude of the stress is proportional to the distance from the center of the bar, with the maximum at the outer edge, and inversely proportional to the area moment of inertia (a measure of the distribution of the section area relative to the center point).

In the case of a human tibia subjected to a torsional loading, the stress distribution of two sections is illustrated in Fig. 1-26. Note that the shear stress generally increases linearly with distance from the neutral axis. The value of the maximum shear stress varies throughout the length of the bone because of changes in the shape of the bone and the distribution of bony material. At the junc-

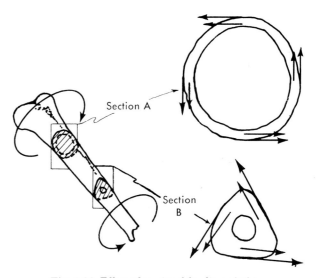

Fig. 1-26. Effect of torsional loading of tibia.

tion of the proximal three fourths and distal one fourth, at section *B* in Fig. 1-26, the cross-sectional distribution produces a stress approximately twice that at the proximal section *A* even though the cortical bone is thicker at the distal section. A torsional fracture of the tibia would be expected to occur at the distal section, as is commonly observed.

If a ferrous alloy rod is twisted until it breaks, the failure plane will be noted to lie perpendicular to the axis of loading, the plane of maximal shear stress.

The cross sections of objects such as cylinders, cylindrical and square tubes, and tibias are termed "closed sections." I beams, channels and C sections all have "open sections." Opening a

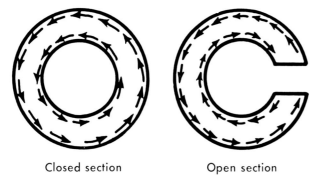

Closed section   Open section

Fig. 1-27. Effect of torsion on closed and open cylinders.

closed section (such as cutting a slot in a tibia) drastically decreases the ability of the structure to carry torsional loads by altering the stress distribution and hence reducing the strength of the section. This can be seen by comparing the stress distributions in closed and open sections subjected to torsion (Fig. 1-27). In the closed section, the stress distribution is such that all stresses have counterclockwise moments about the central axis. Thus they all effectively contribute to the equalization of the applied torque. In the open section, however, the shear stresses are not all similarly directed. The moment produced by the more central shear stresses is in the same direction as the applied torque and is additive. Since the applied torque must be resisted by the net moment of the induced stresses, the stresses along the exterior are greater than those inside. Thus much larger stresses are produced in the open section than in the closed section in resisting the same torque.

As noted previously, shear stresses under torsional loading are associated with equivalent tensile and compressive stresses. In the case of the open section under torsion, large shear, tensile, and compressive stresses are developed in response to the torque. Failures of open sections are noted clinically as fractures of donor tibias or other bones changed to open section structures by cysts and tumors.

Concepts of rigidity including elastic material properties and section and length considerations. We have seen that the section modulus relates the strength of a structure to the distribution of material throughout its cross section. In addition to a consideration of strength, which is a measure of load-carrying capacity, we are also interested in the *rigidity* of a structure. Rigidity is a measure of the amount of load needed to produce deformation

and is related to the area moment of inertia. The rigidity of a beam is the ratio of the deflection and the applied load. Thus the rigidity of a beam might be 5000 N/cm, meaning 5000 newtons are required to produce 1 centimeter of deformation at the center. It might be that the beam would fail at 1000 N of load and 0.2 cm. deflection, but this would not alter our statement of rigidity. The more rigid the structure, the greater the load required to produce a given deformation.

There are several factors that influence rigidity of beams. These are elastic modulus of material, area moment of inertia of the cross section, and length of beam. The area moment of inertia is another measure of the distribution and amount of cross-sectional area. For rectangles it is the base multiplied by the cube of the height divided by 12. Thus a steel orthosis ($E = 207{,}000$ MN/m^2) is more rigid than an aluminum ($E = 70{,}000$ MN/m^2) orthosis of the same size and shape. For the same material, doubling the thickness of a vertical strut (Fig. 1-28) will increase its bending rigidity in the anteroposterior direction by a factor of 2 and in the mediolateral direction by a factor of 8 (because the moment of inertia depends on the cube of the height). If the length of a beam is halved, the rigidity will increase by a factor of 8.

Maximum rigidity is not necessarily a desirable goal, particularly if shock loading must be resisted. If a structure is too rigid, it will not deflect a great deal and therefore will not absorb much energy, before it fails.

Energy concepts in loading
Elastic and plastic strain energy. If the beam is made of ductile material and if a sufficient load is placed on the beam, the load deformation curve obtained is as shown in Fig. 1-29.

The left-hand portion of the curve *(0-q)* represents the familiar reversible linear elastic deflection induced in the material by the bending stresses. Eventually the outermost fibers yield at the section with maximum moment. That is, they continue to deform without any increase in stress, and permanent dislocations occur in the crystalline structure. As the loading is continued, the fibers below the outermost fibers yield. If the load is now removed, a permanent change in shape will be noted. This is the mechanism used by the orthotist to deform a component with bending irons. If the load is increased, eventually a point is reached at which all fibers at this critical section

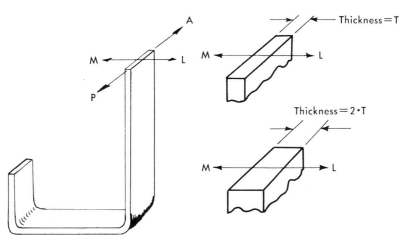

Fig. 1-28. Effect of increasing the thickness of orthosis strut.

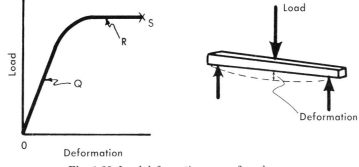
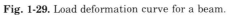

Fig. 1-29. Load deformation curve for a beam.

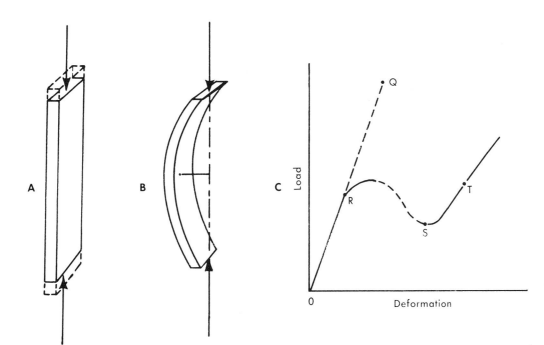

Fig. 1-30. Effect of axial loading on orthosis strut.

yield and, under constant load, the beam continues to deform. This deformation continues until rupture occurs (point s).

The amount of elongation that a simple tension specimen of any material can undergo before rupture is often used as a measure of the ductility of the material. For example, 316 stainless steel elongates 27%, whereas chemically pure titanium elongates as much as 36%.

Influences of energy of failure of columns. Energy concepts are also useful in understanding failures in columnar structures. A *column* is a long slender structure loaded axially. When the identical structure is loaded as a beam (transverse load), the amount of energy that can be absorbed is proportional to the deflection as long as no permanent (plastic) deformation occurs. Columns behave in a nonlinear way. Fig. 1-30, *A*, illustrates the deformation produced by an axial load on the column. The amount of energy absorbed in this manner is also the area under the load-deformation curve. If the column could remain straight, the energy would increase with the load in a linear manner *(0-q)* (Fig. 1-30, *C*). There are other shapes, however, that the column will assume if the load continues to increase. One such shape is illustrated in Fig. 1-30, *B*. The load deformation characteristics for this configuration are reflected in *0-s-t*. The initial straight-line portion *0-r* represents the erect column being loaded axially and remaining in a linear configuration. In region *r-s* the column suddenly bows. At point *s*, the total energy is less than at point *r*. Energy is lost in the damping of vibration when the column snaps from one position to another. Actually, in practical cases, if the column reaches the energy storage level indicated at point *r*, any small disturbance will drastically change its configuration to that at *t*, a state of pronounced bowing.

MATERIALS
Steel

Steel is the general term used to describe a family of alloys produced by removal of impurities from pig iron. It is abundant, is relatively cheap, and can be manufactured in various alloyed and heat-treated states.

The basic advantages that can be incorporated into steel are high strength, high rigidity, considerable ductility, long fatigue life, and ease of fabrication and availability. Among its disadvantages are high density, need for expensive alloying to prevent corrosion, and poor surface wear characteristics in bearings.

Steels may be divided into three classes: carbon steel, low-alloy steel, and high-alloy steel. The carbon steels have a variety of uses, ranging from structural parts to cutting tools. Low-alloy steels are used where higher strength is required, together with moderate ductility. High-alloy steels are used for high-strength applications and are the most corrosion resistant.

Mechanical characteristics

Carbon steel. At low concentrations of carbon (0.05%-0.10%), steel is very ductile but has a low yield strength. As the percentage of carbon increases, the ductility decreases and the yield strength increases. At any particular level of carbon content, appropriate heat treatment can also increase strength at the cost of reducing ductility.

The actual yield strength of carbon steel may vary from 207 MN/m^2 (30,000 psi) to 860 MN/m^2 (125,000 psi) depending on carbon content and heat treatment. The corresponding range in ductility is from approximately 40% to less than 10%.

Low-alloy steel. Steels in this group have mechanical properties that fall between the carbon steels and the high alloy steels. The tensile yields are between 345 and 380 MN/m^2 (50,000-55,000 psi) with ductility of approximately 25%. These steels are not often used for medical products.

High-alloy steels. When corrosion resistance is not a requirement, high-alloy steels can be obtained with extremely high strength-to-weight ratios. These steels are well suited for structures subjected to large, repetitive loads. They are more expensive than low-carbon steels and also more difficult to fabricate. They can be heat treated or cold worked to improve their strength levels even further.

If corrosion resistance is also a requirement for a particular application, there are the following three types of "stainless steels" from which to choose.

HARDENABLE STAINLESS ALLOYS. These alloys contain up to 16% chromium and 0.7% carbon and can be hardened by heat treatment. They are well suited for surgical instruments.

STAINLESS IRON. Members of this family of materials have low-carbon content and can only be hardened by cold-working. The chromium content is usually between 16% and 18% and more chromium is used if resistance to oxidation is required at high temperatures.

CHROMIUM-NICKEL STAINLESS STEEL. The addition of nickel to the stainless iron provides even greater corrosion resistance in all temperature ranges. The alloy cannot be heat treated to increase its hardness or strength, but cold working can be used to accomplish these objectives. An alloy of 18% chromium and 8% nickel (18-8) is the best known of these alloys. When such steels are made with less than 0.03% carbon they are even less vulnerable to corrosion.

Aluminum

Aluminum in both its pure and alloyed forms is a useful metal because of its low density, corrosion resistance, and relatively high strength. Unfortunately, either of the last two properties is usually optimized at the expense of the other. Increased strength often results in decreased corrosion resistance.

Pure aluminum is a very ductile low-strength material (34.5 MN/m², 5000 psi yield) with unlimited uses. Because of the fact that the aluminum oxide that rapidly forms on the surface of aluminum is strongly adherent, progressive oxidation cannot take place. For practical purposes, the pure aluminum is "corrosion resistant." This corrosion resistance is often obtained in the alloys by covering them with pure aluminum (Alclad). However, hydrochloric acid and alkalis dissolve the oxide film on aluminum surfaces and allow rapid material degradation. Therefore, the corrosion resistance of pure aluminum applies only to atmospheric conditions. Aluminum is highly reactive in physiologic solutions.

Aluminum alloys may be divided into two classes, those used for casting and those that are wrought.

Casting aluminum is alloyed with copper, silicon, and magnesium. These alloys have a low-to-moderate strength (131 to 165 MN/m², 19,000 to 24,000 psi yield) and low ductility (0.5% to 1.3%).

Aluminum stock in sheet, bar, tube, or extruded form is known as wrought aluminum. Some members of this class of alloys may be hardened and their mechanical properties may be improved by precipitation of copper at slippage planes often by heat treatment. Such precipitation takes place spontaneously at room temperature for some alloys and at moderate temperatures for other alloys. In some cases such as the 2024 ST alloy often used in orthoses, *high* temperature causes the previously precipitated copper to be dissolved and

allows the crystal planes to slide over each other relatively easily, even for a short time after the aluminum alloy is rapidly quenched. It can be conveniently shaped then rehardened within a few hours at room temperature and more rapidly at moderately elevated temperatures. The copper is again precipitated to "key" the crystal planes, restoring the yield strength and resistance to further deformation. This behavior seems paradoxical to persons familiar only with carbon steels, where heating the steel to high temperatures than rapidly quenching it in water will cause substantial permanent increases in strength and hardness, as in heat-treating a chisel blade.

Cold-working can also be used to improve the mechanical properties of these wrought alloys. These are two groups of wrought aluminum alloys: the Mn-Mg alloys and the Cu-Si-Mn-Mg alloys such as Duralumin. Heat treatment and cold-working of these alloys can produce moderate yield strength (up to 483 MN/m², 70,000 psi) but will result in low ductility at these strength levels.

It is important to note that aluminum and its alloys have an elastic modulus of 69,000 MN/m², whereas steel alloys have an elastic modulus of 207,000 MN/m². For the same shape and loading, aluminum structures will elastically deflect three times more than comparable steel structures. Another basic difference between steel and aluminum is that the former has an endurance limit under repeated or fatigue loading, whereas the latter does not. This means that if the loading conditions are known, a steel structure can be designed so as to allow an infinite life. An aluminum structure is, however, eventually subject to fatigue failure as long as it continues to be loaded. Fortunately, as noted above, at a practical high number of load cycles, a small decrease in stress will allow a tenfold increase in life.

In general, "high-strength" aluminum alloys demonstrate much greater increases in static strength than in strength under fatigue loading at 1 million to 500 million cycles. Furthermore, these "high-strength" alloys are work-hardened to greater hardness and are typically much more sensitive to notches; so they are not as useful in practical orthotics applications as their static strengths might indicate.

Titanium and magnesium

Titanium has been commercially available for only 25 years, yet already it is an extremely important metal. Titanium and its alloys are stronger than aluminum alloys; their strengths are comparable to steel. In addition, titanium and its alloys are considerably more corrosion resistant than aluminum alloys and steels. An added benefit is the fact that titanium is only 60% as dense as steel. Titanium, though, is relatively more difficult to machine.

The elastic modulus of titanium (116,200 MN/m^2) is higher than that of aluminum but only slightly more than one half that of steel. Titanium will absorb about twice the energy before yielding as compared to a comparable strength steel.

Unlike other metals, titanium is structurally useful in its commercially pure form. Depending on heat treatment and working, it is available with yield strength of 210 to 490 MN/m^2 (30,000 to 70,000 psi) with correspondingly inverse ductility of 25% to 15%. As with steel and aluminum alloys, titanium is weldable. Although some steels can be welded in an air atmosphere, both titanium and aluminum alloys must be welded by use of either a tungsten arc with an inert gas (TIG) or a metal arc with an inert gas (MIG) system. In either method, argon or helium is usually the inert gas.

Titanium alloys contain a variety of elements, with Fe, N, Pd, Al, Mn, Sn, Mo, Zr, and V being the most common. Alloying elements are used to increase workability, machinability, and strength. In all cases, however, titanium and its alloys can be formed and fabricated by the same processes used for aluminum alloys and for steel. The major exception to this statement, however, is casting. Titanium is a difficult material to cast.

Magnesium is still lighter than aluminum and its modulus of elasticity is even lower. However, screw threads are likely to strip unless special precautions are taken. When magnesium is machined, the highly flammable chips must be handled cautiously. Magnesium bars or castings are used for some special cases in a variety of industries, but magnesium has had relatively little application in orthotics.

Plastics

There are two major categories of plastics—thermosetting plastics, which require application of heat to cure or harden but which do not soften upon further heating, and thermoplastics, which will soften each time the temperature is raised but harden upon lowering of the temperature.

Thermosetting plastics. The original and still widely used thermosetting plastic is based upon phenol-formaldehyde. The raw material is supplied as a powder and is formed at high temperature (300° F, 149° C) and pressure (13.8 MN/m^2, 2000 psi). The resulting tensile properties will vary with the filler material but range from 27.6 to 82.7 MN/m^2 (4000 to 12,000 psi). For improved structural properties, phenol-formaldehyde may be "filled" with chopped fibers or may be used as a resin to bind materials such as paper or cloth into structural shapes. Such laminates have improved mechanical properties but are also more hygroscopic. Because of the expensive mold needed, this material is best suited for mass production.

A second important class of thermosetting plastics is the urea-formaldehyde resins. Their fabrication and properties do not differ significantly from phenol-formaldehyde except that they are less expensive, may be colored, and are moderately resistant to water. These materials are available in sheet and bar form, but more complex structural shapes must be formed by use of expensive dies and complex molding machinery.

Epoxy resins and the polyesters form a group of low-pressure thermosetting plastics. Because little or no pressure is required to cure these materials, typically as laminates, larger sections can be fabricated with less expensive tools. They are suitable for custom fabrication over a plaster model to fit an individual patient. The low-pressure thermosetting plastics are used either with fillers or as the binding resin in a two-phase laminate material (fiber glass and Dacron stockinet being well-known examples). Epoxy is also used as a very strong glue.

Thermoplastics. The major composition used in the thermoplastics is the group of vinyl resins. These include polyvinyl chloride (PVC), polyvinyl chloride acetate, polyvinyl alcohol (PVA), and polyvinyl acetate. The PVC group consists of tough, hard materials that usually require a plasticizer or softener. Among the uses for these materials are leather substitutes, pipes and tubes, and small complex structural components. All structural fabrications require special tooling and injection-molding equipment. Tube-like shapes may be extruded, but the tooling is also expensive. PVC and PVA sheets and bags are very widely used for plastic laminating in prosthetics and orthotics. Because PVA can be softened by dampening, a conical sleeve can be stretched over a relatively complex plaster model of a stump or limb.

Other important thermoplastic compositions are polyethylene and polypropylene. Both materials are highly stable and are water and solvent resistant. They are easily formed and have many medical uses including polyethylene internal prostheses. Polypropylene also has an indefinitely long fatigue life under repeated loading; so it is useful for orthotic hinge joints. Polyethylene, polypropylene, and recently polycarbonate are being increasingly used for orthotic structures of new designs and for prosthetic sockets. A heated, softened sheet is formed against a plaster model by a vacuum molding process. Polycarbonate has also been used for impact surfaces on tools for surgery.

Nylon is a strong, tough, abrasion-resistant thermoplastic but has the disadvantage of absorbing water. In addition, it is relatively expensive compared with some materials of similar properties. Low-cost nylon washers, though, have been used without lubrication in orthotic joints particularly with aluminum bars.

Rubbers. The term "rubber" refers to the family of natural and artificial elastomers. Included in this grouping with the natural rubber are butyl, polysulphide rubbers, neoprene, nitrile rubbers, and GR-S butadiene-styrene copolymer.

Rubber is used whenever large elastic deformation (up to 300% of the original length of the material) is required, with relatively low force levels. Because most rubbers are almost perfectly elastic, there is only limited energy loss by hysteresis or internal friction. Its nonlinear stress-strain characteristics can provide in a finished structure a large excursion at relative low forces, then more rapidly increasing forces, and finally such large forces as to block further motion. Rubber is a much better elastic energy absorber, on a weight or volume basis, than any metal. Thus rubber can be effective in bumpers, elastic straps, etc.

The skid resistance of cane or crutch tips on wet pavements or ice depends on high flexibility and hysteresis.[29] Natural rubber and some styrene-butadiene compounds, preferably with oil extension of either, would be most suitable around the freezing temperatures of water.

Natural rubber has excellent tensile properties, as well as being resistant to wear. Its resistance to cold, flexing, and aging is also excellent. It is not very resistant to sunlight or to most oils and solvents. Butyl rubber offers resistance to sunlight and solvents but does not have the high tensile strength or wear resistance of natural rubber.

Because of the wide variety of properties that can be produced in rubber by compounding, it is often possible to produce a material that is well suited for a particular application.

Cellular rubbers and plastics. A variety of cellular rubbers and plastics (such as polyurethane) are used in prosthetics and orthotics. The softer grades are primarily used as padding but firmer, more dense varieties are increasingly used for cosmetic covers of endoskeletal prostheses or even as structural elements. Some types have interconnecting pores, allowing absorption and passage of fluids. These open-cell materials may create hygienic problems if perspiration or debris accumulates in the pores. Other types, closed-cell foams, have individual gas-filled cells or "bubbles" that do not interconnect.

When cellular plastic is molded, a smooth and relatively tough skin that is typically formed against the wall of the mold is often an advantage. Blocks cut from cellular material, and perhaps further sanded to a desired shape, have rough surfaces with randomly distributed cavities of remaining pores. In some cases such a surface may be sealed and smoothed by painting with latex. For structural uses one or more layers of plastic laminate may be added.

Sandwich. A still stronger yet light structure may be formed from stiff foam plastic with opposite faces bonded to thin sheets of metal, plywood, or plastic laminate. This concept is an extension and refinement of the familiar corrugated cardboard carton. It is most suitable for simple geometric shapes like flat sheets or tubes. Though it is occasionally suggested for prosthetics or orthotics structures, sandwich construction is not very practical for the custom-shaped three-dimensional structures usually needed.

Porous laminates. Repeated efforts[26,46] have been made to produce practical laminates or sheet plastics sufficiently porous to allow diffusion of insensible perspiration yet either resistant to organic material or easily cleaned. Mechanical or electrical perforation of initially solid material or evaporation of a solvent from a partially gelled "starved" laminate have been attempted. The lack of widespread use is a reflection of some of the major problems with these materials, which include low strength, closing or clogging of pores, and sometimes intolerably rough surfaces.

Leathers. A variety of grades of leather continue to be used in prosthetic and orthotic devices and for orthopaedic shoes. Despite increasing cost, natural variability, and hygienic problems, leathers have a number of attractive properties. This class of materials is discussed in considerable detail in the *Orthopaedic Appliances Atlas,* vol. 1.

Fabrics. Numerous grades of natural and synthetic fabrics are used in orthotic devices. Woven fabrics are typically suited for straps and simple geometric shapes, but they must be tailored to complex three-dimensional shapes, which are much more readily fitted by knitted fabrics. Properties and selection of fabrics likewise are discussed in detail in the *Orthopaedic Appliances Atlas,* vol. 1.

DESIGN CONSIDERATIONS
Practical and economic considerations

In selecting specific materials and components for the various portions of an orthosis, one must consider numerous practical and economic factors. Safety, ease of working, compatibility of prefabricated components, ease of adjustment during fitting or subsequent use and feasibility of attachments are aspects. There also are special considerations when using multiple materials as laminates, as composites or even as assemblies.

In any portion in contact with the body, safety is essential. Lack of toxicity, allergenic tendency, or mechanical irritation is necessary. A material such as glass fiber may be used for reinforcement of a laminate if it is buried in the matrix, but special care must be taken to reseal the fiber ends exposed by grinding during trimming and fitting. Curing of plastics must be complete to avoid toxic or allergic reactions to uncured components of the resin. During initial use of plastic laminates in prosthetics, soon after World War II, a few facilities encountered skin irritation from free monomers left from incomplete curing because of moisture accidentally leaking into certain resins or because of rapid heat loss of exothermic bench-curing resins to a damp, cold plaster model. The characteristic odor of the monomer was readily detected near the supposedly cured laminate. With adequate care, these difficulties were readily overcome. Heating the finished laminate briefly with a heat lamp is effective, if there is any doubt. With the current interest in the forming of pros-

thetic sockets and orthotic devices directly on the patient's body, not only toxicity of base materials, plasticizers or solvents but also workability at tolerable temperatures are factors.

Ease of working with available facilities is an important practical consideration. The necessity to form orthotic structures to fit each individual imposes unusual requirements not typically found in most industrial operations.

Conventional molds, dies, and punches used in mass production of identical parts are sometimes appropriate for prefabricated components of orthotic devices, typically produced in a few stock sizes, perhaps capable of being cut to length or of further slight adjustment of shape. But those parts fitting the body, at least, must be formed to the individual. A wide variety of straps, buckle attachments, and similar parts are available from a few central manufacturers as inexpensive prefabricated elements.

Prefabricated joints such as ankle or knee joints have been available for decades and increasingly widely used after the mid-1950s, partly because of improved control of tolerances and quality. Probably the greatest incentives were the economic savings from reduction in time required of skilled labor and the possibility of more rapid delivery to the patient. In some designs, the "joint head" is a separate element adapted to attachment to a bar or other structural element by screws or rivets. Quite commonly, the joint head is delivered by the manufacturer integral with a relatively long straight bar, which is then formed to shape and cut to the appropriate length for the individual patient by the local orthotics facility.

With the growing use of new designs of orthoses, the conventional prefabricated components of the 1960s will probably decrease in usefulness. Some joints will be replaced entirely by the bending of selected portions of the structure. Other prefabricated components, redesigned to attach readily and securely to plastic laminate, thermoplastic, or composite structures, will continue to cut labor costs and improve service.

Some of the cuffs, shells, or other portions in contact with the body of the individual patient can be prefabricated in a few sizes and shapes. They can then be slightly distorted by straps or laces or more extensively modified (such as with the aid of a heat gun in the case of thermoplastics or postforming thermosetting plastic laminates) to fit the specific patient. Metal bars or similar structures typically are adjusted by using bending irons to strain the metal into the plastic region, leaving a permanent set when this load is removed. In contrast to the common practice prior to 1950, forging of metal bars at high temperature now very seldom occurs in local orthotic facilities.

Simple adjustments during daily wear are preferably provided by Velcro straps.[32] Small adjustments thus are possible in contrast with the substantial steps between successive holes in a belt for a conventional buckle. In addition, even a severely disabled patient frequently can engage and release a Velcro fastening, though he might have considerably more difficulty with a conventional buckle. Preferably a strap should be "snubbed" or passed through a loop fastened by a strap or billet to the opposite structure, laid back on itself, and the loose end attached to the original portion by mating Velcro elements. Just as in a rope-and-pulley system, the load on each end and thus the shear load on the Velcro is thus cut in half compared with a simple overlapping joint of mating straps from opposite sides of the structure.

Buckles with tongues and perforated straps are also widely used. They are reasonably adequate for adjustments requiring substantial steps, but they are especially appropriate for repeated attachment or for opening and closing at a relatively fixed position. Buckles capable of a sliding adjustment along a fabric strap are frequently used to adjust the length of a harness or suspension.

Traditionally the longitudinal bars or uprights of lower-limb orthoses for children have been composed of two portions fastened together by several screws. The length can be increased to accomodate growth in increments of the uniform distance between screw holes in one of the bars. Some newer orthoses lack this adjustability. Thermoplastic materials may allow for some modification of diameter or shape to fit a changing body portion, but such materials do not seem appropriate for accommodating longitudinal growth. Some form of telescoping construction may be needed.

Attachments of orthotic components may be made in a variety of ways. An occasional material like synthetic balata (Orthoplast or Polysar[33,48]) may stick to itself under some conditions, such as when it is hot and wet. Indeed, release agents must be applied to areas that are *not* supposed to stick together when they come into contact during the construction or fitting processes. Metal joint heads may be welded by electric arc or gas flame to give an integral metal bond to adjoining upright bars. Brazing or soldering provides a weaker metal-to-metal connection by a small amount of brazing metal or solder that melts at a much lower temperature than the major structural metal.

Frequently, parts are attached temporarily by a few light screws or rivets before the fitting process. Then more secure connection in the desired alignment is made by additional heavier screws or rivets, or by brazing or welding.

Plastics, leather, or fabric are typically attached to similar materials or to metal structural elements by gluing or by bonding. The goal usually is to attain a very thin layer of glue. Parts must be carefully cleaned and should be clamped together under firm pressure while the glue sets and hardens. The development of epoxy and other improved cements over the last two decades has considerably increased the ease of attachment of parts.

Fabrics typically are sewn together. Leathers may be cemented or sewn together. The type of stitch, size, and material of thread, shape of needle, and spacing will be chosen to suit the materials to be sewn and their thicknesses. Rather close, uniform lock stitching is typically used in orthopaedic appliances.

Composite structures are considerably more complex than those of a single material. It can be demonstrated that there will necessarily be loading directly proportional to the respective moduli of elasticity if two or more different materials are used in parallel with equal deflections. Suppose, for example, that a rigid frame suspends a relatively rigid loading bar by a stiff, high-modulus steel wire and a relatively very flexible, low-modulus rubber band. The steel wire will carry almost all of the load with a very microscopic deflection, whereas the rubber band stretching the same slight amount supports only a trivial share of the total load.

In an important but less dramatic case, a strip of laminate or composite structure under tension carries most of the load on the rather stiff fabric, stiffer fiber glass, or very much stiffer boron or graphite fibers, whereas the low-modulus resin matrix carries relatively little load. The transfer of loads even between two components respectively stiff and flexible, in a single composite material or especially in a more complex structure, may be complicated, involving shearing stresses at the interfaces. One may envision some of these loads by imagining structures of chains and springs connected by bars or beams.

There are also stresses within structures subject to external loading near sudden changes of stiffness. It is well known that there are stress concentrations near notches or holes; it is equally true, though perhaps less obvious, that there are also stress concentrations in the heighborhood of reinforcements, though the relative distributions of tension, compression, and shear stresses will differ between conditions of weakness and reinforcement. Donnell[17] studied the stress concentrations in the vicinity of elliptic discontinuities in edge-loaded sheets. The only condition showing no concentration was that with no discontinuity in stiffness. This analysis also has implication, as Bennett[9][13] has shown, for analysis of stresses in flesh near the brim of a prosthetic socket or an orthotic cuff impinging on the flesh.

The gross properties of a structure, a composite, a laminate, or a foam may be quite different from those of solid samples of the individual component materials and may differ for various types of loading. In a beam, for example, a component with high strength and modulus of elasticity in tension may carry most of the load and determine most of the stiffness on the side loaded in tension; this is a common situation with the steel rods in a reinforced concrete beam. In a plastic composite or laminate, likewise, the graphite or glass fibers may carry most of the tensile or almost all of the compressive loading. The epoxy or polyester matrix, relatively weak when alone, transfers shear loads between fibers and provides lateral support so that the long, thin fibers do not buckle at very low compressive loads as they would as isolated needles or threads when they were raw material before laminating. One of the advantages of Dacron reinforcing fabric is its chemical similarity to the polyester resin matrix, giving it a better shear bond.

In a sponge or foam, especially with thin-walled interconnecting cells, the overall nominal stiffness of the gross material may be very low compared with a solid block of the basic material because under load the thin walls deflect and the cells (whether open or closed) distort readily.

In composite structures and materials there may be practical problems from major differences in thermal expansion, absorption of moisture, or electromechanical properties. Shear stresses will be created between two adhering materials of differing coefficients of thermal expansion if there are changes in temperature. (These differences may be put to use, of course, such as in a bimetallic strip thermometer.) Appreciable differences in absorption of moisture may lead to internal shear stresses, cracking, or delaminating. Early plastic laminates using cotton fabrics, for example, tended to deteriorate if exposed to moisture, especially if the fabric ends were not resealed with resin after trimming of the brim or grinding during fitting. Dacron synthetic fabrics are much more moisture resistant.

Contact between dissimilar metals may lead to electrolytic corrosion in the presence of electrically conducting fluids like perspiration, urine, or blood. Even slight corrosion may accelerate fatigue failure by initiating surface roughness to form stress-raising notches or by facilitating microscopic intergranular corrosion at the bottom of a crack so as to help the crack to progress.

Many of the above examples emphasize the role of shear stress between two materials in a composite or laminate. The interrelationships of shear, tensile, and compressive stresses in most practical loading situations in a single material have already been noted. The ability to transmit shear stresses is especially important, further, in bonding composites and laminates together to make maximal use of the separate properties of each component. Fortunately, epoxy materials (which first came into widespread notice in orthotics as "C-8 resin" at the Second Symposium on Orthopaedic Appliances at Mellon Institute[47] in 1949 and since have been improved) are excellent adhesives when used alone and are very tenacious matrices for composites and laminates.

An especially important precaution with epoxy is to avoid skin contact with uncured resin both in the workshop and in the clinical use of the finished appliance. Appropriate working habits and adequate ventilation are needed in the orthotics facility. Thorough curing is especially crucial with epoxy.

To use composite materials effectively, one should understand the general concepts of stress distribution. If (as in many practical cases and especially during accidents) shock or impact loading is likely, a somewhat resilient or even plastically yielding energy-absorbing material may be preferable to an extremely high strength but very stiff and brittle material. The very stiff fibers in composites will function effectively only if their bonds through the matrix are effective. Therefore the matrix must inherently permit good bonds, the fibers must be clean, and bubbles or films must be avoided. Notches or scratches not only may accelerate fatigue failure but may cut some crucial fibers situated close to the surface where they are especially needed to resist bending.

The evaluation of new materials thus involves much more than a quick comparison of ultimate tensile strength, the values most often quoted in publicity about new material. Compressive, shear, and fatigue strengths, stress-strain characteristics or at least data on yield strength and ductility, impact strength, corrosion properties, thermal expansion, electrochemical properties, and moisture absorption are among the many factors to be considered. For contact with the body, toxic and allergenic properties and dermatologic aspects are crucial. Possibilities of working the material with currently available shop tools and especially for fitting individual patients with three-dimensionally warped cuffs or bars must usually be considered even if the material is used in a prefabricated component. Cost per pound is of negligible concern.

In view of these complexities, it is not surprising that individual relatively small orthotics laboratories tend to be conservative in choices of materials. Innovations have come largely from sponsored research laboratories coordinated by the National Research Council and some large university, government, or private facilities. After substantial clinical trial, the use of these materials has been taught widely through the government-supported prosthetics and orthotics education program.

Special structures

Joints and bearings. Traditional orthotic structures have used numerous joints and bearings to simulate selected motions but prevent others. Obviously restriction of motion leads to stresses. Plantar flexion and dorsiflexion are very often provided by ankle joints opposite the malleoli and on a line usually believed to be at the level of the upper ankle joint but perpendicular to the plane of progression. The desirability of a skewed upper ankle joint axis or an oblique lower axis for the subtalar joint, as emphasized by Isman and Inman,[28] has rarely been accepted.

Often caliper joints below the heel constitute an obvious gross deviation from anatomic position

in the interests of simplicity in donning or removing the appliance and exchanging shoes and of economy. In selected cases with stops preventing significant plantar flexion as well as spasticity or other tightness limiting dorsiflexion, the very limited range of angular motion may cause so little axial "pumping" of the cuffs and bands that the compromise with physiology is acceptable.

Knee joints, typically with locks at least on the lateral bars, have been routinely provided in the leg-thigh orthoses (KAFO). Typically these are provided on a single axis through the approximate center of the femoral condyles, generally a reasonable compromise with the moving instantaneous center of the human knee joint. Fortunately during most of the range of knee motion including sitting positions, the human instantaneous center is near the center of the femoral condyles.[20] Because of the tolerance of tissue to moderate compression and shear, small discrepancies between anatomic and mechanical joints generally can be absorbed, as most clinicians appear to believe, without the complexities of polycentric hinges. The location of the mechanical axis at the joint *space* between femur and tibia, though, is generally criticized as being much too low, a location leading to considerable compression of the band just below the knee joints, against the calf area during sitting, and consequent restriction of return circulation.

Joints traditionally were merely metal against metal. About two decades ago there was great emphasis[44] on the possibility of reducing wear and decreasing squeaking noises by using bushings and washers (such as of nylon) between rubbing surfaces.

Flexible structures as joints. Flexible structures have served as joints for many decades, but new possibilities have arisen with plastics. Coiled wires or cantilever springs have been used as below-knee foot-ankle orthoses or "drop-foot braces" to resist plantar flexion and assist dorsiflexion. Such a device with a leather cuff about the calf was simple and light in weight, but many broke from fatigue failure especially when accidental nicks or scratches from contacts with sharp edges in the environment tended to concentrate stresses. Some designs minimized tendency to slide the cuff axially up and down on the calf, but others caused this irritation.

In recent years plastic laminate rods[25,27] or a helically coiled plastic strip[30] have been used as flexible structures both to resist plantar flexion and to provide some lateral stability. The possible uses for such structures have also been explored for orthoses at levels other than the ankle. The unusually great fatigue resistance of polypropylene plastic as a hinge probably has not been fully exploited.

Lubricants. Lubricants for metal joints have traditionally offered problems because of staining of clothing. The usual oils are generally unsatisfactory. A thin layer of Vaseline reduced wear and squeaking briefly but soon tended to become not only discolored but contaminated with metal particles as well as dirt, tending to act as an abrasive. Subsequent oozing of the lubricant from the joint space then soiled clothing. Experiments with polymolybdenum sulfide and other solid lubricants were only partially satisfactory because of risks of clothing staining and of inadequate lubrication.

Brakes and clutches. Mechanical brakes and clutches and pneumatic or hydraulic resistance have occasionally been suggested to control the ankle, knee, or both.[5,41] Most of these devices have been limited by added bulkiness near an already bulky bony joint structure as well as by added risks of noises or leaks and perhaps by limited understanding of control sources.

Springs. Springs have often been used to resist gravity or to oppose a stronger muscle. Perhaps the most frequent application is to resist plantar flexion and assist return toward dorsiflexion. A simple elastic fabric strap from a garter above the calf to an attachment near the toes—perhaps at the beginning of the shoelaces—will serve many patients, though it is not always acceptable. The Klenzak spring-return ankle joint, with a helical steel spring pressing a ball bearing upon the hardened posterior portion of the top of a stirrup under the shoe, was an early and very widely used prefabricated orthotics component. A screw compressing the upper end of the spring into its housing permitted some moderate adjustment of initial position or torque. Clocklike spiral strip or wire springs are sometimes used at the ankle.

Although helical coils of wire are often used as tension, compression, or torsion springs, many other forms are possible. Beams or cantilever strips of thin metal may be bent; sometimes, as in corset steels, they are attached or inserted into pockets in an appliance, but sometimes these beams are integral parts of another metallic structure. A clock spring is simply a long cantilever beam coiled into a compact spiral.

Simple rubber bands were used in hand orthoses, especially for polio, to allow easy adjustment of the initial tension and spring rate for individual fingers, the thumb, or the wrist. Indeed for certain cases, an ingenious winding of a single rubber band about the thumb and fingers could serve as a simple, inconspicuous combination of opponens and finger orthosis, plus mild spring closing or gripping actuator to be overcome occasionally by extensor muscles.

Metal springs typically have a constant "spring rate" in tension or compression. Beyond an initial linear range, cams or tandem springs may be used to make the force versus excursion curve rise increasingly rapidly. This nonlinear action may produce a desirably smooth action with gradual transition from early large deflection to increasing resistance and ultimate blockage of further motion.

Spring life is particularly affected by fatigue failure. Springs must be carefully designed and manufactured to combine appropriate operating force range, necessary excursion, small size, and adequate fatigue life despite high stresses. All too often the spring is the final element designed after other key elements and dimensions are fixed; then the spring material must be overstressed! As in other fatigue situations early satisfactory life is not necessarily assurance of long endurance. Fortunately substantial improvements are sometimes possible by slight changes in dimensions, materials, or treatment to resist corrosion.

Locks and stops. Locks and stops are elements frequently used in orthotics. Often a joint is free to bend in one direction but is stopped from moving in the opposite direction by a hardened relatively rigid abutment. A hyperextension stop in a knee joint is a typical example. To facilitate fitting and adjustment of alignment, the orthotist may wish to be able to grind the stop surface slightly; yet to resist plastic distortion, the surface should be relatively hard. Occasionally an adjustable screw stop is provided in a joint, but there is seldom room for the broad rubber bumper or piano felt pad used in prosthetics.

Single-plane joints, so commonly used in orthotics, are themselves stops against flexion or rotation about the other axes. Prevention of these other motions, of course, is associated with forces tending to increase friction and wear and to produce clicking or squeaking noises.

Locks are available in a great variety of designs of differing bulk, complexity, durability, and cost. Volume I of the *Atlas*[1] presents numerous varieties, particularly for the knee joint. The drop-ring knee lock, despite many limitations, is still very widely used because of simplicity and low cost. Numerous types of cam or lever locks are frequently used particularly when both medial and lateral joints are to be locked or released simultaneously. Hydraulic locks, though available for placement in the hollow interior of the shank of an above-knee prosthesis, are still generally considered too bulky to control a paralyzed knee by fitting on the outside of a human leg even with atrophied muscles. Although greater understanding of biomechanical requirements as well as of alignment principles for stability may reduce the apparent need for locks, it still seems desirable to explore new types of extension bias means, brakes, and mechanical or hydraulic locks suitable at least for certain applications in orthotics.

External power. External power for orthotics has been studied almost entirely for upper-limb needs,[14,15,21] first for flaccid paralysis and recently for quadriparesis. Bowden cables[38] or hydraulic transmission[23,43] may be used occasionally to transmit power from other parts of the body. The McKibben pneumatic "muscle"[6,40] was widely used for polio cases. Perhaps it was readily accepted because it looked and acted much like a real muscle functioning in tension and because it was sufficiently flexible to allow pronation or supination without interference with a flexor function.

Several designs[22,31] of an electrically driven actuator have been proposed for operation of upper-limb orthoses. These may be controlled by body-operated switches, myoelectric signals from remaining muscles, or small voluntary skin motion moving a magnet with respect to an electrical sensor.[42] Electrical stimulation of paralyzed muscle is growing in importance.[16]

CONCLUSION

A moderate understanding of engineering principles will aid the entire clinic team in selection and wise use of materials and mechanisms to aid the individual patient.

REFERENCES

1. Aldredge, R. H., and Snow, B. M.: Lower extremity braces. In American Academy of Orthopaedic Surgeons: Orthopaedic appliances atlas, vol. 1, Ann Arbor, Mich., 1952, J. W. Edwards; especially axis of knee joint, pp. 365-367, 384, 386, knee-joint locking mechanisms, 388-391.
2. American Society for Testing and Materials: Annual book of ASTM standards, Philadelphia. (Revision issued annually, in some 30 or more parts each containing standards in several fields.)
3. American Society for Testing and Materials: ASTM standards for surgical implants, Philadelphia, July 1973.
4. Anderson, M. H.: In Sollars, R. E., Bray, J. J., Snelson, L. R., and Marmor, L., editors: Upper extremity orthotics, Springfield, Ill., 1965, Charles C Thomas, Publisher.
5. Anderson, M. H,, and Bray, J. J.: The UCLA functional long leg brace, Clin. Orthop. **37**:98-109, 1964.
6. Barber, L. M., and Nickel, V. L.: Carbon dioxide powered arm and hand devices, Amer. J. Occup. Ther. **23**(3):215-225, May-June 1969.
7. Battelle Memorial Institute: Prevention of the failure of metals under repeated stress, New York, 1941, John Wiley & Sons, Inc. (A classic report prepared under the auspices of National Research Council.)
8. Beer, F. P., and Johnston, E. R., Jr.: Vector mechanics for engineers: Statics and dynamics, New York, 1962, McGraw-Hill Book Co.
9. Bennett, L.: Transferring load to flesh, Part II. Analysis of compressive stress, Bull. Prosthet. Res. **10-16**:45-63, Fall 1971.
10. Bennett, L.: Transferring load to flesh, Part III. Analysis of shear stress, Bull. Prosthet. Res. **10-17**:38-51, Spring 1972.
11. Bennett, L.: Transferring load to flesh, Part IV. Flesh reaction to contact curvature, Bull. Prosthet. Res. **10-18**:60-67, Fall 1972.
12. Bennett, L.: Transferring load to flesh, Part V. Experimental work, Bull. Prosthet. Res. **10-19**:88-103, Spring 1973.
13. Bennett, L.: Transferring load to flesh, Part VI. Socket brim radius effects, Bull. Prosthet. Res. **10-20**:103-117, Fall 1973.
14. Committee on Prosthetics Research and Development: Orthotics research and development (a report on a conference), Washington, D.C., 1962, National Academy of Sciences—National Research Council.
15. Committee on Prosthetics Research and Development: The control of external power in upper-extremity rehabilitation (a report on a conference), Publication 1352, Washington, D.C., 1966, National Academy of Sciences-National Research Council.
16. Committee on Prosthetics Research and Development, Subcommittee on Evaluation: Clinical evaluation of the Ljubljana functional electrical peroneal brace, Report E-7, Washington, D.C., 1973, National Academy of Sciences—National Research Council.
17. Donnell, L. H.: Stress concentrations due to elliptical discontinuities in plates under edge forces. In Applied mechanics, Theodore von Kármán anniversary volume, Pasadena, 1941, California Institute of Technology, pp. 293-309.
18. England, C. F., Fannin, R. E., Skahan, J. K., and Smith, H. W.: In Anderson, M. H., and Ellison, M., editors: A manual of lower extremities orthotics, Springfield, Ill., 1972, Charles C Thomas, Publisher.
19. Frankel, V. H., and Burstein, A. H.: Orthopaedic biomechanics—the application of engineering to the musculoskeletal system, Philadelphia, 1970, Lea & Febiger.
20. Frankel, V. H., Burstein, A. H., and Brooks, D. B.: Biomechanics of internal derangement of the knee, J. Bone Joint Surg. **53A**(5):945-962, July 1971.

21. Gavrilović, M. M., and Wilson, A. B., Jr., editors: Proceedings of the Third International Symposium on External Control of Human Extremities, Advances in external control of human extremities, Belgrade, 1970, Yugoslav Committee for Electronics and Automation.
22. Grahn, E. C.: A power unit for functional hand splints, Bull. Prosthet. Res. **10-13**:52-56, Spring 1970.
23. Heather, A. J., and Smith, T. A.: "Helping hand", a hydraulically operated mechanical hand, Orthop. Prosthet. Appliance J. 14(2):36-40, June 1960.
24. Hetényi, M.: Handbook of experimental stress analysis, New York, 1957, John Wiley & Sons, Inc.
25. Hill, J. T.: U.S. Pat. 3,589,359 unidirectional fiberglass *(sic)* composite drop-foot brace, June 29, 1971.
26. Hill, J. T., and Leonard, F.: Porous plastic laminates for upper-extremity prostheses, Artif. Limbs 7(1):17-30, Spring 1963.
27. Hill, J. T., Bensman, A. S., Dozier, A., and Stube, R. W.: Epoxy-fiberglass *(sic)* short-leg brace, Arch. Phys. Med. Rehabil. **52**(2):82-85, Feb. 1971.
28. Isman, R. E., and Inman, V. T.: Anthropometric studies of the human foot and ankle, Bull. Prosthet. Res. **10-11**:97-129, Spring 1969.
29. Kennaway, A.: On the reduction of slip of rubber crutch-tips on wet pavement, snow and ice, Bull. Prosthet. Res. **10-14**:130-144, Fall 1970.
30. Lehneis, H. R.: New developments in lower-limb orthotics through bioengineering, Arch. Phys. Med. Rehabil. **53**(7):303-310, especially p. 322, July 1972.
31. Lehneis, H. R., and Wilson, R. G., Jr.: An electric arm orthosis, Bull. Prosthet. Res. **10-17**:4-20, Spring 1972.
32. Malick, M. H.: Manual on static hand splinting—new materials and techniques, Pittsburgh, 1970, Harmarville Rehabilitation Center. Velcro p. 31; equivalent of p. 36.
33. Malick, M. H.: Manual on static hand splinting—new materials and techniques, Pittsburgh, 1970, Harmarville Rehabilitation Center. Orthoplast described, pp. 30-32.
34. Morris, J. M., and Blickenstaff, L. D.: Fatigue fractures—a clinical study, Springfield, Ill., 1967, Charles C Thomas, Publisher.
35. Murphy, E. F.: Engineering considerations in the design of orthopaedic appliances. In American Academy of Orthopaedic Surgeons: Orthopaedic appliances atlas, vol. 1, Ann Arbor, Mich., 1952, J. W. Edwards; pp. 171-178, especially pp. 176-177 on stress concentration.
36. Paul, J. P.: Forces at the human hip joint, doctoral thesis, University of Glasgow, October 1967.
37. Prosthetic-Orthotic Center, Northwestern University Medical School: Spinal orthotics for orthotists (manual for Orthotics 701) and Lower extremity and spinal orthotics for physicians, surgeons, and therapists (manual for Orthotics 722 and 723), Northwestern University Medical School, Chicago, Ill. (Undated.)
38. Pursley, R. J.: Harness patterns for upper-extremity prosthesis. Chapter 4 in American Academy of Orthopaedic Surgeons: Orthopaedic appliances atlas, vol. 2, Artificial limbs, Ann Arbor, Mich. 1960, J. E. Edwards, pp. 105-128, especially Bowden cable principle, p. 106.
39. Sandor, B. I.: Cyclic stress and strain, Madison, Wisc., 1972, University of Wisconsin Press.
40. Schulte, H. F., Jr.: The characteristics of the McKibben artificial muscle. In The application of external power in prosthetics and orthotics (a report on a conference), Publication 874, Washington, D.C., 1961, National Academy of Sciences—National Research Council, Appendix H, pp. 94-115 (mathematical and experimental analysis of force, length, gas consumption).
41. Scott, C. M., Shaw, N. A., and Amstutz, H. C.: Functional long leg brace research, final report to Social and Rehabilitation Service; University of California, Los Angeles. Prosthetic/Orthotics Education Program, March 1971, hydraulic controls, pp. 39-40; mechanical friction clutch, pp. 41-43.
42. Seamone, W., and Schmeisser, G.: Development and evaluation of externally powered upper-limb prosthesis, Bull. Prosthet. Res. **10-17**:33-37, Spring 1972.
43. Smith, T. A.: Hydraulics for power transmission in prosthetic devices. In The application of external power in prosthetics and orthotics (a report on a conference), Publication 874, Washington, D.C., 1961, National Academy of Sciences—National Research Council, Appendix J, pp. 132-139.
44. Thorndike, A., Murphy, E. F., and Staros, A.: Engineering applied to orthopaedic bracing, Orthop. Prosthet. Appliance J. **10**(4):55-71, Dec. 1956.
45. Timoshenko, S.: Strength of materials, Part I, Princeton, N.J., 1956, D. Van Nostrand Co.
46. Weaver, H. E.: Constructional materials—non-metallic, Part II. Progress report for the month ended December 31, 1948, Sarah Mellon Scaife Foundation Fellowship on Orthopedic Appliances, Mellon Institute of Industrial Research, Pittsburgh, Pennsylvania, pp. 18-21 on perforated plastics as substitutes for leathers.
47. Weaver, H. E., and Young, J. L.: Summary report of Sarah Mellon Scaife Foundation Fellowship on Orthopedic Appliances (November 1, 1949 to August 1, 1951), Mellon Institute of Industrial Research, Pittsburgh, Pennsylvania, especially pp. 15-19 on C-8 resin. See also Anonymous: New resin-fiberglass process builds strong laminates, OALMA J. 4(3):10-12, July 1950.
48. Wilson, A. B., Jr.: A material for direct forming of prosthetic sockets, Artif. Limbs 14(1):53-56, Spring 1970.

PART TWO

The upper limb

CHAPTER 2

Functional anatomy of the upper limb

SHAHAN K. SARRAFIAN, M.D.

The human being, as a living system, functions in relationship to his own body and to his environment. Basically his functional capacities are geared to reach and fulfill definite goals. Through locomotion or other forms of transportation, he determines the placement of his body in the environment. Once translocated, or during the translocation, his functional capacities become extremely varied through the action of the upper limbs. They may work alone or in synchronization with the lower limbs and the spine. The highly specialized organs, the hands, are located at the end of a multisegmented, interconnected system, a system that allows a purposeful placement of the end organs of the body over an element of his environment or simply in space. The precise placement of the hands is usually followed by definite functional activities. These activities can be manipulative, supportive, or expressional.

The functional activities are multitudinous, but the prehensile activities are basically of a power or precision type of pattern. In the power type of grip, there is often a close relationship with the functional activities of the lower limbs; in the precision type of grip, these relations are minimal, absent, or only supportive. The jeweler working on a diamond or the surgeon manipulating microsurgical instruments uses essentially a precision type of grip, with the lower limbs being

immobile. The skier, football player, and bicycle rider coordinate skillfully the power grip with the mobility of the lower limbs. All other intermediary combinations are possible, however, in the infinite variety of daily activities.

The placement of the hand surface, prior to its motor performance, provides a wealth of sensory information through its different transducers. Texture, hardness or softness, shape, temperature, pressure, and dryness or moisture are centrally analyzed by our computer, the brain, and are integrated into a pleasurable, informative, painful, or unpleasant experience. An appropriate motor response usually follows the sensory information. The absence of this sensory phase severely dampens or completely annihilates the motor performance. This sensorimotor relationship is of paramount importance in the planning of a therapeutic program for a problem of functional deficit.

FUNCTIONAL ANATOMY OF SHOULDER

The placement of the hand is accomplished by the shoulder complex supplemented by the action of the elbow and forearm. The shoulder complex is formed by the scapulohumeral, acromioclavicular, and sternoclavicular joints. The last two joints provide the mobility of the scapulothoracic mechanism. The entire system is suspended from the trunk by soft-tissue anchorage, with the only true skeletal articulation being the sternoclavicular joint. For the complex to function adequately, the spine must be stable.

Scapulothoracic mechanism

As the scapula moves over the chest wall, the basic motions involved are elevation and depression, upward and downward rotation, adduction and abduction. During the elevation, the scapula is displaced upward such as in carrying heavy loads or in shrugging the shoulders. Four muscles (Fig. 2-1) responsible for this motion[12] are the *levator scapulae, upper trapezius, rhomboideus major,* and *rhomboideus minor.*

Participation of the *serratus anterior* in elevating the scapula has been controversial. Inman et al.[13] mention the upper digitations of the serratus anterior as elevators. Duchenne,[9] investigating the action through observation and electrical stimulation, concludes that this muscle does not contract while one carries heavy loads on the shoulder. Hollinshead[12] classifies the muscle as a depressor of the scapula.

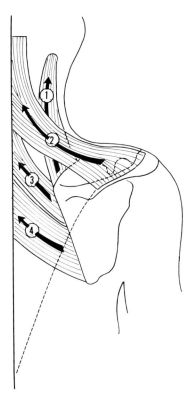

Fig. 2-1. Elevators of scapula. **1,** Levator scapulae. **2,** Upper trapezius. **3,** Rhomboideus minor. **4,** Rhomboideus major.

Depression of the scapula or its caudad displacement, noticed, for example, in crutch walking or in parallel-bar exercising, is actively controlled by the *pectoralis major lower segment, latissimus dorsi,* and *trapezius lower segment*[12] (Fig. 2-2).

The pectoralis major and the latissimus dorsi act as depressors through their downward pull on the humerus. The accessory depressors are the *pectoralis minor* and *subclavius,* and possibly the *serratus anterior lower part.*

Upward rotation occurs when the acromion is elevated and the inferior angle of the scapula is carried forward and outward. The glenoid cavity is directed upward and anteriorly. This scapular rotary motion is provided by a force couple (Fig. 2-3). The upper vector is determined by the action of the *upper* and *middle trapezius.* The lower vector is provided by the *lower trapezius* and *lower digitations of the serratus anterior* (Inman[13]). Upward rotation of the scapula is an important contributor to shoulder-complex action during abduction or flexion of the upper extremity.

As the scapula rotates downward, the acromial process is lowered and the inferior angle is displaced medially. Such motion occurs, for example, when the hand reaches the low back. This rotary motion (Fig. 2-4) is controlled by the combined action of the scapular elevators, which are the *levator scapulae, rhomboideus minor,* and *rhomboideus major,* and the shoulder depressors, which are the *latissimus dorsi, lower segment of the pectoralis major,* and *pectoralis minor.*

Abduction brings the scapula anteriorly and laterally and is controlled by the *serratus anterior* and the *pectoralis minor*[12] (Fig. 2-5). This is an important motion in activating a prosthesis. Adduction displaces the scapula towards the midline. This is brought about by the *middle trapezius, rhomboideus minor,* and *rhomboideus major*[12] (Fig. 2-6). The rhomboidei are elevators and adductors; the latissimus dorsi may act as adductor and depressor. Acting together, elevation is neutralized by depression, and the end result is a pure adduction.

Scapulohumeral joint motion

The motion of the arm will be analyzed in the sagittal plane as flexion-extension, in the frontal plane as abduction-adduction, and around its long axis as internal-external rotation. From a position of maximum extension, the arm can be flexed[12] (Fig. 2-7) by the *anterior deltoid, clavicular head of*

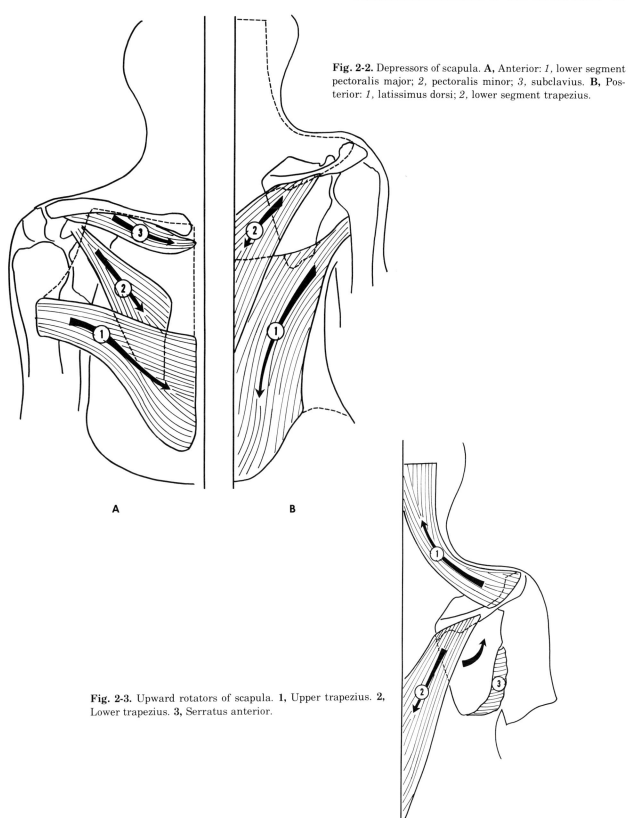

Fig. 2-2. Depressors of scapula. **A,** Anterior: *1,* lower segment pectoralis major; *2,* pectoralis minor; *3,* subclavius. **B,** Posterior: *1,* latissimus dorsi; *2,* lower segment trapezius.

A

B

Fig. 2-3. Upward rotators of scapula. **1,** Upper trapezius. **2,** Lower trapezius. **3,** Serratus anterior.

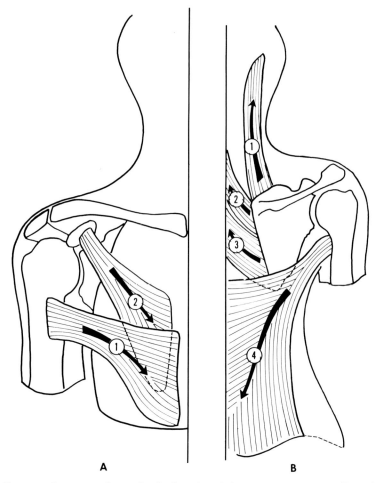

A   B

Fig. 2-4. Downward rotators of scapula. **A,** Anterior: *1,* lower segment pectoralis major; *2,* pectoralis minor. **B,** Posterior: *1,* levator scapulae; *2,* rhomboideus minor; *3,* rhomboideus major; *4,* latissimus dorsi.

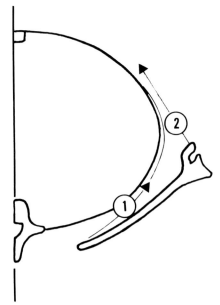

Fig. 2-5. Abductors of scapula. **1,** Serratus anterior. **2,** Pectoralis minor.

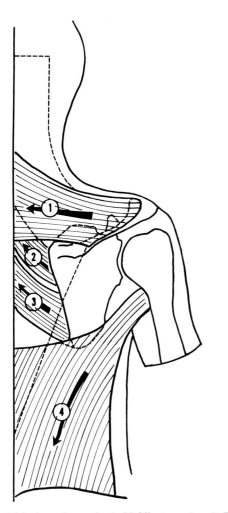

Fig. 2-6. Adductors of scapula. **1,** Middle trapezius. **2,** Rhomboideus minor. **3,** Rhomboideus major. **4,** Latissimus dorsi.

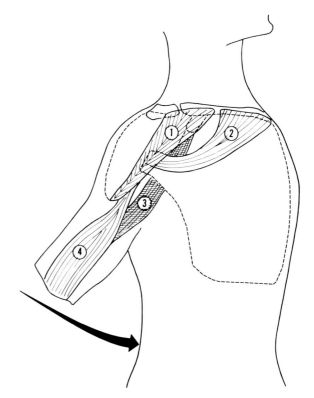

Fig. 2-7. Shoulder flexors. **1,** Anterior deltoid. **2,** Clavicular-head pectoralis major. **3,** Coracobrachialis. **4,** Biceps.

the pectoralis major, sternal head of the pectoralis major, active only until the arm is brought to the side, *coracobrachialis,* and *biceps* (the long head is more active than the short head [Basmajian and Latif[4]]). From a position of full flexion, the arm is extended by gravity unless resistance is offered[12] (Fig. 2-8). Then the following muscles are active: *posterior deltoid, latissimus dorsi, sternocostal portion of the pectoralis major* (until the arm is brought to the side), *teres major,* and *long head of the triceps.* The last two muscles are accessory extensors of the arm. The arm can be adducted anteriorly or posteriorly once the body has been avoided by appropriate flexion or extension. The adductors located anteriorly are the *pectoralis major, anterior segment of the deltoid,* and *coracobrachialis*[2] (Fig. 2-9, *A*). The last two muscles

are accessory adductors. The posteriorly located adductors are the *latissimus dorsi, teres major, posterior segment of the deltoid,* and *long head of the triceps*[12] (Fig. 2-9, *B*). Electromyographically, the posterior fibers of the deltoid are very active, probably to resist the internal rotation that the main adductors (latissimus dorsi and pectoralis major), could produce (Scheving and Pauly[29]).

Rotation of the arm occurs in an external or internal direction (Fig. 2-10). With the arm by the side, it can be rotated internally 80 degrees and externally 60 degrees, whereas, when the arm is in 90 degrees of abduction, the external rotation increases to 90 degrees and the internal rotation decreases to 70 degrees.[1] The internal rotators of the arm at the glenohumeral joint are the *subscapularis, teres major, latissimus dorsi, pectoralis major,* active only with resisted rotation (Scheving and Pauly[29]), and *anterior deltoid.*[12] The external rotators of the arm are the *infraspinatus, teres minor,* and *posterior segment of the deltoid,* as an accessory component.

The arm can be abducted to 180 degrees if com-

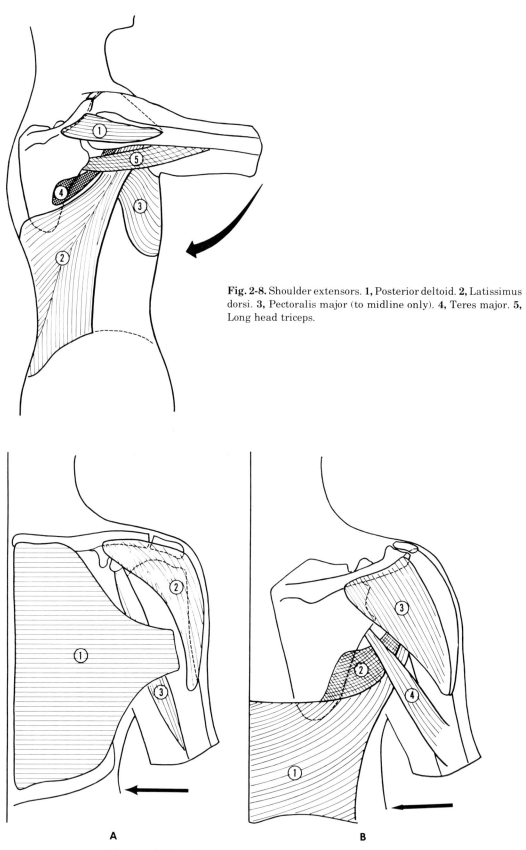

Fig. 2-8. Shoulder extensors. **1,** Posterior deltoid. **2,** Latissimus dorsi. **3,** Pectoralis major (to midline only). **4,** Teres major. **5,** Long head triceps.

A

B

Fig. 2-9. Shoulder adductors. **A,** Anterior: *1,* pectoralis major; *2,* anterior segment deltoid; *3,* coracobrachialis. **B,** Posterior: *1,* latissimus dorsi; *2,* teres major; *3,* posterior segment deltoid; *4,* long head triceps.

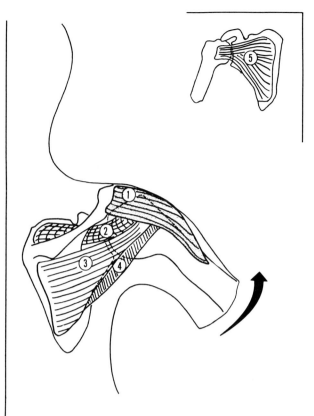

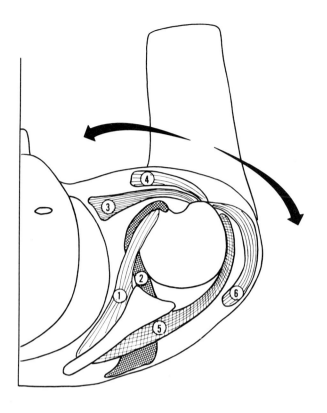

Fig. 2-10. Shoulder rotators. *Internal rotators: 1,* subscapularis; *2,* teres major—latissimus dorsi; *3,* pectoralis major; *4,* anterior segment deltoid. *External rotators: 5,* infraspinatus—teres minor; *6,* posterior segment deltoid.

Fig. 2-11. Shoulder abductors. **1,** Middle segment deltoid. **2,** Supraspinatus, **3,** Infraspinatus. **4,** Teres minor. **5,** Subscapularis.

bined with external rotation. Abduction in full internal rotation is less than 90 degrees; this essential fact was well known to Duchenne.[9] The abductors of the arm (Fig. 2-11) are the *deltoid,* mostly the middle segment, and those in the *rotator cuff,* which are the supraspinatus, infraspinatus, teres minor, and subscapularis (Inman[13] and Van Linge[32]).

The action of these two muscle groups comprise the superior and inferior components of a rotary force couple necessary for arm abduction. This interpretation correlates satisfactorily with the clinical picture of a torn rotator cuff. When the tear is complete, one of the most significant findings is the weakness of abduction from 0 to 90 degrees.

Investigating the prevention of downward dislocation of the humeral head, Basmajian and Bazant[6] explored both electromyelographically and anatomically the factors of vertical stability. All the muscles running vertically—deltoid, biceps, and triceps—were inactive even with a heavy vertical pull. The supraspinatus and posterior fibers of the deltoid, however, were quite active. They concluded that the downward subluxation or dislocation is prevented by the supraspinatus and the superior capsule. This coincides with Duchenne's interpretation of the muscle acting as an "active ligament."

Inman et al.[13] in their extensive exploration of the shoulder physiology clarified the contribution of the four components of the shoulder complex during elevation. When the arm is abducted from 0 to 180 degrees, there is a close relationship between the glenohumeral and the scapulothoracic mechanism. During the initial phase of elevation (from 0 to 30 degrees) the motion is mainly glenohumeral with the scapula being very variable in its action. It may either remain fixed, move laterally or medially, or oscillate as it seeks stabilization. This is called the "setting phase" of the scapula. From 30- to 180-degree abduction, there is a definite relationship between glenohumeral and scapulothoracic motion. For every 15 degrees

of abduction, 10 degrees occurs at the glenohumeral joint and 5 degrees is scapulothoracic
motion. The ratio of contribution is as follows:

$$\frac{SH}{ST} = \frac{\text{Glenohumeral}}{\text{Scapulothoracic}} = \frac{2}{1} = \frac{100 \text{ degrees}}{50 \text{ degrees}}$$

That of the scapulothoracic is 50 degrees, whereas
130 degrees is glenohumeral joint motion.

Upward rotation of the scapula is responsible
for this 50 degrees of arm abduction. Thus the patient with an ankylosed scapulohumeral joint can
still elevate the arm to 50 degrees. A shoulder
fusion, to be optimally successful, must have some
scapular rotators present.

Sternoclavicular and acromioclavicular motion[13]

The clavicle is interposed between the scapula
and the sternum. Scapular motion is present only
if motion is permitted at the acromioclavicular
and sternoclavicular joints. The clavicle is elevated or depressed, protracted or retracted, and
rotated on its long axis. During the first half of
arm elevation, motion occurs at the sternoclavicular joint. For every 10 degrees of abduction, the
clavicle is elevated by 4 degrees. A total range of
36 degrees occurs during the first half of arm elevation. Motion at the acromioclavicular joint is
more limited, being only 20 degrees. It occurs
during the initial (0- to 30-degree) and terminal
(135- to 180-degree) phases of arm abduction.
During the terminal phase of abduction, the clavicle rotates on its long axis approximately 40 to 50
degrees (the posterior border descends). This rotation relaxes the tension of the conoid and trapezoid
ligaments to allow further upward rotation of the
scapula.

FUNCTIONAL ANATOMY OF ELBOW

The forearm moves in a plane of flexion-
extension from 0 to 150 degrees and in a rotary
plane from 90 degrees of pronation to 90 degrees of
supination. Because of the configuration of the
humeral trochlea, the forearm is aligned with the
arm in flexion, but it is slightly abducted (the
carrying angle) in extension. The elbow flexors
(Fig. 2-12) are the *biceps, brachialis,* and *brachioradialis.* The following muscles are considered
accessory flexors: *pronator teres, wrist and finger
flexors,* and *radial wrist extensors.*

The activity of the elbow flexors has been well
analyzed by Basmajian and Latif.[4] The brachialis

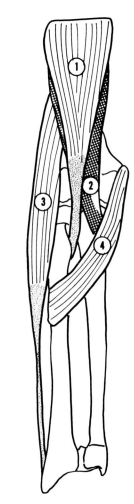

Fig. 2-12. Elbow flexors. 1, Biceps. 2, Brachialis. 3, Brachioradialis. 4, Pronator teres.

is an active flexor at any rotational position of the
forearm and at any speed. The biceps is a flexor of
the unloaded forearm only when it is supinated.
This muscle is deactivated when the forearm is
completely pronated unless heavy resistance is
encountered. In neutral rotation, it becomes active
as a flexor only if a load is lifted.

The brachioradialis is active when a weight is
lifted or when the forearm is flexed rapidly. This
action comes into play best in neutral rotation of
the forearm.

The pronator teres acts as an accessory elbow
flexor only when flexion occurs against resistance
(Basmajian and Travill[5]).

Extension of the forearm (Fig. 2-13) is provided by the *triceps* and *anconeus* acting as an
accessory extensor.

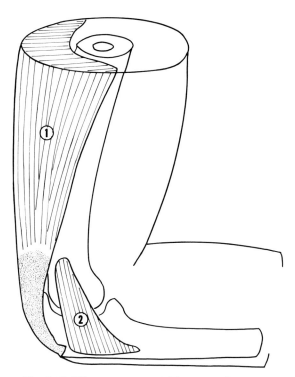

Fig. 2-13. Elbow extensors. 1, Triceps. 2, Anconeus.

According to Travill[31] the medial head of the triceps is the main elbow extensor; it is always active regardless of the resistance applied. The lateral head and the long head of the triceps come into action mainly when resistance is applied to the extension of the forearm.

Forearm rotation (pronation-supination) is 180 degrees only if hand position is the point of reference. With a wrist disarticulation, rotation drops to 120 degrees (Klopsteg and Wilson[17]). This means that a portion of the total rotation range occurs at the radiocarpal and midcarpal joints.

The functional axis of forearm rotation passes from the center of the humeral capitulum through the center of the radial head, the head of the ulna, and the little finger. In this classic interpretation, the distal end of the radius turns around the fixed ulnar head. This view, however, has been seriously challenged by many investigators. Vicq d'Azyr and Winslow detected mobility of the ulna during rotation of the forearm. Duchenne[9] observed that during pronation-supination the distal end of the radius and the head of the ulna trace arcs of a circle in opposite directions, but of equal lengths. Such is true if the hand is kept in constant alignment with the elbow. The first interpretation requires a fixed alignment of the ulna and thus

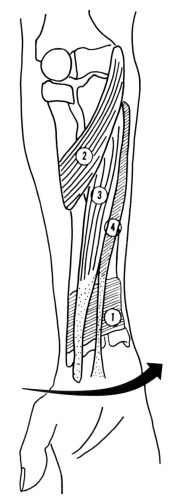

Fig. 2-14. Forearm pronators. 1, Pronator quadratus. 2, Pronator teres. 3, Flexor carpi radialis. 4, Palmaris longus.

allows the hand to displace medially. When the head of the ulna traces an arc of a circle, motion occurs at the humeroulnar joint. According to Duchenne[9] when the forearm is pronating from a position of maximum supination, the ulna is successively extended, laterally displaced slightly, and then flexed. The reverse motion occurs during supination. Poirier and Charpy,[25] investigating the problem of longitudinal rotation, found that the radius and ulna are mobile whereas the distal end of the radius traces a long arc; the head of the ulna turns on itself and traces a smaller arc. More recently, Capener,[8] analyzing the rotational motion, localized the axis in the center of the distal radius but made a point of its variability any place from the radial styloid to the ulnar styloid. Ray et al.[28] described 8 to 9 degrees of lateral abduction of the ulna from full supination to pronation.

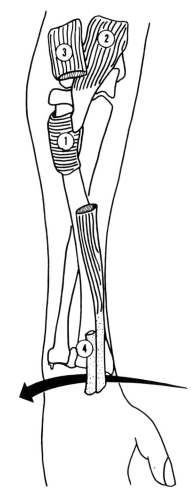

Fig. 2-15. Forearm supinators. 1, Supinator. 2, Biceps. 3 and 4, Extensor carpi radialis longus and brevis.

The proximal radius pivots at the radio-humeral joint. According to Poirier and Charpy[25] the axis that passes through the center of the radial head traces a segment of a spiral, since the contour of the radial head is not a true circle. Furthermore, the radial head is slightly displaced anteriorly during pronation and slightly posteriorly during supination.

The pronators of the forearm (Fig. 2-14) are the *pronator teres* and *pronator quadratus.* The pronator quadratus is effective in any position of flexion-extension of the forearm and therefore is the main pronator (Basmajian[2] and Hollinshead[12]). The pronator teres reinforces the action of the pronator quadratus with resisted or rapid pronation.[2] The accessory pronators are the *flexor carpi radialis* and *palmaris longus,* coming into action in forceful pronation. The supinators of

the forearm (Fig. 2-15) are the *supinator* and *biceps.*[12]

When the elbow is extended the supinator is slightly more efficient, whereas, in flexion the biceps becomes more active (Hollinshead[12]). The biceps reinforces the supinator when supination occurs rapidly or against resistance or when the elbow is flexed in fast unresisted supination (Basmajian[2]). In slow unresisted supination, the biceps is inactive regardless of the position of the elbow. Accessory supinators of the forearm are the *extensors carpi radialis longus and brevis.*

FUNCTIONAL ANATOMY OF WRIST

The wrist can move in flexion-extension and in ulnoradial deviation. By a combination of these motions, it can circumduct to act as an universal joint (Boyes[7]). The wrist joint also contributes to pronation-supination. During activity as in using a hammer, the wrist moves in an oblique plane from extension with radial deviation, to flexion with ulnar deviation. The range of flexion (80 degrees) is slightly greater than that of extension (70 degrees), and the hand ulnarly deviates (30 degrees) more than radially (20 degrees).[1] The ulnoradial deviation is more limited when the wrist is in extension or pronounced flexion. Ulnar deviation is slightly greater when the forearm is fully supinated.

From a functional point of view, the wrist is a key joint. Its stability determines efficient digital performance. The wrist is functionally stabilized in extension during flexion of the fingers. Wrist position also determines grip strength. With hyperflexion of the wrist, the grip is greatly diminished. In the precision grip (pinch) the squeezing power between the thumb and index finger is maximal at 35 degrees of wrist extension. It diminishes as the wrist is flexed or hyperextended.[17] Most finger activities are performed with the wrist at neutral or in slight flexion.

The wrist flexors (Fig. 2-16) are the *flexor carpi radialis, flexor carpi ulnaris,* and *palmaris longus,* when present (this muscle may be absent in 10% to 15% of individuals (Boyes[7]). The accessory wrist flexors are the *long digital flexors* (pollicis, superficialis, and profundus) and *abductor pollicis longus* (Jones[14]). The wrist extensors (Fig. 2-17) are the *extensor carpi radialis longus, extensor carpi radialis brevis,* and *extensor carpi ulnaris.* The *digital extensors* are also very active accessory wrist extensors. Radial abduction of the wrist[12] is

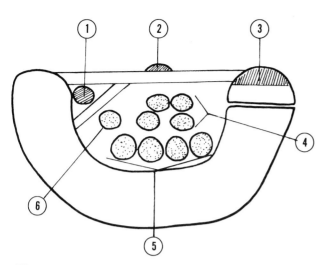

Fig. 2-16. Wrist flexors. 1, Flexor carpi radialis. 2, Palmaris longus. 3, Flexor carpi ulnaris. 4, Flexor superficialis. 5, Flexor profundi. 6, Flexor pollicis longus.

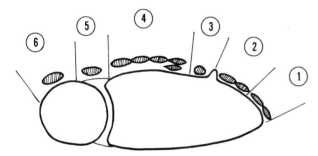

Fig. 2-17. The six compartments on posterior (dorsal) aspect of wrist from right to left: 1, Abductor pollicis longus, extensor pollicis brevis. 2, Extensor carpi radialis longus and brevis. 3, Extensor pollicis longus on ulnar side of Lister's tubercle. 4, Extensor digitorum communis and underneath extensor indicis proprius. All these four compartments correspond to posterior aspect of radius. 5, Extensor digiti quinti located on posterior aspect of radioulnar joint. 6, Extensor carpi ulnaris over head of ulna. The motors in compartments 2 to 6 are the main wrist extensors. The motors located in compartments 3 to 5 are accessory extensors of the wrist.

controlled by the *abductor pollicis longus* and *extensor pollicis brevis*. The accessory radial deviators are the *extensor carpi radialis longus, extensor carpi radialis brevis, extensor pollicis longus,* and *flexor carpi radialis*. The ulnar deviators of the wrist are the *extensor carpi ulnaris* and *flexor carpi ulnaris*.

Relationships between the wrist motors and hand motion have been investigated recently by Radonjic and Long.[26] During closing motions of the fingers, the following wrist extensors are active in a descending order: *extensor carpi radialis brevis,*

extensor carpi ulnaris, and *extensor carpi radialis longus*. As grip power increases, all three extensors participate increasingly. When the grip is lessened, the wrist extensors drop out except for the extensor carpi radialis brevis. During opening motions of the hand, the following wrist ulnar motors are active: *extensor carpi ulnaris* and *flexor carpi ulnaris*. When the opening force increases, the extensor carpi radialis brevis and palmaris longus come into action. The flexor carpi radialis and the extensor carpi radialis longus participate only minimally.

FUNCTIONAL ANATOMY OF HAND

Purposeful placement of the hand is accomplished through the interaction of body and arm motions. If prehensile activities are to follow, a certain sequence of hand actions usually takes place:

1. Opening of digits
2. Positioning over an object
3. Closing of digits
4. Manipulation through arm motion, interdigital interplay, or a combination of both
5. Opening of digits to release object

Nonprehensile hand function may include the act of pushing an object, lifting with the flat hand, or stirring a solution with the open hand or a digit.

Prehensile activities have been analyzed and classified by Napier[23] who divided hand function into two types:

1. Power grip
2. Precision grip

In a power grip, a clamping force is produced by the flexed fingers against counterpressure offered by the palm, thenar eminence, and distal segment of the thumb. To increase grip power, the thumb may be wrapped around the flexed fingers.

In a precision grip, the object is held just between the palmar or lateral aspect of the fingers and the opposing thumb. Stability is gained through only digital interplay. Landsmeer[20] prefers the term "precision handling" instead of "precision grip." He noted that in finger prehension, object manipulation is by the digits, whereas with power grip, object repositioning is done with the wrist and arm.

The type of grip used is determined mainly by the intended activity rather than by its shape (Napier[23]). To unscrew the tight jar lid, one re-

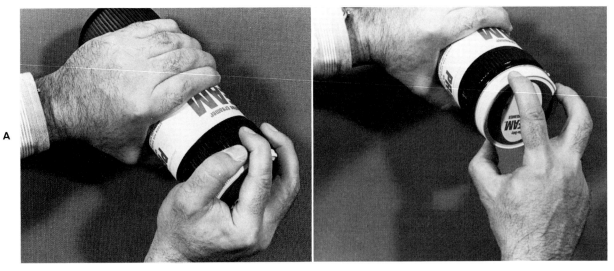

Fig. 2-18. Mixed grip. **A,** Power type of grip used by both hands initially. **B,** As the lid loosens, the right hand adopts a more precision but less powerful type of grip. The shape of the object did not change.

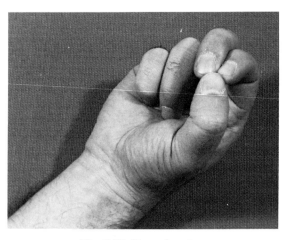

Fig. 2-20. Tip prehension.

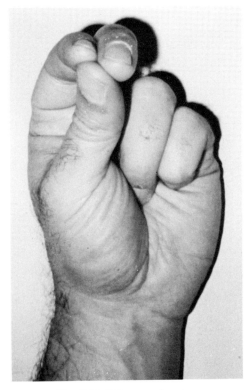

Fig. 2-19. Palmar prehension.

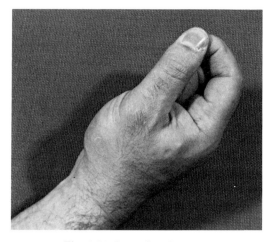

Fig. 2-21. Lateral prehension.

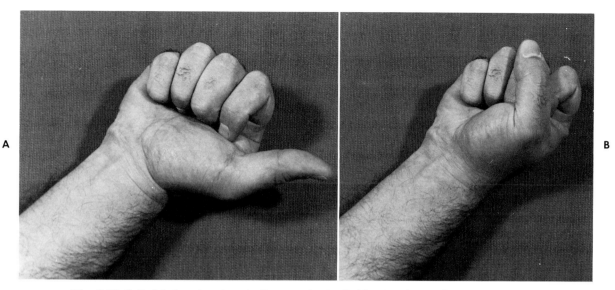

Fig. 2-22. Cylindrical prehension. **A,** Pattern of grip. **B,** The thumb provides counterpressure and adds to the power.

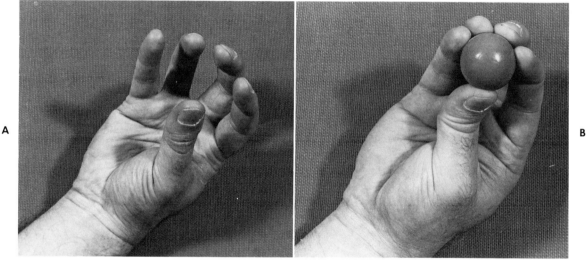

Fig. 2-23. Spherical prehension. **A,** Pattern of grip with average-sized object. **B,** Adducted position of fingers with smaller object.

quires a power grip initially, but as the lid is loosened, the hand adopts a precision grip to complete the task (Fig. 2-18). Keller, Taylor, and Zahm[16] defined the following six major prehension patterns:

1. Palmar prehension: pad of the thumb opposed to the pad of the index and middle fingers (Fig. 2-19)
2. Tip prehension: tip of the thumb opposed to the tip of the corresponding fingers (Fig. 2-20)
3. Lateral or key prehension: pad of the thumb opposed to the lateral aspect of the finger—usually the index finger at the level of the distal segment (Fig. 2-21)
4. Cylindrical prehension: the fingers are flexed at the three joints around the object; the thumb provides the counterpressure and is wrapped around the flexed fingers (Fig. 2-22)
5. Spherical prehension: the fingers are flexed at the three joints and rotated and abducted unless the spherical object is of a small size and the thumb is in a position of opposition (Fig. 2-23)

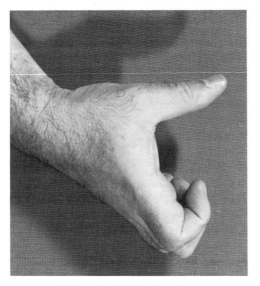

Fig. 2-24. Hook prehension.

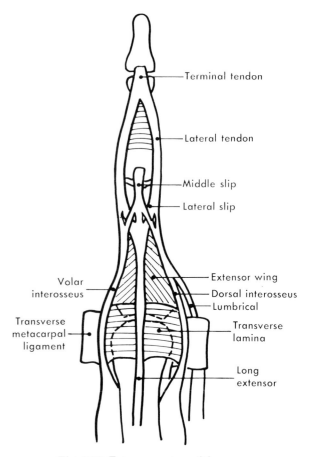

Fig. 2-25. Extensor system of fingers.

6. Hook prehension: the fingers are flexed or hooked at the interphalangeal joints with only slight flexion at the metacarpophalangeal joint (Fig. 2-24)

Using Napier's concept, the above prehensile activities could be grouped into two divisions:

1. Precision grip: palmar, tip, lateral pinch
2. Power grip: cylindrical, spherical, hook grasp

According to Keller et al.[16] palmar prehension is used most frequently among the precision types of grip, both in picking up an object (50% of times) and holding it for use (88%). In palmar prehension, the force of prehension ranges from 15.2 to 31.5 pounds, whereas in the cylindrical prehension it ranges from 64 to 120 pounds (Klopsteg and Wilson[17]).

The five digits, which perform the prehensile activities, must act in coordination relative to each other. A mechanism of coordination among the phalanges of each finger is also necessary.

FUNCTIONAL ANATOMY OF FINGER

The motor control of a finger is determined by the following:

1. Extensor system
2. Intrinsic muscles
3. Long flexor system

Extensor system (Fig. 2-25)

Extension of the fingers is a composite action of extrinsic and intrinsic musculature, with the ten-

dons of these two muscle groups blending into an intricately balanced tendon complex. The primary extrinsic extensor is the extensor digitorum communis, which supplies all four digits. More precise individual control of the index and little fingers is provided by the extensor indicis and extensor digiti quinti muscles respectively. Their tendons join the communis tendons; so each finger has only one basic long extensor tendon.

The main component of the extensor system is the long extensor tendon, which passes dorsally over the center of its corresponding metacarpal phalangeal joint. At this point it is anchored to the phalanx indirectly by fibrous aponeurotic structure, allowing the extrinsic muscles to act primarily on this joint.

Continuing distally on the dorsum of the proximal phalanx, the long extensor tendon trifurcates into middle, radial, and ulnar slips. The middle slip inserts into the base of the middle phalanx. The two lateral slips (radial and ulnar), after receiving contributions from the corresponding intrinsic muscles, continue as the "lateral tendons." Although being relatively lateral, these lie slightly dorsal to the transverse axis of the joint. Over the dorsum of the distal interphalangeal joint the lateral tendons unite to form the "terminal tendon," which inserts into the base of the distal phalanx.

Three intrinsic muscles insert into the middle and lateral slips of the trifurcation of each finger: an interosseus and lumbrical on the radial side and an interosseus on the ulnar side (except for the little finger, which has the abductor digiti quinti). Each intrinsic tendon divides into a medial and lateral band over the dorsolateral aspect of the proximal phalanx. The medial band passes over the lateral slip of the long extensor tendon and unites with the middle slip to form the middle tendon (fasciculus medius, or Poirier's *languette moyenne*). The lateral interosseus band blends with the lateral slip of the long extensor to form the lateral tendon (fasciculus lateralis, or Poirier's *languette latérale*). The tendinous components of this extensor system are held in specific positions by a complex aponeurotic system.

The proximal segment of this aponeurosis is a band, rectangular in shape, with transverse fibers. It originates from the side of the long extensor tendon, wraps around the metacarpophalangeal joint and blends on the volar side with the volar plate, transverse metacarpal ligament, and the fibrous flexor tendon sheath. Through its capsular attachment, the band is functionally connected with the base of the proximal phalanx on the volar side. This aponeurotic band is called the transverse lamina (Landsmeer[19]).

Next to the transverse lamina and in continuity with its distal border is a thin lamina of connective tissue extending from the long extensor tendon to the tendons of the intrinsics. This is called the lamina intertendinea (Landsmeer[18]) or extensor wing, since it covers the dorsolateral aspect of the proximal phalanx like two wings arising from the long extensor. These all serve as the primary extensor of the interphalangeal joints. The extrinsic muscles can complete this action only if by their action the metacarpal phalangeal joint is partially blocked so that some flexion is maintained.

The extensor system is anchored at the level of the proximal interphalangeal joint by the retinacular ligament (Landsmeer[18]) or the lateral

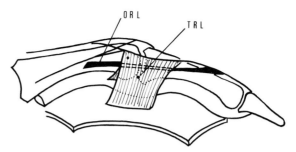

Fig. 2-26. Retinacular ligament system. **ORL,** Oblique retinacular ligament (Landsmeer's ligament, Weitbricht's ligament). **TRL,** Transverse retinacular ligament.

retinacular ligament (Zancolli[33]) (Fig. 2-26). This system has two layers: one superficial and one deep. The superficial layer is a transverse band passing across the proximal interphalangeal joint (Baumann and Patry[6]; Bunnell[7]); it attaches to the flexor tendon sheath (Landsmeer[18]). The deep layer or oblique retinacular ligament (Landsmeer[18]) originates from the lateral border of the proximal phalanx, passes deep to the transverse retinacular ligament, and blends with the lateral fibers of the extensor terminal tendon.

The extensor system can be loaded from a proximal or distal direction. Proximal loading occurs when the long extensor muscle contracts. A pull on the common tendon is transmitted equally to its middle and lateral slips. If hyperextension is available at the metacarpophalangeal joint, the pull of the long extensor cannot efficiently reach the trifurcation. In consequence, the interphalangeal joint cannot be fully extended. Any further proximal displacement of the long extensor tendon is blocked by the transverse lamina, which is now under tension and acts as a check rein. Relaxing the transverse lamina allows the full extension of the interphalangeal joint as shown by Duchenne[9] (Fig. 2-27).

During flexion of the finger, the dorsal perimeter of the finger and actual skeletal length, measured from the metacarpal neck to the tip of the distal phalanx, lengthens (Fig. 2-28). This increase is attributable to the contour of the metacarpal and phalangeal heads (which are not true circles) and the exposure of this bony segment by the volar transposition of the phalanges. If the finger is to flex without encountering progressive resistance from the dorsal structures, the extensor mechanism must then glide distally. This distal displacement occurs, but adaptation is not com-

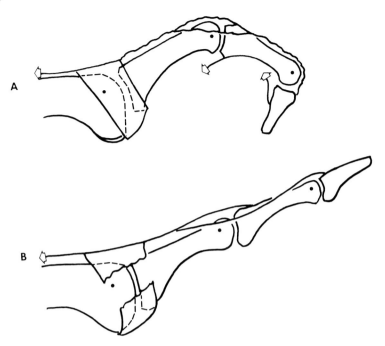

Fig. 2-27. A, Proximal pull of long extensor is partially blocked by transverse lamina, thus limiting extension at interphalangeal joints. **B,** Severance of transverse lamina allows further proximal displacement of long extensor with subsequent full extension at interphalangeal joints.

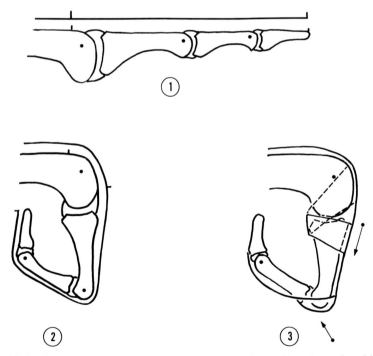

Fig. 2-28. 1, Skeletal length of finger in extension. **2,** Increased skeletal length attributable to noncircular configuration of metacarpal and phalangeal heads. **3,** Adjustment of extensor mechanism to increased skeletal length by distal displacement (partially blocked by transverse lamina) and volar shift of lateral slip.

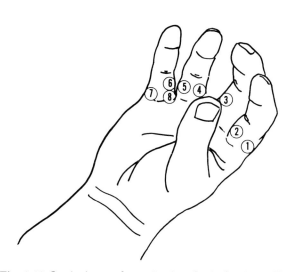

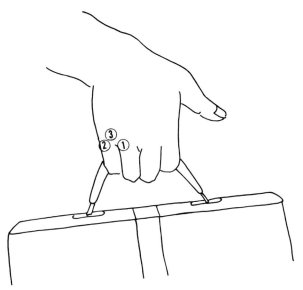

Fig. 2-38. Intrinsic muscles active in spherical grip. 1, First dorsal interosseous. 2, First volar interosseous. 3, Third dorsal interosseous. 4, Second volar interosseous. 5, Fourth dorsal interosseous. 6, Third volar interosseous. 7, Abductor digiti quinti. 8, Fourth lumbrical.

Fig. 2-39. Intrinsic muscles active in hook grip. 1, Fourth dorsal interosseous. 2, Abductor digiti quinti. 3, Fourth lumbrical.

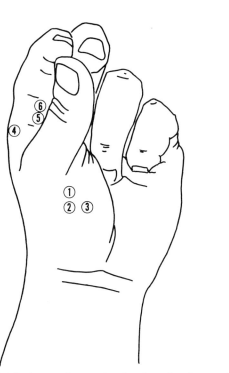

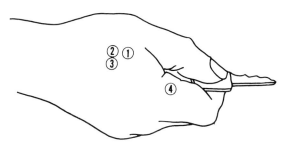

Fig. 2-41. Intrinsic muscles most active in soft lateral grip. 1, Opponens. 2, Short flexor. 3, Adductor. 4, First dorsal interosseous.

Fig. 2-40. Intrinsic muscles most active in soft palmar grip. 1, Opponens. 2, Short flexor. 3, Adductor. 4, First dorsal interosseous. 5, First volar interosseous. 6, First lumbrical.

the index finger only the first dorsal interosseus is appreciably active. There is minimal abductor pollicis brevis activity.

Forrest and Basmajian[11] analyzed the participation of the radial thenar group during the tip-to-tip and key types of grip with soft opposition and firm opposition. With a soft grip, the participation was in a decreasing order from the opponens to the abductor pollicis brevis and the flexor pollicis brevis. The activities were higher for the tip-to-tip grip as compared to the key grip. The participation of the muscular triad increased as the thumb opposed from the index to the little finger. When the force was applied to the opposition, interesting functional shifts occurred in the activity of the triad. The functional pattern became in a decreasing order: flexor pollicis brevis, opponens, and abductor pollicis brevis. Their participation increased as the thumb opposed from the index to the little finger.

REFERENCES

1. American Academy of Orthopaedic Surgeons: Joint motion—method of measuring and recording, 4:83-84, 1969.
2. Basmajian, J. V.: Muscles alive—their functions revealed by electromyography, Baltimore, 1962, The Williams & Wilkins Co.
3. Basmajian, J. V., and Bazant, F. J.: Factors preventing downward dislocation of the adducted shoulder joint: An electromyographic and morphological study, J. Bone Joint Surg. 41A:1182-1186, 1959.
4. Basmajian, J. F., and Latif, A.: Integrated actions and functions of the chief flexors of the elbow: A detailed electromyographic analysis, J. Bone Joint Surg. 39A:1106-1118, 1957.
5. Basmajian, J. V., and Travill, A.: Electromyography of the pronator muscles in the forearm, Anat. Rec. 139:45-49, 1961.
6. Baumann, J. A., and Patry, G.: Observations microscopiques sur la texture fibreuse et la vascularisation de l'ensemble tendineux extenseur du doigt de la main, chez l'homme, Rev. Med. de la Suisse Romande 63:900-912, 1943.
7. Boyes, J. H.: Bunnell's Surgery of the hand, ed. 4, Philadelphia, 1964, J. B. Lippincott Co.
8. Capener, N.: The hand in surgery, J. Bone Joint Surg. 38B(1):128-151, Feb. 1956.
9. Duchenne, G. B.: Physiology of motion, translated by E. Kaplan, Philadelphia, 1959, W. B. Saunders Co.
10. Eyler, D. L., and Markee, J. E.: The anatomy and function of the intrinsic musculature of the fingers, J. Bone Joint Surg. 36A(1):1-9, Jan. 1954.
11. Forrest, W. J., and Basmajian, J. V.: Functions of human thenar and hypothenar muscles. An electromyographic study of 25 hands, J. Bone Joint Surg. 47A(8):1585-1594, 1965.
12. Hollinshead, H.: Anatomy for surgeons. Vol. 3, The back and limbs, New York, 1958, Paul B. Hoeber, Inc., Medical Book Department of Harper & Row, Publishers.
13. Inman, V. T., Saunders, M., and Abbott, L. C.: Observations on the function of the shoulder joint. J. Bone Joint Surg. 26:1-30, Jan. 1944.
14. Jones, F. W.: Voluntary muscular movements in cases of nerve lesions, J. Anat. 54:41, 1919.
15. Kaplan, E. B.: Functional and surgical anatomy of the hand, ed. 2, Philadelphia, 1965, J. B. Lippincott Co.
16. Keller, A. D., Taylor, C. L., and Zahm, V.: Studies to determine the functional requirements for hand and arm prosthesis, Los Angeles, 1947, Department of Engineering, University of California.
17. Klopsteg, P. E., Wilson, P. D., et al.: Human limbs and their substitutes, New York, 1968, Hafner Publishing Co., Inc.
18. Landsmeer, J. M. F.: The anatomy of the dorsal aponeurosis of the human finger and its functional significance, Anat. Rec. 104:31-44, 1949.
19. Landsmeer, J. M. F.: Anatomical and functional investigations of the articulation of the human fingers, Acta Anat. 25(suppl. 24):1-64, 1955.
20. Landsmeer, J. M. F.: Power grip and precision handling, Ann. Rheum. Dis. 21:164-169, 1962.
21. Long, C., Conrad, P. W., Hall, E. A., and Furler, S. L.: Intrinsic-extrinsic muscle control of the hand in power grip and precision handling. An electromyographic study, J. Bone Joint Surg. 52A(5):852-867, July 1970.
22. Mehta, J. J., and Gardner, W. V.: A study of lumbrical muscles in the human hand, Am. J. Anat. 109:227-238, 1961.
23. Napier, J. R.: The prehensile movements of the human hand, J. Bone Joint Surg. 38B(4):902-913, Nov. 1956.
24. Napier, J.: Evolution of the human hand. Seminar at the University of Chicago, Department of Anatomy, Chicago 1965, University of Chicago Press.
25. Poirier, P., and Charpy, A.: Traité d'anatomie humaine, vol. 1, Paris, 1899, Masson & Cie.
26. Radonjic, D., and Long, C.: Kinesiology of the wrist, Amer. J. Phys. Med. 50(2):57-71, 1971.
27. Sarrafian, S. K., Kazarian, L. E., Topouzian, L. K., Sarrafian, V. K., and Siegelman, A.: Strain variation in the components of the extensor apparatus of the finger during flexion and extension, J. Bone Joint Surg. 52A(5):980-990, July 1970.
28. Ray, R. D., Johnson, R. J., and Jameson, R. M.: Rotation of the forearm: An experimental study of pronation and supination, J. Bone Joint Surg. 33A:993, 1951.
29. Scheving, L. E., and Pauly, J. E.: An electromyographic study of some muscles acting on the upper extremity of man, Anat. Rec. 135:239-246, 1959.
30. Strong, C., and Perry, J.: Function of the extensor pollicis longus and intrinsic muscles of the thumb, Phys. Ther. 46(9):939-945, Sept. 1966.
31. Travill, A.: In Basmajian, J. V.: Muscles alive, Baltimore, 1962, p. 112. The Williams & Wilkins Co.
32. Van Linge, B., and Mulder, J. B.: Function of the supraspinatus muscle and its relation to the supraspinatus syndrome, J. Bone Joint Surg. 45B:750-754, Nov. 1964.
33. Zancolli, E.: Structural and dynamic bases of hand surgery, Philadelphia, 1968, J. B. Lippincott Co.

CHAPTER 3

Pathomechanics

JACQUELIN PERRY, M.D.

Purposeful motion occurs when bony segments are moved according to a precisely designed plan. Appropriate muscular contraction to produce the discrete motion is determined by a central control system under the guidance of both volition and sensory feedback from the periphery. This sensorimotor-mechanical loop between brain and performing hand presents a chain of sites selectively susceptible to the different forms of disease and trauma that may occur.

STRUCTURAL INSUFFICIENCY

Loss of joint mobility is the basic concern. It may result from skin rigidity, periarticular adhesions, or destruction of joint surfaces. Each of these tissues is characterized by free interfiber mobility and special gliding surfaces. All have a very limited capacity to regenerate in kind. Consequently, most loss is replaced by scar. Flexibility is correspondingly sacrificed because scar is a mass of nonelastic fibers that lie in all directions and bind to every other fibrous tissue touched.

The severity of such restraint can be lessened by judicious positioning and exercise in the early scar-forming phase. At this time the mass is highly vascular and the fibers are loosely bound, giving the tissue a low density and relative flexibility, which permit it to yield to mobilizing efforts. Response is limited by the primary pathologic condition; so all applied force must be sufficiently subtle to gain motion without tearing, which would only induce more scarring. As the

scar matures, its capillaries recede and fibrous bands become firmer (Fig. 3-1). Clinically this is recognized as whitening and shrinkage of the original mass. Responsiveness to mobilizing efforts is proportionally lessened. By approximately 3 months the mass is rigid and the opportunity to gain motion is lost. This means that measures to assure the basic functional position or to gain a useful range of motion must be initiated early as the opportunity recedes each week.

Periarticular-tissue restraint of joint motion most commonly begins as a reaction to inflammation and distension from edema and synovial overgrowth. This distorts the fine balance between overlying tendons and their capsular attachments; so muscles malfunction. Bony alignment also is lost as the support offered by capsule,

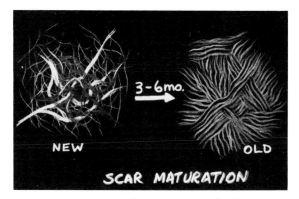

Fig. 3-1. Relative density of new and old scar.

ligaments, and fascial planes is weakened and so the muscles are further made inefficient. Secondary local scarring perpetuates these many problems. This and the later changes of intra-articular damage lead to permanent degrees of dysfunction.

Muscular response is of two types. During the most acute phase there will be splinting of the joint to avoid all motion, so as to lessen pain. As the pain becomes more chronic the pressure of muscular contraction becomes significant. This aggravation is avoided by pain-induced reflex inhibition of all but the mildest muscular action and prevents effective participation in strengthing programs. It has been demonstrated experimentally that the force of muscular contraction is directly transmitted to the intervening joint surfaces (Ford).

Rheumatoid arthritis is the most common cause of the above sequelae today. Because its cause is unknown, the course unpredictable, and therapeutic response unreliable, preservation of optimal function and the prevention of deformity is not entirely successful. The use of orthotics is limited by the chronicity of the disease. Rest in the acute phase is helpful and accepted. Prolonged splinting (that is, for the many years the disease runs its course) so interferes with function that patients do not tolerate the devices. Failure to differentiate between the acute periods, which need protection, and the quiet intervals, which do not, has led to total condemnation of all splinting, yet judicious intermittent orthotic use for the acute periods can both provide pain relief and delay the progression towards deformity.

Skin is the most mobile tissue. It is both rich with elastic fibers and has considerable anatomic redundancy, as evidenced by the natural skin folds about the joints. Other factors in skin mobility are its freedom from the underlying tissues and the layer of subcutaneous fat, which provides a very adaptable base.

Burns, direct trauma, and certain collagen diseases such as scleroderma and dermatomyositis may destroy any or all of these specialized structures and induce secondary scarring. Restriction of joint mobility is the immediate effect because the skin serving as a protective sleeve or glove must move through an arc greater than that of the enclosed joint. Forced idleness soon leads to secondary contractures within the periarticular layers, leading to further loss of mobility.

Being a surface structure, it is the first tissue stretched with any motion. Abrading damage may accompany the minor traumas of daily hand use or the displacement of inadequately fitted orthoses. In addition, skin vascularity is challenged by undue tension or pressure as well as by the scarring itself. Increased susceptibility to stress because of the pathologic skin condition, combined with the necessity to allow segment motion if the hand and arm are to be useful, makes the application of orthoses more difficult than when just deeper structures are involved.

An orthotic program can be successful, however, if these physiologic restraints are given serious respect and special attention is given in the design of apparatus to maintain basic positioning, to assist in the recovery of motion, and to avoid adding more trauma through abrasion.

MOTOR UNIT LOSS

Muscle fibers are the obvious source of motion. When they are healthy and adequate in numbers, strength is good. Otherwise, these patients exhibit a proportional degree of weakness. Because muscle fibers do not survive unless their immediate nerve supply (the lower motor neuron) is intact, these two structures are conceptually linked as a motor unit (Fig. 3-2). Different diseases may specifically attack the individual components of the motor unit. The neuron's cell body lying within the anterior horn of the spinal cord is the selective target of poliomyelitis. Its axon passing within the root and peripheral nerve is subject to infectious neuronitis and trauma. The myoneural

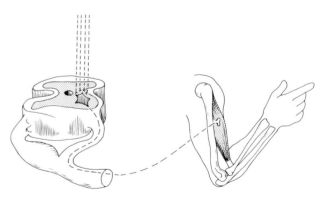

Fig. 3-2. The motor unit extending from anterior horn cell within the spinal cord to include the muscle fibers of the limb. (Modified from Perry, J., and Hislop, H. J.: Principles of lower extremity bracing, New York, 1967, American Physical Therapy Association.)

junction or end plate is specifically involved with myasthenia gravis, and isolated muscle degeneration occurs with muscular dystrophy. The basic characteristics of these diseases have been presented in the chapter on pathologic gait. Upper-limb pathologic conditions tend to fall into two general patterns: systemic diseases, such as poliomyelitis and muscular dystrophy, and localized lesions, of which trauma is the most common.

Because the scope of normal function is so broad, many patients get by despite gross muscular inadequacies. Their motion may appear awkward but remain effective. The patients' ability to substitute so readily is caused by their having selective control and precise sensation. A 20-pound grip and 5-pound pinch can meet all the requirements of self-care. Ability to lift just 1 pound is also minimally adequate.

Versatility in grasp, pinch, or hand placement may be curtailed and substitute motions may appear awkward, but effectiveness will persist. Precision and rapidity of response will be preserved as long as maximum strength is not being challenged.

Efficient use of one's limited strength depends on being able to initiate the action from a position of function rather than from deformed alignment. It also depends on being able to move the segments without intrinsic resistance from contracted periarticular tissues. Hence, prevention or correction of deformity is paramount. Secondly, one needs active antagonists to permit rapid reciprocation so that residual muscle strength can be used. In motor-unit loss, therefore, orthotics serves two functions: prevention of deformity and provision of active antagonist, to provide prompt reciprocation. Total replacement is limited by the scarcity of versatile control sites to activate external power.

Systemic diseases

Severity of the pathologic condition determines whether an individual muscle, a particular group, or total limb musculature suffers partial or complete paralysis. Total motor-unit loss makes an upper limb useless except for cosmetic completeness or to serve as a paperweight. Partial paralysis, however, retains a much higher level of function than one usually anticipates from the muscle-strength test. This occurs because of the ease of substitution. The patient has retained precise sensation and control. Hence, his remaining

motor units can be marshalled accurately and redirected to perform new functions. They change phase at will. A second reason why the upper limb remains functional despite rather extensive paralysis is the little strength needed to perform average self-care and sedentary tasks. A 20-pound grip and 5-pound pinch will meet all the requirements of self-care. Ability to lift just 1 pound permits self-feeding with precut foods. Versatility in grasp, pinch, or hand placement may be curtailed and substitute motions appear awkward, but effectiveness persists.

Efficient use of one's limited strength depends on being able to initiate the action from a position of function rather than from deformed alignment. It also depends on being able to move the segments without intrinsic resistance from contracted periarticular tissues. Hence, prevention of deformity is paramount. Orthoses for this purpose are extremely valuable and well accepted but the patient will not use them for function unless the paralysis is too extensive for effective substitutions. Even then their value depends on the patient having retained sufficient musculature to add versatility to the orthotic effects. Functional orthoses in these patients perform three tasks: Elastic assistance can augment muscles otherwise too weak to perform; stabilization of selected joints will enable remaining musculature to control more distal segments; and provision of antagonistic power will make it possible for a single muscle to move the limb through a more complete arc.

Trauma

Mechanical injury to the peripheral nerves is probably the most common cause of motor-unit loss in the upper limbs. All five of the major motor nerves supplying the arm and hand also contain sensory fibers, but in only one is the sensory loss from injury of functional significance. That one, the median nerve, will be discussed in the section about combined motor and sensory loss. The others are covered here. Orthoses are most often used to prevent deformity. Long-term answers are provided by reconstructive surgery if recovery is not complete.

Axillary nerve lesions. Loss of active shoulder abduction and flexion from deltoid paralysis is the problem. Some patients can marshal other muscles to assist the rotator cuff muscles to raise their arm overhead, but the strength of shoulder control is not functional. Orthotic assistance has not been customary for lack of a readily available device. The pelvic arm support, as a prefabricated shelf item, offers a prompt means for static protection with the hand in a functional and cosmetic position. If long-term disability is anticipated before reconstructive surgery is contemplated, an ambulatory functional arm orthosis should be substituted for the static support.

Musculocutaneous nerve lesions. The biceps and brachialis muscles (supplied by this nerve) are not only the largest elbow flexors, they also have the best leverage. Hence, with a musculocutaneous nerve injury the patient loses all useful elbow-flexor strength. If the other muscles that cross the elbow anteriorly are particularly strong (pronator teres, finger and wrist flexor mass, and the brachioradialis) and can be augmented by momentum from active shoulder control, the patient has a means for independent placement of the unresisted hand.

Orthotic provision of elbow flexion is seldom satisfactory because proximal fixation is generally poor and the functional requirements are high. The tubular shape of the humerus and loss of firm soft-tissue contours with flexor-muscle paralysis offer an unstable base. Indirectly activated ratchet-locking joints do not provide the versatility needed for average everyday tasks, even though, throughout, the full arc and selected stability in multiple positions are available.

Radial nerve. The functional loss associated with injury to this nerve varies according to which of three levels is involved. When the lesion is below the elbow, in the region of the radial head, the extensors, fingers and thumb, and long thumb abductor are paralyzed. Prompt orthotic replacement with elastic extensors maintains hand mobility and use during the recovery period. More is contributed to hand function than passive opening. Electromyographic studies have shown that the finger extensors contract during grasp if the forearm is pronated. Judging from the inaccurate hand use observed when these muscles are even temporarily paralyzed with an anesthetic nerve block, one may consider them to be vital guides for the flexors. It appears extensor tension indicates where the fingers lie in the flexion arc; that is, they complete the proprioception loop.

When the nerve injury is at midhumerus, wrist-extensor paralysis is added to the absence of finger and wrist-extensor control. This greatly exaggerates grasp-and-pinch incompetence because these finger flexors cannot contract sufficiently to make a tight fist if the wrist is flexed. The orthotic need is static support with the wrist in neutral to counteract both the effects of gravity and the pull of the finger flexors as they contract. Later, when the wrist extensor muscles evidence partial recovery (grade 2 or 3 strength), they will overcome the effects of disuse faster if the orthosis is changed to one with elastic extensor assists and a flexion stop. Increased hand versatility is added also.

Axillary-level radial-nerve injuries add triceps paralysis to the previously described finger- and wrist-extensor loss. This deprives the patient of arm depression to stabilize objects or support the body. Deformity is seldom a problem, however, as gravity is active whenever the patient is upright. Hence, protective orthotics is not indicated, nor is there a way to replace the force needed for triceps function because the skin as the intermediary between skeleton and orthosis will not tolerate such stress.

Ulnar nerve. The paralytic pattern presented by injury to this nerve also varies with the level of injury. When the lesion is at the wrist, the conspicuous loss is absent intrinsic muscle action in the ring and little fingers. This results in a claw position of these digits on attempted extension, that is, incomplete interphalangeal (IP) extension and hyperextension of the metacarpophalangeal (MP) joints.

Grasp is also weakened by the loss of direct MP flexion and the usual intrinsic tie between long extensors and flexors. As a result, when one tries to hold an object, the IP joints hyperflex and the MP joints flatten rather than matching the contour of the object being handled. The claw posture of the fingers can be readily corrected with an orthotic MP extensor stop. This allows the intact long extensor muscles to complete IP extension. By setting the MP stop so that the joints are held in 20 or 30° of flexion, one can also improve the grasp. Early and prolonged application of this simple orthosis can induce a mild MP flexion contracture to perpetuate the functional gains. Without orthotic protection the tissues rearrange themselves to create a permanent claw deformity.

As all the interossei and the thumb adductor are supplied by the ulnar nerve, the other digits also display a weak grasp because of loss of direct MP flexion but clawing is prevented by the intact lumbricales in the long and index fingers and abductor pollicis brevis of the thumb.

When the nerve injury is at the elbow, the flexor digitorum profundus muscle bellies to the ring and little fingers are paralyzed in addition to the intrinsics. This deprives the patient of most of his ulnar grasp. The hand is correspondingly weaker, but orthotic needs are not changed.

SENSORY INSUFFICIENCY COMBINED WITH MOTOR UNIT LOSS

To maintain the proper grasp or manipulate an object as it is being used, the hand must repeatedly make minor adjustments in shape and tension. Similarly, the arm continually monitors when it has placed the hand. These motor actions are guided by the intrinsic sensations of position, tension, motion, touch, and spatial relations. When this information is absent, the muscles remain idle. They do not know why, how, or when they should contract. Thus the key to muscle action is sensory feedback. The hand also is a vital source of information as to the character and quality of objects (Fig. 3-3).

Substitution for paralysis presents a higher demand on the sensorimotor system than does normal function. The patient must continue to meet the requirement for successful object control, yet do it in an unnatural way. One muscle can be substituted for another only if the lack of alternate action is accurately known. Without such guidance the remaining musculature is aimless and hence ignored.

In the hand the most critical areas of sensation are the palmar surface of the thumb, index and long fingers, and intervening palm (Fig. 3-4). This is lost if the sensory fibers arising from these areas are interrupted at any point along their path to the brain. The sites of concern are the median nerve, brachial plexus, and the spinal cord at the level of fiber entry.

Median nerve injury causes the most critical loss, since it is the absolute pathway for all the sensory fibers from these critical areas, which also includes the radial side of the index finger. The associated motor loss depends on the level of injury. There are two characteristic sites of injury, wrist and elbow or above. The difference is not one of hand use but of potential control made idle because of sensory loss. Median nerve motor supply includes the thumb's intrinsic muscles and the long flexors of the thumb, index, and long fingers.

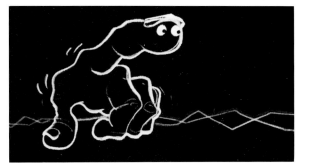

Fig. 3-3. Hand sensation as a source of information.

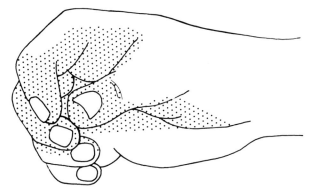

Fig. 3-4. The critical areas of hand sensation are the palmar surface of thumb, index and long fingers, and palm (*shaded areas*).

The latter may have some carryover from the ulnar-supplied ring finger. With injury at the wrist, only the thumb intrinsics (and lumbricales to the index and middle fingers) are paralyzed. Presumably the hand, having the long fingers intact will retain considerable function. Such, however, is not the case because the hand is blind, with the sensory loss being just as profound as with the higher lesion. Orthotic care serves to prevent deformity during the period of recovery, but it will not encourage useful function because of the lack of sensation.

Brachial plexus and spinal cord injuries are less precise in their correlations of sensory and motor loss. Undoubtedly a major factor in this ambiguity is the variation in lesion location. Also the nerve fibers undergo redistribution at several sites. It is inconceivable that this would always occur precisely the same in all individuals.

The brachial plexus, serving as a multilevel interchange, has two sites particularly vulnerable to injury, its trunks and roots. Roots are the structures that extend from the spinal cord to begin formulation of the peripheral nerves. Classically five roots contribute to the brachial plexus: the fifth through eight cervical and the first thoracic (C5, C6, C7, C8, T1). Within a centimeter or two the first two roots (C5 and C6) combine to form the upper trunk. C7 continues as the middle trunk, and the lower two roots (C8 and T1) combine to form the lower trunk. This distinction is clinically significant, since there are two basic patterns of injury that can selectively involve different trunks.

If the patient suffers a downward blow on the shoulder or falls in a manner so as to push the shoulder down and head away, stretch may be placed on the upper trunk causing paralysis of the arm (Erb's palsy). When the damaging force thrusts the arm into abduction, the lower trunk is involved, and hand paralysis may result (Klumpke's paralysis). The seventh root may be included in either. More severe injury may include the entire plexus. Ironically the roots controlling the arm muscles also serve as the pathway for the most critical sensation for the hand. Thus the hand is always disabled.

Sensation for the digits used in precision handling and information gathering, that is, the thumb, index, and long fingers, travels in the upper (sixth root) and middle trunk (seventh root) to enter the spinal cord. Authorities agree that the sixth root supplies thumb sensation and that the seventh root is the dominant of the long fingers, but they differ as to which is responsible for the index finger. More precise knowledge is lacking because such localization data has had to be gained from the patients, and injuries certainly are not exactly repetitious. In contrast to the median nerve the roots supply sensation to both the volar and dorsal surfaces.

With this overlap between the sixth and seventh cervical nerve, root distribution of the degree of sensory impairment varies greatly among patients. Sensory recovery also seems to be better than motor recovery.

Motor innervation of the muscles in the hand tends to be restricted to a single root. Although forearm, arm, and shoulder muscles generally have two and occasionally three roots contributing, the overlap among root supply is such that the trunk formulation creates functional units.

Shoulder elevation, arm external rotation, and elbow flexion are dually innervated by the fifth and sixth roots. Radial wrist extension is pro-

vided by the sixth nerve root. As these two roots combine to form the upper trunk, loss of all these muscles are included in Erb's palsy. The patient with this type of paralysis does well in a functional arm orthosis because it preserves hand use during the period of waiting for available spontaneous recovery, which may be over a 12- to 18-month period. Functional replacement is not sufficiently versatile or spontaneous enough for permanent acceptance. Fortunately reconstructive surgery in the form of arthrodeses and tendon transfers are very effective. They are not undertaken, however, until all chance of recovery has been completed, thus this waiting period needs orthotic supplementation if the patient is to remain two handed in his habits.

If the seventh root is involved, there will be paralysis of the extensors of the fingers and thumb and the ulnar side of the wrist and the elbow. The triceps also has some sixth-root innervation. The extent that this seventh-root injury is combined with upper trunk (or sixth-root) damage dictates whether the hand will be useless because of sensory loss. Orthotic use is then poorly accepted.

The converse picture exists when the injury is localized to the lower trunk of the brachial plexus. This carries the fibers of the eight-cervical and first-thoracic roots. Motor rather than sensory loss is the more significant feature. All the finger flexor and intrinsic muscles are paralyzed. Sensory impairment is limited to the ulnar two fingers. As these digits are neither the components of pinch nor the source of most information, orthotic replacement can be very effective.

Lower-trunk paralysis without involvement of the seventh root (middle trunk) is infrequent. The combination adds paralysis of digital extension; so all hand motion is lost, and it also extends the sensory impairment to include the critical pinch fingers. With available sensation limited only to the thumb, hand precision drops significantly. Unless this is the patient's dominant hand (bilateral lesion), he will make little effort to use it. Function is too inaccurate.

Spinal cord injuries are most often complete transections. As such, they cause loss of all control distal to that level. In the cervical area this means total paralysis of the lower extremities, trunk, and whatever portions of the upper limbs supplied by the segments in and below the lesion. Proximally musculature and sensation are intact. This makes a sharp cleavage plane between loss and preservation. With the loss being so massive, attention is focused on residual control rather than on the loss per se. The patients thus present a picture just opposite that seen in brachial plexus injuries. Also the paralysis is generally bilateral, in contrast to customary unilateral involvement of a brachial plexus injury.

The patient with a functioning seventh segment (C7) will lose all finger flexor power, but retains finger and extension, full wrist, elbow, and shoulder control. He will also have intact sensation in the digits used for pinch. Orthotic replacement of absent finger and thumb flexion is thus very useful.

When the sixth-cervical segment is the lowest level of innervation all finger control is absent, but strong wrist extension, elbow flexion, and shoulder elevation remain. Thumb sensation is intact, but finger impairment varies according to the extent the seventh segment contributes to the index finger. Orthotic replacement must include both flexion and extension of the digits as well as thumb opposition. Acceptance depends on the patient's degree of sensation and his motivation to do things in an effective but awkward manner.

With destruction of the sixth segment, all hand sensation and direct control of finger and wrist are lost. The fifth cervical segment preserves fair elbow flexion and shoulder elevation; so light objects can be handled if orthotic hand control is supplied. The lack of sensation limits the performance to those tasks that can be completed under direct vision.

Except for possible contribution to the fifth root the fourth segment does not provide arm function. It does assure the patient good diaphragm function and neck control. Breathing and thinking are intact, but since arm function depends on replacement of both sensation and versatile motion, functional hand use is not possible today.

CONTROL DYSFUNCTION

Brain and high spinal cord lesions are extremely frustrating to both patients and clinician. By great effort or trick maneuvers the patient may accomplish some motion. It is limited, slow, and resisted by spasticity. This bit of success, however, generates a strong challenge to develop the action to a useful level. Yet patients respond poorly to training. They fail to profit from functional orthoses. Reconstructive surgery is equally limited in extending the patient's function. Cor-

rection of compromising deformity is usually the only gain.

Such a lack of response to intense therapeutic endeavor results from the high requirement of voluntary substitution. Deliberate use of one muscle to replace the function of another demands the same quality of selective control as permits normal function. Yet this is the modality disturbed by a brain or high spinal cord lesion.

Control is the function of the cerebrum. The intactness of this structure determines the patient's ability to selectively move one joint or a desired combination of several segments through a chosen distance and at an elected speed. Whenever the motor or sensory pathways of the upper limb are interrupted, the hand and arm will not move as desired, regardless of the intensity of the command (Fig. 3-5).

A lesion obstructing hand and arm function may lie at some level within the brain or in the most proximal cervical segments of the spinal cord. The effect is isolation of the patient's still normal motor units from their source of central control. Disruption of the cerebral motor pathways also frees primitive sensorimotor centers to initiate independent actions such as spasticity, vestibular posturing, and primitive locomotor patterns.

The vestibular system is a primitive motor pathway present in all humans. It is not active in normal people because it is inhibited by the voluntary (pyramidal) motor system. When there is injury to the cerebral cortex, the vestibular system may be "disinhibited" and may become active. This results in posturing, that is, the patient maintains certain positions of his limbs and trunk.

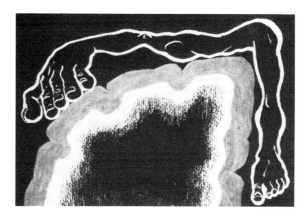

Fig. 3-5. Diagram of distribution of motor area of cerebral cortex (sensory distribution very similar).

These are the sources of laborious motion exhibited by the patient as he attempts to use his arm. They do not represent motion that can be further developed into accurate use. An area of confusion rests with the fact that patients suffering brain trauma may experience spontaneous recovery over a 2-year period. Incomplete spinal cord lesion may improve for 6 to 12 months and patients with cerebrovascular accidents will make neurologic gains for about 3 months. The extent of selective control return determines what function is trainable. Primitive sources of motion are only tantalizing, not trainable.

These primitive patterns, which in the lower limb may enable the patient to walk, are of little use in the upper limb. Stereotype alteration between mass flexion and extension does not permit the arm to accomplish a task more complex than serving as a paperweight. Any voluntary function beyond this is evidence of residual selective control that escaped injury.

Promptness of response is so essential to effective hand function that even mild spasticity is obstructive. Even with good sensation and selective control, the patient will struggle through the resistance offered by spasticity only if the other hand is worse or he has one or two particular tasks that can accommodate a slowly responsive hand.

If the lesion involves the sensory pathways, peripheral reception is lost, through either lack of further transmission or appropriate interpretation at the processing centers. The result is the same as if the damage were peripheral. The limb is ignored. Available musculature is not used, because there is no guidance as to when or how to move.

Thus is created a very frustrating situation. Under direct vision the patient may move his hand fairly promptly and with reasonable accuracy. Yet he fails to use it. There are two probable reasons for rejection. One, he cannot constantly observe his insensitive performing hand and also use his eyes for other purposes. Secondly, effective object control is much more demanding than level of performance accepted by the clinician. To the patient, the frustration of recurrent error is greater than not trying. It really means the patient is more objective than the clinician. Sensory loss is a subtle but very real obstacle to automatic hand use.

CHAPTER 4

Biomechanical analysis system

NEWTON C. McCOLLOUGH III, M.D.
SHAHAN K. SARRAFIAN, M.D.

The upper limb, by design and function, is an extremely complex and sophisticated instrument. Its articulated segments provide for maximum versatility of movement, through the smooth coordination of motor activity, dependent in large measure on the integration of an elaborate sensory feedback system. The basic motor functions of the upper limb in order of their increasing degree of complexity include prehension and release, transfer of objects in space, and manipulation of objects within the grasp. Other motor functions of less importance also exist, such as striking and crawling, but they are not generally considered in the restitution of functional activity in the impaired limb.

The task of restoring the three basic motor functions to the defective upper limb has historically been fraught with difficulty. Gross function of prehension and release, and transfer in space, has been possible to obtain by both prosthetic and orthotic means, but the task of restoring manipulative ability within the grasp has eluded the skill and imagination of many workers over the years. The problem of reduplicating mechanically the highly refined system of joints, levers, and motors present in the normal upper limb is enormous when compared to that in the lower limb. Added to this dilemma is the seemingly impossible task of providing an adequate sensory feedback system to allow coordination of mechanical parts of the degree necessary to restore upper-limb function.

Oddly enough, the prosthetic restoration of an absent upper limb with proximal motor control has been more successful than the orthotic restitution of a severely impaired upper limb at the same level. Design and development of orthotic components to reduplicate upper-limb function is complicated by the presence of intact but functionless anatomy, and the variety of functional loss with which one may be confronted tends to preclude standardization of components as is possible in the design of artificial limbs.

As in the lower limb, the primary function of an orthosis is the *control* of motion of body segments. Additionally, in the upper limb, an orthosis may also *provide* motion through the use of external power sources. An ideal orthosis controls or provides only those motions that are abnormal or absent and permits unrestricted motion in areas where normal function remains. It thus becomes obvious that considerable thought should be given to each level and segment of the limb encompassed by an orthosis in order that the prescribed components, or component types, accurately match the defects present. The basis for orthotic prescription should therefore be an accurate biomechanical analysis of the patient, followed by selection of appropriate components, and finally the creation of an orthotic system from the components selected.

To provide a systematic means whereby a biomechanical analysis of the upper limb can be

TECHNICAL ANALYSIS FORM   LEFT UPPER LIMB   Revised March 1973

Name_____ No._____ Age_____ Sex_____

Date of Onset_____ Cause _____

Occupation_____ Present Upper-Limb Equipment _____

Diagnosis _____

Hand Dominance: Right ☐   Left ☐

Status of other upper limb: Normal ☐   Impaired ☐

1.   Ambulatory status: Normal ☐   Impaired ☐   Walking Aid ☐

2.   Wheelchair ☐   Sitting Position: Stable ☐   Unstable ☐   Reclined ☐   Upright ☐
     Sitting Tolerance: Normal ☐   Limited ☐   Duration_____
     Propulsion: Manual ☐   Motor ☐   Dependent ☐

3.   Cognition: Normal ☐   Impaired ☐

4.   Endurance: Normal ☐   Impaired ☐

5.   Skin: Normal ☐   Impaired ☐

6.   Pain ☐   Location_____

7.   Vision: Normal ☐   Impaired ☐

8.   Coordination: Normal ☐   Impaired ☐   Function: Normal ☐   Compromised ☐
                                                                   Prevented   ☐

9.   Motivation: Good ☐   Fair ☐   Poor ☐

10. Associated impairments: _____

──────────────────────────────── LEGEND ────────────────────────────────

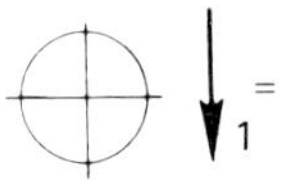

↓₁ = Direction of Translatory Motion (Grade 1,2 or 3)	Volitional Force (V)	Sensation
	N = Normal	N = Normal
	G = Good	= Hypesthesia
	F = Fair	= Paresthesia
60° = Abnormal Degree of Rotary Motion	P = Poor	= Anesthesia
	T = Trace	
	Z = Zero	
30° = Fixed Position		Proprioception (P)
	Hypertonic Muscle (H)	N = Normal
	N = Normal	I = Impaired
	M = Mild	A = Absent
⋀⋁⋀ = Fracture	Mo = Moderate	
	S = Severe	D = Distension or Enlargement

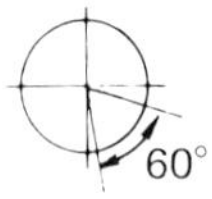

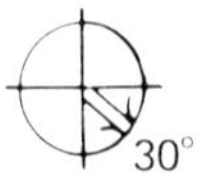

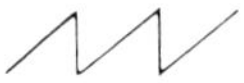

Fig. 4-1

diagrammatically recorded and effectively translated into an orthotic prescription, a technical analysis form for the upper limb has been developed by the Committee on Orthotics and Prosthetics of the American Academy of Orthopaedic Surgeons. The rationale for orthotic prescription is thus reduced to a process of biomechanical matching of modes of external control to functional deficits. The physician is generally knowledgeable regarding the patient's functional loss and the type of control that he would like to impose. He is frequently not knowledgeable, however, with regard to the wide variety of orthotic components available and their physical and mechanical characteristics. The technical analysis form thus serves to provide a bridge of communication between the physician and the orthotist, as well as

providing valuable information for the therapist and engineer. Possibly, there may be times at which no available component exists to provide the desired combination of controls. This method of approach would then serve to point up areas for future research and development.

DESCRIPTION OF UPPER-LIMB TECHNICAL ANALYSIS FORM

The form consists of four pages of appropriate size for inclusion in the patient's hospital record. Separate forms are provided for the right and left upper limbs. The first page (Fig. 4-1) contains spaces for patient data and a summary of major impairments. In general, the impairments noted on this page are those that do not lend themselves to diagrammatic representation. At the bottom of

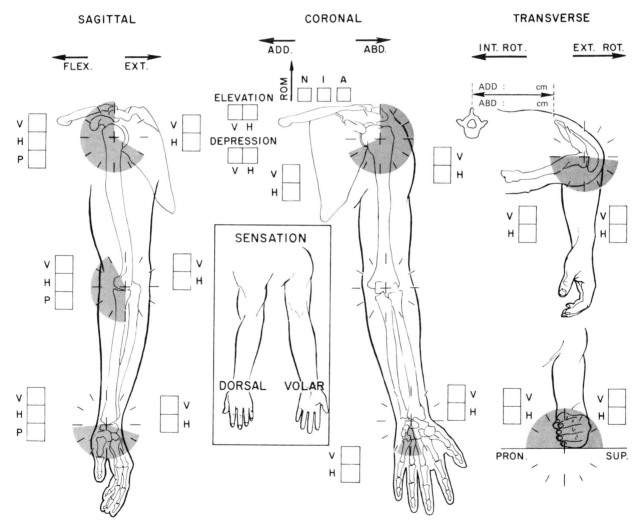

Fig. 4-2

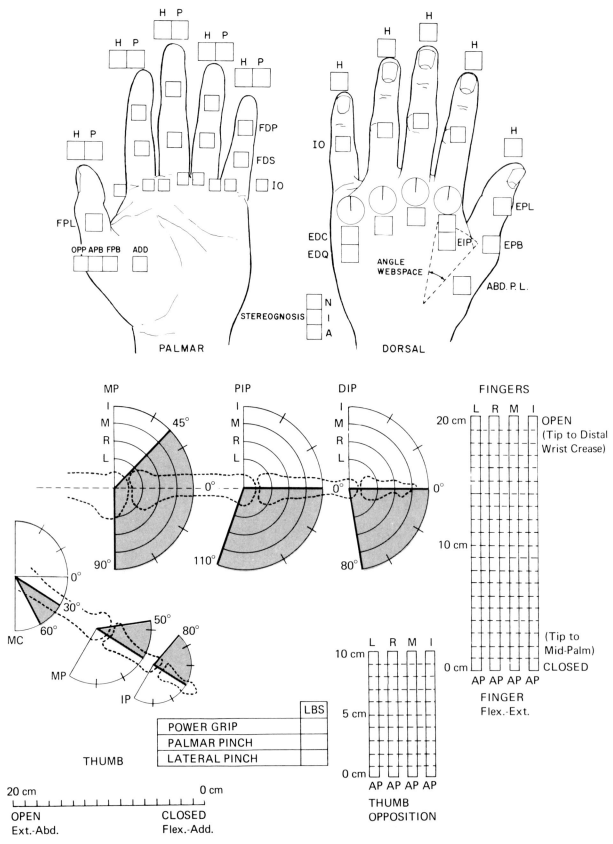

Fig. 4-3

Summary of Functional Disability _____

_____

_____

_____

_____

_____

Treatment Objectives: Prevent/Correct Deformity ☐   Improve Function ☐

                            Relieve Pain ☐   Other _____

ORTHOTIC RECOMMENDATION

UPPER LIMB			FLEX	EXT	ABD	ADD	ROTATION Int.	ROTATION Ext.	AXIAL LOAD
SEWHO	Shoulder								
EWHO	Humerus								
	Elbow								
	Forearm							(Pron.)	(Sup.)	
WHO	Wrist				(RD)	(UD)			
HO	Hand								
	Fingers 2-5	MP							
		PIP							
		DIP							
	Thumb	CM					(Opposition)		
		MP							
		IP							

REMARKS:

_____   _____

Signature   Date

KEY: Use the following symbols to indicate desired control of designated function:

    F = FREE   — *Free* motion.

    A = ASSIST   — Application of an external force for the purpose of increasing the range, velocity, or force of a motion.

    R = RESIST   — Application of an external force for the purpose of decreasing the velocity or force of a motion.

    S = STOP   — Inclusion of a static unit to deter an undesired motion in one direction.

    v = Variable — A unit that can be adjusted without making a structural change.

    H = HOLD   — Elimination of all motion in prescribed plane (verify position).

    L = LOCK   — Device includes an optional lock.

Fig. 4-4

the first page there is a legend for symbols to be used on the limb diagrams. The second page (Fig. 4-2) contains skeletal outlines of the upper limb in the sagittal, coronal, and transverse planes. Overlying the major joints are shaded areas representing the normal ranges of joint motion in each plane and contained within a circle divided into 30-degree segments. Similar smaller circles overlie the midshafts of the long bones for diagramming angular, rotational, or translational deformities of the humerus and forearm. Boxes labeled *V* and *H* are provided to correspond to the location of each muscle group for the purpose of recording volitional muscle strength and degree of hypertonicity, respectively. Boxes labeled *P* are provided at each joint level for the purpose of recording proprioception. A sensation diagram for the upper limb exclusive of the hand is provided in the insert.

The third page (Fig. 4-3) is to be used for the biomechanical analysis of the hand. At the top of the page, dorsal and volar outlines of the hand are to be used for recording sensation according to the symbols in the legend, including proprioception and stereognosis. Also spaces are provided for recording volitional strength and hypertonicity of individual muscles, and angular deformities of the metacarpophalangeal joints. Vertical scales are provided for linear recording of the opening and closing capacity of each finger and the oppositional capacity of each finger to the thumb. A horizontal scale is used to describe the opening and closing capacity of the thumb. A sagittal diagram is provided for recording the goniometric measurements of each digit and thumb. Space is also provided for recording the power of prehension.

The fourth page (Fig. 4-4) contains spaces for summarizing the functional disability and for identifying treatment objectives. The orthotic recommendation chart is also contained on this page along with a key for its use.

INSTRUCTIONS FOR USE OF UPPER-LIMB ANALYSIS FORM
Fig. 4-1

Page one is to be used to record general patient information and data that cannot be readily diagrammed on subsequent pages. It also presents the legend to be used on pages 2 and 3 (Figs. 4-2 and 4-3). Most of the items on the front page are self-explanatory. If the opposite limb is also impaired, space is provided for a brief description

of the functional impairment. If coordination is impaired, function is recorded as being normal, compromised, or prevented.

Fig. 4-2

Page two (Fig. 4-2) presents outlines of the upper limb in the sagittal, coronal, and transverse planes. Overlying the major joints are circles divided into 30-degree segments. The shaded areas within these circles represent the normal ranges of motion present in the unimpaired limb.

Recording motion

The degree of rotary motion or translatory motion is to be obtained from passive manipulation of the joint being examined.

Translatory motion. Linear arrows placed adjacent to the circle indicate the direction of abnormal translatory motion of a joint (subluxation or dislocation). The head of the arrow always points in the direction of displacement of the distal segment relative to the proximal. A number grade of 1, 2, or 3 is placed next to the arrow to indicate the severity of displacement, as indicated in the legend.

> Grade 1 = Subluxation
> Grade 2 = Dislocation that is reducible
> Grade 3 = Dislocation that is irreducible

Rotary motion. The arc of available motion is described by two radial lines drawn from the center of the circle to its perimeter. A double-headed arrow, as illustrated in the legend, is drawn outside and concentric to the circle between the radial lines, and the number of degrees of motion within this arc is recorded adjacent to the arrow. In certain instances, it may be desirable to use two double-headed arrows to describe the joint motion to either side of the neutral joint axis, rather than a single arrow to describe the total range of motion present.

NOTE: If one desires to diagram *active* as well as passive motions, a color code can be used to differentiate the two. Fixed positions or ankylosis of a joint are indicated by a double arrow from the center of the circle to its perimeter, with the position of the joint noted in degrees adjacent to the head of the arrow, as indicated in the legend.

Scapulothoracic motion. In the coronal plane, active elevation of the scapula is indicated as being normal, *N;* impaired, *I;* or absent, *A.* In the transverse plane, abduction and adduction of the scapula are recorded in centimeters from the vertebral border to the spinous process of the thoracic vertebrae along the double-headed arrow.

Recording muscle power and tone

Volitional power is determined by conventional muscle testing, and the letter grade as defined in the legend (Fig. 4-1) for each muscle group (such as flexors and internal rotators) is placed in the box labeled *V* in the appropriate area for that muscle group (Fig. 4-2).

Hypertonicity of each muscle group is graded as follows, and the letter grade placed in the appropriate box for the muscle group labeled *H:*

M = Mild hypertonicity with minimal impairment of function
Mo = Moderate hypertonicity, which compromises but is compatible with function
S = Severe hypertonicity, which is obstructive to function
N = Normal muscle tone

Recording sensation

Proprioception is recorded on the right of the page at the level of each major joint in the box labeled *P,* by use of the key described in the legend.

Tactile sensation of the upper limb, exclusive of the hand, is described on the sensation diagram provided by the inset, according to the key in the legend.

HAND DIAGRAM
Recording motion

Goniometric method. The skeletal outline of a finger and thumb in the sagittal plane is used to record degrees of motion in the small joints of the digits. Concentric arcs about each finger joint are used to plot the range of motion for index, middle, ring, and little fingers. Hatch marks along the outer arc (index finger) are at 30-degree intervals. These ranges may be plotted by use of a dot or mark at the extremes of motion connected by a heavy line or shading. A color code may be used to distinguish active from passive motion. The normal arcs of motion for each joint are defined by the shading between the heavy radial lines numbered in degrees. The joints of the thumb are similarly diagrammed. The angle of the web space of the thumb (in plane of palm) is recorded in the space provided on the dorsal sketch of the hand. Radial or ulnar deviation of the fingers is recorded by means of radial arrows numbered in degrees in

the circles over the metacarpophalangeal joints on the dorsal diagram of the hand.

Linear method. Linear measurements may also be used to describe the opening and closing capacity of the hand.

Fingers. To describe the opening capacity for each finger, measure the distance in centimeters from the tip of the extended finger to the distal flexion crease of the wrist and mark the vertical scale for each finger. Normals are shaded on the respective columns for each finger. Make a mark on the left side of the column for active motion and on the right side for passive motion.

To describe the closing capacity of each finger, measure the distance in centimeters from the tip of the finger to the midpalmar crease and record in a similar manner. The resulting intervals between full opening and full closing for each finger give a diagrammatic picture of finger excursion.

Thumb. To measure the opposing capacity of the thumb, measure the maximum vertical distance in centimeters from the tip of the thumb as it is opposed to each finger to the midpalm and record on the vertical scale for opposition. Active measurements are recorded on the right side of the column for each finger and passive measurements on the left side. To measure the opening and closing of the thumb in extension/abduction–flexion/adduction, measure the distance from the tip of the thumb to the head of the fifth metacarpal in full extension/abduction and full flexion/adduction and mark both measurements on the horizontal scale provided.

Recording muscle power and tone

Volitional power is determined by conventional means, and the letter grade for each muscle (see legend) is recorded in the box provided corresponding to the insertion of each tendon. Interosseous strength for abduction/adduction and metacarpophalangeal flexion is recorded on the palmar diagram; for proximal interphalangeal joint extension, it is recorded on the dorsal diagram.

Hypertonicity of the muscles to each digit is recorded in the box marked *H* at the tip of each finger, both for flexors (palmar diagram) and extensors (dorsal diagram), with the code in the legend being used. If muscle tone is normal, a check mark is made.

Functional motor power of the hand is measured by use of conventional pinch meters and grip dynamometers, and the values are recorded for

TECHNICAL ANALYSIS FORM   RIGHT UPPER LIMB   Revised March 1973

Name _MARGARET   JOHNSON_   No. _948152_   Age _38_   Sex _F_

Date of Onset _1961_   Cause _RHEUMATOID   ARTHRITIS_

Occupation _HOUSEWIFE_   Present Upper-Limb Equipment _NONE_

Diagnosis _RHEUMATOID   ARTHRITIS_

Hand Dominance: Right ☑ Left ☐

Status of other upper limb: Normal ☐   Impaired ☑

---

1. Ambulatory status: Normal ☐   Impaired ☑   Walking Aid ☑

2. Wheelchair ☐   Sitting Position: Stable ☐   Unstable ☐   Reclined ☐   Upright ☐
    Sitting Tolerance: Normal ☐   Limited ☐   Duration_____
    Propulsion: Manual ☐   Motor ☐   Dependent ☐

3. Cognition: Normal ☑   Impaired ☐

4. Endurance: Normal ☐   Impaired ☑

5. Skin: Normal ☐   Impaired ☑

6. Pain ☑   Location _WRISTS_

7. Vision: Normal ☑   Impaired ☐

8. Coordination: Normal ☑   Impaired ☐   Function: Normal ☐   Compromised ☐
                                                                Prevented   ☐

9. Motivation: Good ☑   Fair ☐   Poor ☐

10. Associated impairments: _KAFO – GENU   VALGUM_ Ⓛ

──────────────────────── LEGEND ────────────────────────

= Direction of Translatory
  Motion
  (Grade 1,2 or 3)

= Abnormal Degree of
  Rotary Motion
  60°

= Fixed Position
  30°

= Fracture

Volitional Force (V)
N = Normal
G = Good
F = Fair
P = Poor
T = Trace
Z = Zero

Hypertonic Muscle (H)
N = Normal
M = Mild
Mo = Moderate
S = Severe

Sensation
N = Normal
░ = Hypesthesia
▨ = Paresthesia
▩ = Anesthesia

Proprioception (P)
N = Normal
I = Impaired
A = Absent

D = Distension or
       Enlargement

Fig. 4-5

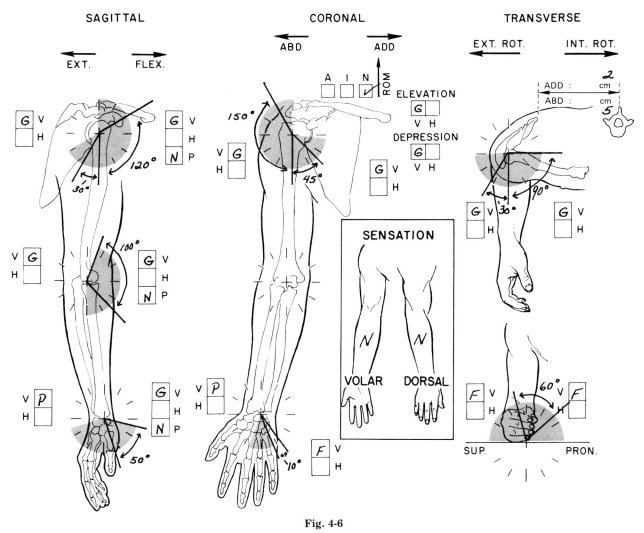

Fig. 4-6

power grip, palmar prehension, and lateral prehension.

Recording sensation

Proprioception is recorded in the box labeled *P* at the tip of each digit, with the code in the legend being used.

Stereognosis is recorded in the space provided as being normal, *N;* impaired, *I;* or absent, *A.*

Tactile sensation is diagrammed as an overlay on the palmar and dorsal hand diagrams according to the key in the legend.

SUMMARY AND RECOMMENDATIONS
(Fig. 4-4)

From the data recorded, a concise summary of the *functional* disability is recorded in the spaces provided, and treatment objectives are identified.

The orthotic recommendation (or prescription) chart is then completed according to the key at the bottom of the page. If the entire upper limb is to be included in the device prescribed (shoulder-elbow-wrist-hand orthosis, SEWHO), one must decide what the requirements are for the components at each joint level and for each movement (flexion, extension, adduction, abduction, rotation, and axial load). Motions that do not apply to specific joints have been blocked out.

ILLUSTRATIVE CASES
Case 1 (Figs. 4-5 to 4-8)

A 38-year-old female was seen for upper-limb involvement secondary to rheumatoid arthritis. Fig. 4-5 provides the basic background information regarding this patient's disability. She is ambulatory with the aid of a knee-ankle-foot orthosis for genu valgum and complains of pain in both wrists.

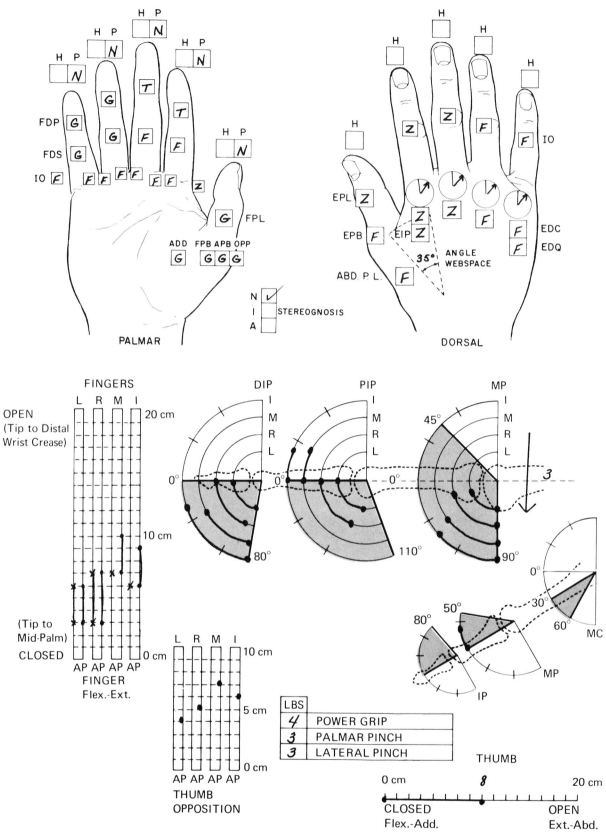

Fig. 4-7

Summary of Functional Disability _WEAK GRASP 2° TO PROGRESSIVE_
DEFORMITY

Treatment Objectives: Prevent/Correct Deformity ☑   Improve Function ☐
                        Relieve Pain ☑   Other _____

ORTHOTIC RECOMMENDATION

UPPER LIMB		FLEX	EXT	ABD	ADD	ROTATION Int.	ROTATION Ext.	AXIAL LOAD
SEWHO	Shoulder							
EWHO	Humerus							
	Elbow							
	Forearm					(Pron.)	(Sup.)	
WHO	Wrist	H -20°		(RD)	H (UD) 20°			
HO	Hand							
	Fingers 2-5 — MP	R	A	A	R			
	Fingers 2-5 — PIP							
	Fingers 2-5 — DIP							
	Thumb — CM			A	R	(Opposition)		
	Thumb — MP							
	Thumb — IP							

REMARKS: _PADDED THERMOPLASTIC DORSAL WRIST SPLINT, 20°_
FLEXION AND 20° OF ULNAR DEVIATION WITH OUTRIGGER
FOR DYNAMIC FINGER EXTENSION AND THUMB ABDUCTION

_____   _10/8/73_
Signature   Date

KEY: Use the following symbols to indicate desired control of designated function:

F = FREE — _Free_ motion.

A = ASSIST — Application of an external force for the purpose of increasing the range, velocity, or force of a motion.

R = RESIST — Application of an external force for the purpose of decreasing the velocity or force of a motion.

S = STOP — Inclusion of a static unit to deter an undesired motion in one direction.

v = Variable — A unit that can be adjusted without making a structural change.

H = HOLD — Elimination of all motion in prescribed plane (verify position).

L = LOCK — Device includes an optional lock.

Fig. 4-8

TECHNICAL ANALYSIS FORM   LEFT UPPER LIMB   Revised March 1973

Name _MANUEL REYNA_   No._848209_   Age_22_   Sex_M_

Date of Onset _11-71_   Cause _AUTO ACCIDENT_

Occupation_ELECTRICIAN_   Present Upper-Limb Equipment _NONE_

Diagnosis _QUADRIPLEGIC   C-5-C-6_

Hand Dominance: Right ☐   Left ☐

Status of other upper limb: Normal ☐   Impaired ☑

---

1. Ambulatory status: Normal ☐   Impaired ☑   Walking Aid ☐

2. Wheelchair ☑   Sitting Position: Stable ☑   Unstable ☐   Reclined ☐   Upright ☑
    Sitting Tolerance: Normal ☐   Limited ☑   Duration _1 ½ HOURS_
    Propulsion: Manual ☑   Motor ☐   Dependent ☐

3. Cognition: Normal ☑   Impaired ☐

4. Endurance: Normal ☐   Impaired ☑

5. Skin: Normal ☑   Impaired ☐

6. Pain ☐   Location_____

7. Vision: Normal ☑   Impaired ☐

8. Coordination: Normal ☑   Impaired ☐   Function: Normal ☐   Compromised ☐
                                                              Prevented ☐

9. Motivation: Good ☑   Fair ☐   Poor ☐

10. Associated impairments: _LOWER LIMB SPASM_

--- LEGEND ---

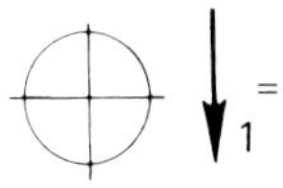

= Direction of Translatory Motion
  (Grade 1,2 or 3)

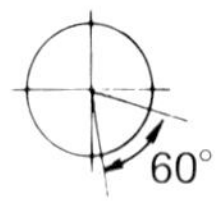

= Abnormal Degree of Rotary Motion
  60°

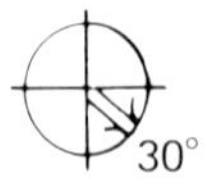

= Fixed Position
  30°

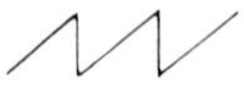

= Fracture

Volitional Force (V)
N = Normal
G = Good
F = Fair
P = Poor
T = Trace
Z = Zero

Hypertonic Muscle (H)
N = Normal
M = Mild
Mo = Moderate
S = Severe

Sensation
N = Normal
= Hypesthesia
= Paresthesia
= Anesthesia

Proprioception (P)
N = Normal
I = Impaired
A = Absent
D = Distension or Enlargement

Fig. 4-9

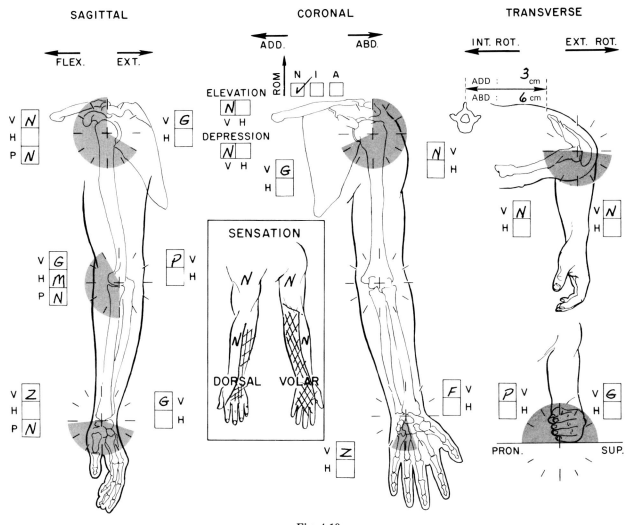

Fig. 4-10

Diagrammatic analysis of the *right upper limb (Fig. 4-6)* exclusive of the hand give a clear picture of the voluntary muscle strength of all muscle groups and the range of motion present in all major joints. In the sagittal plane, one notes absence of the last 60 degrees of forward flexion of the shoulder, as well as inability to achieve the last 30 degrees of shoulder extension. There is a 45-degree flexion contracture of the elbow, and a 20-degree flexion contracture of the wrist. In the coronal plane, there is limitation of the last 30 degrees of shoulder adduction. The wrist is in ulnar deviation with 10 degrees of excessive ulnar deviation possible. Loss of external rotation at the shoulder, and limitation of pronation and supination of the wrist may be visualized in the transverse plane.

Diagrammatic analysis of the hand (Fig. 4-7) indicates the volitional strength of each muscle at its in-

sertion on dorsal and palmar sketches of the hand. Also noted are the ulnar deviation deformities of the digits at the metacarpophalangeal joints, and a contracture of the web-space angle to 35 degrees. Excursion of the joints of each finger is recorded on both linear and goniometric diagrams. Note the flexion contracture of the distal interphalangeal joints and extension contractures of the proximal interphalangeal joints of the index and middle fingers, indicating typical swan-neck deformities of these digits. The metacarpophalangeal joints are noted to be dislocated and irreducible as indicated by the arrow and adjacent numeral *3*. All modes of prehension are noted to be greatly reduced in power, and there is considerable limitation of the opening capacity of the thumb in extension-abduction.

Fig. 4-8 indicates that the primary functional disability is weakness of grasp secondary to progressive

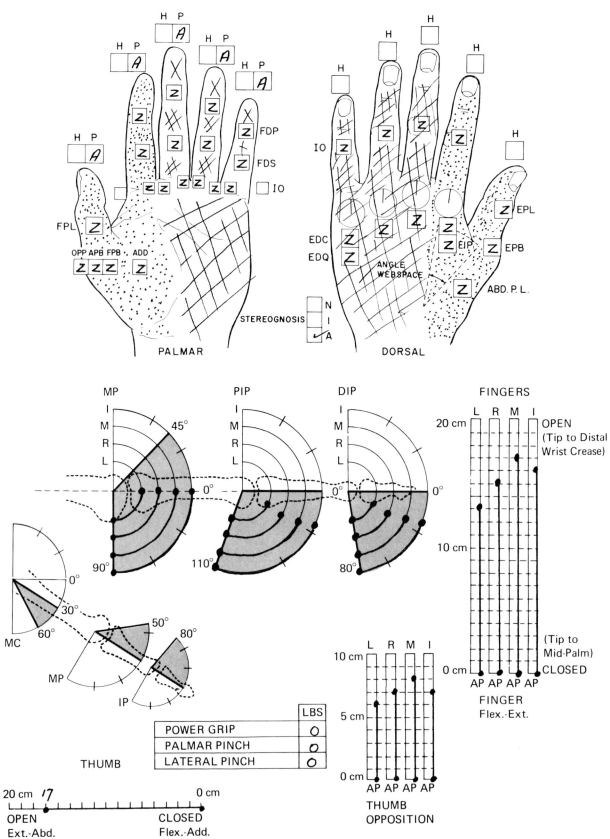

Fig. 4-11

Summary of Functional Disability _No FUNCTIONAL GRASP_

Treatment Objectives: Prevent/Correct Deformity ☐   Improve Function ☑
                        Relieve Pain ☐   Other _____

ORTHOTIC RECOMMENDATION

UPPER LIMB			FLEX	EXT	ABD	ADD	ROTATION Int.	ROTATION Ext.	AXIAL LOAD
SEWHO Shoulder									
EWHO *Humerus*									
Elbow									
Forearm							(Pron.)	(Sup.)	
WHO Wrist			F	F	H (RD) 10°	(UD)			
HO Hand									
Fingers 2-5		MP	F	F	H - 0°	H - 0°			
		PIP	H - 45°	H - 45°					
		DIP	H - 15°	H - 15°					
Thumb		CM			H - 45°		(Opposition)		
		MP	H - 10°						
		IP	H - 10°						

REMARKS: _WRIST EXTENSOR DRIVEN HAND SPLINT - 2ND AND THIRD FINGERS TO THUMB_

Signature _____   Date 8/16/73

KEY: Use the following symbols to indicate desired control of designated function:

F = FREE   — *Free* motion.
A = ASSIST   — Application of an external force for the purpose of increasing the range, velocity, or force of a motion.
R = RESIST   — Application of an external force for the purpose of decreasing the velocity or force of a motion.
S = STOP   — Inclusion of a static unit to deter an undesired motion in one direction.
v = Variable — A unit that can be adjusted without making a structural change.
H = HOLD   — Elimination of all motion in prescribed plane (verify position).
L = LOCK   — Device includes an optional lock.

Fig. 4-12

deformity and pain and that the objective of orthotic treatment is the prevention and correction of deformity and the relief of pain. The orthotic recommendation is to hold the wrist statically in 20 degrees of flexion and 20 degrees of ulnar deviation, to assist metacarpophalangeal extension and to resist metacarpophalangeal flexion, and to assist radial deviation of the fingers and resist ulnar deviation of these digits. It is also desirable to assist the carpometacarpal joint of the thumb in abduction and to resist adduction of this joint. It is suggested that a method of achieving these objectives is to use a padded thermoplastic splint to hold the wrist in the prescribed position with the addition of an outrigger for dynamic finger extension and thumb abduction.

Case 2 (Figs. 4-9 to 4-12)

A 22-year-old male was seen for evaluation of upper-limb disability secondary to spinal cord injury at the C5-C6 level with resulting quadriplegia. Basic background information for this patient is illustrated in Fig. 4-9.

Fig. 4-10 indicates the volitional strength for each muscle group in the upper limb exclusive of the hand and further provides the information that there is no passive limitation of joint movement in the shoulder, elbow, or wrist.

The hand diagram (Fig. 4-11) is shaded according to the code in the legend to indicate anesthesia in the area of the C7 and C8 dermatomes, and hypesthesia in the C6 dermatome. There is no volitional motor power present in the intrinsic or extrinsic muscles of the hand. Proprioception and stereognosis are absent. Goniometric analysis of the fingers indicates a 20-degree flexion contracture of the proximal and distal interphalangeal joints of all fingers. The linear measurement chart also indicates reduced passive opening capacity of the fingers and reduced passive excursion of the thumb into extension-abduction.

Fig. 4-12 indicates that the primary functional disability is that of inability to grasp. The orthotic recommendation is for a wrist-hand orthosis with free flexion and extension of the wrist in 10 degrees of radial deviation, free metacarpophalangeal flexion and extension of digits 2 and 3, immobilization of the proximal interphalangeal joints of digits 2 and 3 at 45 degrees of flexion, and immobilization of the distal interphalangeal joints at 15 degrees of flexion. With regard to the thumb, the carpometacarpal joint is to be immobilized at 45 degrees of abduction and the metacarpophalangeal joint and the interphalangeal joint are to be immobilized at 10 degrees of flexion. Under remarks, it is noted that the orthosis is to be driven by the wrist extensors, providing opposition of the second and third fingers to the thumb.

SUMMARY

The basis for rational orthotic prescription must be a systematic functional appraisal of the impaired limb or body segments. The diagrammatic approach to biomechanical analysis of the upper limb presented here serves to better identify the functional deficits present and forms the basis for appropriate selection of orthotic components. It also serves to identify instances for which adequate components are not available to perform the required tasks, thus indicating areas for further research. In addition to serving as a means for developing a logical approach to orthotic prescription, such a technical analysis provides an improved means of communication between the physician and the orthotist. Although the analysis form itself need not be applied to all patients requiring an orthosis, the concept of a biomechanical approach of this nature is essential to the development of a sound orthotic prescription.

CHAPTER 5

Orthotic components and systems

ARTHUR GUILFORD, C.O.
JACQUELIN PERRY, M.D.

The therapeutic advantage of an orthosis is dependent on its effectiveness in selectively restricting, assisting, or creating motion according to clinical needs. Properly applied, these attributes can contribute very significantly to programs having the following objectives:

1. Prevention or correction of deformity, or both
2. Protection of painful, inflamed, or healing tissues (a recently weakened muscle is one form of healing tissue)
3. Addition of function
   a. Through assistance or replacement of inadequate musculature
   b. Through stabilization of structurally unstable joints

These goals are accomplished by appropriate combinations of static, mobile, and powered orthotic components. Static units are rigid structures contoured to hold the segments in one desired position. A mobile orthosis is articulated to permit motion initiated either by the patient's own muscles or some form of external power. Joint design and alignment determine the planes and arc of motion permitted. Further restriction of arc is possible with stops.

Power is the source of motion. Several external systems are available. Elastic, in the form of rubber bands or springs, is the most convenient. These items are readily available, easily replaced, and automatically activated whenever stretched by the pull of opposing musculature. Although this makes them ready to function as soon as the muscles relax, it also means that antagonistic muscles must have sufficient strength to perform their own task while working against the resistance offered by the elastic units. Also, one must remember that the elastic force remains active until all stretch is lost and that the force decreases as the stretch decreases. Springs offer a more proportional force throughout their range than do rubber bands; otherwise the principles are the same. Thus this type of control is merely expected to move the part through the stretch arc. Any holding function must be accomplished in another way (serrated lock, stops, etc.). Elastic strength is determined by the number and size of rubber bands or springs used. As there is a limitation on tolerable bulk, the potentials for this system are restricted to the provision of light forces.

When patients lack the musculature to activate elastics, an independent power source is required. Harnessing of remote muscles by cabling is tempting. It is a very effective system in prosthetics but does not work in orthotics, since the latter must cope with weight and tissue resistance of paralyzed limbs. Orthotic activation requires a 15:1 power-to-function ratio. Not only is this overly demanding on persons with normal strength, but the majority of patients needing such functional replacement have far less strength to serve as the power source. Hence this system is inappropriate for orthotics.

External power, though still necessitating remote body control for activation, demands only the strength to move a switch. This can be as little as 30 grams if microswitches are used. Lighter ones are available, but they deny the patient necessary feedback information. More independence through better reliability is gained with mechanical switches. Two types of external power are currently employed: carbon dioxide gas and electric motors. A hydraulic system was tried briefly, but efficiency was too low and connecting cables were too susceptible to damage.

The carbon dioxide system creates motion by using the gas to distend a central bladder and thus shorten a woven, nylon, helical sheath (Barber, see reference on p. 129). The sheath is a flexible tube formed by two sets of semivertical fibers wound in opposite directions. This establishes a variable reciprocal relationship between sleeve length and diameter that can be used to operate an orthosis. Gas injection distends the sheath. Since its fibers are not elastic, they accommodate to the diameter change by becoming more horizontal (Fig. 5-1). This brings the two ends of the sheath closer together, thereby creating a contraction force to activate the orthosis. A light spring is used to return the unit to its resting length as the gas is released. By subtle graduation of gas injection and release, a form of proportional control is gained; that is, the effort at gas control provides feedback as to the amount of force being created because it is grossly proportional to the volume of gas within the bladder. Valve design allows the 65 psi line pressure to be operated by light switches without a threat of leakage. These many advantages make the carbon dioxide system very desirable. However, the inconvenience of obtaining the gas in a useful form has been a major deterrent to widespread acceptance. Transfer of the gas from the large storage tanks to patient units has been facilitated by design of special home refill devices, but the techniques remain sufficiently tricky that many families prefer using outside servicing from a fire station or commercial source. Limitations of service outlets has seriously limited this system to only the areas where special servicing can be arranged.

Availability of small motors and rechargeable batteries make use of electricity the next logical step in the development of external power for orthotics. Direct application of this system was not satisfactory because the electric motors responded so quickly that the result was an on-off effect. Although the most able patients could manage it, the majority found the reactions too abrupt for effective orthotic control. The solution has been the design of proportional electrical control. Reliability has been a problem, but that is improving each year.

The standardized biomechanical analysis matrix has been presented in Chapter 4. For the purpose of demonstrating the biomechanical attributes of specific orthoses, only the applicable portions of the matrix will be used.

EXCURSION OF CO$_2$ MUSCLE

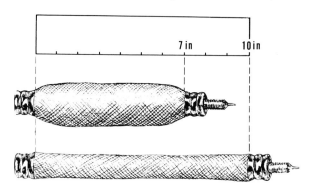

Fig. 5-1. Carbon dioxide "muscle." **A,** Shortening by gaseous distension. **B,** Length available when tube exhausted. (From Barber, L. M., and Nickel, V. L.: Carbon dioxide-powered arm and hand devices, Am. J. Occup. Ther. **23:**215-225, 1969.)

McKibben

Type: HO (hand orthosis)
Name: IP orthosis (finger splint)

H—Hand		Flex	Ext
Fingers 2-5	MP	R	A
	PIP	R	A
	DIP	H	H

Biomechanical: The spring steel strap resists flexion at the metacarpophalangeal (MP) and proximal interphalangeal (PIP) joints. Combined palmar and dorsal encasement of distal phalanx holds the distal interphalangeal (DIP) joint rigid.

Material: Padded ¼" spring steel, steel bands, and webbing wrist strap

Fabrication: Prefabricated

Special considerations: Forces must be balanced so as not to create excessive pressure in any one area.

Type: HO (hand orthosis)
Name: IP flexion assist (finger-bender splint)

H—Hand		Flex	Ext
Fingers 2-5	MP		
	PIP	A	R
	DIP	F	F

Biomechanical: Rubber bands aligned on the volar side produce a flexion force and resist extension.

Material: Looped linked wire frame with rubber bands for flexion force

Fabrication: Prefabricated

Special considerations: Flexor stretch is determined by the number and size of rubber bands used. Total applied force must be less than maximum voluntary extensor strength to permit pressure relief.

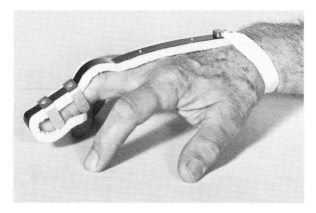

Fig. 5-2

for Fx - static

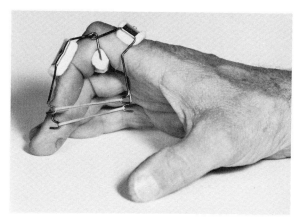

Fig. 5-3

Knuckle bender

Type: HO (hand orthosis)

Name: IP extension assist—dorsal outrigger (reverse finger-bender) (Fig. 5-4, *A*)

H—Hand		Flex	Ext
Fingers 2-5	MP		
	PIP	R	A
	DIP	R	A

Biomechanical: Dorsally positioned rubber bands create an extensor force to pull against flexion deformity. They also resist active flexion.

Material: Looped, linked wire frame with rubber bands for extension force

Fabrication: Prefabrication

Special considerations: The strength of the extensor force is determined by the number and size of the rubber bands used (two sides must balance). Total force must be less than the patient's maximum flexor force to permit stretch relief.

Name: IP extension assist—elastic straps (Fig. 5-4, *B*)

Biomechanical: Dorsal force is applied to finger to assist extension and resist flexion.

Material: Wire frame, metal bands, and strap extensor force

Fabrication: Prefabrication

Special considerations: The DIP joint is usually not influenced.

Name: IP extension assist—coiled spring (Fig. 5-4, *C*)

Biomechanical: A three-point spring-force system is used to assist IP extension. It pulls against the flexion contracture and resists flexion.

Material: Double coiled wire springs, metal bands, and strap

Fabrication: Prefabrication

Special considerations: Dorsal counterforce is applied just proximal to PIP condyles to avoid trauma to dorsal joint structures and to increase pressure tolerance.

REFERENCE

Weniger, H.: (Photographs) H. Weniger, Inc., 70 12th Street, San Francisco, Calif., 1974.

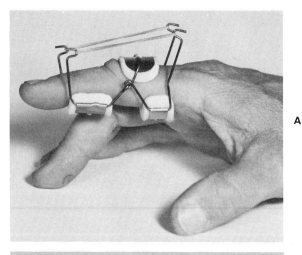

A

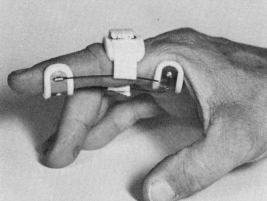

B

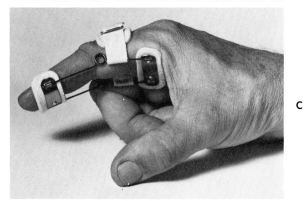

C

Fig. 5-4

Type: HO (hand orthosis)
Name: Basic hand component

Biomechanical: Its purpose is to support the palmar arch, and the component is the foundation for a positional upper-limb orthosis. It serves as an attachment for other components to achieve positioning of the thumb, fingers, and wrist.

Material: Padded metal (Fig. 5-5, *A*) or plastic (Fig. 5-5, *B*) with attachment strap.

Fabrication: It may be preformed and requires patient for final fitting. In most cases, when thermoplastics are utilized, an accurate plaster mold of the hand is necessary.

Special considerations: Hand should be flexible and free from deformity. Excessive edema would be a contraindication.

REFERENCES

Anderson, M. H.: Upper extremity orthotics, Springfield, Ill., 1965, Charles C Thomas, Publisher.

Engen, T. J.: Development of upper extremity orthotics, Parts I and II, Orthotics and prosthetics, March and June 1970, American Orthotic and Prosthetic Association, Washington, D.C.

Nickel, V. L., Perry, J., and Snelson, R.: Handbook of hand splints, Rancho Los Amigos Hospital, Downey, Calif., 1960.

A

B

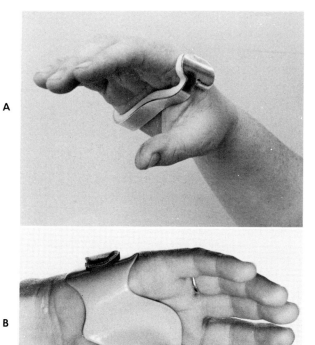

Fig. 5-5

Type: HO (hand orthosis)
Name: Opponens orthosis

		Flex	Ext	Abd	Add	Rotation	
H—Hand						Int	Ext
Thumb	CM	F	S	F	S		
	MP	F	F	F	S	Opposition F	S

Biomechanical: Its purpose is to stabilize the thumb in opposition and to stop extension and adduction at the carpometacarpal (CM) joint.

Material: Padded metal with attachment strap (Fig. 5-6, *A*); plastic with attachment strap (Fig. 5-6, *B*).

Fabrication: It is formed to make total contact with the hand. Attachment is with a leather or Velcro wrist strap. Plastic device consists of the basic hand unit built with integral thumb unit.

Special considerations: It must be shaped to provide total surface contact. The strap should be tight enough to prevent the orthosis from moving distally, but should not interfere with circulation.

REFERENCES

Anderson, M. H.: Upper extremity orthotics, Springfield, Ill., 1965, Charles C Thomas, Publisher.

Engen, T. J.: Development of upper extremity orthotics, Parts I and II, Orthotics and prosthetics, March and June 1970, American Orthotic and Prosthetic Association, Washington, D.C.

Nickel, V. L., Perry, J., and Snelson, R.: Handbook of hand splints, Rancho Los Amigos Hospital, Downey, Calif., 1960.

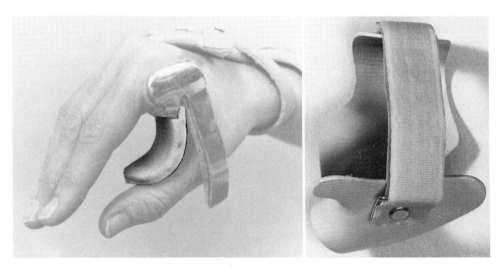

Fig. 5-6

Type: HO (hand orthosis)
Name: Rigid thumb orthosis (thumb post)

H—Hand		Flex	Ext	Abd	Add	Rotation Int	Ext
Thumb	CM	H	H	H	H	Opposition H—I—H	
	MP	H	H	H	H		
	IP	H	H				

Biomechanical: Its purpose is to hold the thumb in position for prehension.

Material: Stainless steel

Fabrication: It is an extension of the metacarpal unit. The distal portion encircles the thumb, but it does not interfere with skin contact between the thumb and fingers.

Special considerations: A tight thumb web space is a contraindication for good function.

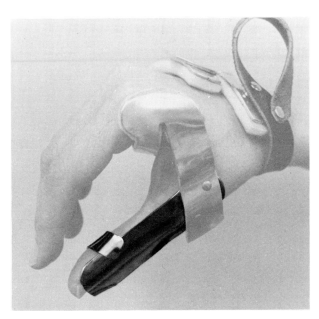

Fig. 5-7

Type: HO (hand orthosis)
Name: Thumb IP extension assist

H—Hand		Flex	Ext	Abd	Add	Rotation Int	Ext
Thumb	CM	R	A/S	A	R	Opposition R—I—R	
	MP	R	A/S	A	R		
	IP	R	A				

Biomechanical: Its purpose is to assist interphalangeal extension of the thumb while stabilizing other thumb joints.

Material: Metal or plastic frame, leather or plastic suspension, and coil spring assist

Fabrication: A short thumb post is extended from the hand unit to prevent hyperextension of the metacarpophalangeal joint. The thumb suspension loop is fitted to the distal phalanx.

Special considerations: The spring tension must be adjusted to balance flexion and extension of the IP joint. This unit may or may not be used with the thumb abduction stop.

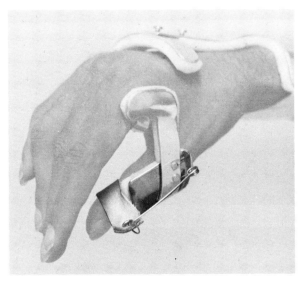

Fig. 5-8

Type: HO (hand orthosis)
Name: Limited MP extension (dorsal lumbrical bar)

H—Hand		Flex	Ext	Abd	Add
Fingers 2-5	MP	F	S	F	F
	PIP	F	F		
	DIP	F	F		

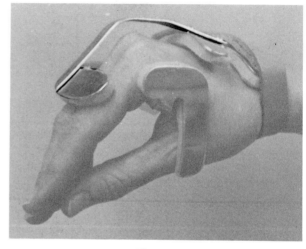

Fig. 5-9

Biomechanical: Its purpose is to stop the MP joints in flexion and to allow extension of PIP and DIP joints. The proximal phalanges are held in a 15-degree flexion so that full extension of the distal phalanges may be obtained by active extrinsic finger extensors.

Material: Metal or plastic basic hand orthosis with metal extension stop

Fabrication: A dorsal finger stop is added to the basic hand unit.

Special considerations: To obtain this position, stop is set in 30 degrees of flexion to allow for slack between orthosis and hand.

NOTE: Illustration also includes a thumb extension stop.

REFERENCES

Anderson, M. H.: Upper extremity orthotics, Springfield, Ill., 1965, Charles C Thomas, Publisher.

Nickel, V. L., Perry, J., and Snelson, R.: Handbook of hand splints, Rancho Los Amigos Hospital, Downey, Calif., 1960.

Type: HO (hand orthosis)
Name: Finger extensor assist

H—Hand		Flex	Ext	Abd	Add
Fingers 2-5	MP	R	S	F	F
	PIP	R	A		
	DIP	F	F		

Biomechanical: Its purpose is to assist IP extension with rubber bands and stop MP extension.

Material: Prefabricated (Fig. 5-10, *A*); padded metal frame, leather or plastic suspension, and rubber band assist (Fig. 5-10, *B*); plastic frame, metal MP exten- sion stop, leather or plastic suspension, and rubber band assist (Fig. 5-10, *C*).

Fabrication: A dorsal MP stop and elastic phalangeal extension assist are added to the hand orthosis. This must be well fitted to distribute pressures evenly over the dorsal portion of the hand.

Special considerations: The stop prevents hyperexten- sion of the MP joints. The rubber bands must be individually adjusted to balance the flexion and ex- tension of each finger. The suspension finger loops may be positioned on the distal phalanges if one wants to influence both proximal and distal IP extension.

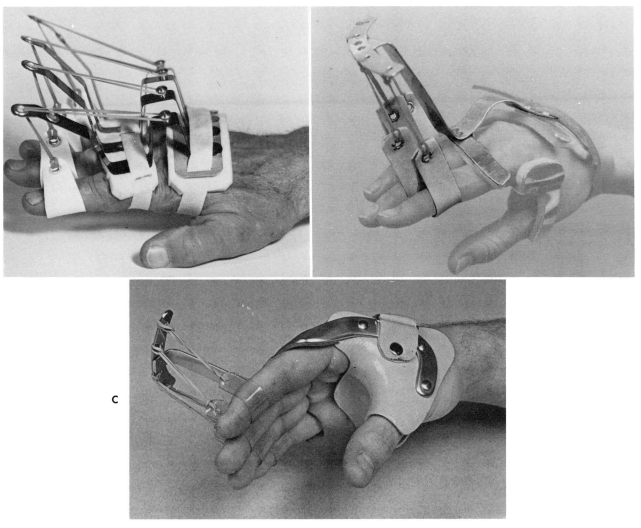

A

B

C

Fig. 5-10

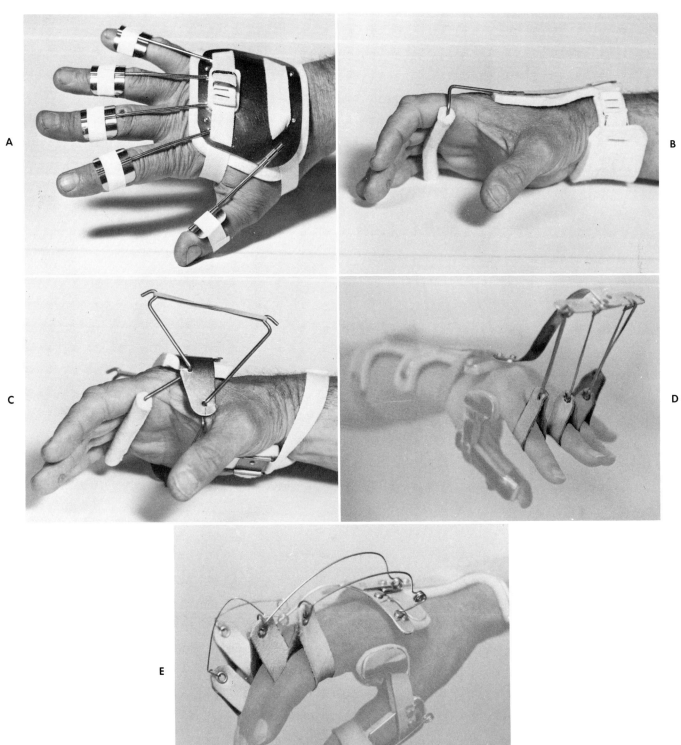

Fig. 5-11

Type: HO (hand orthosis)
Name: MP extensor assist

H—Hand			Flex	Ext	Abd	Add
Fingers 2-5		MP	R	A	F	F
		PIP	F	F		
		DIP	F	F		

Biomechanical: The purpose is to assist MP extension with an external force. (When the assist is attached to the middle phalanx, the patient will also have PIP extension assistance—Fig. 5-11, *A*).

Material: Padded metal and wire frame, metal bands, and webbing wrist-finger straps; this is prefabricated (Fig. 5-11, *A*). Padded metal and wire frame, metal band, and webbing wrist strap; this is prefabricated (Fig. 5-11, *B*). Padded metal and wire frame, metal bands, webbing wrist strap, and rubber bands for extension force; this is prefabricated. A dorsal wrist extension may be used to anchor this type of orthosis (see WHO), (Fig. 5-11, *C*). Padded metal frame, metal extension for extension assist, leather or plastic suspension, and rubber band assist (Fig. 5-11, *D*; NOTE: illustration also includes a thumb post.). Padded metal frame, leather or plastic suspension, and coiled wire springs for extension assist (Fig. 5-11, *E*; NOTE: illustration also includes a thumb extension assist.)

Fabrication: A static or dynamic MP extension assist is added to the basic hand orthosis.

Special considerations: In each orthosis the assist must be individually adjusted to balance the flexion and extension of all MP joints. The suspension finger loops are positioned on the proximal phalanges.

Type: HO (hand orthosis)
Name: Limited MP extension (variable extension stop)

H—Hand			Flex	Ext	Abd	Add
Fingers 2-5		MP	F	S$_V$	S	S
		PIP	F	F		
		DIP	F	F		

Biomechanical: Its purpose is to provide a variable MP stop.

Material: Padded metal frame, radial-ulnar extensions, padded metal dorsal band, wing nuts at MP joints, and leather wrist strap

Fabrication: A dorsal extension is added to the hand orthosis. Must be well fitted over dorsal portion of fingers. An adjustment wing nut is used at the MP joints.

Special considerations: It is used to maintain range obtained by manual stretching. The stop is set to hold MP joints in 5 degrees less than maximum available flexion. It cannot be used to stretch, as patient has no means for periodic escape, that is, no means to relieve skin pressures.

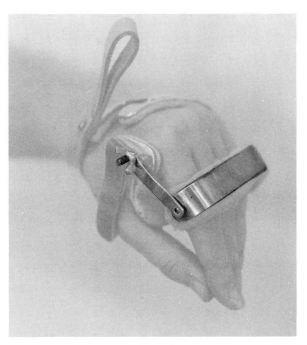

Fig. 5-12

Type: HO (hand orthosis)

Name: Rigid digital and metacarpal orthosis (finger platform orthosis)

H—Hand		Flex	Ext	Abd	Add
Fingers 2-5	MP	H40°	H	H	H
	PIP	H20°	H		
	DIP	H20°	H		

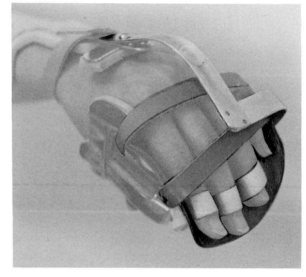

Fig. 5-13

Biomechanical: Its purpose is as a finger flexion hold.

Material: Padded metal frame, metal or plastic dorsal extension, and finger straps.

Fabrication: It is a distal volar extension to the hand orthosis fastened to the dorsal surface.

Special considerations: It is used to maintain the range obtained by manual stretching.

NOTE: A dorsal extension may be used to anchor this type of orthosis (see WHO).

Type: HO (hand orthosis)
Name: Rigid phalangeal orthosis with metacarpal joint
assist (short flexor-hinge orthosis)

H—Hand		Flex	Ext	Abd	Add	Rotation	
						Int	Ext
Fingers 2-5	MP	F	A	H	H		
	PIP	H 2 & 3	H 2 & 3				
	DIP	H 2 & 3	H 2 & 3				
Thumb	CM	H	H	H	H	Opposition H	H
	MP	H	H	H	H		
	IP	H	H				

Biomechanical: Its purpose is to provide prehension by
stabilizing the fingers and thumb. A spring assist is
used for extension of the MP joints.

Material: Padded metal frame, MP joint, thumb post,
finger stabilizers, MP extension spring assist, and
straps

Fabrication: It may be preformed but requires patient
for final shaping and fitting. An accurate plaster mold
may be used for fabrication.

Special considerations: The hand should be flexible and
free from deformity. Excessive edema would be a contraindication. Thumb and fingers are held in functional position.

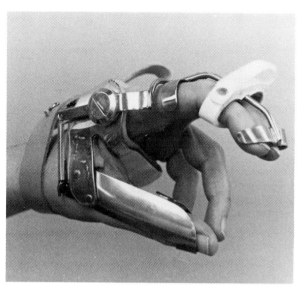

Fig. 5-14

REFERENCES

Anderson, M. H.: Upper extremity orthotics, Springfield, Ill.,
1965, Charles C Thomas, Publisher.

Engen, T. J.: Development of upper extremity orthotics, Parts I
and II, Orthotics and prosthetics, March and June 1970,
American Orthotic and Prosthetic Association, Washington, D.C.

Nickel, V. L., Perry, J., and Snelson, R.: Handbook of hand
splints, Rancho Los Amigos Hospital, Downey, Calif., 1960.

Weniger, H.: (Photographs) San Francisco, Calif., 1974.

Type: WHO (wrist-hand orthosis)

Name: Rigid wrist and limited thumb orthosis (basic long opponens)

	Flex	Ext	Abd	Add	Rotation Int	Rotation Ext
W—Wrist	H	H	H (RD)	H (UD)		
H—Hand						
Fingers 2-5 — MP	S	F				
Fingers 2-5 — PIP						
Fingers 2-5 — DIP						
Thumb — CM	F	S	F	S	Opposition H | H	
Thumb — MP	F	S	F	S		
Thumb — IP	F	F				

Biomechanical: Its purpose is to stabilize the wrist and thumb in the basic position of function.

Material: Padded metal frame with leather wrist and firearm straps (Fig. 5-15, *A*); plastic hand frame with padded metal wrist and forearm section; hand, wrist, and forearm Velcro straps (Fig. 5-15, *B*)

Fabrication: It is shaped to the dorsal or volar side of the hand and forearm and fastened to the basic hand unit.

Special considerations: It must be formed to provide total surface contact. Straps should be tight enough to maintain the orthosis in position, but should not interfere with circulation.

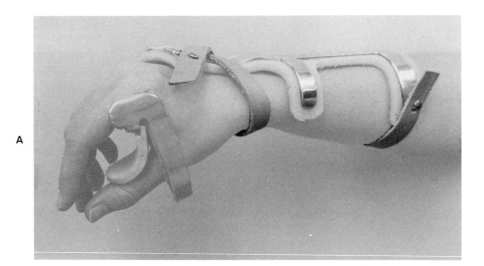

A

Type: WHO (wrist-hand orthosis)

Name: Hand suspensor (prop)

Biomechanical: Its purpose is to provide a suspender support for a wrist-hand orthosis to protect the digits and thumb from painful or deforming pressures of limb weight.

Material: Metal

Fabrication: It is shaped to elevate the hand to relieve pressure on the thumb and allows the fingers to fall into free flexion. This unit is detachable.

Special considerations: Pronation and supination may be adjusted to the desired resting position.

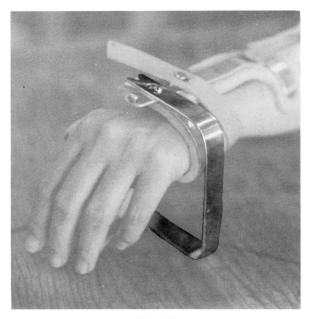

Fig. 5-16

B

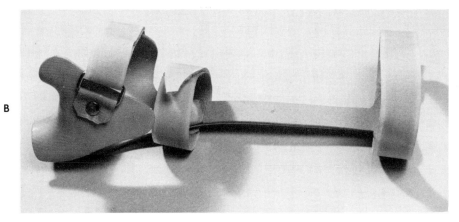

Fig. 5-15

Type: WHO (wrist-hand orthosis)
Name: Wrist-driven flexor hinge orthosis

		Flex	Ext	Abd	Add	Rotation Int	Rotation Ext
W—Wrist		H V	H V	H (RD)	H (UD)		
H—Hand							
Fingers 2-5	MP	A	A	H	H		
	PIP	H 2 & 3	H 2 & 3				
	DIP	H 2 & 3	H 2 & 3				
Thumb	CM	H	H	H	H	Opposition H	H
	MP	H	H	H	H		
	IP	H	H				

Biomechanical: Its purpose is to convert wrist extension motion into finger flexion and extension at the MP joints to provide active prehension.

Material: Plastic hand section, metal finger stabilizer and forearm sections, Velcro straps, and variable grasp opening (Fig. 5-17, *A*); padded metal frame and finger stabilizers, leather and Velcro straps, wrist extension assist, and variable grasp opening (Fig. 5-17, *B*)

Fabrication: It may be preshaped but requires patient for final shaping and fitting. An accurate plaster mold may be utilized for fabrication.

Special considerations: The patient must have some wrist extension. A wrist extension assist may be used until the patient can extend his wrist against gravity. The hand should be flexible and free from deformity. Thumb and fingers are held in functional position.

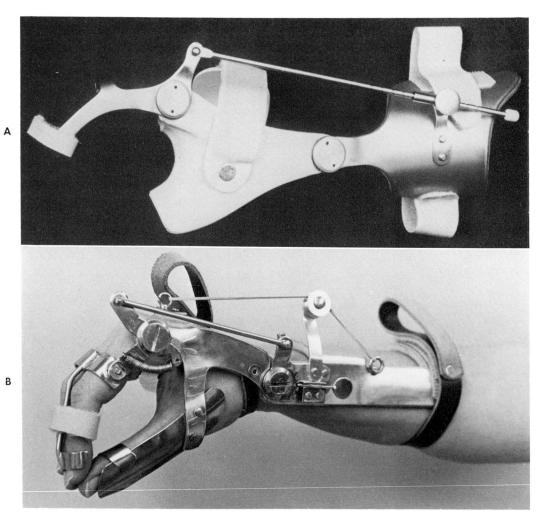

A

B

Fig. 5-17

Type: WHO (wrist-hand orthosis)
Name: Ratchet flexor hinge hand orthosis

		Flex	Ext	Abd	Add	Int	Ext
						Rotation	
W—Wrist		L v	L v	H (RD)	H (UD)		
H—Hand							
Fingers 2-5	MP	L v	A	H	H		
	PIP	H 2 & 3	H 2 & 3				
	DIP	H 2 & 3	H 2 & 3				
Thumb	CM	H	H	H	H	Opposition H | H	
	MP	H	H	H	H		
	IP	H	H				

Biomechanical: Its purpose is to permit passive positioning for effective grasp and release of fingers by use of MP flexion-extension passive lock.

Material: Basic wrist-driven flexor hinge orthosis with (a) ratchet lock, (b) spring for returning fingers to an open position, and (c) prehension compression spring, which maintains constant pressure and eliminates slipping of object that patient is holding

Fabrication: Wrist joint is changed from free to friction. The ratchet unit, which is available in prefabricated form, is added.

Special considerations: The ratchet unit is relatively maintenance free and is an excellent alternative when patients reject use of the more complicated power systems. Thumb and fingers are held in functional position.

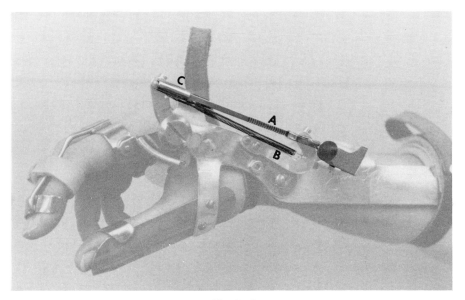

Fig. 5-18

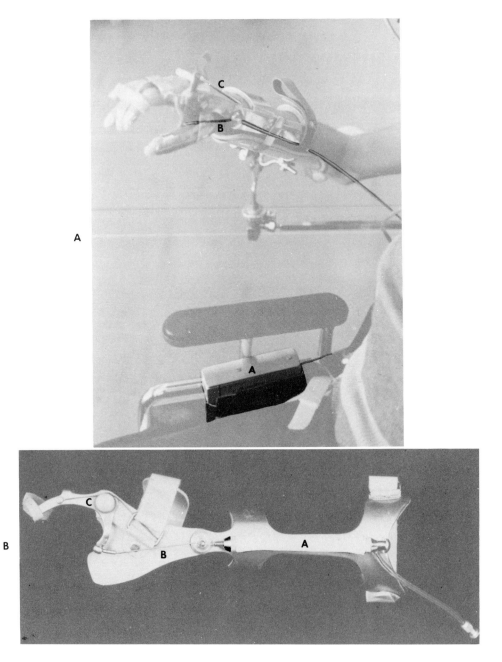

Fig. 5-19

Type: WHO (wrist-hand orthosis)
Name: Externally powered hand orthosis

		Flex	Ext	Abd	Add	Rotation Int	Ext	
W—Wrist		L ∨	L ∨	H (RD)	H (UD)			
H—Hand								
Fingers 2-5	MP	L ∨	A	H	H			
	PIP	H 2 & 3	H 2 & 3					
	DIP	H 2 & 3	H 2 & 3					
Thumb	CM	H	H	H	H	Opposition H	H	
	MP	H	H	H	H			
	IP	H	H					

Biomechanical: Its purpose is to provide external powered prehension by an electric motor or artificial muscle.

Material: Basic wrist-driven flexor hinge orthosis with (A) electric motor and battery pack, (B) control cable for finger flexion, and (C) return spring for finger extension (Fig. 5-19, *A*); basic wrist-driven flexor hinge orthosis with (A) artificial muscle, (B) cable for finger flexion, and (C) return spring for finger extension (Fig. 5-19, *B*)

Fabrication: Wrist joint is changed from free to friction. The external power unit of choice is added. Such units are available in prefabricated form.

Special considerations: Function is dependent on a suitable switch position that will enable the patient to activate the system. Thumb and fingers are held in functional position.

REFERENCES

Anderson, M. H.: Upper extremity orthotics, Springfield, Ill., 1965, Charles C Thomas, Publisher.

Conry, J. E.: Developer of variable grasp opening unit (shown in Fig. 5-17, *B*), Hot Springs, Ark.

Engen, T. J.: Development of upper extremity orthotics, Parts I and II, Orthotics and prosthetics, March and June 1970.

McKenzie, M. W.: The ratchet handsplint, Am. J. Occup. Ther. **27:**477-479, Nov. 8, 1973.

Nickel, V. L., Perry, J., and Snelson, R.: Handbook of hand splints, Rancho Los Amigos Hospital, Downey, Calif., 1960.

Type: EO (elbow orthosis)
Name: Rigid elbow orthosis

	Flex	Ext
E—Elbow	H	H

Biomechanical: It holds the elbow in the desired position.

Material: Padded metal humeral, forearm, and hand cuffs; rigid metal connecting bars at elbow and wrist and webbing straps. It can be made as a custom shell device of leather or plastic.

Fabrication: It may be prefabricated or custom made from measurements.

Special considerations: Metal connecting bars may be adjusted by bending to the desired position. In difficult cases, a plaster mold of the patient's limb may be necessary for fabrication of orthosis. If desired, a variable position lock can be used.

NOTE: Illustration shows additional wrist stabilization device.

Type: SEO (shoulder-elbow orthosis)
Name: Shoulder abduction–assist suspension sling

	Flex	Ext	Abd	Add	Rotation Int	Rotation Ext	Axial Load
S—Shoulder	A/R	A/R	A/R	A/R	A/R	A/R	R
H—Humerus							
E—Elbow	F	F					

Biomechanical: Its purpose is to provide an overhead suspension system that will counteract and balance the forces of gravity acting on a weakened upper limb to allow placement of the hand in a functional location.

Material: The components are (A) wheelchair mounting unit, (B) overhead suspension bar, and (C) suspension springs and leather cuffs.

Fabrication: It is available in prefabricated form.

Special considerations: Usually it is fitted on a temporary basis. Long-term use is unsatisfactory because support must be realigned each time patient is put into the wheelchair.

Fig. 5-20

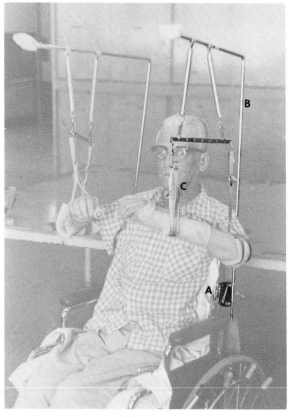

Fig. 5-21

Type: SEO (shoulder-elbow orthosis)
Name: Swivel mobile arm feeder

					Rotation		Axial Load
	Flex	Ext	Abd	Add	Int	Ext	
S—Shoulder	A/R	A/R	A/R	A/R	A/R	A/R	R
H—Humerus							
E—Elbow	A/R	A/R					

Biomechanical: Its purpose is to provide a support system that will counteract and balance the forces of gravity acting on a weakened limb and allow it to become more functional.

Material: Metal frame and ball bearing swivel joints. The components are as follows: (A) wheelchair mounting unit, (B) proximal support link, (C) distal support link (Fig. 5-22, *A*), (D) arm trough, (E) outside rocker, (F) vertical-assist rubber bands (Fig. 5-22, *B*), (G) elevating proximal link—used in place of the standard proximal link as an assist for shoulder abduction; rubber bands are used for the assist (Fig. 5-22, *C*).

Fabrication: The complete unit is available in prefabricated form.

Special considerations: It is usually fitted on a more permanent basis. It is important that the system be accurately balanced to provide the proper amount of assistance to residual shoulder and elbow muscles to achieve maximum range of motion. If rubber band assists are used, adjustments are difficult to maintain.

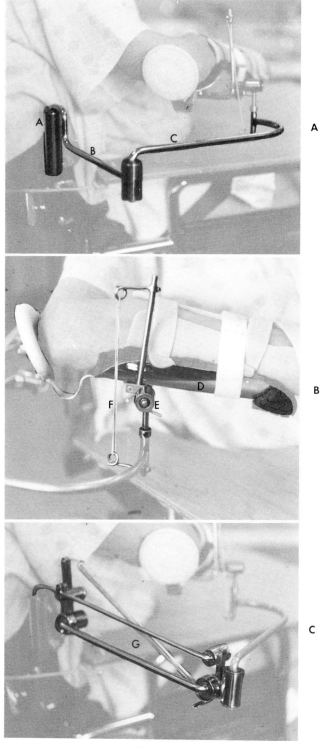

Fig. 5-22

Type: SEO (shoulder-elbow orthosis)
Name: Radial mobile arm support

	Flex	Ext	Abd	Add	Rotation Int	Rotation Ext	Axial Load
S—Shoulder	A/R	A/R	A/R	A/R	A/R	A/R	R
H—*Humerus*							
E—Elbow	A/R	A/R					

Biomechanical: Its purpose is to provide a support system that will counteract and balance the forces of gravity acting on a weakened limb and allow it to become more functional.

Material: Metal frame and ball bearing joints. The components are as follows: (A) wheelchair mounting unit, (B) radial support link, (C) elevation unit (Fig. 5-23, *A*), (D) arm trough, (E) outside rocker, (F) vertical-assist spring, (G) elbow flexion–humerus internal rotation assist (Fig. 5-23, *B*), (H) supination-pronation assist, and (I) wrist-hand orthosis trough clip (Fig. 5-23, *C*).

Fabrication: Complete unit is available in prefabricated form.

Special considerations: It is fitted on a permanent basis. It is important that the system be accurately balanced to provide the proper amount of assistance or resistance to achieve maximum range of motion. Adjustments are permanent and not difficult to maintain.

REFERENCES

Anderson, M. H.: Upper extremity orthosis, Springfield, Ill., 1965, Charles C Thomas, Publisher.

Guilford, A. W.: Design and development presented at orthotic conference, Rancho Los Amigos Hospital, Downey, Calif., 1969.

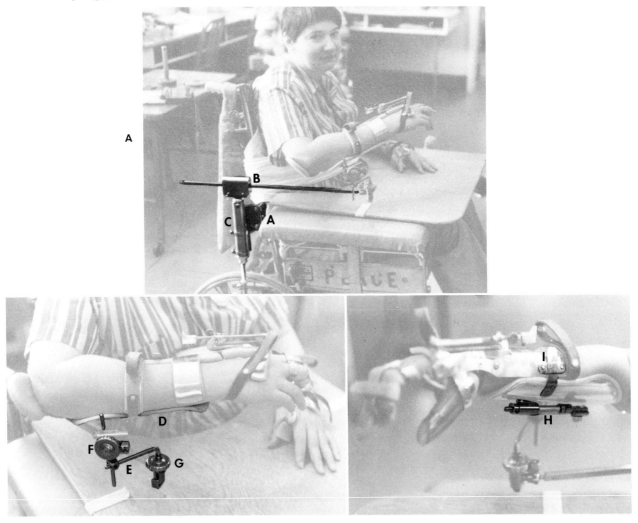

Fig. 5-23

Type: SEO (shoulder-elbow orthosis)
Name: Functional arm orthosis

					Rotation		Axial Load
	Flex	Ext	Abd	Add	Int	Ext	
S—Shoulder	A	S$_V$	R	R	A	R	R
H—*Humerus*							
E—Elbow	F/L$_V$	F/L$_V$					
F—Forearm					(Pron) A/R	(Sup) A/R	

Biomechanical: Its purpose is to support a paralyzed arm and restore independent function for an ambulatory patient.

Materials: The following components are utilized: (A) plastic iliac crest cap, (B) metal hoop to position shoulder joint and transfer the limb load forces to iliac crest, (C) shoulder-joint ratchet, (D) shoulder flexion–assist rubber bands, (E) humeral bar and cuff, (F) shoulder rotation–assist rubber bands, (G) elbow joint—alternating free or locked, (H) plastic forearm cuff, (I) forearm rotation–assist spring (Fig. 5-24, *A*). Joint control is through a cable from a loop that encircles the opposite shoulder. Scapula abduction locks and unlocks the joint components (Fig. 5-24, *B*).

Special considerations: Some hand function is needed to make the orthosis assist useful.

NOTE: Illustrations incidentally include the wrist and hand.

REFERENCE

Anderson, M. H.: Upper extremity orthotics, Springfield, Ill., 1965, Charles C Thomas, Publisher.

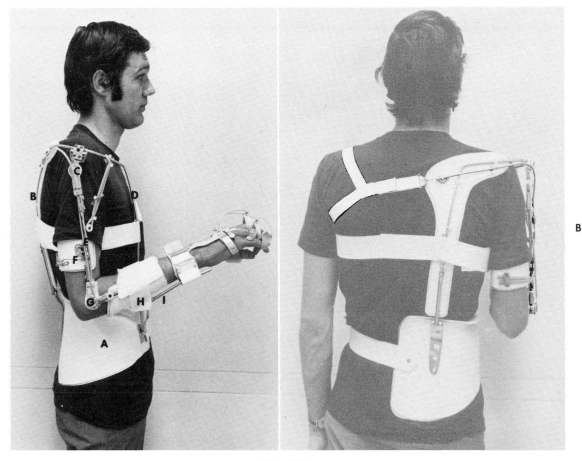

Fig. 5-24

Type: SEWHO (shoulder-elbow-wrist-hand-orthosis)
Name: Electric arm orthosis

	Flex	Ext	Abd	Add	Rotation Int	Rotation Ext	Axial Load
S—Shoulder	A	A	H	H	A	A	R
H—Humerus							
E—Elbow	A	A					
F—Forearm					(Pron) A	(Sup) A	
W—Wrist	A	A	H (RD)	H (UD)			
H—Hand							
Fingers 2-5 MP	A	A	H	H			
PIP	H 2 & 3	H 2 & 3					
DIP	H 2 & 3	H 2 & 3					
Thumb CM	H	H	H	H	Opposition H	H	
Thumb MP	H	H	H	H	H	H	
Thumb IP	H	H					

Biomechanical: A tubular arm frame forms a linkage system for electric motors, which provide six functional motions for a paralyzed upper limb.

Material: Wheelchair mounting unit, aluminum linkage, 12-volt power system, tongue control, and six electric motor components, which are as follows: (1) shoulder rotation, (2) shoulder flexion and extension, (3) elbow flexion and extension, (4) forearm supination and pronation, (5) wrist flexion and extension, and (6) finger prehension (MP flexion and extension)

Fabrication: An arm kit is available in prefabricated form. Linkage must be cut to length and fitted to patient. An orthotist experienced with the upper limb is necessary to provide the required wrist-hand orthosis to complete the system.

Special considerations: The orthosis will fit on any type of wheelchair. Spasticity is a contraindication. Adequate range of motion is necessary. Limb sensation is a vital adjunct. A 2-month training period is required for one to become proficient.

REFERENCES

Barber, L. M., and Nickel, V. L.: Carbon dioxide–powered arm and hand devices, Am. J. Occup. Ther. **23:**215-225, 1969.

Nickel, V. L., Allen, J. R., and Karchak, A., Jr.: Control systems for externally powered orthotic devices, Final Project Report, Rancho Los Amigos Hospital, Downey, Calif., May 1, 1960 to July 31, 1970, Professional Staff Association—Rancho Los Amigos Hospital.

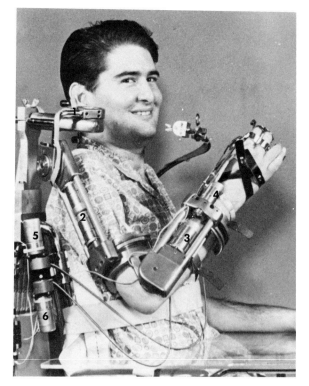

Fig. 5-25

CHAPTER 6

Prescription principles

JACQUELIN PERRY, M.D.

Orthotic designing must give equal emphasis to mechanical efficiency and accuracy of fit, since comfort is critical for acceptance. Smallness of the segments, limitations in soft-tissue padding, and multiplicity of joint motion create high demands, which only a skilled orthotist can meet. Lack of design and fabrication expertise has discouraged the use of upper-limb orthoses in therapeutic programs, even though they could contribute a great deal.

Patients accept hand and arm orthoses only if they have a well-defined therapeutic purpose or if they provide a function that cannot be accomplished in any other fashion. Such reluctance stems from the disadvantages that accompany the wearing of any rigid, insensitive external device.

Interposition of any material between the hand's surface and the object lessens grasp efficiency. Sensation is decreased. Skin friction and subcutaneous contouring (which normally contribute to the grasping ease) are made less available. Lack of mechanical versatility limits the patient's ability to handle with equal ease objects that vary widely in size, shape, and weight. These factors combine to require a greater grasp force and offer less precision than does the naked hand.

The arm, in contrast to the hand, does not present the same problems of surface interference, but it is far more demanding about versatility. One mode of grasp and release by the hand can meet a patient's basic daily needs, but during the same tasks the arm must move through numerous positions. Dressing, body hygiene, feeding, and desk-top activity use very different motions and cover widely scattered areas. All these basic demands cannot yet be met with today's limb orthoses. One further barrier to patient acceptance is the fact that an upper-limb orthosis is conspicuous and hence announces publicly that a disability exists. It also catches on clothes, doorways, and jutting objects.

Countering these limitations is the fact that paralysis, deformity, or pain may make the extremity virtually useless. The contrasting advantages offered by an orthosis become very appealing. Some disadvantages can be minimized by material choice and orthotic design, but they cannot be entirely eliminated. Hence, every upper-limb orthosis is a compromise between gain and loss.

The foremost factor in developing patient acceptance is frank recognition by physician, therapist, and orthotist that a compromise always exists. This approach makes the orthotic plan more realistic. The clinical advantages must outweigh the obstacles. Acceptance also depends on the prescription being functionally appropriate. Patients are quick to sense ineffectiveness, particularly if they are inconvenienced in the process.

This negative view of orthotics has been presented early in the discussion of upper-limb management because failure of the orthotist to consider these factors in making the therapeutic plan or in presenting it to the patient is a major cause of poor acceptance. Sometimes these facts are deliberately omitted for fear of discouraging the patient, but they cannot be ignored. While awaiting the therapeutic benefits to accrue, the various disadvantages will be experienced many times each day. To have these burst through a biased cloud of unrealistic enthusiasm is very disillusioning. Rejection is an almost automatic reaction, which, once initiated, is difficult to reverse.

Guided by these principles, specific orthoses are selected according to the patient's physical need. The therapeutic options currently available will be presented in relation to the basic objectives of upper-limb management, which are deformity control, tissue protection, and restoration of function.

DEFORMITY CONTROL (PREVENTION AND CORRECTION)

Minimization of deformity should always be the first concern in planning a treatment program for any potentially long-term problem. This challenge is particularly acute in the upper limb because even the most basic functions require a considerable range of motion and versatility.

Because deformities develop in such a subtle, creeping manner, preventive measures should be initiated at the time the clinical threat first presents. Only then does the clinician have the opportunity to maintain normal tissue mobility. Situations that undoubtedly will lead to undesirable degrees of deformity unless perfect protection is provided are as follows:

1. Paralysis of muscles that normally counteract the effects of gravity. This is aggravated when there are spastic antagonists.
2. Lesions leading to reactive scarring such as burns, local trauma, and infections involving the joint structures
3. Acute episodes of arthritis leading to pain-induced inhibition of muscular action
4. Asymmetric paralysis, creating a dominant pull to the strong side.

Once the deformity has developed, the normal gliding planes and tissue extensibility have been lost. Now force will be required to tease adhesions loose and to extend contracted fibers. Hence, corrective measures are far more complex than are preventive techniques. Also, their effectiveness is dependent on the reversibility of the tissue state. Unless the deforming changes are mild or have existed only a short time, so that they are semifluid, normal physiologic function may be unrecoverable.

Correction requires a stretching force. If the tissues cannot yield easily they may suffer microtears. This induces further reactive scarring with increased rigidity rather than mobility. Hence, corrective force must be kept within tissue-tolerance levels. If this is insufficient to accomplish the necessary change, further recovery can be gained only by surgical reconstruction. These procedures, however, do not restore normal gliding planes. As a result, some degree of strength or selectivity of control is invariably sacrificed even though a useful range of motion or alignment may be restored.

The standard of adequate joint mobility depends on the patient's potential for recovery. If he is expected to become normal, a full range of motion should be sought. However, if there will be considerable permanent loss of strength or control, less mobility often is preferred. This not only avoids having the treatment directed toward a useless goal, but some contractures are a valuable source of stability.

When muscle strength is lacking and stabilization of a particular joint is the primary requisite rather than provision of motion, a contracture can be an effective substitute. Under these circumstances the therapeutic objective in deformity control is to preserve the useful component of contracture while avoiding further deformation, which would deter function. The result is classed as a functional range of motion rather than normal mobility (Fig. 6-1).

Each anatomic area will be discussed in relation to its own needs for mobility, susceptibility to deformation, potential to profit from functional contractures, and responsiveness to orthotic assistance.

Children are threatened with progressive deformity by structural adaptation throughout their growing years. Concerned families will continue prescribed bracing programs with sufficient regularity to minimize the penalty. For others there will have to be periods of intensive correction to overcome the neglect-induced losses. Results will be correspondingly less good but often adequate. Generally both groups, as soon as is appropriate, are relieved of this practical burden by surgical reconstruction.

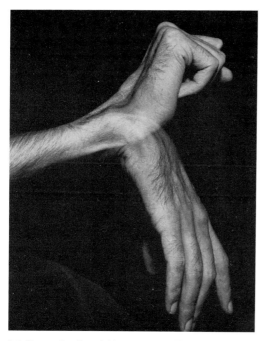

Fig. 6-1. Example of useful contracture. Tightness in extrinsic finger muscles allows active wrist extension to flex fingers, while wrist flexion indirectly pulls the digits into extension.

Protective orthotics

When constant immobilization is required after injury or surgery or to rest inflammed tissues, a plaster-of-paris cast is the ideal agent. However, after partial healing has occurred and protection is not required full time, lighter support and limited arcs of motion are desirable. A well-designed orthosis can hasten the patient's recovery of function at this second stage of protection. Even if stationary posturing is required, an orthosis has the advantages of being removable for hygiene purposes. Also, being both lighter and thinner, it causes less interferences in use of those segments that can be active (Fig. 6-2, *A*).

Selective action can be obtained with mobile units designed to permit only those arcs or planes of motion that are desired (Fig. 6-2, *B*). Force demand can also be lessened by the addition of assistive elastic power. Indications may be recent tendon transfers, arthroplasties, recovering arthritis, or early paralytic states. These techniques aid the healing segment to recover function with-

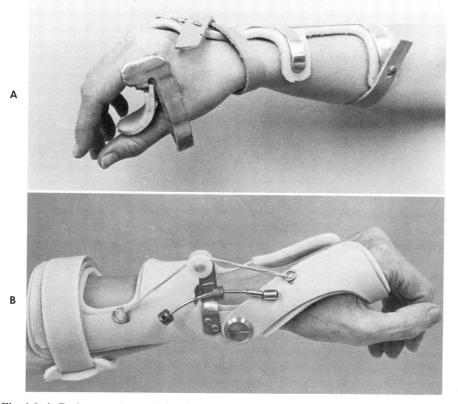

Fig. 6-2. A, Basic protective wrist-hand orthosis. **B,** Mobile protection with elastic extensor assist and stops to limit flexion and extension.

out threat of damage by providing controlled, graduated mobilization, and stress. This permits earlier institution of an activity program that would otherwise be inappropriate. Such a program should include the assistance of a knowledgeable occupational or physical therapist to instruct the patient in his care, to reinforce important guidelines, and to pick up problems in their incipient stage.

Functional orthotics

Orthoses designed to replace lost muscle action or joint stability for the purpose of creating useful function are called "functional orthoses." They are effective only on the relaxed limb. If the artificial force must pull against simultaneously active antagonistic muscles, pressures on the intervening skin quickly exceed tissue tolerance. Also, the delay in action will exceed the patient's patience. Consequently, these devices are seldom of value in persons with central control dysfunctions (upper motor neuron lesions). Spasticity (excess reactions to stretch), reflex posturing, and primitive motion patterns are all sources of uncontrolled antagonistic muscle action at undesirable times. Occasionally the patient with control-dysfunction has a flaccid type of muscle picture and adequate sensation to profit from a functional orthosis. In general, however, these devices are appropriate only for lesions characterized by motor-unit loss.

Sensory impairment severely limits the usefulness of a functional orthosis. One can place and manipulate the hand with just visual direction, but then the entire task must be performed within the line of sight. Also, the lack of automatic feedback requires the person to interrupt his concerns for the task as a whole and focus his attention on the manipulations of the braced limb each time a motion or new position is needed. Patients, consequently, restrict their acceptance of insensitive functional orthotic control to those situations where a portable vise is of value. There are selected vocations where this is an advantage, but they are infrequent.

During normal hand and arm use, the muscles provide two functions:
1. Movement of the segments at varying speeds
2. Stabilization of the joints in a selected posture.

The latter is far more demanding in both force

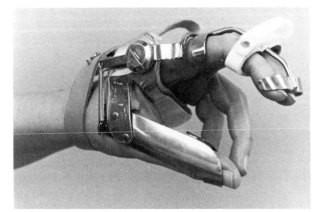

Fig. 6-3. Flail thumb and finger interphalangeal joints held in functional position with static orthotic units. Motion for pinch and release available at metacarpophalangeal joint.

and complexity of action. This is particularly true of the hand, where much of the muscle action consists of prepositioning the segments to permit a particular pattern of single-axis flexion and extension for grasp and release. For effective joint stabilization the patient must have sufficient strength to restrain all planes of motion in order to cope with the weight of the object being handled and the resistance created during the performance of the task (that is, knife pushing against plate).

To simplify both force requirements and control complexity, orthotic posturing, whenever possible, is accomplished with static units set in the one position that has the greatest breadth of application. Areas where this technique is effective are the wrist, forearm, thumb, and finger interphalangeal joints (Fig. 6-3). When positional restraint is needed for only one segment of a motion, arc stops are used. Action at the wrist and metacarpophalangeal finger joints is commonly controlled in this fashion. Serial positioning with a loading ratchet joint is effective at the elbow and shoulder.

Whenever selective motion has to be provided by artificial power, the mode of control has to receive first consideration. Each action must have independent control to meet even the basic requirement of versatility. In addition, the patient must learn to initiate the motion in an unusual way. This is a slow learning process that needs to be taught in organized steps if frustration and disgust are to be avoided.

Training is the key to effective functional replacement. None of the available orthotic techniques match normal versatility; so the patient must adapt to unusual restriction in motion patterns and control mechanisms. The extent to which he can spontaneously accommodate depends on his natural adaptability and on the complexity of the device. Failure to assure that the patient really has attained effective function by both checkout and provision of whatever amount of training is required leads to a very high percentage of device rejection. His performance can be considered effective only when the patient can accomplish the basic tasks with ease. If he must struggle each time, the reward soon ceases to justify the effort. Both training and performance checkout should be conducted by a competent therapist.

HAND ORTHOTICS
The hand

Although the wrist is a separate joint with independent musculature, its posture and control are so critical to hand function that these two areas really constitute one complex functional unit. Hence they are considered together throughout the discussion on orthotics.

Deformity control. Orthotic measures to prevent deformity include both dynamic and static systems. The choice between the two is dictated by the severity and character of the hand dysfunction.

Hand. For any residual control to be effective the thumb and fingers must oppose one another and meet in a secure manner (Fig. 6-4). Also, there must be some degree of mobility to allow an opening and closing arc for grasp and release. Width of this arc, contour of the opposing digits, and the amount of flexion available at the metacarpophalangeal joints determine the size and shape of objects that can be controlled. Stabilization of the wrist in extension (0 to 20 degrees) offers the muscles the optimum resting length. Given these postural advantages, any residual digital flexor muscle strength will have the opportunity to be useful. As strength is gained, its value, of course, increases.

This resting posture of the hand, which constitutes its basic position of function, should be assured by orthotic support if it is not spontaneously available. Hand rolls with loops to hold fingers and thumb are a good emergency measure for severely paralyzed bedfast patients but are not adequate long-term measures for the active

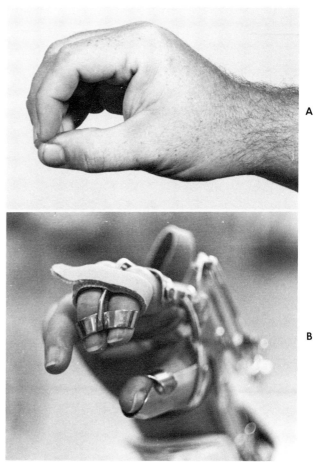

Fig. 6-4. Essential position of thumb and fingers for the most secure pinch. **A,** Normal hand. **B,** Orthotic equivalent.

patient, since they do not control the wrist. Plaster casts used in trauma must meet the same positional requirements.

The basic support to protect the hand from the deforming influences of gravity is a stationary wrist-hand orthosis that holds the wrist in 10 degrees of dorsiflexion, the thumb in neutral opposition, and 35 degrees of abduction and allows the finger metacarpal joints to drop into unobstructed flexion (Fig. 6-2). Thumb position is usually gained with a first metacarpal extension stop (opponens bar) and a −35-degree adduction stop (C bar). To assure free phalangeal flexion of the fingers, one must not allow the palmar bar to overlie any portion of the metacarpal heads (that is, its distal margin must not touch the distal palmar crease). Particular attention must be paid to the fifth finger, as its metacarpal is often considerably shorter than that of the index and long fingers. Failure to curve the palmar bar suffi-

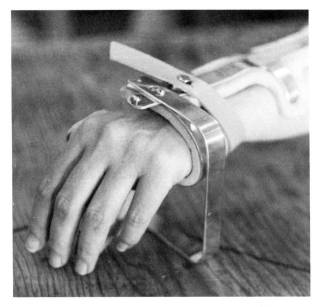

Fig. 6-5. Prop to protect the flaccid hand from the deforming influence of arm weight.

ciently inadvertently splints this joint in extension, with subsequent contracture formation.

A positional complication that too often develops in the totally paralyzed hand is hyperflexion and radial rotation of the more ulnar fingers. This is caused by limb weight pressing against the fingers as the hand rests on the bed, lap, etc. The problem can be avoided by careful positioning of the hand so that the fingers hang freely in midair. But such attention to detail is seldom practiced every minute. A better answer for the patient with arm paralysis so extensive that he cannot protect himself is to add some form of prop to the wrist-hand orthosis (Fig. 6-5).

Active deforming forces, such as vigorously spastic muscles or even ordinary activity of unbalanced musculature, cannot be blocked with an orthosis. The skin is caught between the two forces. Having a poor tolerance for pressure, the skin experiences pain and tissue changes develop quickly, causing rejection of the orthosis.

Correction of a deformity necessitates a stretching force. In the totally paralyzed hand, serial gains can be made in small increments with a variable-hold orthosis (Fig. 6-6, *A*). Each time, it is set so that the joint being treated is held in a position 5 degrees less than that which causes pain. Adjustments are made as the tissues yield. Generally this system serves more to maintain the gains made by therapy than to initiate correction independently.

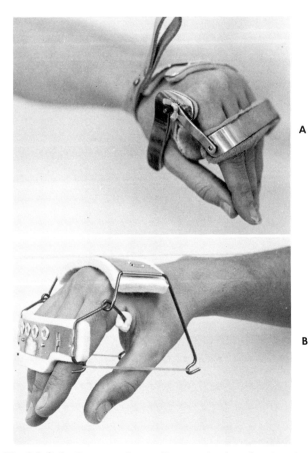

Fig. 6-6. Orthotic means of correcting a contracture (treatment of metacarpophalangeal joint illustrated). **A,** Static variable control unit for paralyzed hand. **B,** Elastic stretch force for patient with active antagonistic muscles (finger extensors) give periodic relief.

For patients with active antagonistic musculature a dynamic system can be used with more rapid results. Rubber bands are generally the stretching force. Their tension is tolerated because the patient has the strength to escape periodically by pulling out of the stretching posture. This means his antagonistic muscle must be stronger than the elastic unit. For example, the patient who lacks MP flexion may be fitted with a "knuckle bender" (elastic MP flexion assist) (Fig. 6-6, *B*). Whenever the stretch becomes uncomfortable, the patient contracts his strong extensor muscles and straightens out the joints for a short time. Comfort restored, he relaxes and the flexing stretch is resumed. If the patient cannot gain this type of periodic relief, the system will not be tolerated for sufficiently long intervals to be effective. A variable-hold system should be selected instead. In both situations progress is most rapid when it is combined with a judicious therapy program to gain both range and strength.

Wrist. A critical threat to hand function is inadequacy of the wrist extensor muscles. Whenever their strength is less than good (grade 4), flexion is the usual resting position. This not only puts the finger flexors at a less competent length but also leads to finger deformity from the tension created on the finger extensors. Unless there are good intrinsic muscles to offer protection, the flexed wrist posture leads to metacarpophalangeal hyperextension and semiflexion of the interphalangeal joints. The resulting posture is a claw hand that, at best, can accomplish only a flat, weak pinch.

Hence prevention of wrist drop is essential. Either a static support or elastic assistance is indicated, depending on the residual strength available (see the section on functional bracing for details).

When central control is disrupted (upper motor neuron lesions) there are three patterns of wrist drop. The most fortunate group of patients have a primitive synergy between wrist extensors and finger flexors. With the hand relaxed, the wrist drops passively. This is corrected by reflex activation of the wrist extensors as the patient closes his hand, even though he does not exhibit any independent voluntary wrist extension. No orthotic support is indicated. If the wrist is maintained in extension, the patient may be unable to relax his hand.

When this synergy is lacking and the forearm is customarily pronated, both gravity and contracting finger flexors act to flex the wrist. These patients quickly develop severe contractures in both wrist and finger muscles if a passive stretch program and orthotic support are not instituted early. Any developing spasticity is aggravated by contractures, since shortened muscles are more readily stretched. A static support is indicated, at least during the patient's early period of disability. Its position will be dictated by the state of the long digital flexors. Fixation of the wrist in extension will draw the fingers and thumb into a tightly flexed posture if these muscles are spastic and contracted because greater flexor muscle length is required to cross the extended wrist than when it is hanging into flexion. In the neglected hand a tight fist may result from just bringing the wrist up to neutral. This position is inappropriate, as it will lead to pain and further digital con-

tracture. Instead, one should support the wrist in whatever flexion is necessary to allow semiopening of the hand. This compromise posture protects the patient from developing further contracture caused by gravity and helps retain the correction gained by physical therapy. Increasing spasticity from change in the patient's neurologic state will not be stopped, but at least the hand is protected from the aggravation of superimposed contracture. In the neglected hand the flexors may be so rigid or so persistently sensitive to stretch that an orthosis cannot be fitted with comfort. Surgical correction is the only answer in this situation.

With upper motor neuron paralysis of both wrist and finger muscles, one should use a static support of the wrist in neutral with the hand free to fall in a functional posture indicated during the early period of his disability. Subsequent management depends on the patient's age and his neurologic course. Some adults maintain this pseudoflaccid state. Those who have pain when their hand dangles will choose to continue their orthotic support indefinitely. The others will discard it eventually, and no harm will result. A majority of patients progress to some stage of spasticity with or without primitive hand-wrist synergies. They should be managed as previously discussed.

Protection. When rest is needed, static orthotic units are selected. Otherwise, the functional devices are used to provide assisted motion in combination with appropriately placed stops to restrict action to the desired arcs.

Functional hand orthotics. Before planning a functional orthosis for the hand, one must assure that there is sufficient arm control to adequately place the hand where it can be effective. Otherwise it will not be used.

Within the hand itself there must be good sensation and mobility. The patient's passive range of motion must permit easy placement of the wrist and digits in the position of function and also allow some further motion for grasp and release.

Minimal sensory requirements are good object and position discrimination in the thumb and index or long finger, preferably both. Although patients do use an anesthetic hand under visual control, they find the combination of paresis and insensitivity overwhelming. Without sensation the patient lacks the cues that permit substitution for his inadequate muscular deficits.

In addition, to be effective, orthotic replacement of lost hand function must assure that all five basic controls are adequate. These are wrist extension stability, grasp force, release, thumb opposition, and finger contouring. The amount and type of apparatus that must be provided to meet these varies with the nature of the paralysis or injury. Each control has several possibilities.

Wrist extension stability. Since most hand activities are performed in pronation, the wrist is consistently subjected to the flexion force of hand weight, object mass, and the contracting long finger flexors. If flexion is not opposed, the patient's grasp force will be weakened and hand placement awkward. Consequently, wrist extensor control is essential during all hand function unless the forearm is supinated. In this one situation gravity provides the extensor force. (See Table 1.)

Whenever strength of the wrist extensor muscles is less than grade 4 (good), orthotic supplementation should be offered. The one exception is the presence of strong finger extensors, flexors, and intrinsics. Normally the long flexors can exert a force four times stronger than their antagonistic extensors. Thus they have the strength to both complete an effective grasp and maintain full metacarpophalangeal flexion (with the help of the intrinsics) despite antagonistic extensor action. This simultaneous muscle activity also enhances the action of the finger extensors at the wrist; so all the functional requirements are met by such a synergy. However, in the presence of lesser strengths in any of these three muscle groups, the patient will be deprived of his most effective grasp unless orthotic wrist support is offered. It is misplaced kindness to omit this assistance.

Wrist extensors with grade 2 or 3 (poor or fair) strength need assistance. An elastic extensor assist (rubber band or spring) gives selective hand placement. This must be combined with a flexor

stop to obstruct the antagonistic force created by the contracting digital flexors and weight of the object being handled.

When there are no effective wrist extensors, a static support is indicated (Fig. 6-2). Support position is dictated by the type of arm control available. Fifteen degrees of dorsiflexion offers more versatility in hand placement, but the patient must have adequate shoulder rotation to substitute for absent wrist flexion. When either paralysis or arthritic ankylosis deprives the patient of adequate shoulder mobility, the wrist should be positioned in 5 or 10 degrees of flexion.

Radial or ulnar deviation are conspicuous deformities that stimulate a strong urge to prescribe an orthosis. Such a device, however, will be effective only if this malalignment is easily corrected manually and is not caused by the pull of contracting wrist or finger muscles during hand use. Otherwise, the deforming force will be greater than the skin can tolerate, causing pain and patient rejection.

Grasp. The ability to handle objects is weakened whenever there is either a loss of flexor muscle strength (grasp force) or the patient lacks intrinsic muscle action to match the contour of his fingers to that of the object being handled. Both thumb and fingers must be adequate, since each represents one side of a pincer mechanism. The orthotic plan is to replace mechanically the essential functions that have been lost.

A. Finger control (grasp force and contouring). With three available flexors, there are seven theoretically possible patterns of pathologic imbalance, but only five are seen clinically. Any one of the muscles may be the sole remaining flexor (that is, only intrinsics, flexor digitorum profundus or flexor digitorum superficialis). There may be isolated intrinsic loss (the intrinsic minus hand) or one may have absence of all active flexion. A further variation is difference of involvement among the four fingers. The index, in particular, seems to respond separately from the others by either being the strongest survivor or the site of maximum impairment.

1. Intrinsic muscle paralysis. In an effort to simplify the details of anatomy, there is a tendency to focus just on the lumbricales, but this is a clinical error. The interossei have the greater bulk and hence offer more strength for the same functions of metacarpophalangeal flexion and interphalangeal extension,

Table 1. Wrist extensor requirements

Muscle grade	Orthotic design
5 or 4 (normal or good)	None
3 or 2 (fair or poor)	Elastic extensor assist with a flexion stop
1 or 0 (trace or zero)	Static orthosis with "hold" set between 5 degrees of flexion and 15 degrees of extension

in addition to providing their abduction and adduction functions. This is best demonstrated with a wrist-level ulnar nerve injury. The index and long finger lumbricales are unimpaired while the interossei are paralyzed. The patient retains his ability to voluntarily assume metacarpophalangeal flexion and interphalangeal extension of these two fingers, but he cannot hold the posture against any resistance. Thus the key fingers really are functionally inadequate for grasp even though unresisted positioning is still possible. Hence, one should consider the intrinsics as a group when making an orthotic plan. Their contribution is digital contouring and selective metacarpophalangeal flexion.

a. Potential deformity: The intrinsic-minus hand, as this pattern of paralysis is often called, demonstrates the residuals of uncoordinated extensor-flexor action (Fig. 6-7, *A*). Unprotected, the hand will develop MP hyperextension and IP flexion contractures, commonly termed a "claw hand." The positioning possible with just lumbrical muscle action will prevent this. Thus in an ulnar nerve lesion only the ring and little finger will claw, but all will be functionally inadequate.

b. Functional loss:
   (1) Lack of specific metacarpophalangeal (MP) flexion and absence of functional coupling between the extrinsic finger flexors and extensors; effect: finger curling and a flat grasp void of selective contouring.
   (2) Lack of lateral contouring (digital abduction-adduction)
   (3) Incomplete interphalangeal extension for release

c. Orthotic plan: Static MP extension stop set in 30-degree flexion prepositions the fingers so that the extrinsic muscles can be effective (Fig. 6-7, *B*). A rigid unit is required because much of the flexor force exerted against the object being handled is reflected as MP hyperextension, which must be restrained. Prepositioning the MP joints in flexion gives the extrinsic flexors a better mechanical advantage to improve their flexor influence at this site. Also, with the MP joints in modest flexion, the tendons of the long finger extensors

are free to act on the interphalangeal joints.

d. Function gain:
   (1) Improved volar finger contouring with greater grasp efficiency by the extrinsic flexors (profundus and superficialis)
   (2) Redirection of the long finger extensors to attain full interphalangeal extension

2. Isolated intrinsic muscle action (intrinsic-plus grasp). When the intrinsic muscles are intact but not the long flexors (that is, flexor digitorum profundus and superficialis), the patient has selective MP flexion accompanied by interphalangeal extension. Although volar contouring is lost, there is firm approximation of the finger's palmar surface against the thumb or any intervening object being handled. Also, lateral contouring (abduction-adduction posturing) is preserved. Thus whatever grasp force is available remains effective. The mass of intrinsic muscles is sufficient to provide a flexor force that meets

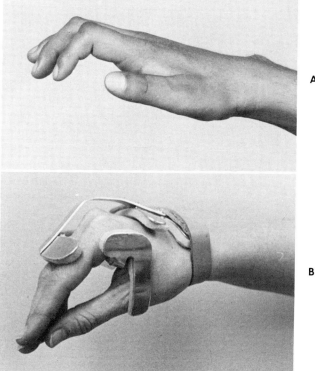

A

B

Fig. 6-7. A, Intrinsic-minus hand with a flat, ineffective posture. **B,** Metacarpophalangeal extension stop to preposition intrinsic-minus finger for function.

average self-care needs. Grasp by this intrinsic-plus hand looks awkward but functions quite well.

    a. Potential deformity: Interphalangeal extension contractures

    b. Functional loss: Selective interphalangeal flexion for contouring about objects or to meet specific functional demands

    c. Orthotic plan: Elastic or variable-hold interphalangeal flexor units to combat deformity; none needed for function; choice depends on strength of the long finger extensors

3. Flexor digitorum superficialis isolated action. Occasionally this muscle is the patient's sole finger flexor. The result is a fairly flat grasp because, as the superficialis muscle acts to flex the proximal interphalangeal joint, it only mildly affects the MP joint, and the distal phalanx is uncontrolled. Stability at this distal joint depends on the integrity of the volar capsular tissues. To the extent that these are lax, the resistance offered by the object being handled will cause passive hyperextension. At times this can be quite disabling.

    a. Potential deformity: Hyperextension of the distal interphalangeal joints

    b. No orthotic plan, because a useful pinch is provided independently and the deformity is not amenable to external support

4. Flexor digitorum profundus isolated action. Despite a potential to exert great strength, this muscle is very ineffective when forced to function alone. Its primary pull is exerted on the distal phalanx with serial activity at the more proximal joints. The effect is to curl the fingers into a fist. This serves to turn the palmar pads away from the object being handled unless it is a slender wand or the object's rough surface prevents the fingers sliding out of position as greater force is exerted.

    a. Potential deformity: There are interphalangeal flexion contractures, "claw hand."

    b. Orthotic plan: Set static interphalangeal units in 45 degrees of proximal joint flexion and 20 degrees of distal joint flexion.

    c. Functional gain: Preset contouring of the fingers so that the flexor digitorum profundus force is directed at the object rather

than having the phalanges slide across its surface.

5. Total finger flexor loss

    a. Potential deformity: There are interphalangeal and metacarpophalangeal extension contractures.

    b. Function loss: Whenever the patient's grasp is less than 0.5 kilogram (1 pound), it is inadequate for any useful function, and orthotic replacement is indicated.

    c. Orthotic plan: The basic unit is a three-digit, single-hinge orthosis that aligns the thumb, index, and long fingers in the palmar pinch position. It is often called a "flexor hinge hand." The fingers are held in semiflexion (45 degrees at the proximal interphalangeal joints and 20 degrees distally). Metacarpophalangeal motion is guided by a single hinge, which stops lateral motion but allows free flexion and extension. The thumb is held in opposition with neutral extension of the phalanges (Fig. 6-8, A). Artificial flexion power is then applied to this orthotic system according to the strength of the patient's finger and wrist extensors.

There are two patterns of alignment that are very critical to the effectiveness of the flexor hinge orthosis. One is the relationship among the digits. The other is the transverse correlation between the orthotic and anatomic axes of the wrist and the metacarpophalangeal joints. The thumb, index, and long fingers must meet in a three-jaw chuck fashion, with the thumb pad contacting the middle of the area formed by the two fingers. Longitudinally, they should be positioned so that the two fingers protrude about 3 mm beyond the end of the thumb. This is most easily done by first fixing the opposed thumb in 35 degrees of abduction with the metacarpophalangeal and interphalangeal joints at zero extension and then flexing the fingers until the desired relationship exists. The purpose is to facilitate picking up objects from a flat surface. Transverse compatability at the wrist metacarpal joints prevents the digital segment from migrating distally as the wrist is extended (and vice versa with flexion). When such does occur the palmar pads

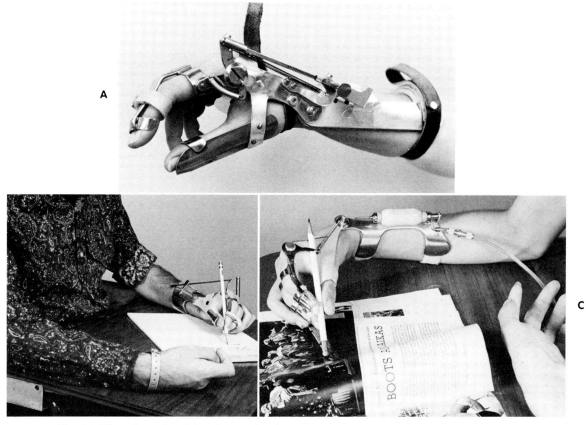

Fig. 6-8. Flexor hinge hand. Single hinge hand orthosis is the basic unit. Wrist component is static or hinged, depending on source of finger control. **A,** Passive ratchet orthosis has a static wrist. **B,** Wrist extensor tenodesis orthosis. **C,** Externally powered orthosis.

are blocked from participating in grasp and metal-to-metal gives poor object control.

(1) Elastic flexor assist (rubber bands or springs). The maximum flexion force that can be provided is limited to the amount of resistance the long finger extensor muscles can accept as they extend the metacarpophalangeal joints. As they are not large muscles, and they must act on a hinged orthosis as well as lift the fingers, the resulting pinch force is seldom effective—rarely 0.5 kg. Consequently, the indication for this type of flexor replacement should be restricted to patients with a resolving lesion who need only temporary assistance. It is not adequate otherwise.

(2) Wrist extensor tenodesis orthosis (Fig. 6-8, *B*). Active wrist extension can be

harnessed to provide voluntary finger flexion (and hence a grasp force) through bar linkage of the forearm and digital units across an intervening palmar segment. Preferably the wrist extensors should be grade 4 or better. Patients with less strength may exhibit an extensor lag but still profit; that is, they cannot complete the full extension range but can accept resistance through a shorter arc. These patients find the tenodesis orthosis an advantage if the final grasp is 1 to 2 kg. Often they supplement their weakened control with gravity aided by forearm supination.

Release of grasp is gained by flexion of the wrist. Patients who have retained wrist flexor action can do it directly. They have more precise control because they can alternate between grasp and release in any forearm position. When direct wrist flexion is missing, the patient uses gravity by relaxing wrist extensors with the forearm pronated. For good control an easy passive range of 45 degrees is necessary in both wrist flexion and extension.

Effectiveness of this system depends not only on total wrist extensor strength but also on the relative contribution of the two radial wrist extensor muscles: longus and brevis. This differentiation relates to the relative amount of radial deviation that accompanies the extensor effort. When the extensor carpi radialis brevis is strong, the pull is in neutral and 75% of the extensor force is realized as grasp. Independent longus action creates so much radial deviation that the resulting grasp force is only one third of available wrist extension strength. The difference in power loss relates to having the wrist travel an oblique path while the orthotic tenodesis must be aligned longitudinally to match the axis of wrist and metacarpophalangeal joints.

(3) Passive ratchet-bar orthosis (Fig. 6-8, A). Passive prepositioning of the hand for grasp is useful because the basic functions in self-care and desk-top activities employ a sustained grasp rather than frequent positional alterations. Ratchet orthoses offer the patient, devoid of direct-control sources, this type of hand function, without the complexities of external power.

For grasp, the finger unit is pushed toward the thumb post by hitting it with the opposite heel of the hand, forearm, or other part. This position is then held by the ratchet until it is loosened by a quick tap on the spring release. The basic requirement for operation, thus, is light contralateral arm control to activate both ratchet and release.

(4) External power. The requirements for attaining habitual use of an externally powered orthosis are stringent. Both carbon dioxide gas (Fig. 6-8, C) and electric motor systems need periodic repair. Unless this can be provided with such promptness or interchangeable parts included so that the patient experiences no significant interruption in his daily pattern of performance, he will not rely on the device. Instead he settles for that which is consistently reliable. Often the alternate is quite primitive, such as the use of a mouth stick.

The relative merits of the two systems of external power have already been discussed in the general presentation on this subject. Application to the hand directly follows the basic rules.

Operation of a powered system depends on the patient learning to use unusual control sites and different forms of feedback to gain better object manipulation. Not all patients are capable of this. They may not be sufficiently aware of how they move to learn new methods of performance ("motor morons" versus "motor athlete"). Many also lack future goals that depend on having optimum precision or versatility of grasp.

The complexity of power control calls for ingenuity, persistence, and gadget tolerance to learn how and then to continue practicing until device management attains the semiautomatic level. One must also allow a period of time for device refinement to meet the needs of the individual. It requires the closely coordinated effort of the occupational therapist, orthotist, and patient to attain optimum alignment of hinges and digital components, the best force for the switch activator and reliability of components. Only when the device is efficient and the patient has attained semiautomatic control will it become part of the patient's habit plan. Even to get started in the control-learning process, the patient must have a formal training program by a knowledgeable occupational therapist. Unless the patient has the opportunity to approach this unique way of handling objects in an organized fashion, the experience of success will be so delayed that frustration will replace ambition and the device will be rejected.

Thus external power is not for every patient. There are specific personality and intellectual requirements. The need for fairly regular servicing means that the patient must live in an area where this is available and have the initiative to seek it promptly. Lastly, there has to be available both a formal training program and some follow-up refresher opportunity.

Experience has also taught that bilateral fitting with external power is too complex for most patients. By the time they sort the two control systems the total demand is more than doubled. Thus it is therapeutically wise to equip only one side (usually the dominant or strongest) with power and rely on the other extremity for a control site. This is not a matter of economy, but concession to reality.

Control sites may be any place where a lever or switch can be made sufficiently secure that the patient can reliably activate it each time. Patients with scattered paralysis often can call on residual toe, thigh, or even contralateral finger musculature. When there is segmental loss such as with spinal injury, the available control sites are limited to residuals in the other arm, the head, or the tongue.

Release. Cessation of flexor muscle action and passive rebound of the tense extensors are the basic components of grasp release. Opening of the hand for unobstructed withdrawal from (or approach to) the object is provided by the combined action of the intrinsic and long extensor muscles.

1. Intrinsic paralysis. These muscles contribute to interphalangeal extension in two ways. They can independently extend these joints. In addition, their flexor action at the metacarpophalangeal joint redirects the pull of the long extensor muscles so that they too can exert an effective force across the interphalangeal joints. The combined pull of the two

muscle groups (intrinsic and extrinsic) is a much stronger action.
   a. Potential deformity: There may be a "claw hand" that leads to interphalangeal flexion and metacarpophalangeal extension contractures.
   b. Functional loss: There is incomplete interphalangeal extension during attempted hand opening.
   c. Orthotic plan: Use a static metacarpophalangeal stop set in 30 degrees of flexion to redirect the pull of the long extensor tendons so that this muscle can complete interphalangeal extension. Because of the flexibility of the "stop" the final position is about 15 degrees of flexion. The purpose is to avoid neutral extension or hyperextension.
   d. Functional gain: With this orthotic assistance, full opening of the hand is possible.
2. Long extensor muscle paralysis (extensor digitorum communis, extensor indicis, extensor minimi digiti). These muscles are the sole source of metacarpophalangeal extension. They add strength to the interphalangeal extension.
   a. Potential deformity: Metacarpophalangeal joint flexion contractures are present.
   b. Functional loss:
      (1) Lack of metacarpal-phalangeal extension.
      (2) Positional feedback to the flexor muscles for precise hand use.
   c. Orthotic plan: Elastic extensor assists for the metacarpophalangeal joint are used with the finger slings applied to the proximal phalanx.
   d. Functional gain: The hand opens moderately. In addition, because of the associated metacarpophalangeal flexor action of the intrinsic muscles as they contribute interphalangeal extension, the effect of the elastic pull is usually incomplete. Selection of stronger elastics (or springs) to avoid this limitation is undesirable, however. They would hold the metacarpophalangeal joints in hyperextension when the hand was at rest, leading to an unacceptable deformity.
3. Combined long extensor and intrinsic muscle loss. Release of grasp by flexor muscle relaxation is still possible, but the patient cannot

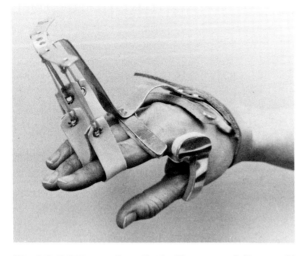

Fig. 6-9. Extensor assist orthosis. Placement of sling provides both interphalangeal and metacarpophalangeal extension. Metacarpophalangeal stop avoids hyperextension.

open his hand efficiently to approach or withdraw from objects.

a. Potential deformity: There are flexion contractures of metacarpophalangeal and interphalangeal joints.

b. Functional loss: Hand cannot open.

c. Orthotic plan: Elastic extensor assists with the force applied to the middle phalanx and metacarpophalangeal extension stop set in 30-degree flexion (Fig. 6-9). Theoretically, one should place the finger slings on the distal phalanx to gain full extension. However, as the fingers curl into a fist, the position of the last phalanx changes so drastically that effective alignment of the elastics (or springs) is lost. For example, the composite flexion of the three phalangeal joints during palmar pinch moves the distal phalanx from a horizontal to a vertical position. Further flexion, as occurs with a cylindrical grasp, carries the distal phalanx past the vertical into a new horizontal line with the tip facing the palm. Elastics pulling from a position dorsal to the hand similarly have their relationship changed from one that acts to extend to one that would flex the fingers. With a tight fist, this loss of extensor alignment also occurs with the slings on the middle phalanx.

Thumb

For the thumb to meet its obligation as one half of the prehension system, it must be able to easily assume a posture opposite the fingers, with the space wide enough to handle large as well as pin-sized objects. Consequently, a basic requirement is adequate joint mobility.

Deformity control. To avoid disabling contractures, one needs to give specific attention to three areas. Of prime concern is sufficient mobility of the first web-space tissues to allow 35 degrees of abduction between thumb and index finger metacarpal joint. Loss of this width limits the size of objects that can be handled. The first web space contains two powerful muscles (first dorsal interosseus and adductor pollicis). Incidental to their prime functions, they tend to pull the two metacarpals together. As each of these muscles has a dense fascial covering that develops easily, narrowing of the space will be perpetuated if an abduction force is not available.

The second concern is flexion at the carpometacarpal joint to permit the thumb to assume a position opposite the fingers. This range is adequate only when, with just light fingertip pressure, the thumb metacarpal can be placed in the plane that falls between the index and long fingers.

The third requirement is neutral extension of the metacarpophalangeal and interphalangeal joints. This allows the full palmar pad to contact the objects. The patient's limited grasp force is thereby augmented by the holding qualities of the fat pad's contouring about the object and the friction of the overlying skin. Flexion at either joint correspondingly lessens the area of pad contact against the object. This nail offers a particularly poor holding surface unless the object is so small (such as a pin) that only hairline contact is needed.

Protection. Protection of the thumb muscles and joint structures embodies the same principles as functional replacement and so will not be discussed separately.

Functional replacement. The three basic controls that require orthotic replacement whenever they are insufficient are opposition, grasp force, and release. Holding force is the prime concern for the first two functions, as the thumb must be able to withstand the flexing force of the fingers during prehension. Release requires only accommodation to thumb weight.

Opposition. Of the three motions comprising opposition (abduction, flexion, and rotation), only the first two are provided with an orthosis. This means that although the thumb can be placed opposite the fingers with sufficient spacing for good prehension, contact will be made with the

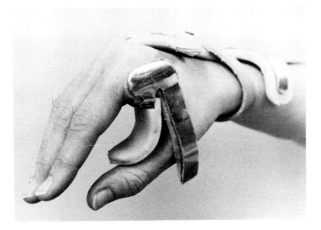

Fig. 6-10. Basic opposition orthosis with metacarpal extension and adduction stops.

side of the thumb more than by its palmar pad. A large amount of the pressure is thus exerted against the side of the nail bed, limiting the patient's tolerance of the prehension force. Usually a 2 or 3 kg force still is accepted without undue discomfort or skin irritation.

The act of opposition is performed at two levels of endeavor. Positioning requires little effort, but holding the thumb in opposition against the flexor force of the fingers demands good strength. Early attempts to maintain versatility by using mobile and spring-assist systems merely deprived the patient of effective grasp because of lack of thumb stability. Consequently, all orthotic replacement of opposition now is done with static components. An extension stop (radial bar) supports the thumb in flexion, whereas an adduction stop (C bar) maintains grasp in thumb abduction (Fig. 6-10). The other end of each motion arc is unrestricted to permit further gain, if possible.

Placement of the extension stop (radial bar) is critical. Three forces work against the thumb metacarpal stop. These are the flexing force of the fingers, thumb extensor muscle action, and weight of the arm when the hand is resting on the table. Maximum leverage would be gained at the metacarpal head, but this is an irregular surface that gains weight poorly. Hence, a compromise just proximal to this area must be accepted. In attempts to gain leverage, some orthotists erroneously try placing the extension stop on the phalanx. This induces metacarpophalangeal flexion without controlling the metacarpal. It obstructs rather than helps thumb function.

Effective positioning of the adduction stop (C bar) also presents difficulties. If the web tissues

are contracted, they overlap and obscure the metacarpophalangeal joint, causing the adduction stop to act on the phalanx rather than the metacarpal, leading to metacarpophalangeal hyperextension without correcting metacarpal alignment. Physical therapy stretching maneuvers or surgery are needed to alter metacarpal placement directly.

Grasp force. The ability to hold objects depends on having sufficient thumb flexion and adduction to push against the flexing fingers. Hence, strength rather than versatility is a basic requirement. Varying patterns of paralysis present four clinical pictures, but only the two more severe problems respond well to orthotic management.

Interphalangeal flexor loss. Isolated flexor pollicis longus loss is not an incapacitating handicap unles the volar capsule of this joint is lax. Then the interphalangeal joint collapses into pronounced hyperextension under the opposing forces of grasp. When this is the sole functional lack, there is no means of providing orthotic replacement without interfering with other available function.

Carpometacarpal adduction–metacarpophalangeal flexion loss. The adductor pollicis muscle not only serves to move the metacarpal toward the opposing fingers during prehension but also acts as the prime thumb metacarpophalangeal flexor. When this muscle is paralyzed, stability of the metacarpophalangeal joint depends on the volar capsule. When it is lax, the joint will collapse into hyperextension. Substitution attempts by the long thumb flexor merely results in an undesirable degree of interphalangeal flexion without offering useful metacarpophalangeal stabilization. The resulting grip is weak. If this is an isolated loss, as with an ulnar nerve lesion, the other functions of the hand are too good to make orthotic assistance acceptable.

Complete intrinsic muscle loss. Lacking opposition and carpometacarpal adduction, the best a patient can accomplish is a weak fingertip pinch against just the index finger. It is ineffective because the actions of the long thumb flexor and extensor muscles combine to overflex the metacarpophalangeal and interphalangeal joints while hyperextending the carpometacarpal joint. Hence the thumb can only reach the index finger and tends to pull away from it in the process of pinching.

An effective orthotic answer is the addition of a phalangeal extension stop to the opponens replacement orthosis. This positions the thumb

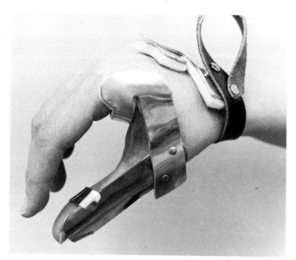

Fig. 6-11. Thumb post. Static unit to position paralyzed thumb for function.

opposite the fingers, allows the extrinsic muscle to continue acting at the interphalangeal joint, and prevents metacarpophalangeal collapse into hyperextension as opposing finger forces are met.

Total thumb muscle loss. When both the intrinsics and long flexor muscles are inadequate, the patient has no thumb grasp force. Function can be restored with an orthosis that holds the thumb in its basic position, that is, the interphalangeal and metacarpophalangeal joints in neutral extension and the carpometacarpal joint in opposition (Fig. 6-11). Literally, the thumb is made into an opposing post against which the finger flexors can act to create grasp. The one difficulty is the need for the orthotic component to overlap the palmar pad in order to stabilize the distal phalanx. Material in this area must be kept to a minimum if the device is to be effective.

Release. Replacement of absent extrinsic extensor and abductor action requires little force because one need contend only with the weight of the digit. A simple elastic unit is adequate, though awkward, because one must provide a projecting fulcrum for the rubber bands. In accordance with the common assumption that the long thumb extensor is solely responsible for the interphalangeal extension, it is customary to place the sling around the distal phalanx. This interferes with palmar-pad usage for sensation and grasp assistance. It also overlooks the anatomic fact that the small muscles of the thumb have the same anatomic arrangements as do the fingers. Thus, in addition to their stated abductor and adductor

action, they also provide combined metacarpophalangeal flexion–interphalangeal extension. Although they are not as efficient an interphalangeal extensor as is the finger system, they are functionally adequate, particularly when there is resistance to metacarpophalangeal flexion. Using this principle, the problem of palmar pad obstruction can be avoided by locating the sling at the proximal phalanx and relying on intrinsic muscle action for interphalangeal extension.

ARM ORTHOTICS

For the arm to meet its obligation of appropriate hand placement so that it can function effectively, there must be composite action at the shoulder, elbow, and forearm. In addition, there is a significant body mass with considerable leverage to be controlled. These factors greatly complicate the use of orthotics as a therapeutic aid in arm-disability management.

Deformity management

Neither the shoulder nor the elbow has a basic position of function, though there is one for the forearm. Instead, the goal is to maintain a wide range of motion. Consequently, positional orthoses do not have a prominent role in the control of arm deformity, as was described for the hand. In selected instances, special units are used to recover specific segments of the function arc. Otherwise the emphasis is on passive and active exercise by nurse, family, and physical therapists.

A functional arm orthosis helps to maintain midrange mobility by the repeated positional changes that accompany performance of various tasks throughout the day. They also make passive ranging for the rest of the arc easier.

Shoulder. At the shoulder the functional range of motion includes 90 degrees of flexion and abduction, full internal rotation, and 20 degrees of external rotation. The awkwardness of having one's arm supported in extreme elevation or external rotation and the discomfort induced by the orthotic forces needed to sustain arm weight in such alignment have discouraged clinicians from employing orthoses to prevent deformity. As a result, "Statue of Liberty" braces and "abduction splints" are rarely used. They represent an era before the value and possibilities of deformity prevention through early mobilization were realized.

Elbow. No limitation of flexion of motion is

acceptable, as full range is required to get the hand to the face. Extension criteria depend on whether the patient needs to use his arms for body support or transfer. When this is not so, weak elbow flexor muscles are aided by 20- to 30-degree flexion contracture, which offers a more efficient starting position from which to raise the hand and the objects it holds. More force is required to flex the elbow at 30 degrees than at higher angles.

A person dependent on crutches or assistance of his arm to stand or to transfer in and out of a wheelchair needs a full range of extension. Body transfer-force requirements quickly exceed triceps strength if the elbow is even slightly flexed. This is an area of arm function that is generally overlooked in the acute phase of disability but should receive a critical review, particularly with the type of paralysis being seen today. Restoration of full elbow extension is a strong challenge, as the flexor muscle mass is large, closely wrapped about the joint, and well endowed with fibrous tissue. For these reasons an intensive short-term program with serial plaster-of-paris casts is often preferred to regain range of motion. However, variable hinged, removable orthotic shells that fit with comparable security offer the advantage of selected periods of activity. This allows a functional training program to accompany the deformity correction effort.

Recovery of lost arcs of motion with an orthosis is difficult. Although the long leverage offered by the humerus and forearm would seem ideal, neither the olecranon or the antecubital area are able to tolerate sufficient pressure to provide an effective counterpoint. An alternate system is to use broad, carefully contoured cuffs with side hinges to which a corrective force has been applied. Extreme care must be taken to align the orthotic joints with the transverse axis of the elbow, or the cuffs will tilt and cause intolerable levels of local pressure. Efforts to simplify alignment by substituting swivel cuffs merely dissipate the corrective force; so there is no effect. In either system the tubular contour of the humerus and softness of overlying tissues make stable fixation difficult.

Elastic corrective forces are tolerated only if the patient has antagonistic muscles of adequate strength to overpull the elastic periodically for relief. The tissues are intolerant of constant stretch. When the patient lacks this means of self-protection, the corrective orthosis is one having

serially adjustable stops to hold the gain accomplished by a formal therapy program. Recently, the Rancho Los Amigos Hospital staff has found that when the contracture is dense or spasticity is one component of the deforming force, a motorized orthosis with a very slow motion pattern can be effective when other efforts have failed (Fig. 6-12). In the spastic patient, rate of travel must be so slow that neither the length or velocity sensors within the muscle spindle are stimulated. Also, there must be a force cutoff so that no tissue tearing occurs. Similar slowness of motion is needed when one attempts to recover range after operative release, to accommodate the highly viscous state of the tissues. Lengthy rest periods are interspersed between intervals of the graduated stretch. The sequence is gradual stretch, hold,

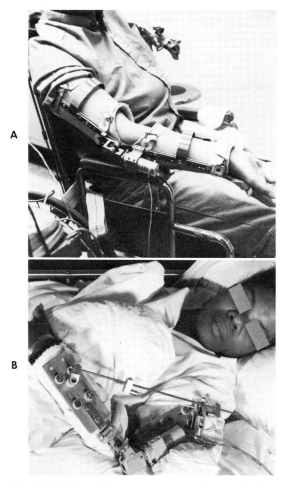

Fig. 6-12. External power to correct elbow contractures. **A,** Power unit attached to plastic orthosis designed to accommodate spasticity. **B,** Power unit attached to arm and forearm cast fitted with range stops to control exercise arc.

relax, and rest. The Rancho powered elbow exerciser was designed to operate on a 10-minute cycle. Moving at 1 degree per second, stretch is induced for about 22 seconds. Then maximum tension is released by having the motor reverse for 8 seconds. The joint is subsequently held in this corrected position for the remainder of the cycle to avoid excessive stretch. The motor was designed to stall whenever joint resistance was 70 inch-pounds. During the stall condition, this torque continues to be exerted on the joint structures without motion occurring. As the contracture yields, the device moves further in the stretch direction, thereby always operating at the outer limit of range of the joint. Such systems are still very experimental but have proved effective when well controlled. Vigorous force by any means merely causes loss of range by creating microtears, which induce reactive scarring and even heterotopic ossification.

Forearm. A position within the interval between midpronation and full pronation is critical if the hand is to approach and manipulate objects on a table top with optimum ease. In contrast, supination contractures are a major deterrent to function, since they turn the hand away from the work area. A single orthotic position of midpronation is a compromise that does not significantly interfere with hand use. Given the option, neutral rotation is generally used when one limb serves as an assistant to the other. Although full pronation is commonly preferred for unilateral hand function, it is also essential when extensive hand bracing is required. An unopposed biceps (common with many of the paralytic patterns seen today) rapidly leads to a supination contracture, as the forearm is so rotated every time the elbow is flexed. These deformities are very resistant to correction because the entire interosseus membrane is shortened, as well as the tissues about each radioulnar joint. Hence an early program to prevent deformity is much more effective than one designed to gain correction. The soft tissues of a child usually are sufficiently mobile to respond to a corrective orthosis. Such is not true of adults unless the deformity is of very recent origin.

To create a rotating force on the forearm without distorting the wrist, the orthosis must firmly grasp the radius and ulna directly. Yet only the distal 2 inches are sufficiently subcutaneous to provide a stable purchase. Then it can only be accomplished if the cuff is accurately contoured to the surfaces available. If one erroneously chooses the hand for the distal area of fixation because of its convenient anatomy, all the corrective force will be applied to the wrist. This multiarticulated area will yield, resulting in severe distortion among the carpals without any change occurring in the forearm. For proximal fixation one must flex the elbow and grasp the humerus.

The orthosis will be tolerated only during periods of rest or light activity, as otherwise it must work against active biceps pull. Excessive pronation can be managed in a similar fashion, though seldom is this deformity a functional deterrent unless extreme.

Protective orthotics

The shoulder presents a special orthotic challenge, that is, to assume the weight of the arm so as to avoid harmful (or painful) stretch of an injured brachial plexus or paralyzed glenohumeral musculature. Although the agent most frequently employed is an arm sling, its effectiveness is limited by the amount of weight the base of the neck can accept comfortably. Often this is insufficient to meet clinical demands. In the past, a customary alternative was an abduction splint. However, rarely is this acceptable because poor fixation on the trunk makes the orthosis unstable. Also, the arm is held in an awkward, nonfunctional posture. A second device is the functional arm brace. The new designs offer stability and comfort, but the device is more elaborate and costly than one can justify when assisted arm function is not the goal. Just recently a better answer has been introduced by the Rancho Los Amigos Hospital staff. It is a static arm support comprised of a forearm trough supported on a molded plastic iliac cap (Fig. 6-13). The arm is held in a cosmetically pleasing pose, and the hand is available for use, making early recovery functional. The orthosis is easy to put on, and full unloading of arm weight is accomplished. The iliac arm support can be made in predetermined sizes for immediate fitting, thereby closing the previously lengthy gap between sling and functional arm orthosis. In those very select circumstances where it is necessary to hold the arm in abduction, orthotic stability can be improved with a similarly molded iliac cap.

Elbow and forearm. Protective orthotics is rarely employed in these areas. When needed, modification of functional orthoses serve well. At

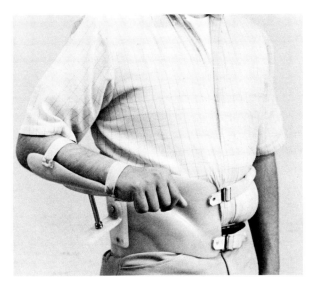

Fig. 6-13. Static arm support orthosis.

the elbow, a previously valuable technique was the use of a hinged orthosis to induce joint stability by guiding scar maturation after resection arthroplasty. This need has now been largely replaced by the development of implantable artificial joints.

Functional orthotics for arm

Because the basic purpose of arm motion is to position the hand, the prime requisite for a functional arm orthosis is a useful hand, though it need not be normal. Other requirements are good proprioception and a range of motion that permits easy placement within the functional area. Also, somewhere there must be a source of control to selectively move the arm in a productive manner. This may be weak muscles within the arm that only need assistance, or it may be remote sites that are used to operate switches.

The many combinations of shoulder, elbow, and forearm motions can be grouped into two fundamental action patterns: elevation and depression. Elevation is involved in the functions of reach, carry, and lift. Light elevation activities are reproducible with an orthosis. Vigorous effort is obstructed by the difficulties of attachment, the need to exert all positioning forces through the skin, and the few control sources available. Depression is used for object stabilization and body transfer. These are forceful events that cannot be reproduced with functional orthoses.

All functional arm orthoses have two basic

obligations: (1) assumption of arm weight and (2) provision of controlled motion.

Both tasks are much more difficult to accomplish in the ambulatory than in the wheelchair-dependent person. Upper-limb weight is 5% of the total body mass. Inconsequential when the arm is hanging limp at the side, it becomes very significant as the arm is raised. With the shoulder flexed (or abducted) 90 degrees and the elbow extended, the limb presents (in a 70 kg person) a 102 kg/cm demand for support. If both joints are flexed 45 degrees the support requirement drops to 73 kg/cm. Requirements are less if only elbow motion is used, but this correspondingly shortens the patient's reach.

This load, plus the weight of the orthotic components applied to hand and arm, must rest on whatever base is available. In ambulatory patients the body is the only source. Wheelchair-dependent persons can use the chair's frame. The sturdier base makes it possible to provide much more versatile control and more effective forms of power. Consequently, replacement of the lost arm function is far better for the person sitting in a wheelchair than for his otherwise better endowed ambulatory brethren. In selected instances it is appropriate to effect a compromise by attaching a wheelchair type of orthosis to a stationary site (chair or table edge). The ambulatory person with paralyzed arms can then function at his desk or dining table. Although this meets his needs in that one situation, the patient remains nonfunctional elsewhere.

Ambulatory functional arm orthosis

Initially the orthosis was suspended from the shoulder because this is an effective prosthetic practice. However, limb weight for the two situations is dramatically different. Also shoulder girdle stability is much less in the paralyzed patient. Anatomically, the only point of skeletal fixation between upper limb and trunk is the sternoclavicular joint, a flat, nearly vertical articulation that offers no weight-bearing capability. Hence the limb is suspended by soft tissues. With paralysis, muscle strength is lost and the supporting fascial planes are stretched by unrelieved stress. Without these supports, arm weight can drag on the brachial plexus, leading to further paralysis and loss of sensation. Pain may be an added penalty.

To avoid such complications (and they may not be reversible), Schottstaedt and Robins directed

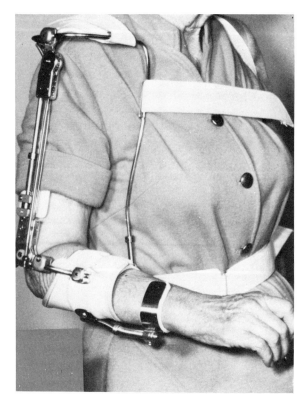

Fig. 6-14. Ambulatory functional arm orthosis (elastic powered).

the load to the pelvis[6] (Fig. 6-14). For their poliomyelitis patients a padded band was sufficient. However, the more vigorous patients with brachial-plexus injury require better fixation on the pelvis. The current answer is an iliac cap carefully contoured for comfort during sitting as well as standing. A movable link between base and thoracic frame allows the trunk to move without causing loss of orthotic alignment. These modifications have not only improved brace comfort, but also enhanced its use and hence its acceptance because they permit the patient to substitute trunk motion for unavailable arm control.

The minimum requirements for useful hand placement are 45 degrees active shoulder flexion, full selective elbow flexion, and forearm fixation in midpronation. Shoulder abduction is not essential, as the ambulatory patient can substitute by turning his body to appropriately redirect his flexion. The quoted degree of shoulder flexion is an important component of reach and self-feeding. Because of the high force requirements, shoulder flexion is usually accomplished passively through trunk flexion. A lock holds the shoulder position. It is released when the elbow is fully extended.

Elbow-flexion control is the most demanding. In the course of daily hand use, one employs the full range from 140 degrees flexion to complete extension. Any limitation requires awkward substitution. This means that selective control through the entire arc must be provided. An effective compromise is active prepositioning and lock fixation. Because control sources are so restricted, one is tempted to call on the other normal limb. However, the patient does not tolerate having it so encumbered. This approach means he must interrupt whatever his good arm is doing to position a second extremity that, at best, offers only limited function. The inconvenience is too great for the reward. Quickly the braced limb is ignored and the orthosis is soon discarded. Hence, to be accepted, the orthosis must include its own means of active elbow flexion.

Active elbow flexion can be accomplished with rubber bands in sufficient numbers to lift the forearm and hand, an alternating locking ratchet joint, and a remotely operated lock to maintain the desired position. Contralateral shoulder abduction is an effective and accepted control of the lock. Return of the arm to an extended position requires unlocking the orthotic joint and triceps actively. Poor (grade 2) stretch is sufficient. This is not available if C7 root damage accompanies the injury to C5 and C6.

When the triceps is not adequate, capabilities of the functional arm orthosis are greatly curtailed. The elastic force must now be slightly less than that required to lift the arm so that elbow extension is still available. To attain the desired degree of flexion, the patient has to find some additional mechanical substitute. It may be the pendulum effect of quick trunk rotation while the elbow is unlocked, leaning against a table edge, or pushing the forearm up with the thigh. All these techniques are awkward and thus lower the functional capabilities of the orthosis and consequently its acceptance. Therapeutic indications must be strong.

TOTAL UPPER-LIMB PARALYSIS
Wheelchair functional arm bracing

With the chair frame as a stable base, orthotic designers have had much more latitude in the amount of apparatus they could consider. This has led to development of three characteristic designs: (1) balanced arm slings, (2) mobile arm supports, and (3) powered orthoses.

Balanced arm slings. These devices, by suspending the arm from an overhead bar attached to the wheelchair, offer an immediate means for arm motion by weak muscles. Height and alignment dictate the function possible. This potential can be increased with springs and balance bars.

The occupational therapists use balanced arm slings to initiate arm function, particularly for exercise and to maintain a range of motion. The arm slings may be selectively positioned to assist in the prevention and correction of shoulder and elbow deformity.

The pivotal character of the suspension, though allowing a range of relatively effortless motion, also tends to pull the arm back to the neutral point. Thus the slings offer very little selectivity as to the motions they assist or resist. Alignment must be reset with each use, since one needs to turn the overhead bar out of the way each time the patient transfers out of the wheelchair. For these several reasons, balanced arm slings are classed as an exercise aid that should be replaced with a mobile arm support if a device is needed for increased function. Mobile arm supports are more compact, specific as to functions aided, and permanent in adjustment.

Mobile arm supports. The fundamental function of the mobile arm support is to assume the weight of the arm so that very weak muscles (poor, and even trace) can provide useful motion. When there is a significant difference of strength between opposing muscle groups, the axis of the ball-bearing support is tilted so that gravity can assist the weaker group or even provide total replacement. To use gravity as a functional force, the opposite muscle group must have sufficient strength to perform its needed task while working against this added resistance.

Initially there was such enthusiasm for this device that great effort was made to use the head and trunk as control sources for arm motion. However, the results were too inaccurate and too costly of energy to be effective. Experience with a variety of paralytic pictures has led the occupational therapists to establish the following rules. A patient cannot gain effective, independent arm function with a mobile arm support unless his shoulder and elbow exhibit some muscles of grade 1 or 2 (trace or poor) strength. There must also be sufficient range of motion to allow passive placement of the hand near the mouth and across a lapboard surface. Lengthened handles can be used as a training

device but are an unacceptable long-term answer.

A stable sitting posture is another essential for effective arm function. Of first concern is a well-fitted wheelchair. If mechanical trunk supports are necessary, they should allow slight lateral mobility. Until the patient has established at least 2 hours of wheelchair-sitting tolerance and adequate health for continuity of effort, training is unsatisfactory.

Use of the mobile arm support requires a well-defined purpose. Strengthening of recovering muscles is an objective patients accept readily. To be effective, however, there must be repeated use throughout the day. This will occur only if the patient is able to do activities that are meaningful to him. Hence the patient's activity goals determine the success of the program as much as proper fitting and equipment selection. Both the swivel and radial arm devices serve well as temporary training aids.

Although it is very desirable to reestablish bilateral activity, counteracting balance requirements and a common need to use different types of substitutive motion with each area adversely complicate control. As a result, better function actually is gained by fitting the patient with only one mobile arm support.

There are currently two structural patterns available: swivel and radial arm. Though they provide many functions in common, each has certain advantages over the other.

Swivel mobile arm support orthosis (Fig. 6-15). The system now designated as a swivel mobile arm support represents the original approach to functional arm bracing introduced by the Warm Springs, Georgia, Foundation staff in the 1940s.[1] Their design was so effective it has persisted with only minimal change. To simplify the method of adapting lever length and alignment according to individual patient requirements, a shaft-bending technique has been substituted for the earlier collection of interchangeable parts. A second modification, designed by the Rancho Los Amigos Hospital staff, was the addition of an elevating proximal arm segment to assist shoulder abduction. The swivel system offers an unobstructed arc of horizontal motion the full length of the patient's arm, and vertical reach up to his head. How much of this potential range can be used by any one patient depends on the balance needed for the bidirectional control. Holding forces are minimal. The ball-bearing fulcrums give the

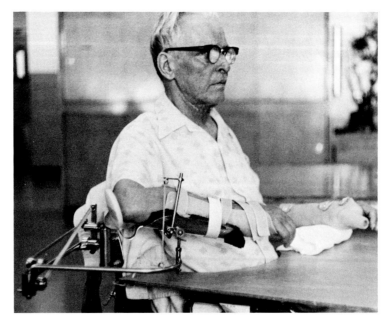

Fig. 6-15. Balanced arm slings.

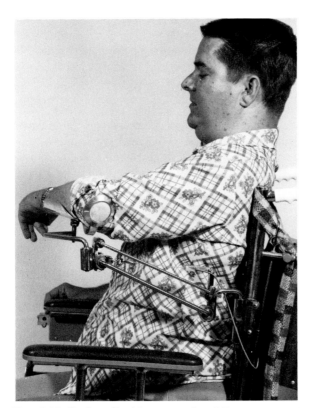

Fig. 6-16. Carbon dioxide–powered mobile arm support orthosis.

patient greater mobility for versatile hand placement but little or no reinforcement of strength for lifting. Only light objects can be managed.

Other advantages of the swivel mobile arm support system are its availability and ease of patient fitting. The unit, including the elevating proximal arm, is a commercial item. Guidelines that enable occupational therapists to independently assemble and adjust the units have been published. The system can be positioned so that it does not interfere with objects on the lapboard. The elevating arm is a specific aid for strengthening the shoulder abductor muscles. For patients with inadequate abductor force, a power unit can be added (Fig. 6-16).

One can also give a limited amount of assistance to selected muscle groups by adding rubber bands. Elastic does deteriorate rather rapidly, however; so this approach is for training rather than for long-term use.

Swivel mobile arm supports have two important disadvantages. They are conspicuous and they protrude to the side unless the patient accommodates by reaching across his body or far forward. The width of this protrusion makes it impossible to go through doorways without repositioning one's arms. This is a particular inconvenience if the patient is operating an electric wheelchair.

Radial-arm mobile arm support. This was spe-

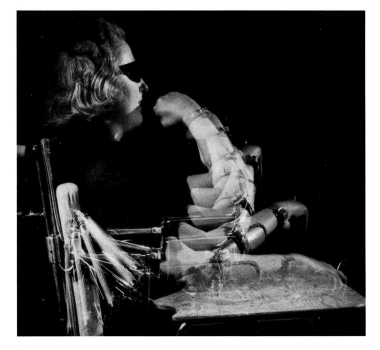

Fig. 6-17. Powered elevating proximal arm for swivel mobile arm support orthosis.

cifically designed to avoid lateral protrusion of the swivel levers with customary posturing. There are also several other assets to the design. It is less conspicuous and has fewer parts. The latter asset makes the unit less formidable for assembly at home. These advantages alone have led patients with a spinal injury to prefer the radial-arm system to the swivel design for long-term use. A further gain is the fact that patients with mild spasticity or limited range of motion also can use it, because there is better vertical motion and horizontal mobility is more stable.

Unfortunately, the radial-arm style also has its disadvantages. The bar protrudes behind the chair as the shoulder is extended. Free arm motion may be interrupted by the bar's hitting the body when the hand is brought to the center of the work area (a recent addition of a horizontal spring may have solved this latter problem). Also, the bar's surface tends to nick, leading to jerky arm motion after a period of use.

Availability presents other limitations. The radial-arm system is still not a commercial item. Guidelines for adjustment and assembly have yet to be written. Lacking a clear explanation of the system, occupational therapists are unable to make many of the adjustments needed to meet individual patient requirements. These latter barriers, of course, have practical solutions.

Powered arm orthosis. When patients lack even the minimal controls of trace shoulder and elbow musculature, external power must be substituted. Power systems have not been difficult to design, but effective control mechanisms remain a stumbling block for most patients. The problems are twofold: Arm function almost invariably requires simultaneous selective motion at both the shoulder and elbow to move the hand along the appropriate diagonal path. This is difficult to accomplish with control sites outside the arm. As a result, the patient usually has to exercise a sequence of motions by alternating between two to six control sites until the hand has finally arrived at the desired destination. When this mode of control is compounded by a lack of sensation, the patient is unsure of the hand's exact position and thus cannot make the fine adjustments needed for accurate function. The latter situation is common to most of the patients seen today. As a result, though powered arm orthoses should remain available to fulfill the needs of selected patients, the major effort today is in the development of environmental control systems that completely bypass the paralyzed, insensitive upper limb.

Carbon dioxide mobile arm support (Fig. 6-17). As many as six power units (artificial muscles or pistons using carbon dioxide) have in the past been added to a mobile arm support of standard configuration. The possibilities of adding assistance in this manner to segments of a mobile arm support are multiple. However, the problems of control and maintenance are significant. An effective compromise mixes mechanical and powered units to enhance the function of persons who have retained partial arm control.

Two artificial muscles using carbon dioxide are now applied by Engen to the swivel mobile arm support, with a spring-assisted elevating proximal arm to give abduction and elbow flexion combined with forearm supination.[3,4] It is considered appropriate for patients who, though lacking arm musculature, have retained scapular elevation. Control sources are selected from those areas retaining active musculature.

The elevating proximal arm has a coil spring assist to lessen the power requirements. A short swivel arm with its fulcrum posterior to the olecranon joins the humeral and forearm sections.

In addition to the two sources of positive control, the system permits free horizontal motion at the junction between humeral and forearm segments. If the patient has voluntary pronation or supination, he is free to rotate within the forearm trough. This segment can also serve as a fixation point for the hand orthosis. By combining the free and powered motions, a degree of versatility is gained.

Another example of selected carbon dioxide–powered assistance is the use of one unit to activate the elevating proximal arm. The other components of the mobile arm support are under voluntary control (Fig. 6-17).

Electric arm orthosis (Fig. 6-18). To provide a more positive control of a larger series of functions, an anthropomorphic orthosis was designed with 6 degrees of freedom. The unit is more anatomic because it is suspended from a proximal point on the chair opposite the shoulder and thus is comparable to normal arm, trunk relationships. Control is provided by six two-way electric switches operated by the tongue. The tongue switch unit can be moved to or away from the face with a second switching unit operated by the head or shoul-

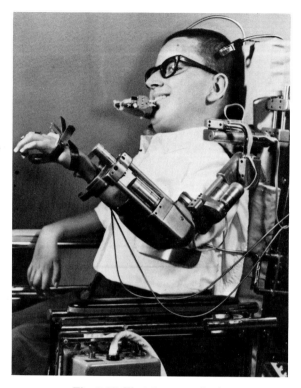

Fig. 6-18. Electric arm orthosis.

der. Feedback is dependent on the sensation within the limb or by the patient's vision. Fitting has been greatly simplified by the development of adjustable limb segments so that a single basic design is appropriate for older children and adults. One limitation in the orthosis being used as envisioned is the difficulty in the obtaining of normal diagonal motion. About 30 motions are required to get a single bit of food from plate to mouth. Experience has demonstrated that the postpoliomyelitis patient who has retained normal sensation despite his paralysis has good control, whereas the patient more commonly seen today with spinal-cord injury lacks the necessary feedback for effective performance.

SUMMARY

Arm and hand orthoses can make major contributions to the management of dysfunction when properly selected, designed, and fitted, but the requirements are exacting. There is no place for casual orthotic service; either it is good, or it is an unacceptable waste.

REFERENCES

1. Bennett, R. L., and Stephens, H. R.: Care of severely paralyzed upper extremities, J.A.M.A. **149:**105-109, 1952.
2. Britt, L. P., and Bennett, R. L.: Care of the aftereffects of
   poliomyelitis (forearm and hand), Arch. Phys. Med. Rehabil.
   31:646-653, 1950.
3. Engen, T. J.: Development of upper extremity orthotics,
   Orthot. Prosthet. **24:**12-29, March, 1970.
4. Engen, T. J.: Development of upper extremity orthotics,
   Orthot. Prosthet. **24:**1-31, June 1970.
5. McKenzie, M. W.: The ratchet hand splint, Am. J. Occup.
   Ther. **27:**477-479, Oct.-Nov. 1973.
6. Schottstaedt, E. R., and Robinson, G. B.: Functional bracing
   of the arm. II, J. Bone Joint Surg. **38A:**841-856, 1956.

PART THREE

The lower limb

CHAPTER 7

Normal human gait

JOHN H. BOWKER, M.D.
†CAMERON B. HALL, M.D.

Each person's unique pattern of walking represents his solution to the problem of how to get from one place to another with minimum effort, adequate stability, and acceptable appearance. The inability to walk with reasonable facility and to stand with adequate security are the principal handicaps felt by individuals with lower-limb incapacities. Restoration of these deficiencies as completely as possible is the first goal of lower-limb rehabilitation.

One cannot overestimate the importance of fully understanding the elements of the rehabilitation process including orthotic engineering and design, surgical procedures, orthotic prescription practice, and training in the use of these devices.

If we are to apply assistive or restrictive orthoses that will correct aberrant limb function, then it is obvious that complete comprehension of the elements of normal gait and their relationship to the abnormal is essential to realization of these goals.

Faced with a large number of handicapped individuals with malfunctioning lower limbs, a research team combining the talents of electrical and mechanical engineers, physicians, physiologists, orthotists, and prosthetists was assembled under the Advisory Committee on Artificial Limbs, National Research Council, at the University of California at Berkeley during World War II.

_____
†Deceased.

The report of this group provides an "analysis of the magnitudes, directions, and rates of change of translations, rotations, and forces in the lower extremity and pelvis with respect to three coordinate axes in space." Capitalizing on work already accomplished, proceeding with innovative techniques, and combining the multiple talents of the team, they were able to obtain findings that comprise the cornerstone of our knowledge of human gait.

THE GAIT CYCLE

This analysis is confined to the movement of the body below the level of the umbilicus, though we recognize that trunk sway, arm swing, and head motion play an extremely important role in normal gait. For ready comprehension, the human locomotor system is reduced to its simplest possible form: a series of articulated sticks assembled to resemble the limb segments of man, stripped of muscles, but moving with the same pattern in response to the many forces involved. These forces are gravity acting on the body mass, counteractions of the floor, muscular effort generated within the limb segments, and resultant forces from the potential and kinetic energy developed in this moving mass. The movements of the limb segments have been arrested, as by a camera, at certain constantly recurring critical incidents in the gait cycle to allow study of the activity and relationships of the segments in normal walking as

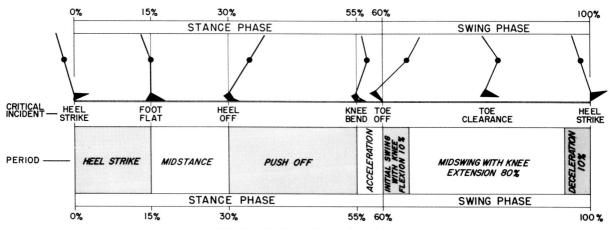

Fig. 7-1. Analysis of a single stride.

compared to altered patterns created in abnormal locomotion.

Viewed from the side, stroboscopic photographs of suitably marked thigh, leg, and foot segments resemble articulated sticks moving through space, allowing one to focus his attention on one limb at a time. One can see that the limb repeats its movements for each step, progressing through a sequence of standing on the ground followed by swinging through the air. By convention, the start of a complete gait cycle is that instant at which the swing-limb heel strikes the ground. Following a progression of events, the cycle ends when that particular heel again strikes the ground. Hence heel strike indicates both 0 and 100% of the gait cycle.

Careful review of still photographs taken sequentially throughout the gait cycle reveals certain generally accepted divisions and events. The gait cycle is seen to consist of two phases. *Stance,* which comprises 60% of the entire cycle, is followed by *swing,* the remaining 40%. The resulting overlap of phases, when both limbs are weight bearing, is *double stance.* The two phases are subdivided into periods by events known as *critical incidents* (Fig. 7-1).

Stance phase implies support of the body weight. The stance limb assumes increasing amounts of this weight transferred from its mate soon after *heel strike,* the first critical incident. This first 15% period of the gait cycle, known by the same term, heel strike, terminates at *foot-flat,* the second critical incident. It is followed by that period between 15% and 30% known as *midstance.* During this period the person is balanced on his stance limb, and his body continues to move

forward to the critical incident of *heel-off,* terminating the midstance period and initiating the push-off period. The mass of the body is now on the downhill portion of its undulating path, adding potential energy by its movement as it falls through the next 25% of the cycle known as *push-off.* This starts with the initial critical incident of heel-off, which is an interval of single limb support, and continues to *knee bend,* where the stance knee is seen to bend as hip and knee flexion prepare the limb for the swing phase. At this time 55% of the entire gait cycle has been completed.

Shortly before knee bend, the opposite limb has completed its swing phase, contacted the ground and started to prepare for the transfer of weight to the new stance limb. This shift of weight from the old stance limb has prompted many individuals working in the orthotic and prosthetic fields to consider the true stance phase terminated at about this time (55%) even though the "original" stance foot is still in contact with the ground. Careful consideration of all factors, however, allows one to suggest that it is best to retain the older designation while recognizing that the original stance limb is supporting a rapidly decreasing portion of the body weight during the final 10% of stance phase. The final 5% of stance phase, known as *acceleration,* extends from knee bend at 55% to the final critical incident of toe-off, marking the completion of stance phase and the beginning of the swing phase at 60% of the full gait cycle.

The *swing phase,* occupying the last 40% of the cycle, is divided into three periods; initial swing, midswing, and deceleration. The first 10% of swing phase is known as *initial swing* and begins with the critical incident of *toe-off* and continues as the foot rises in an arc responding to flexion of the knee and continued forward motion of the limb well started by hip flexion in stance acceleration period. *Midswing,* which represents 80% of swing phase, begins as the swing limb passes its stance counterpart, the knee extends and the path of the foot reverses to fall in a forward swinging arc. During this period, the foot is actively dorsiflexed by the anterior leg muscles to avoid stubbing the toe at the bottom of the pendulum swing (toe clearance). During the final 10% of swing phase, *deceleration* occurs. The rapidly moving swing limb, now out in front of the body, is smoothly braked by gravity and the limb musculature to conclude the full sequence at 100% of the gait cycle with ground contact at *heel strike.*

It is evident that the foot is in contact with the ground through 60% of the cycle and is swinging forward in the air to pass its stationary mate during 40% of the cycle. It is also obvious that an overlap of stance phases must occur if each foot is to have ground contact for 60%. Observation reveals that the swing foot hits the ground before the opposite stance foot is lifted. The period during which both feet are weight bearing is termed "double stance." It is of greatest duration while a person walks slowly and is of least duration while one moves rapidly. Double stance must occur with each sequence; should the swing foot fail to contact the ground prior to the departure of the stance foot at toe-off, the individual will momentarily have both feet off the ground at the same time and will be trotting, leaping, or running. The striding, energy-conserving gait of man is characterized by this double-stance phase in his walking pattern.

The cycle is continually repeated, with feet alternating as the individual walks over level ground. It is important to recognize that this sequence is observed only in normal limbs moving over level surfaces at a normal walking speed. Ramps, inclines, stairs, or uneven ground, jogging or running, will sharply alter this smooth, repetitious cadence.

The energy requirements of stance phase result from muscular activity of (1) the hamstrings and glutei maximi, in decelerating the swing limb through the last milliseconds prior to heel strike and their continued activity as hip stabilizers during the initial part of stance; (2) the quadriceps femoris, in stabilizing the knee and absorbing shock by eccentrically contracting to allow the knee to flex under increasing loading; (3) the anterior leg muscles, in eccentrically contracting to absorb the shock of heel strike and thereafter to lower the forefoot to foot-flat; (4) the paraspinous and trunk musculature, in balancing the torso at foot flat; (5) the contraction of the triceps surae through most of the stance phase; and (6) the contraction of the hip abductors to stabilize the pelvis throughout the stance phase.

Analysis of muscle function during swing reveals that (1) hip flexors initiate acceleration of the stance limb and continue to provide support throughout swing; (2) knee extensors dampen knee flexion to prevent excess heel rise after toe-off; (3) knee flexors aid in lifting the toe from the ground; (4) foot dorsiflexors elevate the forefoot during swing to prevent toe stubbing; (5) hip extensors decelerate the swing limb prior to heel strike; and (6) hamstrings decelerate both knee extension and hip flexion.

To understand the effect of the articulated lower limb on the moving mass of the human body, we shall use a well-understood, constantly employed reference point used to study bodies in motion—the center of gravity (CG). The center of gravity of a body, volume, area, or line is that point at which it would be perfectly balanced in any position. In the upright human, the center of gravity lies just anterior to the second sacral vertebra within the true pelvis. Seen from the front, this is just above the symphysis pubis; from the side, just above the tip of the greater trochanter. By studying the reactions of the CG to certain situations, we can often predict or analyze what the body as a whole is doing. By substituting the CG as an entity for the complex form of the trunk with limbs attached, the human figure can be reduced to a lump much as the complex thigh and leg were reduced to the sticks employed to analyze a single forward stride. Utilizing the concept of a single mass moving in space, one can then apply the laws of physics to understand some of the peculiarities of human gait.

Newton's first law of motion states that a body set in motion will continue in a straight line until compelled by impressed force to alter its path. However, Newton's first law of motion in itself is not so important in studying walking and what it costs to walk as is this corollary. A body in motion following a crooked path has numerous impressed forces acting to alter its pathway, at an increased cost of energy consumption. Thus the study of a CG path moving in space provides some comprehension of energy expenditure. Human center-of-gravity movement may be effectively recorded on a photograph produced by an open-shuttered still camera in a darkened room exposed to a pinpoint source of light marking the CG while the person walks. Such photographs taken from the side, above, and in front of the subject will produce a streak of light, wavering across the film. From the side, matching the vertical rise and fall of the CG, this streak describes a sine wave rising and falling a total of only 2 inches. The summit of this rise appears at midstance when balanced on one limb and the low point when both feet are on the ground in the double-stance phase. Thus, as a person walks, he rises and falls a total of 2 inches with each step. His energy expenditure is proportional to his weight and is measurable in foot-pounds of work. In addition to his rising 2 inches when he is balanced on one foot in midstance, his body moves laterally over that foot to place his CG in true balance while he is on one limb. On taking the next step, he moves to the opposite side, and the light streak on the photograph taken from above shows the total lateral shift of the human CG from left to right to again be approximately 2 inches. An individual moving with a limp might drop his CG a full 4 inches instead of 2 inches and shift to the side 4 inches at a greatly increased cost in energy. It becomes apparent, therefore, that a limp is not only cosmetically undesirable but functionally demands a much higher expenditure of energy than does a smooth, normal gait, and it follows that everything possible must be done to eliminate the limp from the gait of an orthosis wearer.

BASIC DETERMINANTS OF GAIT

With the conviction that man, for all his complexity, is a structure capable of undergoing mechanical analysis, an attempt was made to devise a mechanical model for more exact engineering studies of gait. A simple pylon of average limb length was fitted with a nonarticulated foot. Instead of the sine-wave pattern of the human subject with its energy-conserving, smooth reversal from stance to swing phases, the tracing of the CG path was a series of connected arcs with sharp reversal points. The arc described by the moving CG at the tip of the artificial greater trochanter, given an average stride length, was found to produce a 3-inch vertical displacement from heel strike to midstance. The 3-inch CG shift of the

model would produce a 50% greater expenditure of energy in elevating the body weight with each step than normal. To identify the critical features in human gait that differ from the mechanical model, a detailed study was made of thousands of enlarged prints from high-speed motion pictures of individuals walking while fitted with identifying targets to show translatory and rotary motion of the several limb segments. The elements of human lower-limb function that account for the smooth sinusoidal CG path with vertical and horizontal displacement of only 2 inches have become known as the basic determinants of gait.

There are six determinants, but they apply only if the individual is walking across a level surface at normal speed. The effect of arm swing, shoulder rotation, trunk flexion and extension, and head bob all contribute to the final molding of the human pattern of gait, but they do not affect the path of the center of gravity.

First determinant of gait—pelvic rotation
(Fig. 7-2)

The pelvis (Latin, 'a basin') can be pictured as a bowl supported by two legs. At the start of double stance with the swing foot at heel strike and the stance foot at heel-off, the pelvis is supported by a bipod, forming an isosceles triangle, the apex of which establishes the CG height from the ground, and the sides of which intersect the plane of the floor at a given angle. The center of gravity of the bowl is at the lowest point of its undulating path. Photographs taken by overhead cameras of living subjects reveal that the pelvis rotates in the horizontal plane 4 degrees forward with the swing limb and 4 degrees to the rear with the stance limb, thereby spreading apart the apex of the isosceles triangle, propping up the leaning bipod legs, and consequently elevating the center of gravity ⅜ inch. By horizontal pelvic rotation alone, the theoretical 3-inch amplitude of CG displacement had now been cut by ⅜ inch to 2⅝ inches total. Orthotic devices that do not permit this rotation of the pelvis may be producing rather than diminishing a portion of a patient's limp.

Second determinant of gait—pelvic tilt
(Fig. 7-3)

Study of gait photographs taken in front and to the rear of the walking subject reveal that the pelvis normally tilts down 5 degrees from the stance limb at midstance. This lowers the CG in

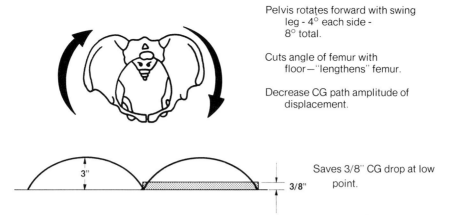

Pelvis rotates forward with swing
leg - 4° each side -
8° total.

Cuts angle of femur with
floor—"lengthens" femur.

Decrease CG path amplitude of
displacement.

Saves 3/8" CG drop at low
point.

Fig. 7-2. First determinant: pelvic rotation. (Courtesy U.C.L.A. Prosthetics-Orthotics Education Program, Los Angeles, Calif.)

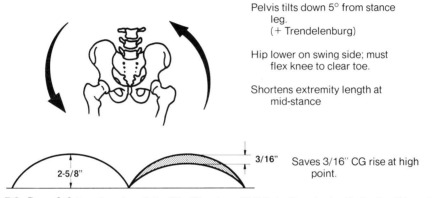

Pelvis tilts down 5° from stance
leg.
(+ Trendelenburg)

Hip lower on swing side; must
flex knee to clear toe.

Shortens extremity length at
mid-stance

Saves 3/16" CG rise at high
point.

Fig. 7-3. Second determinant: pelvic tilt. (Courtesy U.C.L.A. Prosthetics-Orthotics Education Program, Los Angeles, Calif.)

the center of the pelvis and also lowers the hip joint on the swing side. The person is therefore required to flex the knee of the swing limb to prevent toe stub during swing. The lowering of the CG at the crest of the summit has been found to be about 3/16 inch, reducing the amplitude of vertical displacement from 2 5/8 to 2 7/16 inches.

Third basic determinant of gait—knee flexion after heel strike (Fig. 7-4)

The mechanical model, a pylon with a nonarticulated foot, would seem an adequate reproduction of the normal limb during the stance phase up to the point of knee bend. However, careful review of published data reveals that the human knee is flexed twice within the gait cycle. It first begins to flex in response to heel strike, serving to absorb shock under the control of the eccentrically contracting quadriceps femoris until foot-

flat. This first knee flexion also allows a diminution in the rise of the CG summit by 7/16 inch, resulting in the final CG amplitude of displacement of 2 inches. The knee then progressively extends to assist stretching the triceps surae, in preparation for heel-off. Shortly thereafter, the knee flexes again to lift the toe from the ground. The locked knees of orthoses would seem to contribute to, rather than prevent, a limp.

A summation of the first three determinants of gait reveals that pelvic rotation, pelvic tilt, and knee flexion after heel strike together provide the 1-inch reduction of the mechanical model's 3-inch vertical amplitude of CG displacement to the 2-inch total seen in the normal human lower limb. However, they do not reproduce the center of gravity's smooth, undulating sine-wave path. Further actions are necessary to avoid an abrupt direction change at the low point with a cor-

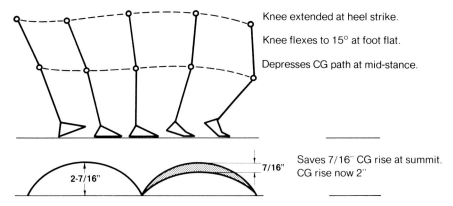

Knee extended at heel strike.

Knee flexes to 15° at foot flat.

Depresses CG path at mid-stance.

Saves 7/16" CG rise at summit.
CG rise now 2"

Fig. 7-4. Third determinant: Knee flexion occurring after heel-strike. (Courtesy U.C.L.A. Prosthetics-Orthotics Education Program, Los Angeles, Calif.)

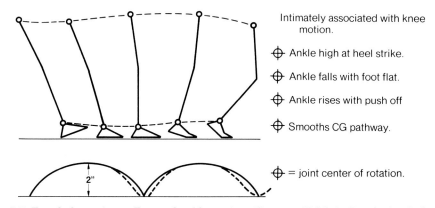

Intimately associated with knee motion.

⊕ Ankle high at heel strike.

⊕ Ankle falls with foot flat.

⊕ Ankle rises with push off

⊕ Smooths CG pathway.

⊕ = joint center of rotation.

Fig. 7-5. Fourth determinant: Foot and ankle motion. (Courtesy U.C.L.A. Prosthetics-Orthotics Education Program, Los Angeles, Calif.)

responding acute energy expenditure. These actions are found in the next two determinants.

Fourth determinant of gait—foot and ankle motion (Fig. 7-5)

In producing the desired CG reversal pattern it is best to consider the fourth determinant, foot and ankle motion, and the fifth determinant, knee motion, as being intimately related.

The center of rotation of the ankle joint, roughly a point on the axis connecting the tips of the medial and lateral malleoli, rises and falls over a small but definite arc formed by the lever arm of the calcaneus from heel strike to foot-flat. At heel strike, the ankle center is elevated, whereas through midstance the foot is flat on the ground and the center of rotation remains at a fixed height. Soon after midstance, however, the heel lifts from the ground, causing the center of rotation of the ankle to rise again, and the total effect is to round off the sharp reversal of the CG at its low point. Well-engineered shoe modifications to accommodate locked ankles are needed to reproduce this determinant in therapeutic devices.

Fifth basic determinant of gait—knee motion (Fig. 7-6)

As mentioned above, knee motion is intimately associated with the fourth determinant, foot and ankle motion. The interplay serves to achieve the final baseline reversal pattern of the CG path. For convenience, one may consider the joint center of rotation to be a point on the axis connecting the greatest prominences of the femoral condyles, recognizing that the knee actually has a moving center of rotation. In response to heel strike, the knee begins to flex and, as noted above, the ankle center of rotation falls until the foot reaches the foot-flat position. Then the knee reverses its action to one of extension while the ankle level remains stationary. During this period of time the limb has become progressively more vertical. The con-

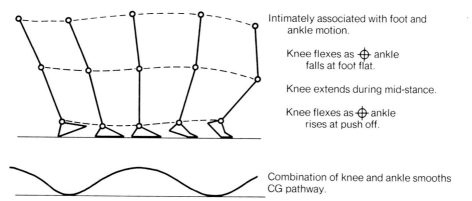

Intimately associated with foot and ankle motion.

Knee flexes as ⊕ ankle falls at foot flat.

Knee extends during mid-stance.

Knee flexes as ⊕ ankle rises at push off.

Combination of knee and ankle smooths CG pathway.

Fig. 7-6. Fifth determinant: Knee motion. (Courtesy U.C.L.A. Prosthetics-Orthotics Education Program, Los Angeles, Calif.)

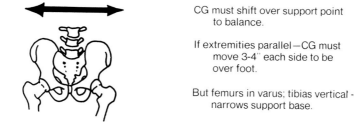

CG must shift over support point to balance.

If extremities parallel—CG must move 3-4" each side to be over foot.

But femurs in varus; tibias vertical - narrows support base.

Total lateral motion 1.75".

Fig. 7-7. Sixth determinant: Lateral pelvic motion. (Courtesy U.C.L.A. Prosthetics-Orthotics Education Program, Los Angeles, Calif.)

current knee and ankle actions serve to produce further smoothing of the body's center of gravity path that otherwise would have included an abrupt reversal point. With heel-off, the ankle rises and compensates for the accompanying loss in limb verticality. Further heel rise is counter-balanced by accompanying knee flexion; so the CG level change is again smoothed.

The combination of these five determinants—pelvic rotation, pelvic tilt, knee flexion after heel strike, foot and ankle motion, and knee motion—results in a smooth, undulating CG path with its 2-inch amplitude of vertical displacement. The final determinant is concerned with lateral movement of the center of gravity.

Sixth determinant of gait—lateral pelvic motion (Fig. 7-7)

In order to balance on one foot, it is not suffi-cient to simply raise the other. By so doing a person will immediately fall to the unsupported side. To remain upright, he must shift his body to the side of the supporting foot, bringing his CG directly over his support point to establish equilibrium.

In a similar fashion, man's alternating bipedal gait demands that the CG be shifted over the stance foot in order to balance while the swing limb is being carried forward. It has been said that walking is a series of falls and recoveries, allowing one to move along the line of progression.

The CG is in the center of the pelvis just ante-rior to the second sacral vertebra. Some 4 or 5 inches to either side lie the hip sockets. Fortunate-ly, the femoral and tibial axes do not drop verti-cally from the hip joints. Instead, the femoral shafts are adducted in varus and the tibial shafts are vertically aligned in valgus at the knee joint. This effectively narrows the base of support so that, to be sufficiently secure, one must move the CG only 1 inch laterally toward the stance foot.

This action is reversed when weight is trans-ferred to the other foot, resulting in a total CG dis-placement of 2 inches per gait cycle. The trunk is not completely centered over the support foot by this displacement. Instead a mixture of momen-tum and displacement are used for security. As lateral momentum abates, and the trunk tends to fall toward the other side, that limb is already preparing to accept body weight.

The final combination of all six determinants—pelvic rotation, pelvic tilt, knee flexion after heel strike, foot and ankle motion, knee motion, and lateral pelvic motion—allows the center of gravity to rise and fall as well as to move from side to side within a 2-inch square box providing man with his efficient and unique gait.

AXIAL ROTATION OF LEG SEGMENTS

Viewed from above, the anatomic components of the lower limb do not swing forward and backward, well aligned in the sagittal plane. Actually, there is considerable rotation of the various segments of the limbs about their long axes.

In general, there is a progressive, serial internal rotation of the lower limb that starts in swing phase and progresses to foot-flat, followed by an abrupt reversal of direction into external rotation as the foot prepares to leave the ground. At the conclusion of swing phase, the hip, with the pelvis swung forward on this side, is in relative external rotation. At heel strike, with the foot in neutral rotation, the tibia rotates internally to align the ankle with the foot. This motion occurs in the subtalar joint. Rotational forces are reversed as foot-flat is completed, after which strong external rotation occurs against the still fixed foot. This brings the foot into the last vestiges of internal rotation to stabilize it during push-off. The moment the foot leaves the ground, it is externally rotated and the limb prepares for heel strike by again internally rotating.

The pelvis rotates forward 4 degrees during swing and backward 4 degrees with stance, producing a total pelvic rotation of 8 degrees. At the same time, the swing femur externally rotates about 5 degrees as the stance femur internally rotates 3 to 4 degrees, giving a total femoral rotation of 8 to 9 degrees during the full gait cycle. The tibia rotates a total of 9 degrees on the femur. The magnitude of rotation of the various limb segments is of considerable interest in the design of orthotic devices.

MUSCLE ACTIVITY IN GAIT CYCLE

For simplification of initial analysis, the lower limb has been considered a structure of articulated skeletal levers operating in space without sources of power. Muscles are now added, grouped about the joints as primary flexors, extensors, abductors, adductors, and internal or external rotators. Some span only one joint, whereas others cross two or more. Some may act as flexors in one limb position while serving as abductors or external rotators in another.

In general, muscles accelerate, decelerate, or stabilize limb segments. They may act, therefore, while contracting, lengthening, or remaining the same length. For the most part their function during walking will require short periods of activity and allow longer periods of relaxation during each individual complete single stride. The pendulum-like action of the limb and momentum perform great service in the movement of the limb or its components.

Motors

As motors, muscles perform work in a mechanical sense, lifting, moving, pushing, or twisting a certain mass with a certain force for a certain distance, allowing the calculation of work performed. Muscles utilize concentric contraction in this type of activity. Concentric contraction implies a shortening of the distance between the origin and the insertion of the muscle. The force exerted can be readily measured.

Shock absorbers

Absorption of shock by deceleration of a moving limb segment is possibly the major function of the great bulk of muscles in the lower limb while walking. This function is performed by eccentric contraction, which allows the distance between the origin and the insertion of the muscle to progressively increase. Contrary to the concept that a muscle is at rest while being lengthened, these muscles are performing significant work while being elongated as they are resisting the passive forces tending to create motion in an opposite direction.

Stabilizers

As stablizers, muscles perform work in a biologic sense. They serve basically as guy wires to hold a limb in a certain fixed position by locking the joints. They move no mass through no distance and the mechanical evaluation of their function is difficult. Isometric contraction is utilized for this function, and the muscle, although working hard, does not shorten the distance between its origin and insertion. These muscles perform increasing magnitudes of work without visible motion as the load supported increases.

Measurement of muscle activity

The most accurate measurement of muscle activity remains the wire electromyograph even

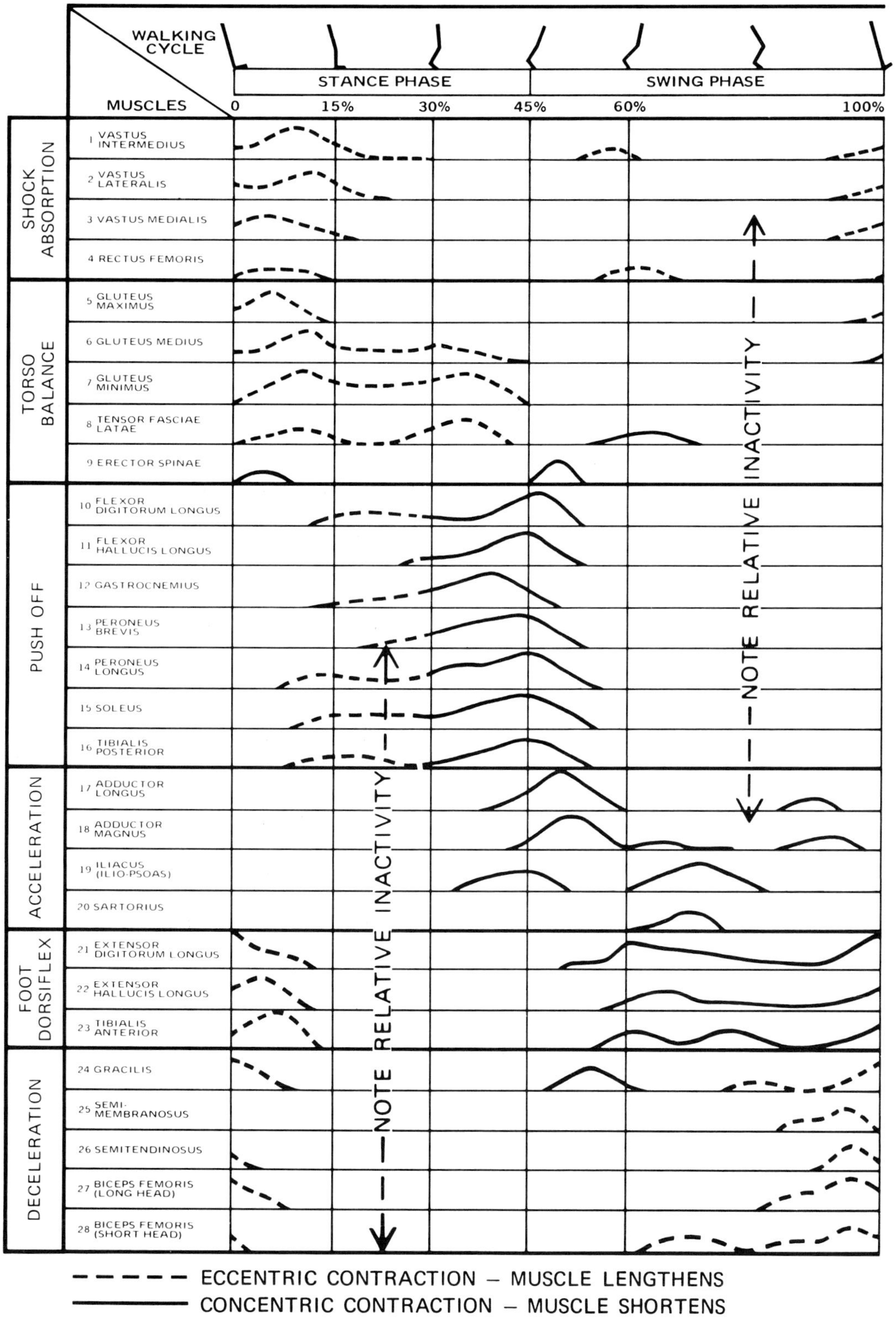

Fig. 7-8. Electromyograph of lower limb during walking. (From Dr. Charles O. Bechtol, Los Angeles, Calif.)

though it records only the electrical signals brought by the motor nerves from the brain and tells us little about the actual force, amplitude, or type of contraction of the muscles themselves. The electromyograph is extremely useful in the determination of when a particular muscle is being signaled by the brain to contract, but the recording of this signal cannot tell us whether this muscle is requested to contract concentrically, eccentrically, or isometrically. For that reason the analysis of the following electromyograph taken of each muscle during a single stride is quite revealing. The chart itself has been arranged to follow the usual single-stride sequence with muscles grouped, as much as possible, to show their major effect on the limb segment. They are chronologically arranged in order of their appearance as the stride progresses. The curves of their electrical potential have been altered to identify concentric or eccentric contraction.

Electromyograph of lower limb during walking (Fig. 7-8)

A muscle found active at heel strike is the quadriceps femoris, which is found to be in full contraction at the start of the stance phase, showing good activity potential. It is contracting eccentrically, lengthening to act as a shock absorber by allowing controlled flexion of the knee to 15 degrees by foot-flat. The duration of quadriceps activity is extremely brief, originating in the last 10% of the swing phase to stabilize the knee and ceasing at the end of the initial 15% of stance. The rectus and vastus intermedius portions fire again briefly after toe-off to dampen excess heel flexion, again contracting eccentrically.

The muscles comprising the hip abductor, pelvis balancer, and torso supporter groups begin activity at heel strike and complete their function by heel-off. Like the quadriceps, these muscles are contracting eccentrically, allowing the pelvis to drop 5 degrees into a Trendelenburg sign from the stance hip. The small tensor fasciae latae contracts concentrically after toe-off to slightly abduct the limb in initial swing, placing it in a better position to initiate hip flexion.

The next set of muscles to become active is the triceps surae and posterior tibial group. During initial firing just after foot-flat they are stretched in eccentric contraction to stabilize the tibia and permit knee extension. Near the end of midstance, they contract concentrically to return the ankle from 10 degrees of dorsiflexion to neu-

tral. It is a moot point as to whether they are actually shortening or isometrically holding. Regardless of interpretation, the force demands on the soleus and gastrocnemius are high. Some investigators believe that these muscles primarily act to lock the ankle, with heel rise and the registered push-off force resulting from the anterior angulation of the tibia combined with the body mass being far forward of the supporting foot.

The hip accelerators, which are fairly massive muscles, contract concentrically. The iliacus begins its action in terminal stance and continues into early swing, while the other flexors, which include sartorius, gracilis, adductor longus, and tensor fasciae latae, trade off throughout swing.

The foot dorsiflexors are made up of the three principal anterior leg muscles. They contract eccentrically after heel strike to allow smooth descent of the forefoot to the ground. Their concentric contraction in swing phase is minor and of low magnitude, simply providing enough force to dorsiflex the unloaded foot to prevent toe stub.

The hamstrings are in the last stages of eccentric contraction at the time of heel strike and rapidly assume a rest phase until they again eccentrically contract in the last stages of swing to decelerate the swing limb just prior to heel strike. Their brief action at initial contact is essential for limb stability. During initial swing, the short head of the biceps contracts to flex the knee and allow toe clearance.

In summary, a number of interesting observations can be made. The first is that the electromyogram cannot tell us whether muscles are contracting, lengthening, or isometrically stabilizing. The recordings are all identical.

The second finding is that the three really massive muscle groups of the lower limbs—the gluteals, the quadriceps and the soleus—all contract eccentrically during normal walking over level ground.

The third finding, derived by observation of the amount of muscle activity during the midstance period, while a person is theoretically supporting all his mass in the upright position, is that muscle activity is recorded only in the ankle plantar flexors. This would appear to be a state of equilibrium with conservation of energy for the more proximal muscles.

The fourth finding of interest is derived by similarly checking midswing, at which time the mass of the limb is being moved through the greatest distance at the greatest velocity. Al-

though considerable muscle activity occurs at initial swing, during midswing only scattered muscle activity is found. The conservation of energy is remarkable and possibly further substantiates the extreme efficiency that man has developed in his locomotion patterns. The smooth sinusoidal path of his CG is shown to be an efficient design for elevating and depressing his body weight. From a mechanical standpoint the drop of the center of gravity down the slope from midstance to double stance will be exactly balanced by the rise from that point to again achieve midstance on the summit of the opposite slope. The kinetic energy lost in descending this slope is equal to the potential energy gained by achieving the summit. Even with this saving, man uses approximately 38% of his energy-producing capacity in level walking at 3 miles per hour.
walking at 3 miles per hour.

REACTIONS BETWEEN FOOT AND FLOOR

The foregoing demonstrates the pattern of the production and the application of forces within the body. These power systems may or may not result in efficient locomotion, dependent on the factors of gravity and friction.

Without gravity, ground contact is undependable and adequate functional stabilization of the foot for acceleration and deceleration would be absent. The magnitude, direction, and extent of these factors can be measured by a force plate, a complex device upon which a subject may stand or walk. The plate will measure the amount and direction of the forces of vertical loading, fore and aft shear, medial and lateral shear, and internal and external torque. Vertical force is shown to increase steadily from heel strike to foot-flat, exceeding body weight momentarily as the descending mass of the CG loads the new stance foot. A subpeak representing 60% of body weight occurs immediately after heel strike, well before the maximum at foot flat. It has been suggested that the heel-strike phase be divided into two subphases, initial contact and contact response, eliminating the term "heel strike" completely, since many handicapped individuals, such as spastics with their equinus gait, never strike the heel at any time. Through midstance the vertical loading may drop below the body weight as the CG passes over the summit with the vertical forces rising again as the forces of heel-off are added. Heel-off for the same lack of descriptive accuracy in other than

normal gaits might well be termed "terminal stance." Vertical loading drops rapidly in the final stages of stance as the opposite foot contacts the floor and assumes the support of the falling CG mass.

Fore and aft shear recordings demonstrate a forward peak immediately after heel strike. This is quickly reversed as the foot pushes back on the floor with the acceptance of body weight as the CG climbs to its summit on the stance leg, after which the falling mass again pushes backward on the foot after heel-off with a resultant thrust to the rear by the push-off foot.

Lateral and medial shear recordings reveal the initial adducting forces secondary to the swing foot striking the ground followed by a shift to lateral pressure as the CG applies a bending moment to the hip joint resisted by the hip abductors. The effect of the pelvic stabilizing group returns to near equilibrium as the CG comes directly above the support foot through midstance. With heel off, the CG is shifting to the opposite side in its 2-inch lateral excursion and the lateral forces rise as a result through the push-off phase.

SUMMARY

This brief introduction to the study of normal gait should assist in the initial understanding of the basics of how we walk. It is in no way intended to be an exhaustive or authoritative treatise on any aspect of gait technology. It is intended to stimulate students in the many specialties concerned with the care of the handicapped to seek the excellent technical material published by their respective professions.

READINGS

1. Inman, V. T.: Conservation of energy in ambulation, Bull. Prosthet. Res. 10-9:26-35, Spring 1968, Veterans Administration, Washington, D.C.
2. Murray, M. P., Drought, A. B., and Kory, R. C.: Walking patterns of normal men, J. Bone Joint Surg. 46A(2):335-360, March 1964.
3. Peizer, E., Wright, D. W., and Mason, C.: Human locomotion. Bull. Prosthet. Res. 10-12:48-105, Fall 1969, Veterans Administration, Washington, D.C.
4. Peizer, E., and Wright, D. W.: Human locomotion. In Murdock, G.: editor: Prosthetic and orthotic practice, London, 1969, Edward Arnold, Ltd., pp. 15-35.
5. Saunders, J. B. DeC. M., Inman, V. T., and Eberhart, H. D.: The major determinants in normal and pathological gait, J. Bone Joint Surg. 35A(3):543-558, July 1953.
6. Sutherland, D. H.: An electromyographic study of the plantar flexors of the ankle in normal walking on the level, J. Bone Joint Surg. 48A(1):66-71, Jan. 1966.

CHAPTER 8

Pathologic gait

JACQUELIN PERRY, M.D.

The strength, joint mobility, and coordination needed for walking represents only a fraction of normal lower-limb potential. Running, climbing, dancing, and lifting are far more vigorous activities that also are readily performed by the ordinary person.

When paralysis or tissue damage restricts the patient's physical ability, he spontaneously draws on this reserve for the simpler task of walking. Only when the loss exceeds his ability to adapt, or the effort becomes too strenuous, does he display a visible abnormality in his gait. Thus it is useless to admonish a patient to do better, as his reserve has already been exhausted. Capability to respond more than just momentarily (if even that) is lacking. Instead, if there is to be lasting improvement in the patient's gait, the clinician must accurately identify and correct the deficit. As the disparity between loss and substitution capability increases, walking becomes more precarious. The extent to which this gap may be lessened by an orthosis or other therapeutic procedures depends on both the nature and extent of the patient's pathologic condition.

At one time one needed only to memorize a list of typical limps. Such an approach no longer will suffice, for clinical concern now includes a widely disparate span of pathologic abnormalities—cerebral palsy, myelodysplasia, strokes, brain and spinal injury, muscular dystrophy, a miscellany of other neuromuscular lesions, more severe levels of arthritis, the consequences of multiple trauma, and a variety of congenital abnormalities.

Gait abnormalities have become correspondingly more complex. No longer can one call on a short list of limps from which to derive an effective therapeutic plan.

Instead, it is necessary to identify the actions of each body segment (trunk, pelvis, hip, knee, ankle, and foot) and to note their deviation from the normal pattern during the individual phases of gait. These observations are then related to the patient's physical findings (sensation, range of motion, and muscle strength) and the etiology of his disability. From this bank of information one deduces which abnormal actions represent the primary loss and which are volitional substitutions. The ability of the patient to substitute is defined both by the extent and the biomechanical characteristics of his pathologic condition.

When few pathologic conditions were being managed, it was customary to identify gait deviations by diagnosis. With the broader concerns of today, this would result either in an endless list or omissions of many significant but less common lesions. Both disadvantages are avoided with a biomechanical approach that classifies the diseases by the components of motion they disrupt. This system permits use of the more common forms of pathologic conditions for illustration while offering a means for consideration of every other type of lesion as well. Familiarity with the

Table 2. Components of walking

Source of motion	Motor unit (muscles)
Articulated levers	Bones and joint
Awareness of need and action	Sensory system
Control of motion	Central motor system
Energy	Cardiopulmonary system

functional characteristics of the different types of disease and injury that involve the locomotor system not only provides a means of identifying the proper therapeutic plan, but also permits definitions of its potential to effect change, that is, the possibility for recovery and adaptation.

Walking, like every other physical task, has five functional requirements (Table 2). Each is provided by a specific anatomic system that can be selectively damaged by certain types of abnormality. These are as follows:

Source of motion. In man, the source is the muscles. However, the muscle fibers are so intimately dependent on their immediate nerve supply that a functional classification must consider the two structures as one. As a result, the human source of motion is the "motor unit," a functional composite of lower motor neuron, myoneural junction, and the muscle fibers that a neuron commands.

Levers to translate motion into desired action. The skeleton and its complex articulation provide the leverage to define what effect a contracting muscle will have. Joint anatomy determines the direction in which motion can occur. Bone length proportionally magnifies the motor unit's actions.

Awareness of quality of motion needed. The velocity, extent, force, and direction of motion and its effects on the body are sensed by the peripheral nervous system's receptors. This information is then carried to and through the tracts of the central nervous system to centers where it is interpreted and transformed into appropriate instruction to the motor system.

Control source to provide desired motion. The quality of motion that is produced is directed by the upper motor neurons. Their action is a response to the feedback from the sensory system, as much as it is an expression of the patient's will.

Energy to move. The patient must have sufficient energy both to walk and to perform the desired task on arrival at his destination. Availability of adequate energy is dependent on the cardiopulmonary system's ability to provide appropriate amounts of oxygen to the muscles and their supportive tissues.

The anatomic site of a patient's disease or injury dictates which of these components of walking are disrupted. Patterns of loss fall into the following categories:

1. Structural insufficiency (leverage loss)
2. Motor unit insufficiency
3. Combined motor unit and peripheral sensory impairment
4. Central control dysfunction (control and feedback impairment)
5. Energy insufficiency

A generic terminology, which has been in development over the past 5 years is used to describe the phases of gait. This approach allows identification of the appropriate phases without dependence on normal performance to provide the distinguishing critical events. Seven phases of gait are identified in this fashion. They are initial contact, contact response, midstance, terminal stance, and preswing for the stance period, after which the swing period is divided into initial swing, midswing, and terminal swing.

Initial contact is normally a heel strike, but may also be accomplished with the flat foot or forefoot (toe).

Contact response refers to the reaction of the limb segments to being loaded under the circumstance dictated by its mode of initial contact. With a heel strike the foot normally falls forward quickly into a flat-foot posture. If the toe made contact first, the motion may be reversed.

Midstance is the period of stationary foot support. It is the beginning of single stance. The normal person's foot remains flat on the ground and the body advances by progressive dorsiflexion of the ankle and extension of the knee. Disability may lead to either inadequate or excessive motion at this joint, with reflections on higher segments as well. Also, there may never be a flat-foot posture even though there is a period of stability.

Terminal stance applies to the single stance period when the body is forward of the supporting foot. Normally it is signaled by heel-off. The disabled person may maintain heel contact or never have it. A disabled patient may maintain flat-foot contact throughout the weight-bearing interval, with heel rise merely being part of the total limb lift for swing, or the heel may never have contacted the ground.

Preswing refers to the final moments of stance. It is normally characterized by rapid knee flexion and increased ankle plantar flexion. These actions are often lost with disability. The significance is lack of readiness for the swing phase.

Initial swing begins with movements directed toward picking up of the foot and advancing of the unloaded limb. Normally there is a sharp increase in knee flexion, and the toe clears the ground. With disability, the toe may drag and knee flexion may be inadequate. Both events often induce well-characterized substitutions.

Midswing refers to the actions that occur after the swing limb is forward of the supporting limb. This is a period of progressive, though passive, knee extension, while the hip continues to flex actively and the ankle dorsiflexes. A point is reached where both hip and knee are in 30-degree flexion.

Terminal swing is the final period of knee extension that is an active event controlled by the quadriceps. During this same period, hip extensors are decelerating hip flexion; so it remains at 30 degrees. As the knee approaches 5-degree flexion, the hamstrings also decelerate knee extension in preparation for the initiation of stance.

Any of these events may be inadequate in a variety of combinations if the person is disabled. More specific error in gait, which is a characteristic of the different types of disability, will be presented in the ensuing sections. A key to accurate interpretation of a person's limp is close attention to all the body segments (trunk, pelvis, hip, knee, ankle, foot, and toes). Allowing oneself to focus only on the most conspicuous event leads to many errors in treatment planning and functional prediction.

STRUCTURAL INSUFFICIENCY

With each step, the swing limb is actively advanced while the trunk and stance limb passively move over the supporting foot. The ease with which this is accomplished depends on the mobility of the lower-limb joints and the amount of weight and jarring they can accept. Deformity and pain are the limiting factors. These, in turn, are dictated by the quality of one's articular cartilage, flexibility of the periarticular soft tissues, and the contour of the supporting skeleton.

Each has specific modes of abnormality that one must understand if the mechanics of abnormal gait caused by skeletal and articular lesions and the contribution of orthotics are to be understood.

Skeletal malformation

The contours of the articular skeleton and supporting shafts may become deformed at any age through disease or trauma, but the most susceptible period is the years of growth. Wolff in 1892 observed that changes in the use of a bone are followed by certain definite changes in its internal architecture.[2]

Although initially the patient may not appear abnormal, continued performance in the presence of deformity is costly. Adults, lacking the adaptability of growing tissues, react to excessive stress by developing degenerative changes that lead to pain. Malaligned joints display such changes much earlier than is seen with normal aging. Children respond not with pain but by growing into progressive degrees of deformity as their constantly changing tissues respond to abnormal stresses. From birth until maturity the bones are undergoing two patterns of change that make them particularly susceptible to malaligned weight-bearing. The constant remodeling that accompanies the longitudinal and circumferential growth can easily be distorted (Fig. 8-1). The articular ends as well as the epiphyseal plates remain cartilaginous during much of the growth period. This softer tissue is quite responsive to stress (Fig. 8-2). Asymmetric forces on either the joint surfaces or the epiphyseal plates discourage new growth on the compressed side while inducing overdevelopment contralaterally.[8] Structural asymmetry results. Weight-bearing on this now malaligned joint accentuates the problem, leading to further deformity. Progression is subtle but persistent.

Soft-tissue restrictions

In addition to direct attack on joint structures, the pain induced by the abnormality may be a vigorous deforming mechanism. Pain is a physiologic signal of harm. As such, it initiates reflex muscular inhibition. Thus failure to hold oneself in proper alignment, or exercise to gain necessary strength, is initiated at the reflex, not volitional, level.

This has been dramatically demonstrated by DeAndrade and colleagues in an experiment where the knee was progressively distended with sterile plasma[4] (Fig. 8-3). As intra-articular tension was increased, the subject's quadriceps extensor force correspondingly decreased. Finally, a point of no response was reached. At this time the joint was anesthetized with a local agent. Full

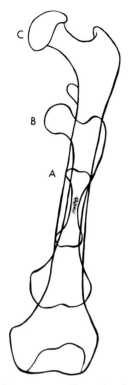

Fig. 8-1. Remodeling process of growing bone. A, Newborn model. B, Young child. C, Final adult form. (Adapted from Grant, J. C. Boileau: A method of anatomy, Baltimore, 1944, The Williams & Wilkins Co.)

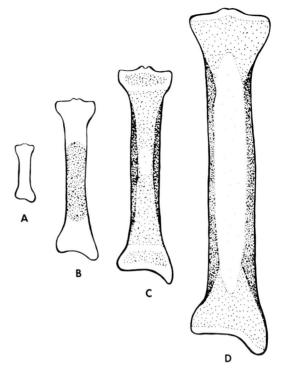

Fig. 8-2. Bone ossification scheme. A, Fetal model. B, Primary ossification center. C, Epiphyseal ossification centers and early staff modeling with cortex and medullary canal. D, Final adult form: all ossification centers united into one bone, cancellous bone restricted to metaphyseal areas, shaft characterized by dense cortex and medullary canal. (Adapted from Arey, L. B.: Developmental anatomy, ed. 7, Philadelphia, 1974, W. B. Saunders Co.)

quadriceps strength promptly returned. Hence, the previous failure to vigorously extend the knee was not one of mechanical obstruction, but an example of reflex inhibition induced by the pain of distension.[4] Another pain avoidance mechanism is the semiflexed posture initially assumed by swollen joints (Fig. 8-4). This is the position where intra-articular pressures are least.[5] Further deformity is evidence of idleness in an overly protective position and the lack of exercise or splinting to correct malalignment.

Knee-flexion deformity. Weight-bearing in the presence of deformity increases the compressive force on the joint by the requirement of greater muscular action for support. This has been measured experimentally at the knee by use of an articulated cadaver limb instrumented to identify the tibiofemoral, patellofemoral, and quadriceps holding forces.[7]

With the knee fully extended, no quadriceps

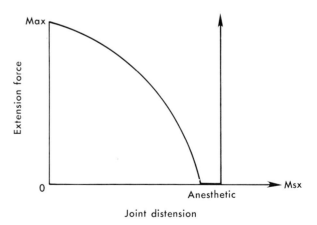

Fig. 8-3. Reflex inhibition of a knee extensor force induced by joint distension. (Adapted from DeAndrade, M. S., Grant, C., and Dixon, A. St. J.: Joint distention and reflex muscle inhibition in the knee, J. Bone Joint Surg. **47A:**313-322, 1965.)

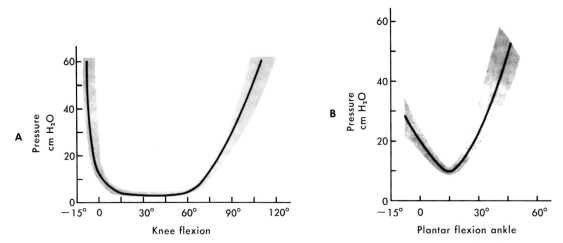

Fig. 8-4. Influence on joint distension on knee and ankle position. **A,** Knee. Note minimal tension is between 15 and 45 degrees of flexion. **B,** Ankle. Note minimal tension is in 15 degrees of plantar flexion. (Adapted from Eyring, E. J., and Murray, W. R.: The effect of joint position on the pressure of intraarticular effusion, J. Bone Joint Surg. **46A:**1235-1241, 1965.)

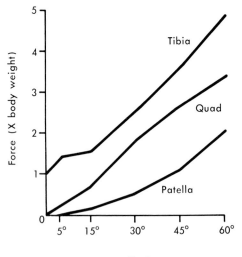

Fig. 8-5. Forces on flexed knee induced by weight bearing. (Adapted from Ford, W. R.: Analysis of knee joint forces during flexed knee stance. University of Southern California—Rancho Los Amigos Hospital Resident Papers, **V:**135-137, 1972.)

force was required and the tibiofemoral joints experienced only "body" load. Flexion of 5 degrees needed a holding force equivalent to 3% of body weight. The knee-stabilizing requirement rose to a force equivalent to 75% of body weight, with the knee flexed 15 degrees. The 30-degree position tripled the force demand (Fig. 8-5). Greater angles required correspondingly higher supporting forces.

The forces registered on the tibial plateaus equaled the quadriceps value plus the basic load of the limb. Hence, with a 20-degree knee flexion deformity, the tibiofemoral junction is experiencing a load twice that of body weight. Patellofemoral compression reflected similar but smaller responses.

A companion study that used kinetic electromyography to measure muscle action during standing and walking with the knee in different degrees of flexion confirmed the preceding findings. The knee-flexion deformity increased the demand not only on the quadriceps but also on all the extensor support muscles.[11]

Clayton observed that patients with rheumatoid arthritis seek orthopedic help when their knee deformities are between 10 and 20 degrees of flexion.[3] This observation coupled with the research data suggests that the effects of sustained quadriceps action equivalent to 1 times body weight is more than the tissues can accept. One can equate this to similar levels of deformity in the other joints of the lower limb.

Valgus deformity. Because body weight is medial to the supporting limb when the other foot is off the ground, the trunk normally is shifted toward the support side with each step. This creates a valgus thrust at the knee with an average 11 degrees of motion.[10] During this time the tibia remains erect.[15] Normally the muscles that cross the joint medially, particularly the vastus medialis, offer protection. However, the arthritic patient with a swollen, painful knee minimizes his quadriceps action to avoid compressing his swollen, sensitive joint structures. This leads to more deformity as the patient walks without adequate muscular support. Orthotic support of such a deformed knee, therefore, must accommodate two forces—that needed to contain the malalignment, and the valgus thrust of each step. Hence, the area of support must be large.

When the patient also has a painful hip, the valgus thrust at the knee is accentuated. To lessen the compressive action of the abductor muscles, the patient, with each step, excessively shifts his weight laterally. Normally the abductors contract vigorously to counterbalance the unsupported, medially aligned trunk. Consequently, the hip is subjected to a compressive force 2.5 times body weight during each period of single stance. This load can be decreased to just body weight if the trunk is shifted laterally so that the body weight is aligned over the hip joint. Then no abductor muscle action is needed as a counterbalance, but this shift occurs primarily at the knee, increasing its stress. A crutch to assist the hip may solve the knee problem as well.

The knee may be similarly stressed indirectly by deformity of the foot, for during each step the body must be aligned over whatever base of support is available. With a varus (inversion) deformity at the subtalar joint, only the lateral side of the foot is available for weight-bearing. Standing now strains the lateral ankle structures as well as tending to increase the deformity. The patient can lessen his stress by positioning his leg to the side so that weight is borne on a valgus knee. In time the knee may actually become the more painful site and the focus of attention. Correction of its alignment, however, should be first directed to the offending foot. The foot support will have two purposes—realignment to whatever extent joint laxity will allow and medial support to broaden the base available for standing. Provision of a medial wedge to fill in the space between the deformed foot and the floor allows the patient to move his body weight more medially; in other words, to use more of his foot for support. This redirects body weight so that it acts as a corrective rather than a deforming force at the foot, ankle, and knee.

Ankle plantar flexion deformity (Fig. 8-6). A 15- or 20-degree contracture is often considered advantageous to the patient because it helps

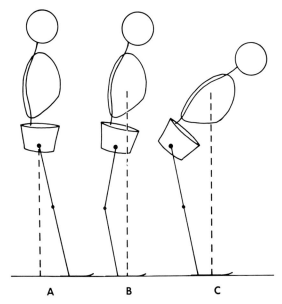

Fig. 8-6. Influence of ankle plantar flexion on standing posture. A, Without postural adaptation, fixed-ankle plantar flexion would place trunk mass behind the area of support provided by the foot and so the patient is too unstable to stand independently. B, Stability can be gained by hyperextension of the knee. C, Lacking hyperextensive knee stability may be gained by flexing the hip. This is possible only if extensors are sufficiently strong. (Adapted from Perry, J.: Kinesiology of lower extremity bracing, Clin. Orthop. Related Res. **102:** 18-31, 1974, Philadelphia, J. B. Lippincott Co.)

stabilize the knee by thrusting the tibia back. Although this is true during the first moments of stance, it can be a major obstacle after that. The stance limb must yield into slight dorsiflexion if the other limb is to accomplish an effective step. Not only does the body have to move forward over the stance limb, the supporting foot also must roll to a heel-off position. Both depend on anterior ankle mobility. An alternate is for some part of the limb to substitute the ankle motion lost through a plantar flexion contracture. The first area that tends to respond is the knee. Its natural range of hyperextension is readily available. The growing child will continue to stretch until the knee range equals the amount needed for an effective contralateral step. If the foot remains flat on the ground throughout stance, the resulting recurvatum can be 40 degrees or more. Even adult knees will eventually stretch this much if there are no protective muscles active.

Hip flexion is the second means of substituting for poor ankle posture. This is tolerated only if the patient has adequate hip extensors. Otherwise, an unstable stance posture is induced. This situation is created by every knee-ankle orthosis that locks the knee in extension and either sets the ankle at neutral or accommodates the existing plantar flexion contracture without the addition of a heel lift. Unless the ankle can be placed into slight dorsiflexion, the patient does not have a stable standing posture. Crutches obviously help but do not provide the same security available when each bone is aligned vertically on the one below.

When these substitutions (knee hyperextension or knee flexion) are not available, the length of the contralateral step is correspondingly shortened. Often the patient can accomplish only a "step-to" gait on that side. Hence plantar flexion deformities at the ankle are subtle sources of knee deformity and poor walking.

One can thus see from these examples that to meet the patient's problem attention cannot be restricted to just the area of complaint. Instead, one needs to analyze both the walking and standing posture of all the segments of the extremity to learn how trunk weight is being accepted.

MOTOR INSUFFICIENCY

Normal motion will not occur unless the appropriate muscle is active. This, in turn, is dependent on the health of its motor units (Fig. 8-7). Each motor unit consists of a lower motor neuron

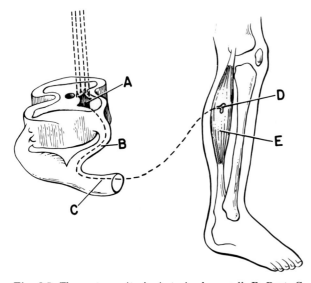

Fig. 8-7. The motor unit. A, Anterior horn cell. B, Root. C, Axon of peripheral nerve. D, Myoneural junction. E, Muscle. (Courtesy of Perry, J., and Hislop, H. J.: Lower extremity bracing, New York, 1967, American Physical Therapy Association.)

and the muscle fibers it activates. These vary in number according to the size and precision of the muscle. Destruction of any segment within the motor unit totally disrupts its function as it performs on an all-or-none basis.

The lower motor neuron is the final common pathway that translates all neurologic instructions into motion. It is comprised of a cell body that lies within the anterior horn of the spinal cord and an axon traversing the peripheral nerve. These two structures in combination with the motor end plate (myoneural junction) and the muscle fibers present four discrete sites within a motor unit that can be selectively injured by different pathologic entities. The anterior horn cells are selectively destroyed by poliomyelitis. Disruption of the axon or its roots occurs with infectious polyneuritis (Guillain-Barré syndrome). Muscle fiber degeneration is the consequence of muscular dystrophy. Myoneural junction failure is the pathomechanism of myasthenia gravis. The clinical differences that make these diseases seem so distinct are their varying potential for recovery, the patterns of muscle involvement, and their tendency to develop contractures.

Poliomyelitis is an acute infectious disease that selectively damages anterior horn cells. The cell bodies that are not completely destroyed gradually recover, with the major gain occurring in the first 6 months. Further improvement in the subsequent 6 to 12 months primarily represents strength gain from overcoming disuse atrophy and function adaptation to permanent deficits. Of the total eventual strength to be recovered, 95% occurs within the first year.[12]

There is no typical pattern of paralysis. A few widely scattered muscles may be weakened, there can be total paralysis of all four extremities, or any of innumerable combinations of partial and complete loss may exist. Within this highly varied picture, one does see several groups of muscles that may be simultaneously disabled. Sharrard explained this with his microscopic mapping of anterior horn cell destruction in patients who had valid muscle tests before their deaths. He found that muscles are supplied by one-to-three segment long columns that overlap and entwine in a fashion that makes several muscles susceptible to the same local lesion.[12]

Muscular dystrophy is a bilaterally symmetric, progressive degeneration of muscle fibers. There are several different patterns of involvement, each with a characteristic age of onset. The most common is called pseudohypertrophic (Duchenne's) because of the disproportionately enlarged calf muscles. Traditionally, this has been considered as an unexplained artifact of the disease. More recently it is believed to represent work hypertrophy, since these muscles are used with all available vigor to stabilize the knees despite weakened quadriceps and hip extensor muscles. Genu recurvatum is not pronounced in these patients because the stress occurs in the later growth years. Also, the intramuscular fibrosis encourages flexion-contracture formation. As the disease progresses, all muscles are involved, leading to characteristic gait deficits and similar substitution techniques. They are less effective, however, as the substituting muscles are also losing motor units through muscle-fiber degeneration. Parallel involvement of the upper limbs and respiratory muscles limit the patient's opportunity to substitute with crutches.

Guillain-Barré syndrome is a rapidly progressive, self-limiting inflammatory disease of unknown etiology that involves the neurons at the root level. After a period of paralysis the disease resolves to full recovery in the majority of instances, but not all. Although sensory involvement is considered part of the syndrome, it is usually inconsequential or not even identifiable. The motor loss is very similar to that of poliomyelitis, except for its bilaterality and the spontaneous resolution. Recovery starts proximally and progresses to the periphery. Clinical experience has demonstrated that the rate of recovery can be obstructed by early overuse of the weakened muscles. The lower limb muscles most susceptible to such strain are the soleus and gluteus medius. Both must be grade four (good) to meet the demands of stance during walking.

Strength requirements

The functional significance of the impairment depends on the number of motor units lost within a muscle as well as the number and identity of the muscles involved. Large muscles with gross function, such as the gluteus maximus, have about 1000 muscle fibers per motor unit, whereas muscles with more discrete actions have smaller units.[6]

Functional demands on muscles differ. The hip abductors and triceps surae (soleus primarily) must have good (manual grade 4) strength for a

Muscle strength (Beasley)	%
Normal	
Real	100
Manual	75
Good	40
Fair	15
Poor	5

Fig. 8-8. Relationship between manual muscle test grade and actual strength as a percent of normal.

patient to walk without a limp; whereas the hip extensors need be only fair (grade 3) and the quadriceps may be poor to zero.

Beasley quantitated the strength of poliomyelitis patients with varying degrees of paralysis and related these values to the findings in a group of normal children in the same age group.[1] (Fig. 8-8). He found grade four (good) was only 40% of normal, fair 15%, and poor 5%. Sharrad, approaching the question from the viewpoint of motor unit density, arrived at very similar values for the manual muscle test grades.[14] In a group of patients who died from poliomyelitis, he compared actual anterior horn cell count to their manual-strength grade. Hence the least evidence of weakness by manual test means the patient has only about 40% of average normal strength. The fact that patients can walk with grades two and three (poor and fair) is indicative of the low demand made by walking in comparison to normal total locomotor potential.

Respiratory impairment from diaphragm paralysis is another potential limitation of the patient's ability to walk. If the lower limbs are normal, a vital capacity of 20% of normal is adequate; otherwise, the demands are high because of the extra energy consumed by an abnormal gait.

Gait characteristics

Despite their differences in etiology and clinical course, patients with pure motor unit loss (poliomyelitis, muscular dystrophy, and Guillain-Barré syndrome) have a strong common bond. They have a tremendous ability to substitute.

With both selective motor control and sensation intact, the remaining musculature can be marshalled to perform with maximum advantage. Being acutely aware of even minor position changes, they are able to respond promptly and automatically with the proper adaptation. This allows them to alter the timing of their muscle action so that they can absorb considerable loss without limping. Further paralysis necessitates substitutive posturing. Orthoses are accepted as functional aids either to lessen a cosmetic limp or to provide function when the patient is too paralyzed (or deformed) to effectively substitute.

Spontaneous awareness of the alignment needed to maintain stance stability or clear the floor during swing in the presence of specific motor loss leads to characteristic limp patterns. They are employed by all patients with sufficient selective control and proprioception to sense and create these substitutive motions. Hence these limps are a model of motor-control efficiency, which can be used to judge, in other types of disability, how much of the functional impairment is the influence of sensory or central control loss; that is, if the musculature is present, one would expect the characteristic limp unless these other disabling factors exist.

The patient's first response is to establish a stable standing posture. When muscle strength is minimal, trunk weight is aligned so it will act as a holding force on one side of the joint while simultaneously tensing an opposing ligament for contralateral support. Both the hip and knee have a dense ligament on one side so that any degree of hyperextension offers weight-bearing stability. This is not available at the ankle. Thus the patient has to rely on active control, a useful contracture or extreme posturing, as the normal stance position is in midrange. To be balanced, body weight must be aligned over the middle of the foot. This point is anterior to the ankle at the naviculocuneiform junction. Normally this places the ankle in slight dorsiflexion (Fig. 8-9). Without direct control by the soleus or a useful restraining contracture, the joint is unstable and the tibia will fall forward, causing knee flexion. To minimize this threat, the patient chooses knee hyperextension and passive ankle plantar flexion (Fig. 8-10). This alignment offers stance stability, but in the growing child the drive for this secure alignment encourages progressive ligamentous stretch and the development of severe hyperextension deformities (useful in childhood, painful in adults).

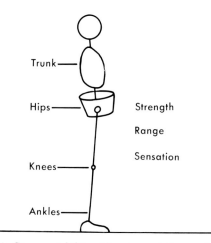

Fig. 8-9. Stance stability. (Courtesy of Perry, J.: Cerebral palsy gait. In Orthopaedic aspects of cerebral spastic, London, 1974, International Medical Publishers.)

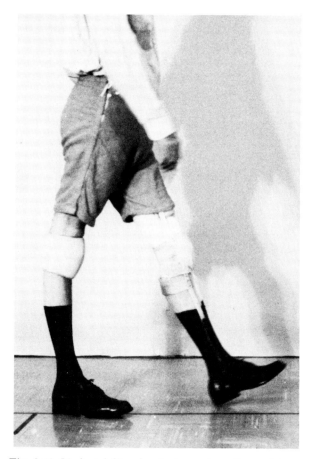

Fig. 8-10. Limb stability, despite trace strength, quadriceps, and soleus, is maintained by sustained ankle plantar flexion and knee hyperextension.

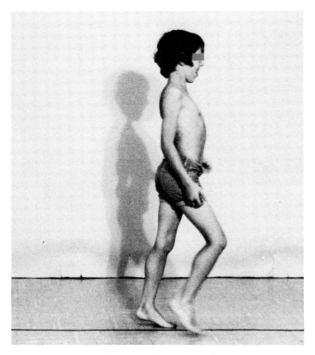

Fig. 8-11. Steppage gait.

During walking the patient's gait is a mixture of postural substitutions that accomplish an effective swing and secure stance. The characteristic substitutions are as follows:

1. Steppage gait (Fig. 8-11). Excessive hip and knee flexion to lift a drop foot when the ankle dorsiflexor muscles are paralyzed.
2. Circumduction gait. Pelvic hiking with a circumferential or a forward flip easily advances the limb when hip and knee flexors are inadequate.
3. Flat foot contact. There is active ankle plantar flexion just before the foot contacts the ground to lock the tibia, and hence the knee is stabilized despite a paralyzed quadriceps. A moderate degree of genu recurvatum may develop in the growing child.
4. Genu recurvatum. There are two mechanisms:
   a. Accommodation to a fixed-ankle plantar flexion contracture (Fig. 8-6).
   b. Paralysis of soleus and quadriceps (Usually there is also severe hip extensor weakness.). The patient stabilizes his limb by active hip extension using residual gluteus maximus, friction between foot and floor, and tension on a mildly tight iliotibial band. (The latter is made taut either by its gluteus maximus attachment or through trunk posturing.) Rapid trunk motion can substitute for gluteal lack.

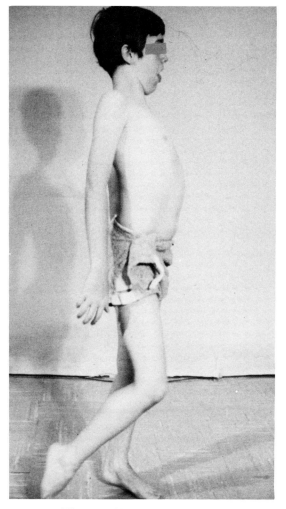

Fig. 8-12. Gluteus maximus limp.

With the knee hyperextended, the tibia is angled posteriorly, thereby locking the ankle in plantar flexion as well. Whatever quadriceps exists assists in the hyperextension maneuver. If this gait is used early in childhood, severe deformity will result. Pain is the sequel in adults.

5. Gluteus maximus limp. Trunk hyperextension to lock hip when extensors are poor (Fig. 8-12).
6. Gluteus medius limp. Lateral deviation of trunk to substitute for inadequate hip abductors (Fig. 8-13).

MOTOR INSUFFICIENCY COMBINED WITH PERIPHERAL SENSORY IMPAIRMENT

Superimposition of sensory impairment on a motor unit loss sharply extends the patient's disability because it curtails his opportunity to

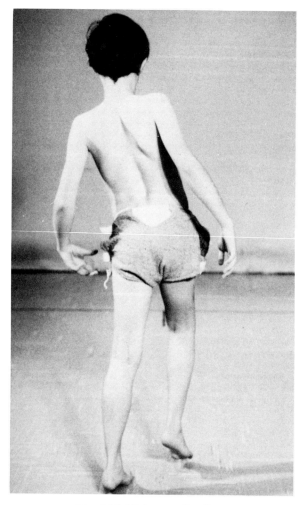

Fig. 8-13. Gluteus medius limp.

substitute. The most common causes are spinal cord injury involving either or both the lumbar and the sacral segments and its congenital equivalent, myelodysplasia. Other causes are cauda equina injury, toxic peripheral neuritis, and peripheral nerve damage (sciatic or posterior tibial, particularly).

Penalties of sensory loss

These patients with the same degree of motor unit loss as the person with poliomyelitis will not walk nearly as well. In the areas of sensory loss, the patient does not know the position of his joints or precisely when or where his feet are contacting the floor; nor are alternate sources of information wholly satisfactory. To see one's feet, the patient must lean over, but this requires hip extensor

control and trunk stability that may not exist. Neither is the sensory input from still innervated proximal body segments a satisfactory substitute for distal loss. The distance between floor and reaction point is so great that postural imbalance occurs more quickly than the body can respond. Consequently, compensatory efforts are initiated too late to be effective or demand more strength than is available. Loss at even one joint (the ankle) presents a measurable impairment and a challenge to limited muscle strength. With greater areas of involvement, the disability rapidly exceeds the patient's ability to compensate sufficiently to walk. Orthotic support of paralyzed, insensitive limbs adds stability but offers no sensory input unless the appliance extends onto an innervated area. So the patient continues to lack the information necessary to know where and how much to move with ease.

When the sensory impairment is an irritative one (as seen in toxic neuritis), pain, tingling, and other unpleasant sensations add to the problems of sensory loss. Standing and walking are discouraged because the soles of the feet, being the most sensitive areas, are irritated by the weight and motion, which abrade the surface.

Lumbosacral spinal cord injury

Whether acquired (trauma) or congenital (myelomeningocele), a lesion in this area results in a flaccid paralysis not unlike poliomyelitis. There is motor loss from damage to the anterior horn cells. Gait will not be as efficient, however, because the sensory fibers in the area are also destroyed. The total pathologic picture is a mixture of root, cell, and tract injury. Occasionally the most distal segments of the cord escape injury, creating areas of spasticity (see discussion on central cord loss for details).

Distribution of motor innervation to the lower limb muscles relates specific muscles within each neurologic segment. As a result, characteristic patterns of paralysis are seen at the different levels of spinal cord injury (Fig. 8-14). When the loss is less than the retained function, classification of the patient's disability focuses on the lesion, that is, an L5-S1 lesion. However, when the loss is dominant, it is customary to focus on the residual ability and speak of functional levels such as L3-L4 and L1-L2.

L5-S1 Lesion (Fig. 8-15). The first and second sacral segments, variably augmented by L5, are

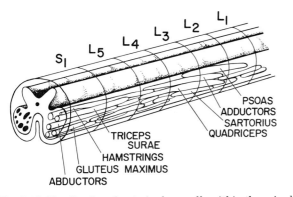

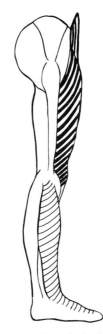

Fig. 8-14. Distribution of anterior horn cells within the spinal cord. Note clustering of hip flexors and abductors and quadriceps in L2-L3 area and the hip abductors, extensors, and ankle plantar flexors at S1. (Adapted from Sharrard, W. J. W.: The distribution of the permanent paralysis in the lower limb in poliomyelitis, a clinical and pathological study, J. Bone Joint Surg. **37B**:540-558, 1955.)

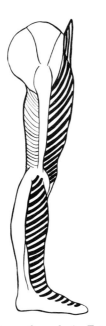

Fig. 8-15. L5-S1 pattern of paralysis. Total paralysis of gluteus maximus hip abductors and triceps surae *(clear areas)*. Weak hamstrings *(light shading)*. Normal hip flexors, quadriceps, and ankle dorsiflexors *(dense shading)*.

Fig. 8-16. L3-L4 pattern of paralysis. Normal hip flexors and quadriceps *(dense shading)*. Weak ankle dorsiflexors *(light shading)*. Total paralysis, hip abductors and extensors, and ankle plantar flexors.

the prime innervation of the gluteus maximus, gluteus medius, soleus, and gastrocnemius. Their loss decreases the patient's hip extensor and ankle plantar flexion stability during stance. If these muscles also have considerable L5 innervation, the patient will be able to substitute well with his normal quadriceps. Then only foot deformities, particularly varus, will be of concern. With associated L5 damage, or if the patient happens to have

more isolated innervation of his hip abductor/extensor musculature and ankle plantar flexors, instability during stance is significant. There will be a major knee flexion thrust each time the limb is loaded. This leads to a serious calcaneus deformity that is aggravated by the still strong action of the tibialis anterior. The limited subtalar support also leads to foot deformities. Sensory deprivation, limited to the soles of the feet, is not critical, as there are active muscles still crossing every joint. Orthotic stabilization of the ankle to restrict dorsiflexion will allow the patient to use trunk lordosis to lock his hips. Crutches are generally needed for lateral stability. Community-level ambulation is the usual accomplishment, though the patient's gait is not normal. Often, surgical tendon transfers or tenodeses replace the orthoses.

L3-L4 functional level (Fig. 8-16). The fourth and fifth lumbar segments are the major nerve supply to the hamstrings and tibialis anterior. The fourth segment also contributes to the quadriceps. When both these segments as well as the sacral ones are damaged, all foot control and hip extension are lost. Thus, a drop foot has been added to the previous picture. Foot and ankle sensation (proprioception in particular) is severely im-

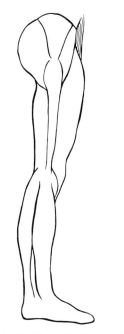

Fig. 8-17. L1-L2 paralysis. Weak hip flexors *(light shading)* complete paralysis, otherwise clear areas.

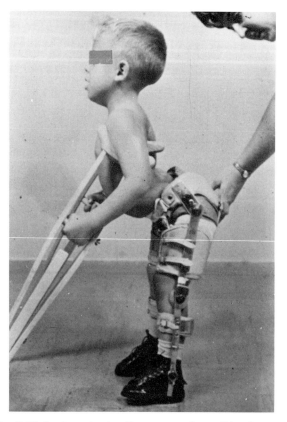

Fig. 8-18. Inadequate standing posture for walking because trunk cannot be aligned over feet. Note that even with full trunk weight on crutches, assistance by a therapist is required for balance. This child does not have the capacity to walk through the combined effects of deformity and paralysis.

paired, if not totally absent. Standing and walking is rarely possible without orthotic support of the ankles. The quadriceps are not strong enough, nor is there adequate position sense between the tibia and foot. Escape of the fourth root preserves the quadriceps and thus improves the patient's potential. The critical factor will be freedom from obstructive contractures (hip and knee flexion, ankle plantar flexion), for they must be able to passively stabilize their hips by postural alignment.

The child with myelomeningocele is also threatened with dislocating hips because the hip adductors are still strong while the abductors are paralyzed. Lacking dorsiflexors and sitting more than they stand, such children commonly develop plantar flexion contractures and foot deformities.

L1-L2 functional level (Fig. 8-17). The first lumbar segment represents the highest neurologic level contributing motor and sensory function to the lower extremities. In combination with the second, third and fourth segments it innervates the hip flexors. There is a basic anatomic rule that a joint is innervated by the same neurologic level as the muscles crossing it. Available hip proprioception can thus be judged by the strength of the patient's hip flexors.

When this muscle group is totally paralyzed,

one should not expect an adult to accomplish useful walking. Children with their shorter leverages do much better, particularly if they are started early. With all position sense lost at the hip as well as more distally, the patient will have to use quite exaggerated posturing to assure stance stability at the hips. The adult may accomplish the motions, but the effort will be so costly that it serves only as exercise, not useful locomotion. Any degree of hip, knee, or ankle deformity that denies the patient easy access to postural stance stability will deny him all possibility of walking or standing. These patients should not be expected to use their arms for physical support during standing, as these arm muscles are also their only means of taking a step. To accomplish either a swing-through or swing-to gait, they will have to work vigorously. No muscle will repeatedly tolerate this level of exertion unless there is an adequate rest period between

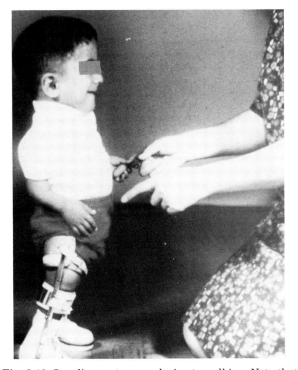

Fig. 8-19. Standing posture conducive to walking. Note that despite complete lower-limb paralysis, trunk is centered over hips so that arm support is not required, just one finger contact for balance. Knee-ankle orthoses are set in sufficient dorsiflexion to allow the patient to lock his paralyzed hips by hyperextension. No pelvic band is necessary.

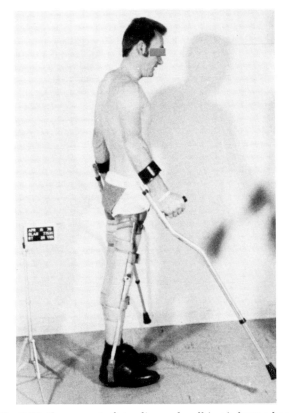

Fig. 8-20. Energy cost of standing and walking is least when minimal trunk lordosis is required to lock hips.

efforts. If the arms are used to support the trunk during standing as well as to lift the body during swing, such a rest is unavailable (Fig. 8-18). Hence the basic requirement is easily attained passive hip extension (Fig. 8-19). This, of course, means the absence of any obstructive flexion (contracture or spasticity). A second requirement is that the amount of lordosis needed to stabilize trunk and hips be minimal (Fig. 8-20).

Early standards of pelvic control by fair-strength trunk muscles' being adequate if the patient were contracture free to have proved to be unrealistic. In fact, the latest review of patients with spinal cord injury who are independent walkers on a daily basis showed they not only have hip flexor muscle action (and hence sensation) but also have active control of at least one knee.[9]

CENTRAL CONTROL DYSFUNCTION

Spinal cord injuries in the thoracic area and lesions involving the brain paralyze patients through loss of central control. Their motor units are still intact, but the patients can no longer dictate how they move. Instead, they respond to a variety of stimuli, leading to involuntary motions commonly grouped under the term "spasticity" (Fig. 8-21).

The intact nervous system provides selective control, habitual control, and suppression of primitive motor responses. Selective control allows the individual to move one joint independently of the other and to elect the direction, intensity, and duration of the action. Habitual control is the source of routine actions by which the normal person automatically carries out his daily tasks. These two types of control operate on a background of primitive stretch and motion patterns created by lower centers of sensorimotor exchange. Under normal conditions the actions of the lesser centers are inconspicuous because they are subdued and integrated by the extrapyramidal cerebral pathways. With a high spinal cord injury or brain damage, the suppressive influence of the

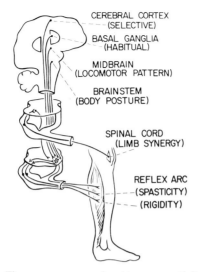

Fig. 8-21. The seven sources of motion are available through normal and primitive control mechanisms.

cerebrum is removed. Unmasked, the lesser centers of sensorimotor exchange become the instigators of raw action. These may still be useful if their timing and strength are not too inappropriate, otherwise they are obstructive. Destruction of the cerebral cortical or basal ganglia centers or their tracts thus not only deprives the patient of his mechanisms for initiating normal motion, but also exposes to varying extent the five types of primitive motion. Four of the primitive motions represent automatic responses to slow stretch, fast stretch, limb position, and body position. The fifth is a form of voluntary limb action constituting a primitive locomotor pattern.

Quick stretch is the stimulus for true spasticity. The reaction is clonus. It represents the response of velocity-sensitive receptors within the muscle spindle.

Slow stretch will elicit a sustained muscle action that is customarily misinterpreted for contracture. This represents a response of the length change sensors of the muscle spindle and should be called rigidity. A quick stretch also creates a change in muscle length and hence can stimulate these sensors, thereby initiating rigidity as well as spasticity. Rigidity can be differentiated from contracture only with a neurologic suppressive agent such as an anesthetic or icing or by relaxing neuromuscular facilitation or fatigue.

Limb position alters the tone of the limb muscles, thereby setting their sensitivity to stretch. With the hip and knee extended, the basic exten-

sor muscles (gluteus maximus, quadriceps, and, in particular, the ankle plantar flexors) become tense. They are relaxed when these joints are flexed. Similarly, the flexor muscles including the ankle dorsiflexors are primed by limb flexion. The 45-degree position is roughly the dividing line; that is, when the knee is extended for walking or standing, the hip will also extend and the ankle will be pulled down into plantar flexion. (With flexion of the knee, these muscles are relaxed and readily permit dorsiflexion.)

Both the soleus and gastrocnemius are activated; hence, posturing at the foot is not merely a passive response of a contracted gastrocnemius as is generally assumed. Nor is it spasticity; that is, the muscle was not stretched but underwent a change in tone because of a difference in total limb position.

Release of the vestibular system in the brainstem makes the tone of the limb muscles highly responsive to body position. Extensor tone in the lower limbs is increased whenever the patient is erect. This is most conspicuous at the triceps surae. (In the upper limb the response is flexion.) The examiner may also find that the patient is incapable of voluntarily moving his limb while supine, yet when standing he had sufficient control to walk. This means weak control signals, inadequate in the lying position, were enhanced by the upright posture. Because the purpose of the orthotic program is to attain optimum posture for walking, his needs must be determined with the patient standing. Otherwise, the problem will be underestimated and hence inadequately managed.

A locomotor center within the midbrain offers a means for primitive gait when the patient's cerebral pathways have been damaged. This center permits the patient to voluntarily use the extensor and flexor mass patterns in a reciprocal fashion for walking; that is, he can, at will, take a step or stand still, but when he chooses to move all three joints (hip, knee, and ankle), they will move simultaneously and in a set fashion, which he cannot moderate. For example, during the latter part of swing, one normally reaches for step length by extending the knee while maintaining hip flexion and ankle dorsiflexion. The patient dependent on his primitive locomotor center will not be able to hold these flexed postures. Instead, the hip will extend and the ankle will plantar flex as he extends his knee. Conversely, in taking

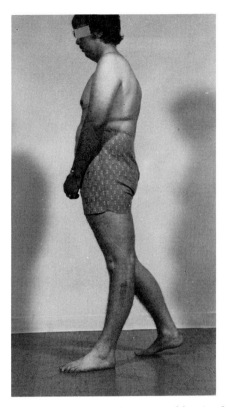

Fig. 8-22. Extensor pattern is characterized by simultaneous hip extension, knee extension, and ankle plantar flexion.

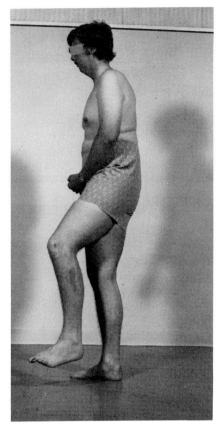

Fig. 8-23. Flexor pattern. Simultaneous hip flexion, knee flexion, and ankle dorsiflexion.

a step, hip and knee flexion and ankle dorsiflexion occur together. The extensor pattern is equivalent to the midstance standing posture with an element of excess ankle plantar flexion (Fig. 8-22), whereas the flexor pattern abruptly brings the limb into a position midway between initial and terminal swing (Fig. 8-23). This recovers the limb from its trailing positon and advances it slightly ahead of the supporting limb, with the knee remaining semiflexed. If the patient is totally dependent on locomotor patterning for limb control, as he extends his knee in preparation for stance, a complete extensor response is initiated. The hip retracts from its flexed position, and the foot is pulled down into plantar flexion.

Not all step length is lost, however, because the normal motion of the uninvolved limb has allowed the body to advance; hence the new vertical position is still somewhat ahead of the sound supporting foot. Only the more severely involved patients have this much difficulty.

High spinal cord injury

Thoracic and cervical levels of injury present different potentials for walking because of the type of residual possible.

The relative inflexibility of the thoracic spinal cord and its narrow vertebral canal tend to translate all injuries at this level into complete transections. These patients have no residual of normal selective or habitual control, yet they are subject to the motion reflexes present within the cord. Their lower-limb neuron are free to react to slow and fast stretch and to the mass influences of limb posture. Lesions in the T9-T6 range are particularly tantalizing. The patient is usually young, has active control of a major segment of his trunk, and has normal upper limbs with which to operate crutches. Fitted with appropriate knee-ankle orthoses, he can always stand by propping himself on his crutches. The more vigorous will also accomplish a swing-to or swing-through gait. But the energy expenditure is too demanding for more than an exercise experience. There are basic deficits that prohibit making the task easier with training or devices. These are the absence of both sensation and active control of pelvis and hips and the presence of primitive spinal motor responses. For a stable stance he must lock his lumbar spine and hips by aligning his trunk in extreme lordosis. Stretch on the hip flexors may cause them to react and pull him out of this safe posture. Of course, any hip flexion contracture is prohibitive. To take a step, he must maintain his precarious lordotic alignment while lifting his crutches, advance them, and then lift his body and swing it forward. The amount he can move his crutches forward will be dictated by the degree of stance stability he was able to attain and on whether he can move his crutches ahead faster than his trunk will fall if he leans forward. Advancement of the body is also extremely challenging as his lack of lumbar and hip control means the motion must occur entirely at his shoulders. This makes the body one rigid lever with considerable weight distally because of the orthotic mass that is required to control limb "spasticity" and accept the thrusts of abrupt loading from a swing-through gait. The addition of a spinal component to the lower-limb orthoses does provide lumbar and hip stability for stance, but it also increases the weight and rigidity, which the patient must manage. The result is that the disadvantages outweigh the advantages.

Coupled with these mechanical barriers are the effects of lost sensation. The patient is no longer automatically aware of his limb position in any plane (sagittal, coronal, transverse). Hence, malalignments are not corrected locally while they are still minor. Instead, postural errors are not appreciated until they disturb the upper trunk or head. By this time, great effort is required to restore balance. Each step recreates this situation. With knees and ankles rigidly locked, the body and limbs must be lifted and swung in one large motion rather than by a sequence of controlled position changes at each joint. This makes the margin between stability and falling very narrow. The energy cost of walking in this fashion is so great that it is a strenuous athletic feat that leaves the person exhausted, even when performed by powerful, healthy young men. Such walking is not a useful means of locomotion. The patient cannot travel far enough and is too tired to be effective when he has arrived. Exceptions

to this experience are too rare to justify considering walking a practical goal for the patient with a complete thoracic lesion. As part of his upper-limb training for easy body transfer, however, he may be provided adequate temporary orthoses to try walking so that he can experience its inefficiency and choose the wheelchair as his preferable mode of travel.

Cervical spinal cord anatomy allows a greater tolerance for motion extremes. This, coupled with modern emergency care, is limiting many acute injuries to incomplete lesions. As a result, the patient retains some of his normal selective and habitual motor control and sensation (Fig. 8-30). Superimposed on this will be the action of uninhibited lower motor neuron reacting to stretch and primitive limb synergies. The exact picture will depend on the areas of spinal cord damage and the severity of the loss. There are three basic patterns of incomplete injury. Hemisection is called a Brown-Sequard lesion. Because of the

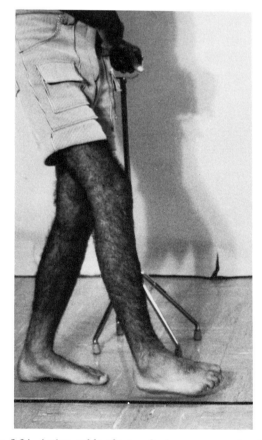

Fig. 8-24. Active ankle plantar flexion accompanying knee extension as a residual of extensor pattern.

crossing of the sensory tracts the patient retains motor control on one side and sensation in the opposite limb. Anterior cord injury will impair motor control in both limbs but preserve sensation bilaterally. There is also a central cord lesion that generally is quite profound, but in less severe situations there is selective segmental sparing. The sacral tracts, being most peripheral, are preserved best and the cervical tracts are most damaged. Thoracic and lumbar tracts have correspondingly intermediate positions and sensitivity to injury.

The basic ability of the patient to walk will depend on how much sensation and normal motor control remains. Bilateral involvement is far greater than just twice unilateral impairment, as the patient cannot call on one limb to substitute for the other. The overlay of primitive stretch reflexes and limb synergies will make the gait awkward and less efficient but, by themselves, do not dictate whether the patient can walk. Their

gait deficits are comparable to bilateral adult hemiplegia.

Adult hemiplegia

A cerebrovascular accident, trauma, or any other form of pathologic condition that is localized primarily on one side of the brain may cause hemiplegia at any age. The resulting control is a composite of altered sensation, impaired-to-absent selective control, primitive locomotor patterns, erect postural reflexes, limb posture tone, spasticity, and rigidity. A hemiplegic patient's ability to walk depends on the presence of voluntary limb control (selective or patterned), adequate proprioception, and intact body balance. Selective control provides the normal sequential, asynchronous yet posturally related changes at the hip, knee, and ankle during both stance and swing. This allows a smooth, continuous flow from one step to the next. In contrast, the primitive locomotor patterns

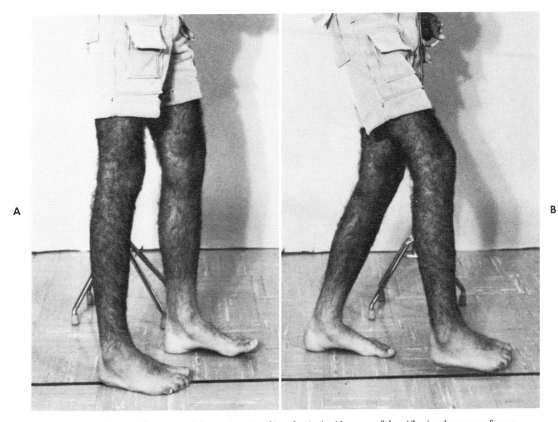

A   B

Fig. 8-25. Late midstance ankle motion (trailing foot). **A,** Absence of dorsiflexion because of overactivity of the ankle plantar flexors at the presence of toe clawing in the hemiplegic limb advancement of stance limb and body is restricted with corresponding amount of shortening of the step by the sound limb. **B,** Exaggeration of normal dorsiflexion by his sound limb. This is used to extend step length of his hemiplegic limb, which lacks full knee extension.

consist of abrupt simultaneous extension (or flexion) of hip, knee, and ankle in a single mass movement.

The subtle interplay of these primitive control mechanisms is readily demonstrated by the variations in the severity of a patient's equinovarus foot deformity by examinations conducted under different situations. During walking the deformity may appear extreme and feel very rigid when manual correction is attempted with the patient standing. The problem represents a mixture of stretch reactions, limb extensor tone, erect posture tone, and the extensor locomotor pattern. If the examination is conducted with the patient sitting, the deformity will feel much less rigid than was anticipated because the flexion of the hip released limb extensor tone. With the patient supine, there may be very little resistance to manual correction, for the vestibular and locomotor pattern are no longer active.

The extensor pattern, though providing limb stability during stance, also creates performance obstacles for both limbs. The prime deterrent is

excessive ankle plantar flexor muscle action. This deprives the patient of a heel-strike (Fig. 8-24). Instead, his initial floor contact will be made with the flat foot. During midstance he will be denied the yielding action that normally allows slight dorsiflexion, which permits the body to pass ahead of the stationary foot (Fig. 8-25). The sustained plantar flexion also holds body weight back on the heel during terminal stance, thereby depriving the patient the opportunity to roll onto his forefoot (heel off) during terminal stance. The sequel to this is the loss of knee flexion in his preswing posture (Fig. 8-26). The culminations of these motion limitations is a restriction of trunk advancement and corresponding shortening of the step length by the other limb (Fig. 8-25, A). Inability to shift his weight forward onto his forefoot and the subsequent loss of knee flexion in his preswing posture restricts his ability to gain adequate knee flexion for toe clearance during swing; that is, the 35 degrees usually gained passively is lost, so that an automatic 35-degree arc of active flexion by itself is inadequate. Sev-

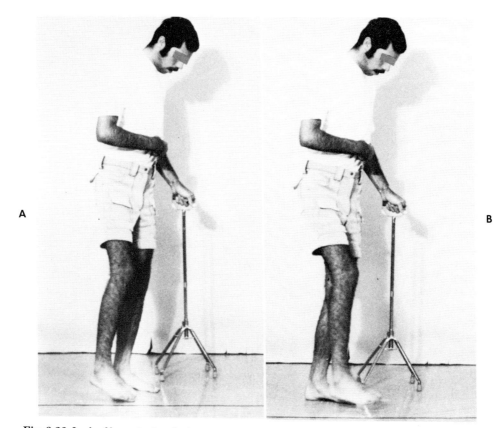

Fig. 8-26. Lack of knee flexion during swing. **A,** Initial swing. **B,** Midswing (toe clearance gained by hiking his pelvis).

enty degrees of flexion normally is required. This need is lessened with a shorter step by the other limb.

Excessive foot and ankle muscle activity also causes varus during stance (Fig. 8-27). The prime offender is the soleus. Its insertion on the os calcis is far medial of the subtalar joint axis. Other contributors are the tibialis posterior and the two

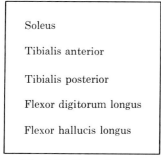

```
Soleus

Tibialis anterior

Tibialis posterior

Flexor digitorum longus

Flexor hallucis longus
```

Fig. 8-27. Sites of varus.

long toe flexors (hallucis and common). Often, tibialis anterior muscle activity persists through stance as a stretch reaction, adding another varus mechanism. The seriousness of this posturing depends on the severity of the muscle action. If postural correction is accomplished easily, orthotic restraint can be flexible. If considerable force is required, then the orthotic device must be rigid.

When the primitive extensor pattern is inadequate, the greatest loss occurs in the soleus and hip extensors. The quadriceps generally survives best of the three areas. Soleus weakness deprives the patient of tibial stability during stance. Without adequate restraint by this muscle the impact of initial floor contact thrust the tibia forward, causing the knee to flex (Fig. 8-28, A). Such flexion is reflected at the hip as well. Thus a small amount of uncontrolled motion at the ankle, which most observers tend to ignore, can have major impact

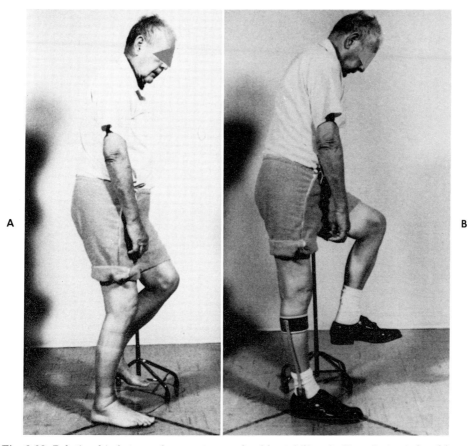

Fig. 8-28. Relationship between knee posture and ankle stability. **A,** Knee flexion induced by a weak soleus, allowing tibia to fall forward. **B,** Knee extension accomplished by an ankle-locking orthosis to replace the absent soleus.

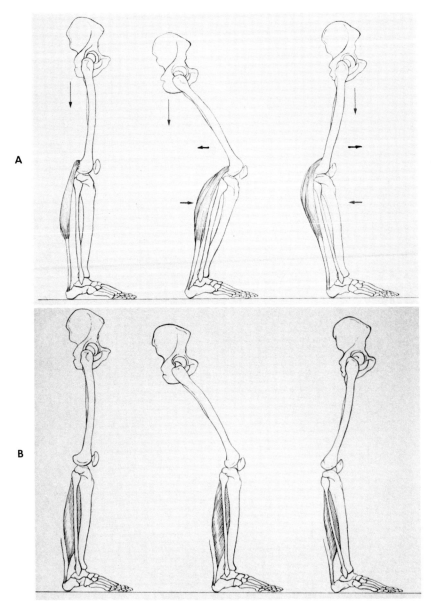

Fig. 8-29. Independent action of the triceps surae muscles. **A,** Gastrocnemius. *Left,* Normal alignment with the gastrocnemius relaxed. *Center,* Knee flexion induced by contraction of the gastrocnemius. *Right,* When knee is locked by passive hyperextension, gastrocnemius action is directed to ankle. **B,** Soleus. With origin entirely on the tibia, soleus has no direct effect on the knee. Hence ankle position can be maintained independently of knee posture. *Left,* Normal alignment. *Center,* Knee flexed, ankle unchanged. *Right,* Knee hyperextended.

on total limb stability. If there is accompanying hip extensor weakness, the patient will be unable to walk unless an orthosis is provided to restrict ankle dorsiflexion. (Fig. 8-28, *B*). An adjustable locked ankle orthosis is the item of choice. The presence of a gastrocnemius is not an effective substitute. To the contrary, contraction at the

time of initial floor contact will cause greater knee flexion because its origin is in the femur. Patients have to prevent this by deliberate knee hyperextension (Fig. 8-29). This is possible only if there is adequate proprioception and selective control.

Moderate hip weakness can be effectively supplemented with a cane, but more severe loss denies the patient all opportunity to walk. The observed gait errors are excessive knee flexion and a forward drop of the trunk (Fig. 8-28, A). Theoretically the knee can be held with a locking orthosis, but this prevents the patient using the flexion pattern to take a step. Also, there is not the selective control to align the trunk for stability. The flexion pattern provides a means of taking a step. Simultaneous hip flexion, knee flexion, and ankle dorsiflexion accomplish two needed actions. The limb is picked up sufficiently for the toe to clear the ground. It also is advanced from its former trailing position to a point slightly ahead of the stance limb. However, if the patient is totally dependent on primitive locomotor patterns, further step length is not available. Instead, as the patient extends his knee to reach ahead, he will lose his hip flexion because a complete extensor pattern will be activated, causing hip extension. The ankle plantar flexion component of the extensor pattern also deprives the patient of his previous dorsiflexed posture; so initial floor contact will lack heel strike.

A second concern with the prestance foot positioning is varus. The tibialis anterior is the only ankle dorsiflexor that participates in the flexor pattern. In addition, it may be augmented by active toe flexors or the tibialis posterior's contracting out of phase. See list below:

> *Sources of varus*
> Soleus
> Tibialis posterior
> Flexor hallucis longus
> Flexor digitorum longus
> Tibialis anterior

Often the flexor pattern is incomplete. The most common failure is lack of ankle dorsiflexion, leading to a drop foot during midswing and terminal swing and the lack of heel strike at the initiation of stance. By itself, a drop foot is not the cause of toe drag during initial swing. Knee flexion is the key. If the patient has this control, he will merely step higher to clear the floor. (Fig. 8-30). Other substitutions, such as circumduction, pelvic hiking, and leaning far to the side, appear to be means of accommodating for a drop foot, but really they are replacing absent knee flexion. When the equinus during swing merely represents absent dorsiflexor action and not a contracture or nonphasic plantar flexor muscle action, a flexible orthosis is very effective. However, even with the

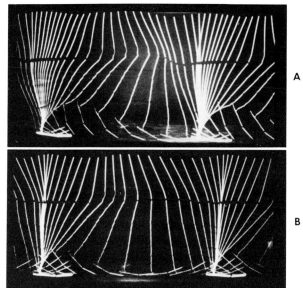

Fig. 8-30. Strobe light record of hemiplegic patient with passive drop foot. **A,** Unaided drop-foot gait. **B,** Normal limb action with ankle dorsiflexion activated by an implanted electronic stimulation of the peroneal nerve (Rancho-Medtronic unit).

ankle stabilized at neutral there will be a noticeable toe drag during initial swing if the patient lacks knee flexion. This problem disappears as the swing limb proceeds ahead of the stance limb.

If the patient has both deficiencies, that is, absent knee flexion and ankle dorsiflexion, there will be a severe toe drag throughout swing, making advancement of the limb very difficult, particularly from its initial trailing position.

Knee flexion may also be blocked by quadriceps spasticity. At times it is just the rectus that has changed phase, making its hip flexor action dominant. Unfortunately, this also obstructs knee flexion.

Lack of hip flexion will prevent the patient from walking because he cannot take a step. Few persons have sufficient trunk control to substitute with pelvic hiking when inadequate hip flexion is their problem. Impairments of hip and knee flexion generally signify rather severe lesions with trunk deficits as well.

To provide a clear picture of the hemiplegic mechanisms influencing a patient's gait, the complete lesion was described. This presented total dependence on locomotor patterns and responsiveness to all the primitive reflexes. Partial loss is a more common event. Each patient demonstrates a slightly different mixture of residual (or recovered) selective and primitive mechanisms. These mixtures are evidenced in two basic ways. Some patients display selective control of poor to fair strength on muscle test; yet when walking, they employ primitive patterns of greater strength. This is one example of the inability to make a functional interpretation from a static test in the patient with an upper motor neuron lesion. Other patients have sufficient control to moderate the abruptness of limb action during gait. Generally the break in primitive pattern dominance occurs first at the hip. This permits the patient to maintain hip flexion during terminal swing and at the same time extend his knee. However, the foot continues within the pattern and is pulled into plantar flexion as the knee extends, even though during earlier knee flexion there was good ankle dorsiflexion.

When one is treating patients with brain damage (stroke and brain trauma, in particular), cognition is an additional factor to weigh during the evaluation of a disabled person's ability to walk. Cognition is the collective term for all the functions of the mind. Those that relate to walking are initiative, imagination, adaptability, comprehension, judgment, and memory. Any disabled gait is more difficult than normal function. A person must be motivated to put out this extra effort. Also, he must be able to develop effective substitutes either through his own adaptability or by the teachings of others. To profit from the teaching of others, he must comprehend their instructions and be capable of remembering them. Lastly, if failure to perform in an appropriately adapted fashion threatens his safety, he must use judgment in the tasks he attempts and wisely accept the security offered by an orthosis or various other walking aids.

Sensory loss may consist of impaired proprioception in the limb (common at the foot; may involve the knee) or a disturbed body image. If the patient has good position sense at the hip and active patterns, an orthosis that locks the ankle will provide enough indirect feedback for an effective and safe gait. Impaired body image denies the patient awareness of that side of his body. As a result, he fails to appropriately align his trunk mass to stand erect. Instead, the patient tends to fall toward the hemiplegic side (Fig. 8-31). One's natural tendency is to blame the hemiplegic limb for not providing support, yet the amputee does very well with no limb at all.

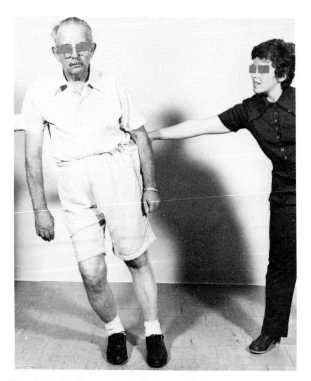

Fig. 8-31. Patient with body image failing to accommodate for lack of support by the hemiplegic limb. Note lack of concern on his face.

Cerebral palsy

Cerebral palsy is a difficult entity to describe because it neither represents one cause nor one syndrome. Instead, the term refers to a group of motion disorders resulting from brain damage occurring in the formative periods of fetal development, birth and early infancy. Within the common denominator of control dysfunction are included the two basic patterns: spastic paralysis and dyskinesia. Each has several subdivisions.

Spastic paralysis. Deficient selective control, primitive responses, and impaired sensation characterize the actions of these patients. Depending on the limbs involved, their disability is subclassified as hemiplegia, diplegia, and quadriplegia.

Hemiplegic children are always effective walkers, even though limb function on the involved side is far from normal. The typical gait deficits of cerebral palsy hemiplegia are very similar to those of the adult picture, with minor exceptions. They generally have some selective control and, as a result, their hip abductors are active. Proprioceptive deficits are less severe and body image is intact. Orthotic concerns focus on the foot, with equinovarus being the characteristic challenge.

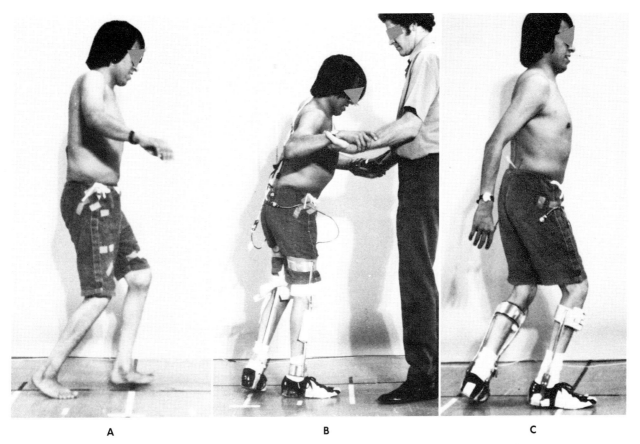

A   B   C

Fig. 8-32. Diplegic gait. The patient had gastrocnemius and adductor muscle releases several years ago. **A,** Free gait. Note patient's ability to advance himself by using his forefoot as a rocker. **B,** Loss of stride length when knee orthosis is used to correct his knee flexion posture. **C,** Stride length also shortened by ankle orthosis that blocks foot-rocker action.

The diplegic child is characterized by "spastic" impairment of both lower limbs. Mild upper limb involvement is not uncommon, and some authorities say that there is always some, though a very precise examination may be needed to display it.

Characteristically, these patients walk and stand in a crouch with hips and knees flexed and weight borne only on the forefeet. Their gait is largely dependent on primitive locomotor patterns with superimposed influences of hypertonicity and later contractures. Gastrocnemius contracture is such a prominent finding that all "toe stance" tends to be attributed to errors at the ankle. However, flat-foot support cannot be accomplished unless either the knees are straightened or the ankles are put into excessive dorsiflexion. The latter posture is a common sequel of surgical gastrocnemius release. Freed from the restraints of a contracture, the ankle yields to the

dictates of the knees. Generally this accommodation is not complete, so there is now a mixture of knee flexion, the heel-off stance, and a visible degree of ankle dorsiflexion (Fig. 8-32).

Orthotic assistance is often sought to correct this unsightly posture. Any attempt to counteract the excessive ankle posture with ankle-foot orthoses without lessening the knee posture shortens the patient's step. It deprives him of the tibial tilt needed to move his body forward over the supporting foot. Straightening of the knees with locked orthoses is a much more severe restraint of the patient's ability to walk because it blocks the primitive flexion pattern needed to take a step. Indirect control can be gained by influencing the femur at the hip. The adductor muscles, in addition to causing scissoring, are also hip flexors. If their spasticity or contracture levels are not too severe, orthoses that place the limb in less adduction also can decrease the pull of these muscles. Loss of their flexion action allows the femur to assume a more vertical posture with corresponding improvement in knee alignment. Free flexion is still available at both hip and knee; so primitive locomotor patterns can still be used to take steps. Contracted muscles, however, fight such restraint. In these instances, surgical release must precede the use of training orthoses (if such are indicated).

Poor balance results from body image impairment, proprioceptive loss, and the fact that these children lack a normal side to provide compensatory action. Hence, precarious gait or total inability to walk is a likely state. These patients must be assessed carefully so that assessment of their potential is realistic.

Quadriplegia (really a bilateral hemiplegia) not only represents grossly equal involvement of all four limbs, it is consistently a more severe lesion. Scissoring, equinus, and difficulty balancing are the primary gait characteristics.

Dyskinesia. The involuntary motions that characterize these patients may be alternating (tremor), writhing (chorea form), or random (athetosis). Athetosis is by far the most commonly seen disorder in this group. More often it is mixed with spasticity rather than presenting in a pure form. Although the muscles are relaxed when the child is resting in a well-supported position, any voluntary act or postural demand promptly sets off widely random, involuntary movements. The strength and scope of these actions increase as the patient exerts greater effort. Thus attempts to willfully restrain oneself only exaggerate the response. This makes the customary forms of orthoses not only ineffective but a handicap. There is no fixed pattern to control. Also the natural interplay between limb segments during walking means that adjacent joints must increase their action when one is abnormally restrained. The basic pathophysiologic abnormality causing the problem is not known. Neither strength nor sensation are lacking. A recent concept is that the children experience inappropriate proprioception.

ENERGY INSUFFICIENCY

Energy consumption is no concern when one is dealing with young, healthy individuals with mild to moderate impairment. However, the broader range of pathologic condition that is receiving attention today requires one to consider both the amount of energy the disabled gait will demand and the total energy productivity of the patient. Restraints are related to the cardiovascular and pulmonary systems, as the basic need is transportation of sufficient oxygen to the muscles. Myocardial infarction, other types of heart failure, diabetes, emphysema, bronchitis, or other forms of chronic pulmonary obstructive disease are common findings in the age groups of patients subject to strokes. Hence the medical history must become a significant factor in the gait plan.

REFERENCES

1. Beasley, W. C.: Quantitative muscle testing: Principles and applications to research and clinical services, Arch. Phy. Med. **42**:398-425, 1961.
2. Bick, E. M.: Source book of orthopedics, New York, 1968, Hofner Publishing Co.
3. Clayton, M.L.: Surgery of the lower extremity in rheumatoid arthritis, J. Bone Joint Surg. **45A**:1517, 1963.
4. deAndrade, M. S., Grant, C., and Dixon, A. St. J.: Joint distension and reflex muscle inhibition in the knee, J. Bone Joint Surg. **47A**:313-322, 1965.
5. Eyring, E. J., and Murray, W. R.: The effect of joint position on the pressure of intraarticular effusion, J. Bone Joint Surg. **46A**:1235-1241, 1964.
6. Feinstein, B., Linderard, B., Nyman, E., and Wholfart, G.: Morphologic studies of motor units in normal human muscles, Acta Anat. **23**:127-142, 1955.
7. Ford, W. R.: Analysis of knee joint forces during flexed knee stance. In Resident Papers, University of Southern California, Rancho Los Amigos Hospital **5**:135-137, 1972.
8. Haas, S. L.: Retardation of bone growth by a wire loop, J. Bone Joint Surg. **27A**:25-36, 1945.
9. Hussey, R. W.: Ambulation in spinal cord injury patients. In Resident Papers, University of Southern California, Rancho Los Amigos Hospital **5**:215-219, 1972.
10. Kettlekamp, D. B., Johnson, R. S., Smidt, G. L., Chao, E. Y. S., and Walker, M.: An electrogoniometric study of knee motion in normal gait, J. Bone Joint Surg. **52A**:775-790, 1970.
11. Roby, P. J.: Kinesiology of knee flexion deformity using electromyography. Doctoral dissertation, 1973, Loma Linda University, Loma Linda, Calif.
12. Sharrad, W. J. W.: Muscle recovery in poliomyelitis, J. Bone Joint Surg. **37B**:63-79, 1955.
13. Sharrad, W. J. W.: The distribution of the permanent paralysis in the lower limb in poliomyelitis, J. Bone Joint Surg. **37B**:540-558, 1955.
14. Sharrad, W. J. W.: Correlation between changes in the spinal cord and muscle paralysis in poliomyelitis, Proc. Roy. Soc. Med. **40**:346, 1953.
15. Wright, D. G., Desai, S. M., and Henderson, W. H.: Action of the subtalar and ankle joint complex during the stance phase of walking, J. Bone Joint Surg. **46A**:361-382, 1964.

CHAPTER 9

Biomechanical analysis system

NEWTON C. McCOLLOUGH, III, M.D.

An accurate biomechanical analysis of the lower limb is fundamental to proper orthotic prescription. Until relatively recently, there has been no organized or systematic approach to analyzing and recording basic information relating to an impaired lower limb for the purpose of prescribing an orthosis. More often than not, the physician will perform an examination, do some mental calculating, and then write a "prescription," based upon a rather meager knowledge of orthotic components. Frequently little thought is given to analyzing specific biomechanical defects present in a given limb with the aim of translating this information into an appropriate mechanical substitute. Even when this is done, all too often the device prescribed impairs to some degree the normal biomechanical functions that coexist in the same limb. For example, an orthosis prescribed for genu recurvatum may also limit normal knee flexion during swing phase and restrict motion of the subtalar joint as well.

The primary function of an orthosis is the control of motion of certain body segments. An ideal orthosis controls only those motions that are abnormal or undesirable and permits motion where normal function can occur. It is apparent, then, that considerable thought should be given to each level of the limb encompassed by an orthosis in order that the prescribed components or component types accurately match the defects present. The basis for orthotic prescription should be an accurate biomechanical analysis of the patient, followed by selection of appropriate components, and finally the creation of an orthotic system from the components selected.

To provide the means by which a biomechanical analysis of the lower limb can be diagrammatically recorded and effectively translated into an orthotic prescription, a technical analysis form has been developed by the Committee on Orthotics and Prosthetics of the American Academy of Orthopaedic Surgeons. This approach to orthotic prescription eliminates any preconceived ideas regarding appliance types such as those associated with specific disease entities or eponyms. The rationale for orthotic prescription is reduced to a process of biomechanical matching of modes of external control to functional deficits. The physician is knowledgeable regarding the patient's functional loss and the type of control that he would like to impose. He is frequently not knowledgeable, however, with regard to the wide variety of orthotic components available and their physical characteristics. The technical analysis form thus serves to form a bridge of communication between the physician and the orthotist as well as providing valuable information for the therapist and engineer. It is conceivable that there may be times at which no available component exists to provide the desired combination of controls. This method of approach would then serve to point up areas for future research and development.

DESCRIPTION OF LOWER-LIMB TECHNICAL ANALYSIS FORM

The form consists of four pages of appropriate size for inclusion in the patient's hospital record. The first page (Fig. 9-1) contains spaces for patient data and a summary of major impairments. In general, the impairments noted on this page are those that do not lend themselves to diagrammatic representation. At the bottom of the first page there is a legend for symbols to be used on the extremity diagrams. The second and third pages (Figs. 9-2 and 9-3) contain skeletal outlines of the right and left lower limbs respectively in the sagittal, coronal, and transverse planes. Overlying the major joints are shaded areas representing the normal ranges of joint motion in each plan and contained within a circle divided into 30-degree segments. Similar smaller circles overlie the midshafts of the long bones for diagramming angular, rotational, or translational deformities of the femur and tibia. Boxes labeled *V* and *H* are provided and correspond to the location of each muscle group for the purpose of recording volitional muscle strength and degree of hypertonicity respectively. Boxes labeled *P* are provided at each joint level for the purpose of recording proprioception. The fourth page (Fig. 9-4) contains spaces for summarizing the functional disability and for identifying the treatment objectives. The orthotic recommendation chart is also contained on this page along with a key for its use.

INSTRUCTIONS FOR USE OF THE LOWER-LIMB TECHNICAL ANALYSIS FORM

Most of this portion of the form is self-explanatory (Fig. 9-1). Abnormal *bone and joint* conditions may include such entites as osteoporosis, Paget's disease, and coxa vara.
Limb shortening is recorded as follows:
Anterosuperior spine to sole of heel
Anterosuperior spine to mediotibial plateau
Mediotibial plateau to sole of heel
In leg-length discrepancies exceeding one-half inch, x-ray studies of leg length may be indicated and an appropriate space is provided for this measurement.

Under the heading of *ligament,* checkboxes are provided for the major ligaments of the knee and ankle to indicate abnormal laxity. The sections on *sensation, skin,* and *vascular* impairments cover considerations that may influence orthotic design and are self-explanatory.

Balance is either normal or impaired, and if impaired, the extent of impairment is indicated by the type of walking support used.

Gait deviations are not readily diagrammable. Major dynamic gait abnormalities should be described in the spaces provided.

Other impairments should also be noted, such as upper-limb involvement or significant systemic disease.

Legend and limb diagrams (Figs. 9-2 and 9-3)

Two terms must first be defined:
1. *Translatory motion* is motion in which all points of the distal segment move in the same direction, with the paths of all points being exactly alike in shape and distance traversed.
2. *Rotary motion* is motion of a distal segment in which one point in the distal segment or in its (imaginary) extension always remains fixed.

The symbols described in the legend are used in conjunction with the right- and left-limb diagrams according to the following rules:
1. Rules pertaining to recording motion:
   a. *Diagramming motion.* The degrees of rotary motion or centimeters of translatory motion are to be obtained from passive manipulation and are to reflect passive, not active, motion at the site being examined. In the lower limb, joints are to be observed during weight bearing, and if the degree of joint excursion is greater under conditions of loading than by passive manipulation, this figure is diagrammed rather than the smaller figure (such as recurvatum of the knee).
   b. *Translatory motion.* Linear arrows horizontally placed below the circle indicate the presence of (abnormal) translatory motion at one or more of the six designated levels of the lower limb listed on the left side of the form. The head of the arrow always points in the direction of displacement of the distal segment relative to the proximal segment. Linear arrows vertically placed on the right side of the circle indicate (abnormal) translatory motion along the vertical axis at the site indicated.
   c. *Rotary motion.* Normal ranges of rotary motion about joints are preshaded on

TECHNICAL ANALYSIS FORM   LOWER LIMB   Revised March 1973

Name _____ No. _____ Age _____ Sex _____

Date of Onset _____ Cause _____

Occupation _____ Present Lower-Limb Equipment _____

Diagnosis _____

_____

_____

Ambulatory ☐   Non-Ambulatory ☐

MAJOR IMPAIRMENTS:

A. Skeletal
    1. Bone and Joints: Normal ☐   Abnormal _____
    2. Ligaments: Normal ☐   Abnormal ☐   Knee: AC ☐   PC ☐   MC ☐   LC ☐
                                                      Ankle: MC ☐   LC ☐

    3. Extremity Shortening: None ☐   Left ☐   Right ☐
        Amount of Discrepancy: A.S.S.-Heel _____   A.S.S.-MTP _____   MTP-Heel _____

B. Sensation: Normal ☐   Abnormal ☐
    1. Anesthesia ☐   Hypesthesia ☐   Location: _____
        Protective Sensation: Retained ☐   Lost ☐
    2. Pain ☐   Location: _____

C. Skin: Normal ☐   Abnormal: _____

D. Vascular: Normal ☐   Abnormal ☐   Right ☐   Left ☐

E. Balance: Normal ☐   Impaired ☐   Support: _____

F. Gait Deviations: _____

_____

G. Other Impairments: _____

_____ LEGEND _____

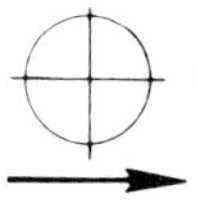

= Direction of Translatory Motion

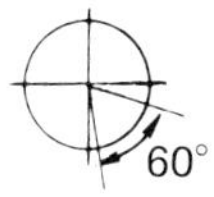

= Abnormal Degree of Rotary Motion   60°

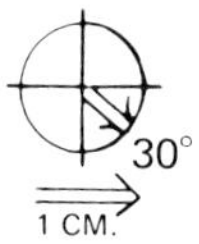

= Fixed Position   30°

1 CM.

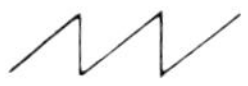

= Fracture

Volitional Force (V)
N = Normal
G = Good
F = Fair
P = Poor
T = Trace
Z = Zero

Hypertonic Muscle (H)
N = Normal
M = Mild
Mo = Moderate
S = Severe

Proprioception (P)
N = Normal
I = Impaired
A = Absent

D = Local Distension or Enlargement

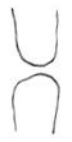

= Pseudarthrosis

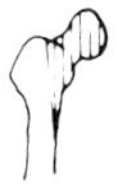

= Absence of Segment

Fig. 9-1

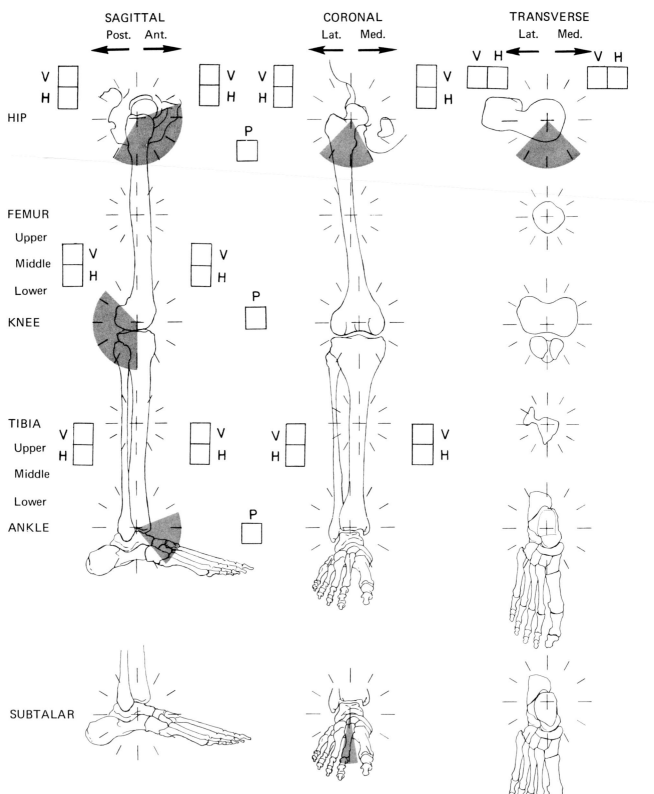

Fig. 9-2

RIGHT

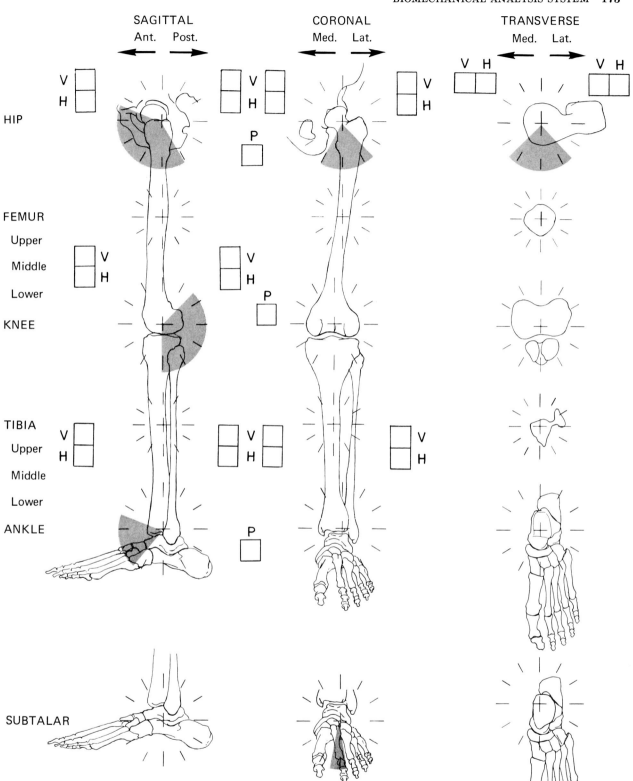

Fig. 9-3

Summary of Functional Disability _____

_____

_____

_____

_____

_____

Treatment Objectives:

Prevent/Correct Deformity ☐   Improve Ambulation ☐

Reduce Axial Load   ☐   Fracture Treatment ☐

Protect Joint   ☐   Other_____

ORTHOTIC RECOMMENDATION

| LOWER LIMB | | FLEX | EXT | ABD | ADD | ROTATION | | AXIAL LOAD |
						Int.	Ext.	
HKAO	Hip							
KAO	Thigh							
	Knee							
AFO	Leg							
	Ankle	(Dorsi)	(Plantar)					
	Subtalar					(Inver.)	(Ever.)	
FO Foot	Midtarsal							
	Met.-phal.							

REMARKS:

_____   _____

Signature   Date

KEY: Use the following symbols to indicate desired control of designated function:

F = FREE — *Free* motion.

A = ASSIST — Application of an external force for the purpose of increasing the range, velocity, or force of a motion.

R = RESIST — Application of an external force for the purpose of decreasing the velocity or force of a motion.

S = STOP — Inclusion of a static unit to deter an undesired motion in one direction.

v = Variable — A unit that can be adjusted without making a structural change.

H = HOLD — Elimination of all motion in prescribed plane (verify position).

L = LOCK — Device includes an optional lock.

Fig. 9-4

the diagram. Abnormal rotary motion, either as limited or as excess motion, is indicated by double-headed arrows placed outside and concentric to the circle, to indicate the extent of available motion present in the affected joint. In certain instances, it may be more meaningful to use two (2) double-headed arrows in order to describe the range of motion to either side of the neutral joint axis, rather than a single arrow that describes the total range of motion present. If one head of an arrow fails to reach the preshaded margin, limitation of joint motion is denoted. Conversely, if one head of an arrow projects beyond the preshaded margin, excess motion is designated. Numbers in degrees are placed adjacent to the arrows to indicate the arc described. In addition, radial lines drawn from the center of the circle and passing through its perimeter at the tips of the double-headed arrow are to be used for more graphic representation of the arc of available motion. At sites where rotary motion does not normally occur (such as the knee joint in the coronal plane), the presence of abnormal rotary motion is similarly designated by a double-headed arrow with adjacent numerical value in degrees.

    d. *Fixed position.* Double radial arrows indicate a fixed joint position and describe in degrees the deviation from the neutral joint position in translatory sense, and the extent of abnormal translation is indicated in centimeters adjacent to the arrow (such as subluxed tibia in a knee of a hemophiliac).

2. Rules pertaining to muscle:
    a. *Volitional force.* Volitional force of muscle groups (such as hip flexors) is determined by conventional means on the examining table. The legend symbol corresponding to muscle strength is recorded in the box labeled *V* adjacent to the skeletal outline at the proper location for each muscle group. The letter grades correspond to the standard muscle grading system used in poliomyelitis. A check mark is used if muscle strength is normal.

    b. *Hypertonicity.* Hypertonicity is further identified in the legend as *H.* The symbol (such as mo) for muscle group tone is to be placed adjacent to the skeletal outline in the box labeled *H* at the proper location for each muscle group. Hypertonic muscle estimates are to be made with the patient in the functional position for the lower limb, that is, observation during standing and walking. The letter grades for hypertonic muscle are as follows:

    m indicates a mild degree of hypertonicity, functionally insignificant.

    mo indicates a moderate degree of hypertonicity sufficient for useful holding quality, or with some functional value.

    s indicates severe hypertonicity, obstructive in terms of function.

(Muscle groups in a patient with spastic paralysis may also be graded according to volitional force, such as dorsiflexors of the foot in a hemiplegic person.)

3. Rules pertaining to proprioception:
A box labeled *P* is provided at each of the major joint levels. The appropriate symbol for proprioceptive loss is placed in the box according to the legend.

4. Rules pertaining to fracture or bone deformity: All translatory or rotary motions at the fracture on the shaft of a long bone are diagrammed on the circle located at the midshaft of each bone. The actual fracture site is indicated by the fracture symbol. All bony deformities such as valgus angulation of the shaft are likewise diagrammed on the circle located at the center of the shaft, regardless of the position of the angular deformity. The location of the deformity is designated by circling the appropriate level of the left-hand side of the chart.

Summary of functional disability (Fig. 9-4)

This summary is intended to be a concise analysis of the factors that are significant in producing functional impairment and for which orthotic control is desirable.

Treatment objectives (Fig. 9-4)

The objectives of orthotic treatment are identified here by checking the appropriate boxes. There

TECHNICAL ANALYSIS FORM   LOWER LIMB   Revised March 1973

Name _W.S._____   No._608213_ Age _22___ Sex _M_____

Date of Onset___1952_____   Cause _POLIOMYELITIS_____

Occupation _STUDENT_____   Present Lower-Limb Equipment _AKO - KNEE LOCK 90°_
                                                              PLANTAR STOP

Diagnosis _PARALYSIS (L) LOWER LIMB_____

_____ _3-9-70_

Ambulatory ☑   Non-Ambulatory ☐

MAJOR IMPAIRMENTS:

A. Skeletal
    1. Bone and Joints: Normal ☐   Abnormal _OLD TRIPLE ARTHRODESIS (L) FOOT_
    2. Ligaments: Normal ☐   Abnormal ☑   Knee: AC ☐   PC ☐   MC ☑   LC ☐
                                                    Ankle: MC ☐   LC ☐

    3. Extremity Shortening: None ☐   Left ☑   Right ☐
        Amount of Discrepancy: A.S.S.-Heel _1 3/4"_ A.S.S.-MTP _3/4"_ MTP-Heel _1"_

B. Sensation: Normal ☑   Abnormal ☐
    1. Anaesthesia ☐   Hypesthesia ☐   Location:_____
        Protective Sensation: Retained ☐   Lost ☐
    2. Pain ☑   Location:_____(L) ANKLE_____

C. Skin: Normal ☑   Abnormal:_____

D. Vascular: Normal ☑   Abnormal ☐   Right ☐   Left ☐

E. Balance: Normal ☑   Impaired ☐   Support:_____

F. Gait Deviations: _GLUTEUS MEDIUS LURCH (L)_
    _CIRCUMDUCTION (L) LIMB_____

G. Other Impairments:____0_____

─────────────────────── LEGEND ───────────────────────

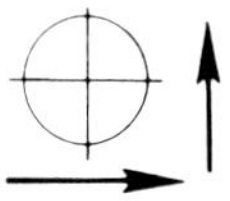

= Direction of Translatory
  Motion

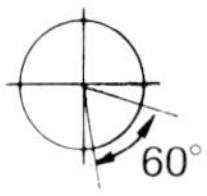

= Abnormal Degree of
  Rotary Motion   60°

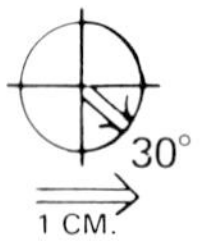

= Fixed Position   30°
1 CM.

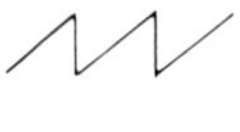

= Fracture

Volitional Force (V)
N = Normal
G = Good
F = Fair
P = Poor
T = Trace
Z = Zero

Hypertonic Muscle (H)
N   = Normal
M   = Mild
Mo = Moderate
S   = Severe

Proprioception (P)
N = Normal
I = Impaired
A = Absent

D = Local Distension or
     Enlargement

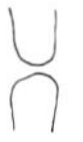

= Pseudarthrosis

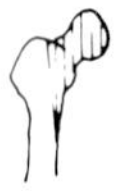

= Absence of Segment

Fig. 9-5

may frequently be more than one objective treatment.

Orthotic recommendation (Fig. 9-4)

The level of orthotic application is selected on the basis of the information obtained. A full lower-limb orthosis to include the hip is identified in the chart as an *HKAO,* or hip-knee-ankle-orthosis, whereas an appliance designed to control only the ankle-foot complex would be designated as *AFO.*

For each joint to be encompassed or controlled by the device, the type of control in each direction of movement is inserted in the blanks provided, abbreviated according to the "key" at the bottom of the page. Thus, the types of control to be provided, and not the specific components to be used, form the basis of the orthotic recommendation. Under the section concerning remarks, more exacting recommendations as to components or special considerations in fabrication can be recorded.

ILLUSTRATIVE CASES
Case 1 (Figs. 9-5 to 9-7)

This 22-year-old male was seen for residual paralysis of the left lower limb because of poliomyelitis. Fig. 9-5 provides basic background information regarding this patient. His present orthosis was of the conventional above-knee type with drop-ring knee locks and a 90-degree plantar stop at the ankle. It is noted that he had had a previous triple arthrodesis of his left foot. The medial collateral ligament is noted to be lax, and there is 1¾ inch shortening of the left lower limb. Pain is present about the left ankle, and his gait is characterized by a gluteus medius limp and circumduction of the limb.

Diagrammatic analysis of the limb (Fig. 9-6) gives a clear picture of the voluntary strength of all four muscle groups indicated by letter grade. In the sagittal plane one may note loss of 30 degrees of hip extension, 20 degrees of hyperextension of the knee, and limitation of dorsiflexion of the ankle to the neutral position. In the coronal plane, a 15-degree valgus excursion of the knee is observed, as well as approximately 10 degrees of abnormal inversion and eversion of the ankle joint, secondary to old triple arthrodesis of the foot, indicated by the fixed position of the subtalar joint. In the transverse plane, one may note 20 degrees of external tibial torsion. Proprioception is of course normal throughout the limb.

The summary of this patient's functional disability (Fig. 9-7) and the objectives of treatment are self-explanatory.

The orthotic recommendation (Fig. 9-7) indicates that it is desirable to allow free knee flexion and stop hyperextension of the knee. At the ankle, the combination of a dorsiflexion stop and resistance to plantar flexion is recommended to achieve knee stability by creating an extension moment at this joint during stance phase. It is also desirable to stop inversion and eversion of the foot (in reality occurring at the ankle joint), since this is a source of pain. Under the section concerning remarks, it is suggested that the orthotic requirements can be met by use of the "UCLA functional long leg orthosis" in combination with a "UCB" type of shoe insert.

Case 2 (Figs. 9-8 to 9-10)

This 63-year-old male was seen for residual paralysis of the left lower limb secondary to cerebral thrombosis. Fig. 9-8 illustrates the basic background information and the areas of major impairment in this patient. His present orthotic equipment consists of a conventional below-knee orthosis with a 90-degree plantar stop. It may be noted that some hypestehsia exists on the left side of the body and that his balance is impaired to the extent that he must use a cane in ambulating. The patient's gait is characterized by inversion and drop foot during swing phase, and hyperextension of the knee at midstance.

Diagrammatic analysis of the limb (Fig. 9-9) gives a clear picture of the volitional strength of the major muscle groups. In addition, one may note a mild degree of spasticity in the adductors of the hip and the plantar flexors and invertors of the foot and ankle. Proprioception is seen to be impaired distally, but normal at the knee and hip joints. In the sagittal plane, one may note a 25-degree excursion of the knee and limitation of dorsiflexion of the ankle to the neutral position.

The summary of the patient's functional disability and the objectives of treatment are self-explanatory (Fig. 9-10).

The orthotic recommendation (Fig. 9-10) indicates that free dorsiflexion and a plantar-flexion stop 10 degrees above neutral are desirable to aid in preventing hyperextension forces at the knee during stance phase. Also, resistance to inversion and free eversion at the subtalar joint are indicated. Elimination of all flexion-extension motion in the tarsal and midtarsal joints is recommended

Text continued on p. 183.

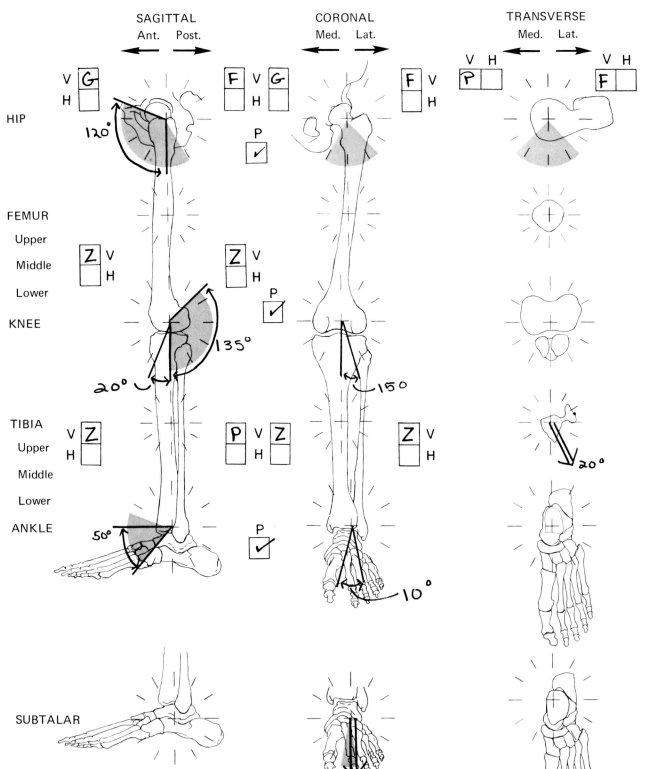

SAGITTAL
Ant. Post.

CORONAL
Med. Lat.

TRANSVERSE
Med. Lat.

HIP

FEMUR
Upper
Middle
Lower

KNEE

TIBIA
Upper
Middle
Lower

ANKLE

SUBTALAR

Fig. 9-6

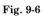

LEFT

Summary of Functional Disability *Unstable knee stance phase →
recurvatum; drop foot c̄ inadequate
foot clearance. Circumduction with
present equipment →
↑ energy expenditure
Ankle motion in M-L plane → pain*

Treatment Objectives:

Prevent/Correct Deformity ☑	Improve Ambulation ☑
Reduce Axial Load ☐	Fracture Treatment ☐
Protect Joint ☑	Other _____

ORTHOTIC RECOMMENDATION

LOWER LIMB			FLEX	EXT	ABD	ADD	ROTATION Int.	ROTATION Ext.	AXIAL LOAD
HKAO Hip									
KAO *Thigh*									
Knee			F	S					
AFO *Leg*									
Ankle			S (Dorsi)	R (Plantar)					
	FO Foot	Subtalar					S (Inver.)	S (Ever.)	
		Midtarsal	F	F					
		Met.-phal.	F	F	F	F			

REMARKS: *UCLA functional long leg brace; UCB insert
to control M-L motion at ankle
1½" heel and sole lift* Signature _____ Date 5/30/72

KEY: Use the following symbols to indicate desired control of designated function:

F = FREE — *Free* motion.
A = ASSIST — Application of an external force for the purpose of increasing the range, velocity, or force of a motion.
R = RESIST — Application of an external force for the purpose of decreasing the velocity or force of a motion.
S = STOP — Inclusion of a static unit to deter an undesired motion in one direction.
v = Variable — A unit that can be adjusted without making a structural change.
H = HOLD — Elimination of all motion in prescribed plane (verify position).
L = LOCK — Device includes an optional lock.

Fig. 9-7

TECHNICAL ANALYSIS FORM   LOWER LIMB   Revised March 1973

Name E. L. _____   No. 819644   Age 63   Sex M

Date of Onset 3/18/72   Cause CEREBRAL THROMBOSIS _____

Occupation Post Office Clerk   Present Lower-Limb Equipment BKO - 90° STOP

Diagnosis Left Hemiplegia _____

_____ 5-20-72

Ambulatory ☑   Non-Ambulatory ☐

MAJOR IMPAIRMENTS:

A. Skeletal
    1. Bone and Joints: Normal ☑   Abnormal _____
    2. Ligaments: Normal ☑   Abnormal ☐   Knee: AC ☐   PC ☐   MC ☐   LC ☐
                                             Ankle: MC ☐   LC ☐

    3. Extremity Shortening: None ☑   Left ☐   Right ☐
        Amount of Discrepancy: A.S.S.-Heel _____   A.S.S.-MTP _____   MTP-Heel _____

B. Sensation: Normal ☐   Abnormal ☑
    1. Anaesthesia ☐   Hypaesthesia ☑   Location: (L) Upper + Lower Limb
        Protective Sensation: Retained ☐   Lost ☐
    2. Pain ☐   Location: _____

C. Skin: Normal ☑   Abnormal: _____

D. Vascular: Normal ☑   Abnormal ☐   Right ☐   Left ☐

E. Balance: Normal ☐   Impaired ☑   Support: CANE

F. Gait Deviations: INVERSION AND MILD DROP FOOT - SWING
    PHASE   HYPEREXTENSION KNEE AT MID STANCE

G. Other Impairments: _____
    MYOCARDIAL INFARCT - 2 years ago
    ———————————— LEGEND ————————————

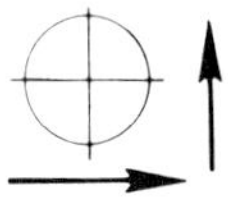

⊕↑ = Direction of Translatory Motion

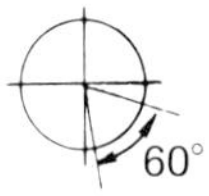

Volitional Force (V)
N = Normal
G = Good
F = Fair
P = Poor
T = Trace
Z = Zero

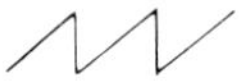

Proprioception (P)
N = Normal
I = Impaired
A = Absent

⊕ 60° = Abnormal Degree of Rotary Motion

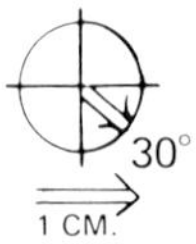

D = Local Distension or Enlargement

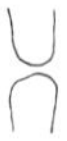

⊕ 30° = Fixed Position

1 CM. ⇒

Hypertonic Muscle (H)
N = Normal
M = Mild
Mo = Moderate
S = Severe

= Pseudarthrosis

= Fracture

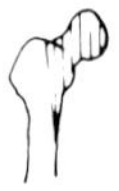

= Absence of Segment

Fig. 9-8

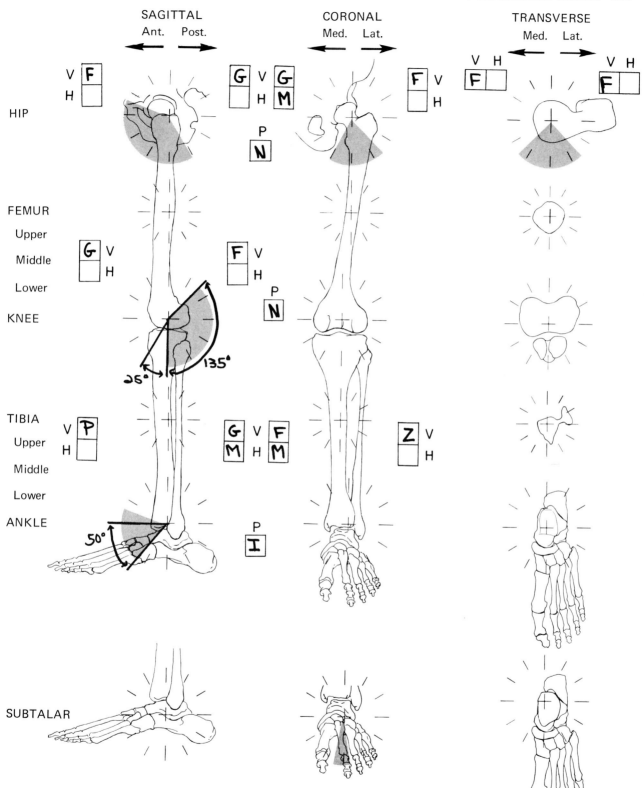

Fig. 9-9

Summary of Functional Disability *Unable to clear foot during swing phase 2° to inadequate dorsi flexion; Instability at foot contact 2° to inversion of foot during swing phase; Recurvatum of knee during mid-stance 2° to spastic heel cord*

Treatment Objectives:

Prevent/Correct Deformity ☑   Improve Ambulation ☑
Reduce Axial Load ☐   Fracture Treatment ☐
Protect Joint ☐   Other _____

ORTHOTIC RECOMMENDATION

LOWER LIMB		FLEX	EXT	ABD	ADD	ROTATION Int.	ROTATION Ext.	AXIAL LOAD
HKAO	Hip							
KAO	Thigh							
	Knee							
AFO	Leg							
	Ankle (V)	F (Dorsi)	S- ↑ 10° (Plantar)					
	Subtalar					R (Inver.)	F (Ever.)	
FO Foot	Midtarsal	H	H					
	Met.-phal.	H	H	F	F			

REMARKS: *Adjustable plantar flexion stop set at 10° above neutral to control genu recurvatum.*
Lateral "T" strap
Extended stirrup and march bar

_____   _____
Signature   Date

KEY: Use the following symbols to indicate desired control of designated function:

F = FREE   — *Free* motion.
A = ASSIST — Application of an external force for the purpose of increasing the range, velocity, or force of a motion.
R = RESIST — Application of an external force for the purpose of decreasing the velocity or force of a motion.
S = STOP   — Inclusion of a static unit to deter an undesired motion in one direction.
v = Variable — A unit that can be adjusted without making a structural change.
H = HOLD   — Elimination of all motion in prescribed plane (verify position).
L = LOCK   — Device includes an optional lock.

Fig. 9-10

to effect a right foot-lever system for the purpose of transmitting a flexion moment to the knee through the calf band at heel strike. Under the section concerning remarks, specific suggestions are made with regard to the components of this system.

SUMMARY

The basis for rational orthotic prescription must be a systematic functional appraisal of the impaired limb or body segment. The diagrammatic approach to biomechanical analysis of the lower limb presented here serves to better identify the functional deficits present and forms the basis for appropriate selection of orthotic components. It also serves to identify instances for which adequate components are not available to perform the required tasks; thus areas for further research are indicated. In addition to serving as a means

for developing a logical approach to orthotic prescription, such a technical analysis provides an improved means of communication between the physician and the orthotist. Although the analysis form itself need not be applied to all patients requiring an orthosis, the concept of a biomechanical approach of this nature is essential to writing the orthotic prescription.

REFERENCES

1. Committee on Prosthetics Research and Development, Report of the Seventh Workshop Panel on Lower Extremity Orthosis of the Subcommittee on Design and Development, National Research Council—National Academy of Sciences, March 1970.
2. McCullough, C., III: Introduction to lower extremity orthotics, Instructional course lectures of the American Academy of Orthopaedic Surgeons 20:116-124, 1971.
3. McCollough, C., III, Fryer, C. M., and Glancy, J.: A new approach to patient analysis for orthotic prescription, Artif. Limbs 14:68, 1970.

CHAPTER 10

Orthotic components and systems

ANTHONY STAROS, M.S.M.E., P.E.
MAURICE LeBLANC, M.S.M.E., C.P.

In 1956, Thorndike, Murphy, and Staros[22] enumerated the many limitations of current orthopaedic appliances, stressing patient dissatisfaction with the devices. They specified remedies and offered suggestions for application of engineering principles to the future design of orthoses.

Since the time of that paper, certain improvements in metal orthoses recommended by Thorndike and associates have been forthcoming, including prefabrication of orthotic components and better quality control. Complaints of excess bulk, weight, noise, and rigidity are still common because metal orthoses suffer inherently from these problems.

Licht[11] in 1966 and Perry and Hislop[16] in 1967 thoroughly reviewed the state of the orthotic "art," and since then, distinct changes have been noted.

The trend has been one of gradual improvement, aided by the efforts of the Committee on Prosthetics Research and Development.[3-6] We have witnessed the transition from "bracemakers" forging their own metal parts from carbon steel to orthotists assembling orthopaedic appliances from prefabricated, mass-produced parts of various metals. More recently, learning from their colleagues in prosthetics, orthotists have begun making some appliances of thermosetting plastics (Fig. 10-1), which permit them to employ some of the material long used in prosthetics. The use of these materials also allows greater flexibility in

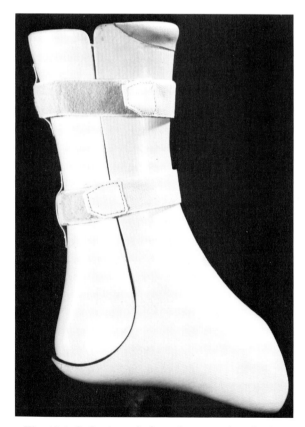

Fig. 10-1. Orthosis made from thermosetting plastics.

184

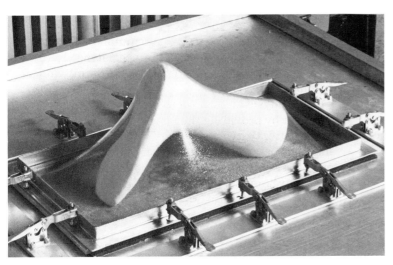

Fig. 10-2. Forming AFO by use of vacuum.

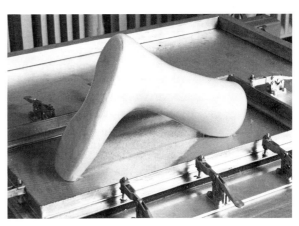

Fig. 10-3. Vacuum-formed AFO before trimming.

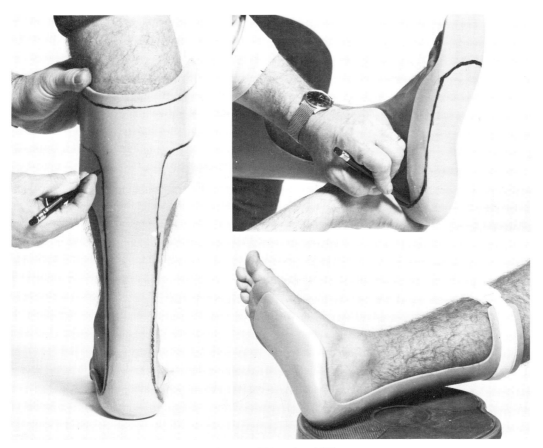

Fig. 10-4. Trimming AFO.

design and adjustment, lower appliance weight, and improved cosmesis.

Rubin[17] recently noted the trend away from metal orthoses, as more completely plastic systems are becoming useful.[23] Often mentioned for the future are composites such as boron or graphite with epoxies or other plastics. By strategic design, inexpensive and easy-to-use thermoplastics of various types can be expected to meet adequately many functional and structural demands without excessive weight, bulk, noise, or over-bracing.

The orthotist now usually bases fabrication and fitting on a plaster cast impression of the limb to be served. He may use vacuum forming techniques (Figs. 10-2 and 10-3) to construct the appliance over the model taken from the cast impression.[2,13] In many instances plastic orthoses can be mass produced in an adequate number of sizes, with modifications suiting the special needs to each patient, achieved by heat post-forming and trimming (Fig. 10-4).

The physician and the clinic team assist the orthotist by providing the biomechanical analysis of the patient's dysfunction.[14] This data along with information about edema, spasticity, etc., and the orthotist's own assessment of weight, comesis, etc., then may be employed by the orthotist to design an

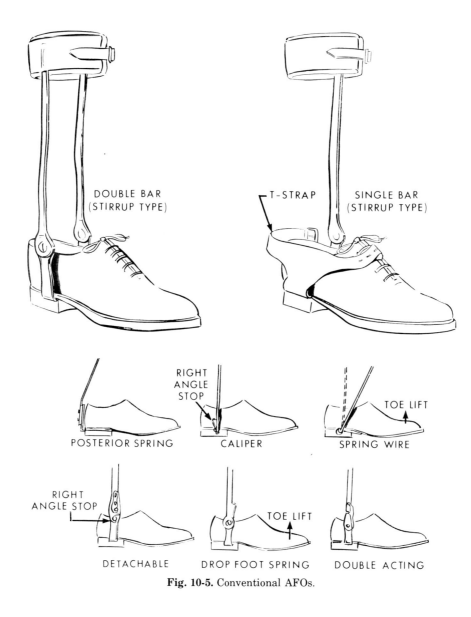

Fig. 10-5. Conventional AFOs.

appliance of an appropriate material to provide those biomechanical functions needed by the patient.

TERMINOLOGY IN ORTHOTICS

Harris[8] has summarized the work of the Committee on Prosthetics Orthotics Education* (CPOE) and others[20] to clarify terminology in orthotics. The use of "orthosis" is encouraged rather than the use of such terms as "brace," "splint," and "caliper." An orthosis usually is defined as a device applied on the exterior of the body to restrict or enhance motion, or reduce the load on a body segment.

It was recommended by CPOE that orthoses "be described by the joints they encompass," to eliminate such terms as "long leg brace" and "short leg brace" as well as confusing eponyms. Acronyms such as "knee-ankle-foot orthosis" (KAFO), or "ankle-foot-orthosis" (AFO), are therefore employed in this chapter. Used to describe the function designed into an orthotic system are the terms as "free," "assist," "resist," "stop," "hold," and "lock," which clearly present the na-

*National Academy of Sciences—National Research Council.

ture of the controls in the three planes of motion for all joints and limb segments.

DESCRIPTIONS OF LOWER-LIMB ORTHOSES

This section describes both typical components and lower-limb orthotic systems that are commonly used. Each device is described in biomechanical terms.

Examples of plastic orthoses for the lower limb are given, as well as conventional metal components (Figs. 10-5 and 10-6).

The authors have chosen to detail only commonly used orthoses. These serve as a model from which custom designs can be devised to suit individual patient needs as identified by the clinic team. Therefore the contents of this chapter constitute but a guideline on design principles for the physician, therapist, orthotist, and other members of the clinic team to formulate a general description to which the orthotist can appropriately respond.

FABRICATION AND FITTING OF LOWER-LIMB ORTHOSES

Staros[18] refers to the "new orthotics" as a system based not only on new terminology and new

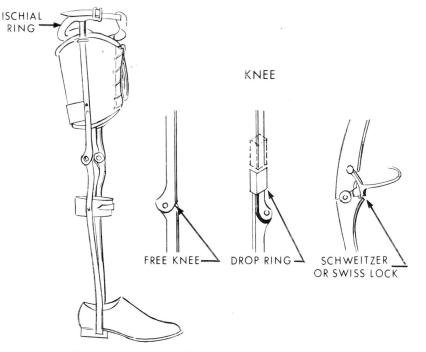

Fig. 10-6. Conventional lower-limb orthotic components.

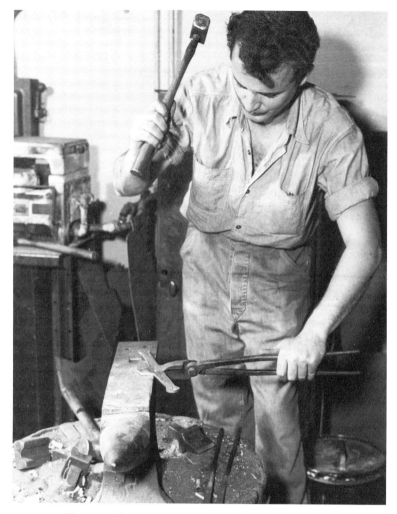

Fig. 10-7. Forming of conventional lower-limb orthosis.

designs and materials but also as a system displac-ing routine fabrication processes from the ortho-tist's fitting laboratory. Although metal orthoses will continue to be used, even these should not be formed or even assembled in the fitting area where patients are received. The hammer and anvil days (Fig. 10-7), when metal parts were so formed to provide braces, are certainly receding. Mass-production of these parts and such recent innova-tions as bending fixtures for shaping metal braces to limb tracings (Figs. 10-8 to 10-10) should consti-tute only interim steps. We have thus progressed from the art of tracing and bending to the technol-ogy of casting and thermal forming of orthoses.

The techniques used for working with the dif-ferent materials used in orthoses, both of the con-ventional metal design and those using plastic structures, are described in the *Orthopaedic Appliances Atlas*.[1]

Casting procedures for lower-limb orthotics are also well described in the above-mentioned volume. Modifications will take place in casting procedures as new types of orthoses are designed. The PTB weight-bearing orthosis requires cast-ing technique much like the casting procedure used for the PTB below-knee prosthesis. The knee (KO) and knee-ankle-foot (KAF) orthoses using a supracondylar suprapatellar socket design re-quire casting procedures that are not yet routine in orthotics. The various manuals that have been referenced for each of these kinds of appliances should be consulted by the orthotist before casting.

Lusskin[12] and Lehneis[10] have indicated in some detail the sometimes poorly understood need for

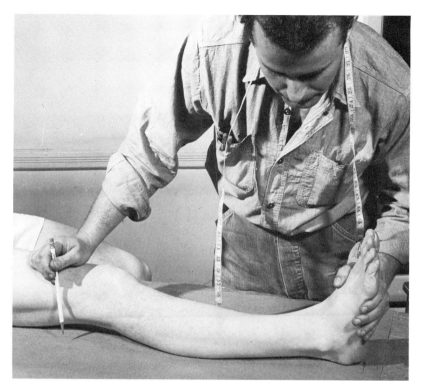

Fig. 10-8. Tracing lower-limb contours.

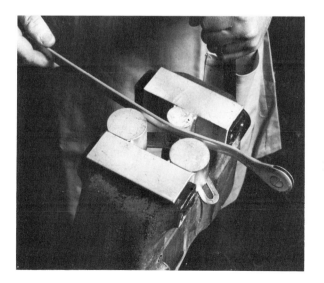

Fig. 10-9. Bending metal uprights.

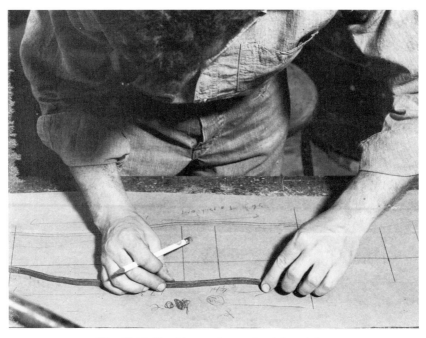

Fig. 10-10. Checking contours of metal uprights.

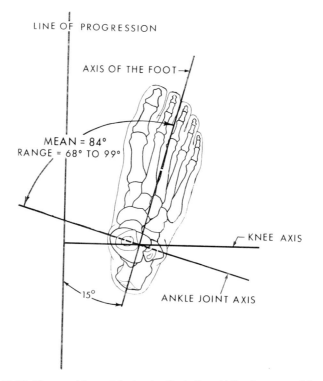

Fig. 10-11. Knee, ankle, and foot axis of rotation. (After Inman and Inman.)

accurate alignment when mechanical joints are used in orthoses. The accommodation of "tibial torsion" recognizes the deviation that exists between the transverse plane orientation of the knee axis and the talocrural (ankle) axis (Fig. 10-11). Similarly it is necessary for the orthotist, when aligning mechanical joints, to accommodate the difference between the ankle and foot axes and deviations of the long axis of the limb.

REFERENCES

1. American Academy of Orthopaedic Surgeons: Orthopaedic appliances atlas, vol. 1, Braces, splints, shoe alterations, Ann Arbor, Mich., 1952, J. W. Edwards, Publisher.
2. Artamonov, A.: Vacuum-forming techniques and materials in prosthetics and orthotics, Inter-Clinic Information Bull. **11**:10-9-18, 30 July 1972.
3. Committee on Prosthetics Research and Development, National Academy of Sciences: A clinical evaluation of four lower-limb orthoses, Report E-5, 1972, Washington, D.C.
4. Committee on Prosthetics Research and Development, National Academy of Sciences: Clinical evaluation of a comprehensive approach to below-knee orthotics, Report E-6, 1972, Washington, D.C.
5. Committee on Prosthetics Research and Development, National Academy of Sciences: Eighth workshop panel on lower-limb orthotics, Report of Workshop held October 2-4, 1972, Washington, D.C.
6. Committee on Prosthetics Research and Development, National Academy of Sciences: Seventh workshop panel on lower-extremity orthotics, Report of Workshop held on March 9-10, 1972, Washington, D.C.
7. Committee on Prosthetics Research and Development, National Academy of Sciences: Clinical evaluation of the Ljubljana functional electrical personal brace, Report E-7, 1973, Washington, D.C.
8. Harris, E. E.: A new orthotics terminology—A guide to its use for prescription and fee schedules, Orthot. Prosthet. **27**(2):6-19, June 1973.
9. Isman, R. E., and Inman, V. T.: Anthropometric studies of the human foot and ankle, Bull. Prosthet. Res. BPR **10-11**:97-129, Spring 1969.
10. Lehneis, H. R.: Orthotics alignment in the lower limb, Proceedings of the 1st International Congress on Pros-
11. Licht, S.: Orthotics etcetera, Baltimore, 1966, Waverly Press.
12. Lusskin, R.: The influence of errors in bracing upon deformity of the lower extremity, Arch. Phys. Med. Rehab. **47**:520-525, 1966.
13. Lyons, C.: Vacuum-formed upper extremity splints, Inter-Clinic Information Bull. **11**:10-19-23, July 1972.
14. McCollough, N. C., III, Fryer, C. M., and Glancy, J.: A new approach to patient analysis for orthotic prescription. Part I. The lower extremity, Artif. Limbs **14**(2):26-80, Autumn 1970.
15. Mooney, V., and Snelson, R.: Fabrication and application of transparent polycarbonate sockets, Orthot. Prosthet. **26**(1):1-13, March 1972.
16. Perry, J., and Hislop, H. J.: Principles of lower-extremity bracing, New York, 1967, American Physical Therapy Association.
17. Rubin, G., and Dixon, M.: The modern ankle-foot orthoses (AFO's), Bull. Prosthet. Res. BPR **10-19**:20-41, Spring 1973.
18. Staros, A.: Functional analysis of lower-limb orthoses, Proceedings of the 1st International Congress on Prosthetics Techniques and Functional Rehabilitation **2** (Paper II-75):215-219, 1973.
19. Staros, A.: Joint designs in prosthetics and orthotics, Prosthet. Int. 3(10):1-20, 1970.
20. Staros, A.: Nomenclatures and classification of orthotic components. In Murdoch's Prosthetic and orthotic practice; a report of a conference in Dundee, Scotland, June 1969, London, 1970, Edward Arnold Ltd., pp. 484-488.
21. Staros, A., and Peizer, E.: The clinical engineer, American Society of Mechanical Engineers, Winter Annual Meeting, Nov. 1973.
22. Thorndike, A., Murphy, E. F., and Staros, A.: Engineering applied to orthopaedic bracing, Orthop. Prosthet. Appliance J., pp. 55-71, December 1956.
23. Yates, G.: A method for the provision of lightweight aesthetic orthopaedic appliances, Orthopaedics 1(2):153-162, 1968.
24. Veterans Administration (United States), Program guide, G-2, M-2, Part IX, Braces, lower-extremity, Washington, D.C., February 27, 1956, Department of Medicine and Surgery, Veterans Administration.

thetics Techniques and Functional Rehabilitation, Paper IV-109, **4**:73-79, 1973.

Type: Hip joint
Name: Free-motion hip joint

		Flex	Ext	Abd	Add	Rotation	
						Int	Ext
Hip		F	F	H	H	H	H

Biomechanical purpose: To prevent abduction-adduction while allowing flexion-extension in a defined plane of motion. By the nature of the design, it will also prevent internal-external rotation.

Material and design: Aluminum, stainless steel, carbon steel, or chrome molybdenum steel; *A* is the leather protector, *B* is the pelvic band, *C* is the upper bar, *D* is the joint pivot, and *E* is the lower bar.

Fabrication: Comes prefabricated; is easily attached to pelvic band and distal portions or the orthosis.

Special consideration: Requires proper alignment to permit free hip flexion and extension.

Type: Hip joint
Name: Hip joint with positive stop

		Flex	Ext	Abd	Add	Rotation	
						Int	Ext
Hip		F	S∨	H	H	H	H

Biomechanical purpose: To prevent hip extension while permitting flexion. The angle of the extension stop can be adjusted.

Material and design: Aluminum, stainless steel, carbon steel, or chrome molybdenum steel.

Fabrication: Comes prefabricated; can be easily assembled to the pelvic band and distal brace hardware.

Special consideration: Must be properly aligned to permit unimpeded hip flexion.

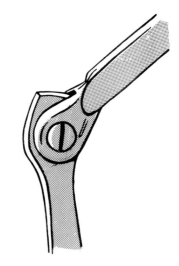

Fig. 10-13

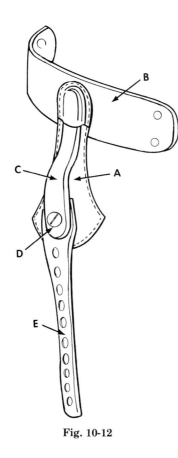

Fig. 10-12

Type: Hip joint
Name: Hip joint with lock

					Rotation	
	Flex	Ext	Abd	Add	Int	Ext
Hip Lock Mode	H	H	H	H	H	H
Unlock Mode	F	S$_V$	H	H	H	H

Biomechanical purpose: To prevent flexion and extension during ambulation (the lock mode). The unlocking mode for sitting is manually operated; then the joint will stop extension at variable angles yet permit flexion. It holds both abduction and adduction as well as internal and external rotation.

Material and design: Aluminum, stainless steel, carbon steel, or chrome molybdenum steel. Can be either level or drop-ring lock design.

Fabrication: Comes prefabricated; is easily assembled to the pelvic band and distal components of an orthosis.

Special consideration: Proper alignment is necessary to permit unimpeded sitting.

Fig. 10-14

Type: Hip joint
Name: Hip joint with extension stop, abduction and/or adduction hinge

					Rotation	
	Flex	Ext	Abd	Add	Int	Ext
Hip	F	S$_V$	S$_V$	S$_V$	H	H

Biomechanical purpose: To permit hip flexion while providing variable stop to hip extension. Abduction and/or adduction can also be limited in a variable manner. Holds rotation.

Material and design: Carbon steel.

Fabrication: Comes prefabricated and can be easily assembled to pelvic band and distal joint components.

Special consideration: Careful alignment must be applied to permit unimpeded hip flexion.

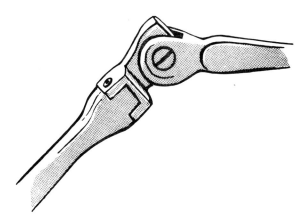

Fig. 10-15

Type: Hip joint

Name: Hip joint with lock and abduction and/or adduction hinge

	Flex	Ext	Abd	Add	Rotation	
					Int	Ext
Hip Lock Mode	H	H	S$_V$	S$_V$	H	H
Unlock Mode	F	S$_V$	S$_V$	S$_V$	H	H

Biomechanical purpose: To prevent flexion-extension in the lock mode, permit free flexion while stopping extension at variable angles in the unlock mode. It provides controlled limits on abduction or adduction or both, at the same time holding against internal-external rotation.

Material and design: Carbon steel or stainless steel. Can be either plunger (Fig. 10-16, *A*) or drop-ring lock design (Fig. 10-16, *B*).

Fabrication: Comes prefabricated and can be easily assembled to pelvic band and distal joint components.

Special consideration: Anteroposterior alignment is critical to permit unimpeded sitting.

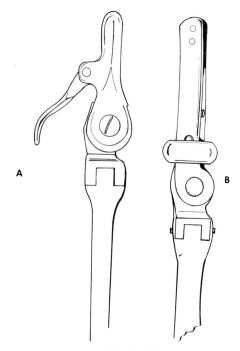

Fig. 10-16

Type: Suspension system

Name: Silesian belt

	Flex	Ext	Abd	Add	Rotation	
					Int	Ext
Hip	F	F	R	R	R	R

Biomechanical purpose: To provide a suspensory function and resist internal and external rotation and abduction-adduction of the hip while permitting free flexion-extension.

Material and design: Metal and fabric.

Fabrication: Made from webbing of measurements taken from the patient.

Special consideration: Attachment joints on orthosis and waist belt must be carefully placed to provide proper control.

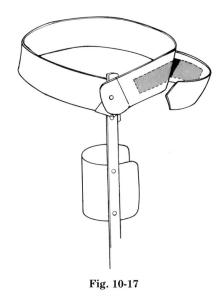

Fig. 10-17

Type: Knee joint
Name: Free-motion knee joint

					Rotation	
	Flex	Ext	Abd	Add	Int	Ext
Knee	F	F	H	H	H	H

Biomechanical purpose: To hold against valgum/varum permitting free flexion and extension. Will also hold against rotation.
Material and design: Aluminum, stainless steel, carbon steel, or chrome molybdenum steel.
Fabrication: Comes prefabricated; is easily attached to rest of orthosis.
Special consideration: Requires proper alignment to provide unimpeded flexion and extension.

Type: Knee joint
Name: Knee joint with extension stop

					Rotation	
	Flex	Ext	Abd	Add	Int	Ext
Knee	F	S $_V$	H	H	H	H

Biomechanical purpose: To stop extension at any angle while permitting flexion. Motions in other planes are held.
Material and design: Aluminum, stainless steel, carbon steel, or chrome molybdenum steel.
Fabrication: Comes prefabricated; is easily attached to rest of orthosis.
Special consideration: Requires proper alignment to permit free flexion for comfortable sitting.

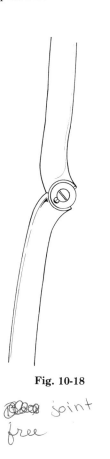

Fig. 10-18

joint free

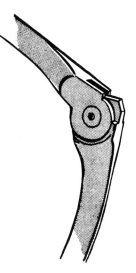

Fig. 10-19

Box joint

Type: Knee joint
Name: Knee joint with lock

					Rotation	
	Flex	Ext	Abd	Add	Int	Ext
Knee Lock Mode	H	H	H	H	H	H
Unlock Mode	F	S V	H	H	H	H

Biomechanical purpose: To prevent flexion and extension in the lock mode; in the unlock mode, flexion is permitted, with a variable stop on extension. An essential purpose is to hold against valgum and varum. Will hold against rotation.

Material and design: Aluminum, stainless steel, carbon steel, or chrome molybdenum steel. Can be plunger (Fig. 10-20, *A*), lever (Fig. 10-20, *B*), or drop-ring (Fig. 10-20, *C* and *D*) lock designs.

Fabrication: Comes prefabricated; is easily attached to the rest of orthosis.

Special consideration: Requires proper alignment to permit free flexion for comfortable sitting.

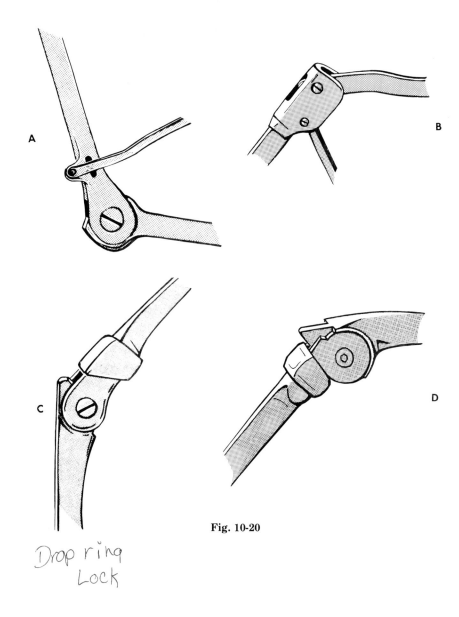

Drop ring Lock

Fig. 10-20

Type: Knee joint
Name: Polycentric knee joint

					Rotation	
	Flex	Ext	Abd	Add	Int	Ext
Knee	F	S$_V$	H	H	H	H

Biomechanical purpose: To provide simulation of "true" knee center permitting free flexion and with a variable stop on extension. Motions in other planes are held.

Material and design: Aluminum or stainless steel with two mechanical centers of rotation.

Fabrication: Comes prefabricated; is easily attached to rest of orthosis.

Special consideration: Requires proper alignment to provide good simulation of true knee center.

Type: Knee joint
Name: Knee joint with adjustable dial (or turnbuckle)

					Rotation	
	Flex	Ext	Abd	Add	Int	Ext
Knee	S$_V$	F	H	H	H	H

Biomechanical purpose: To provide progressive knee extension through an adjustable stop that prevents knee flexion; motions in other planes are held.

Material and design: Carbon steel or stainless steel.

Fabrication: Comes prefabricated; is easily attached to rest of orthosis.

Special considerations: Alignment critical to permit sitting.

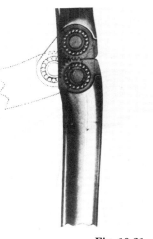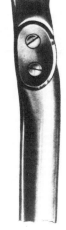

Fig. 10-21

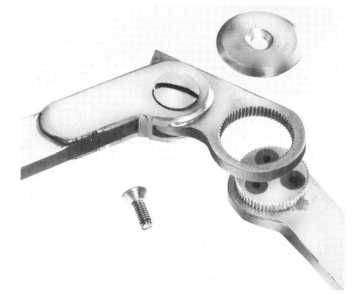

Fig. 10-22

Type: Ankle joint
Name: Free-motion ankle joint

	Flex	Ext	Abd	Add	Rotation	
					Int	Ext
Ankle	(Dorsi) F	(Plantar) F				
Foot Subtalar			S	S	(Inver) S	(Ever) S

Biomechanical purpose: To permit free ankle flexion and extension while the orthosis serves as an anchor for a pad or strap to control valgum or varum; may also be used with KAFO when free ankle motion is desired.

Material and design: Side bar and joints: aluminum, stainless steel, carbon steel, or chrome molybdenum steel.

Fabrication: Comes prefabricated with stirrup; is easily attached to other parts of orthosis.

Special consideration: Alignment of joints is important to accommodate tibial torsion.

Type: Ankle joint
Name: One-direction positive stop ankle joint

	Flex	Ext	Abd	Add	Rotation	
					Int	Ext
Ankle	(Dorsi) S$_\vee$ or F	(Plantar) F or S$_\vee$				

Biomechanical purpose: To stop plantar flexion or dorsiflexion at some prescribed position while permitting motion in the opposite direction.

Material and design: Side bars and joints (Fig. 10-24, *A*): aluminum, stainless steel, carbon steel, or chrome molybdenum steel. Stirrup (Fig. 10-25, *B*): stainless steel or carbon steel. Stirrup can either contain lower ride bar as in Fig. 10-24, *A* or the easily detachable caliper type of shower in Fig. 10-24, *C* might be used.

Fabrication: Comes prefabricated with stirrup; is easily attached to other parts of orthosis.

Special consideration: Alignment of joints is important to accommodate tibial torsion.

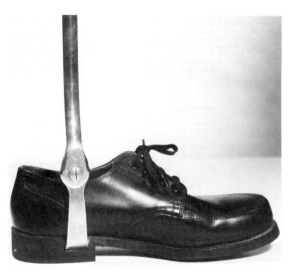

Fig. 10-23

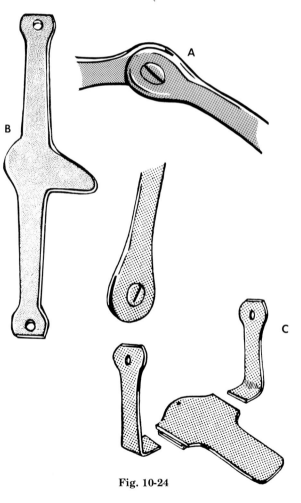

Fig. 10-24

Type: Ankle joint
Name: Two-direction positive stop ankle joint

					Rotation	
	Flex	Ext	Abd	Add	Int	Ext
Ankle	(Dorsi) S∨	(Plantar) S∨				
Foot Subtalar					(Inver) S∨	(Ever) S∨

Biomechanical purpose: To provide stops in both directions at the ankle (or can also be used posteriorly, at the subtalar).

Material and design: The side bars and joints are aluminum; the stirrup is stainless steel.

Fabrication: Comes prefabricated with stirrup; is easily attached to other parts of orthosis.

Special consideration: Alignment of joints is important to accommodate tibial torsion, when used at the ankle.

Type: Ankle joint
Name: One-direction spring-loaded ankle joint

					Rotation	
	Flex	Ext	Abd	Add	Int	Ext
Ankle	(Dorsi) R or A	(Plantar) A or R				
Foot Subtalar					(Inver) H	(Ever) H

Biomechanical purpose: To assist dorsiflexion and resist plantar flexion, but can be reserved.

Material and design: Side bars and joints: aluminum, stainless steel, carbon steel, or chrome molybdenum steel. Stirrup: stainless steel or carbon steel.

Fabrication: Comes prefabricated with stirrup; is easily attached to other parts of orthosis.

Special consideration: Alignment of joints is important to accommodate tibial torsion.

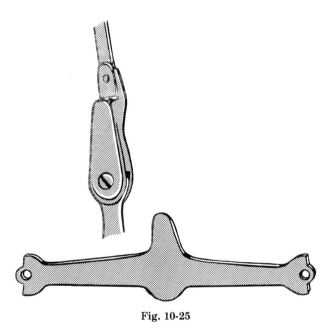

Fig. 10-25

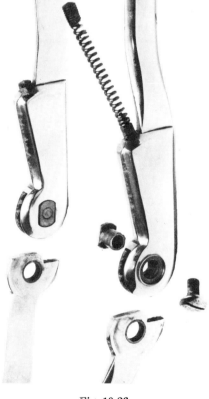

Fig. 10-26

Type: Ankle joint
Name: Two-direction spring-loaded ankle joint

					Rotation	
	Flex	Ext	Abd	Add	Int	Ext
Ankle	(Dorsi) R	(Plantar) R				
Foot Subtalar					(Inver) R	(Ever) R

Biomechanical purpose: To provide resistances in both directions at the ankle (or can be also used posteriorly, at the subtalar)

Material and design: The side bars and joints are aluminum; the stirrup is stainless steel.

Fabrication: Comes prefabricated with stirrup, is easily attached to other parts of orthosis.

Special consideration: Alignment of joints is important to accommodate tibial torsion, when used at the ankle.

Type: Ankle joint
Name: Solid ankle

					Rotation	
	Flex	Ext	Abd	Add	Int	Ext
Ankle	(Dorsi) H	(Plantar) H				
Foot Subtalar					(Inver) H	(Ever) H

Biomechanical purpose: To restrict all motion at ankle and subtalar joint.

Material and design: Carbon steel or stainless steel; usually used with foot plate to restrict motion in foot joints.

Fabrication: Comes prefabricated; no serious problems in assembly.

Special consideration: Usually requires shoe-modifications (soft heel and rocker bar) to simulate ankle motion.

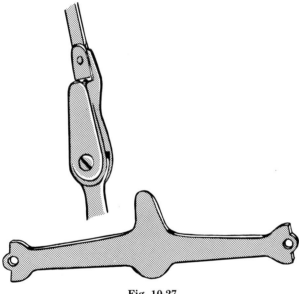

Fig. 10-27

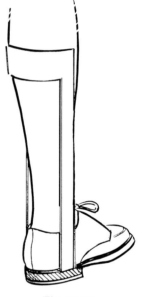

Fig. 10-28

Type: Ankle joint
Name: Single-bar plunger ankle joint

					Rotation	
	Flex	Ext	Abd	Add	Int	Ext
Ankle	(Dorsi) R or F	(Plantar) F or R				
Foot Subtalar					(Inver) F or R	(Ever) F or R

Biomechanical purpose: To provide resistance to either plantar flexion or dorsiflexion, yet permit transverse rotation around long axis of side bar. Vertical displacement of side bar (piston-cylinder arrangement) can be resisted by spring.

Material and design: Stainless steel or aluminum.

Fabrication: Comes prefabricated with stirrup; is easily attached to other parts of orthosis.

Special consideration: Used when subtalar motion can be permitted, or under slight resistance.

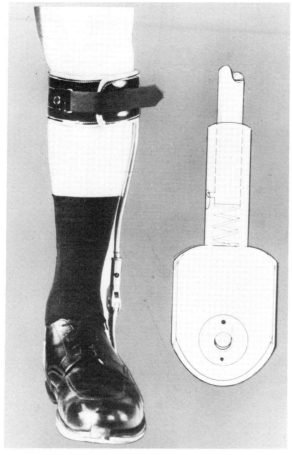

Fig. 10-29

Type: Shoe modification
Name: Sach heel and rocker bar

		Flex	Ext
Ankle		R*	R*
Foot	Subtalar		
	Midtarsal	F*	F*

*Simulated

Biomechanical purpose: To provide low resistance deformation of heel, at heel contact, *simulating* plantar flexion and with the rocker bar, a roll-over *simulated* dorsiflexion. Some subtalar motion will result.

Material and design: Sponge rubber laminae in heel, between thinned regular heel and leather heel base and leather rocker bar.

Fabrication: Requires replacing regular shoe heel with sponge rubber section and thinned out regular rubber, leather, or neoprene heel. Rocker bar is shaped from leather and nailed and glued in place.

Special consideration: Useful in AFOs where normal ankle function is restricted (see AFO-7 and AFO-10).

REFERENCES

Lindseth, R. E., and Glancy, J.: Polypropylene lower-extremity braces for paraplegia due to myelomeningocele, J. Bone Joint Surg. **56A**(3):556-563, April 1974.

McIlmurray, W. J., and Greenbaum, W.: The application of Sach foot principles to orthotics, Orthop. Prosthet. Appliance J. **13**:209-214, 1959.

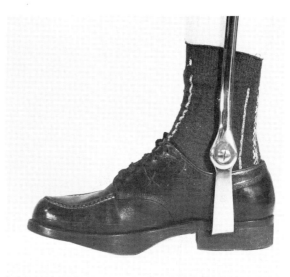

Fig. 10-30

Type: Accessory

Name: Anterior kneecap or infrapatellar strap

	Flex	Ext	Abd	Add
Knee	R	F	F	F

Biomechanical purpose: To provide posteriorly directed horizontal force at knee to prevent flexion of the knee.

Material and design: Leather or plastic sheet and fabric.

Fabrication: Comes prefabricated; must be assembled to rigid (metal) orthosis.

Special consideration: None.

Type: Accessory

Name: Valgus or varus corrective kneecap or pressure pad

	Flex	Ext	Abd	Add
Knee	F	F	R or F	F or R

Biomechanical purpose: To provide medially or laterally directed horizontal force at knee to resist valgum or varum.

Material and design: Leather or plastic sheet and fabric.

Fabrication: Comes prefabricated; must be assembled to rigid (metal) orthosis.

Special consideration: None.

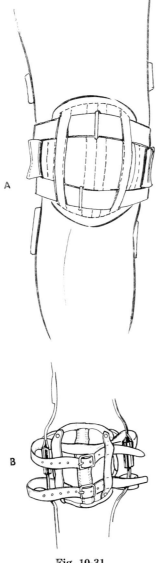

Fig. 10-31

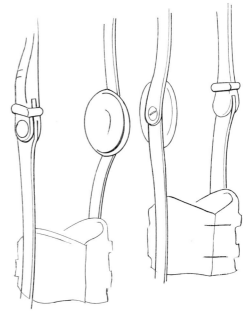

Fig. 10-32

Type: Accessory

Name: Valgus or varus corrective ankle strap (Fig. 10-33, *A*) or pressure pad (Fig. 10-33, *B*)

					Rotation	
	Flex	Ext	Abd	Add	Int	Ext
Ankle	(Dorsi) F	(Plantar) F				
Foot Subtalar					(Inver) R or F	(Ever) F or R

Biomechanical purpose: To provide medially or laterally directed horizontal force at ankle to resist valgum or varum.

Material and design: Leather or plastic sheet and fabric.

Fabrication: Comes prefabricated; must be attached to rigid orthosis.

Special consideration: None.

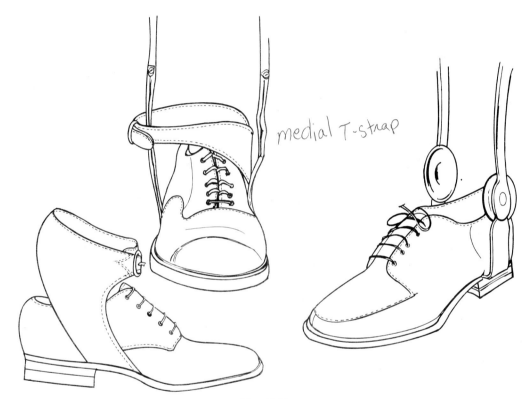

medial T-strap

Fig. 10-33

Type: FO (foot orthosis)

Name: Molded insert FO (University of California Biomechanics Laboratory)

	Flex	Ext	Abd	Add	Rotation	
					Int	Ext
A-Ankle						
F-Foot Subtalar					(Inver) R or H	(Ever) R or H
F-Foot Midtarsal	H	H	H	H	H	H

Biomechanical purpose: To hold foot in position of function in the shoe; can be used in conjunction with higher level orthoses to serve as foot attachment. See molded insert AFO (AFO-3).

Material and design: Molded plastic

Fabrication: Requires plaster cast model of foot and plastic laminating or vacuum forming of thermoplastic.

Special consideration: May need a size wider shoe.

REFERENCES

Committee on Prosthetics Research and Development, National Academy of Sciences: A clinical evaluation of four lower-limb orthoses, Report E-5, 1972, Washington, D.C.

Henderson, W. H., and Campbell, J. S.: UC-BL shoe insert casting and fabrication, Bull. Prosthet. Res. **10**(11):215-235, Spring 1969.

Inman, V. T.: UC-BL dual axis ankle-control system and UC-BL shoe insert: Biomechanical considerations, Bull. Prosthet. Res. **10**(11):130-145, Spring 1969.

Mereday, C., Dolan, C. M. E., and Lusskin, R.: Evaluation of the UC-BL shoe insert in "flexible" pes planus, New York University Medical Center, Sept. 1969.

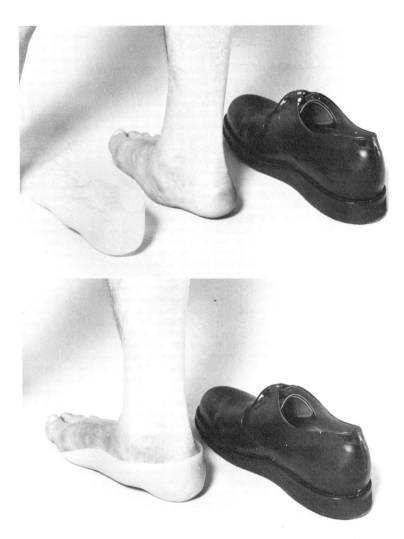

Fig. 10-34

Type: FO (foot orthosis)
Name: Bilateral shoe clamp FO (Denis Browne splint)

		Flex	Ext	Abd	Add	Rotation	
						Int	Ext
A-Ankle		(Dorsi) F	(Plantar) F				
F-Foot	Subtalar					(Inver) Hv	(Ever) Hv
	Midtarsal	H	H				
	Met Phal	H	H	H	H		

Biomechanical purpose: Axial limb rotation is determined by position of foot plate on bar. Abduction of entire limb by length of bar. Subtalar foot position depends on curve of bar, with apex of curve proximal producing a varus foot position, whereas, if the apex of the curve is distal, it produces a valgus position of the feet.

Material and design: Primarily metal

Fabrication: Prefabricated splint is easily attached to shoes.

Special consideration: Can interchange shoes, but should use high-top shoes.

REFERENCE

American Academy of Orthopaedic Surgeons: Orthopaedic appliances Atlas. Vol. 1. Braces, splints, shoe alterations, Ann Arbor, Mich., 1952, J. E. Edwards.

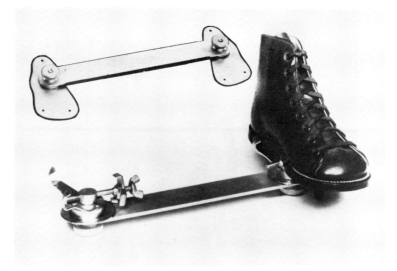

Fig. 10-35

Type: AFO (ankle-foot orthosis)
Name: Double Bar AFO (conventional short leg orthosis)

					Rotation	
	Flex	Ext	Abd	Add	Int	Ext
A-Ankle	(Dorsi) A	(Plantar) S/R				
F-Foot Subtalar					(Inver) H	(Ever) H

Biomechanical purpose: To provide dorsiflexion assistance during swing phase or to stop or limit plantar flexion. Joints can be varied.

Material and design: Metal uprights and shoe attachments, metal band, with leather or plastic accessories. Uses single channel, single-axis ankle joint.

Fabrication: Components are commercially available; bending to conform uprights to leg shape and location of ankle axis are critical. Requires fixed shoe attachment.

Special consideration: Uncontrolled motion may occur inside shoes. Straps are often added to limit varus or valgus at the ankle joint.

REFERENCE

American Academy of Orthopaedic Surgeons: Orthopaedic appliance atlas. Vol. 1. Braces, splints, shoe alterations, Ann Arbor, Mich., 1952, J. W. Edwards, p. 410.

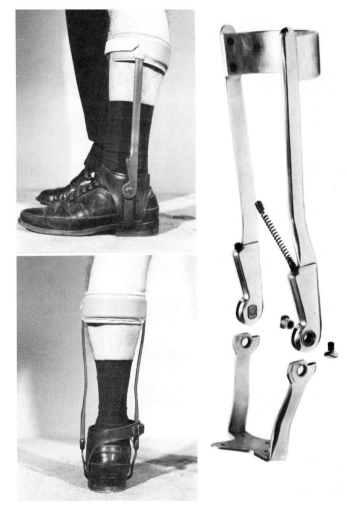

Fig. 10-36

Type: AFO (ankle-foot orthosis)
Name: Single bar orthosis

					Rotation	
	Flex	Ext	Abd	Add	Int	Ext
A-Ankle	(Dorsi) A	(Plantar) R				
F-Foot Subtalar					H	H

Biomechanical purpose: To provide dorsiflexion assistance during swing phase, or limit, or stop, plantar flexion.

Material and design: Metal upright and shoe attachment, metal or plastic band, with leather or plastic accessories, uses ankle joint (A-4).

Fabrication: Components are commercially available; bending to conform upright to leg shape and location of ankle axis are important. Requires fixed shoe attachment.

Special consideration: Subtalar motion occurs to a greater degree then with a double bar brace. Transverse rotation may be provided with special VAPC joint (A-8).

REFERENCES

Evaluation—VAPC modular single-bar braces, Bull. Prosthet. Res. **10**(9):152-153, Spring 1968.
VAPC draft manual, Single-bar leg and leg-thigh braces, September 15, 1970.

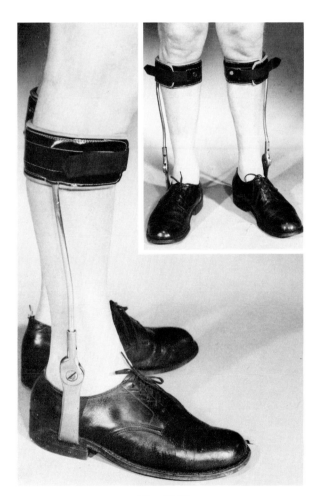

Fig. 10-37

Type: AFO (ankle-foot orthosis)

Name: Molded insert (New York University)

					Rotation	
	Flex	Ext	Abd	Add	Int	Ext
A-Ankle	(Dorsi) F/A/S	(Plantar) F/R/S				
F-Foot { Subtalar					(Inver) H	(Ever) H
{ Midtarsal	H	H				

Biomechanical purpose: To provide a strong medio-lateral stabilization of the subtalar joint and foot; effect on ankle motion as determined by type of ankle joint selected.

Material and design: Plastic or plastic laminate insert with metal uprights, metal or plastic band, with leather plastic accessories. Ankle joints may provide free, stop, or dorsiflexion assist motion.

Fabrication: Requires plaster cast model of foot and plastic laminating or vacuum forming of thermoplastic insert. Metal components are commercially available. Bending to conform uprights to leg shape and location of axis is critical.

Special consideration: Interchangeability of shoes with same heel height possible, but the use of inserts may require wider shoes.

REFERENCES

Committee on Prosthetics Research and Development, National Academy of Sciences: A clinical evaluation of four lower-limb orthoses, Report E-5, 1972, Washington, D.C.

Dolan, C. M. E., Mereday, C., and Hartmann, G.: Evaluation of NYU insert Brace, New York, July 1969, New York University Medical Center.

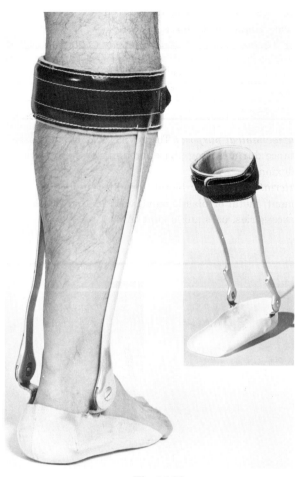

Fig. 10-38

Type: AFO (ankle-foot orthosis)

Name: Double rod (epoxy-fiberglass upright and conventional steel wire systems)

					Rotation	
	Flex	Ext	Abd	Add	Int	Ext
A-Ankle	(Dorsi) A	(Plantar) R				
F-Foot Subtalar					(Inver) R	(Ever) R

Biomechanical purpose: To provide dorsiflexion assistance during swing phase with a very minimum of mediolateral stabilization.

Material and design: Rods are made of spring steel wire or epoxy-fiberglass. Calf band may be metal or plastic; shoe attachment is metal.

Fabrication: Rods and other parts are commercially available. Requires assembly of rods to a band and the use of a metal shoe attachment.

Special consideration: These two orthosis represent lightweight AFO for light load dorsiflexion assistance.

REFERENCES

Evaluation: AMBRL fiberglass-epoxy drop foot brace, Bull. Prosthet. Res. **10**(9):153-155, Spring 1968.

Hill, J. T., and Stube, R. W.: The USAMBRL fiberglass dropfoot brace, Prosthet. Int. **3**:9-25-28, 1969.

Hill, J. T., and Stube, R. W.: Manual for the USAMBRL lateral rod drop-foot brace, United States Army Medical Bioengineering Research and Development Laboratory Tech. Rep. 7004, August 1970.

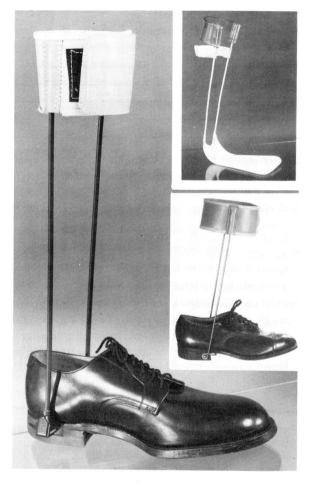

Fig. 10-39

Type: AFO (Ankle-foot orthosis)
Name: Shoe clasp (Veteran's Administration Prosthetics Center)

	Flex	Ext	Abd	Add	Rotation	
					Int	Ext
A-Ankle	(Dorsi) A	(Plantar) R				
F-Foot Subtalar					(Inver) R	(Ever) R

Biomechanical purpose: To provide dorsiflexion assistance during swing phase while providing slight mediolateral stability.

Material and design: Posterior bar made of epoxy-fiberglass material. Clasp is made of stainless steel; band can be metal or plastic.

Fabrication: Parts available commercially in kit form. Requires careful fitting of clasp to shoe heel counter and assembly of other parts to posterior bar.

Special consideration: Uses sliding attachment on cuff to reduce chafing. Orthosis is light-duty, lightweight, inexpensive device that allows interchangeability of shoes with same heel height. Low quarter Blucher type of shoes with firm heel counter required. Slightly longer shoes may be needed.

REFERENCES

Committee on Prosthetics Research and Development, National Academy of Sciences: Clinical evaluation of a comprehensive approach to below-knee orthotics, Report E-6, 1972.

Greenbaum, W.: VAPC equinus-control ankle-foot shoe-clasp orthosis (draft manual), New York, 1971, Veterans Administration Prosthetics Center.

Rubin, G., and Dixon, M.: The modern ankle-foot orthoses (AFOs), Bull. Prosthet. Res. **10-19:**20-41, Spring 1973.

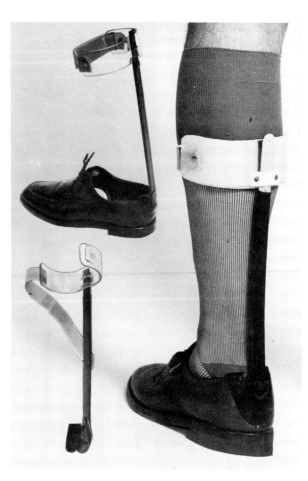

Fig. 10-40

Type: AFO (ankle-foot orthosis)

Name: Posterior bar (Army Medical Bioengineering Research and Development Laboratory)

	Flex	Ext	Abd	Add	Rotation	
					Int	Ext
A-Ankle	(Dorsi) A	(Plantar) R				
F-Foot Subtalar					(Inver) R	(Ever) R

Biomechanical purpose: To provide dorsiflexion assistance during swing phase while providing only a slight amount of mediolateral stabilization.

Material and design: Posterior bar is either epoxy-fiberglass or spring steel; calf band shoe (heel) attachment are metal, although band may be plastic.

Fabrication: Bar and other parts are commercially available; requires assembly of bars to band and shoe heel and modification of shoe heel.

Special consideration: A lightweight AFO for light-load dorsiflexion assistance. Plastic bars will be slightly more durable than is spring steel.

REFERENCES

Hill, J. T., and Fenwick, A. L.: A contoured, posterior, fiberglass-Epoxy Drop-Foot Brace, United States Army Medical Bioengineering Research and Development Laboratory Tech. Rep. 6805, May 1968, Forest Glen, Md.

Hill, J. T., and Stube, R. W.: An improved manufacturing technique for the USAMBRL fiberglass-epoxy drop-foot brace, United States Army Medical Bioengineering Research and Development Laboratory Tech. Rep. 6910, July 1969, Forest Glen, Md.

Hill, J. T., and Stube, R. W.: Manual for the USAMBRL posterior bar drop-foot brace, United States Army Medical Bioengineering Research and Development Laboratory Tech. Rep. 7003, August 1970, Forest Glen, Md.

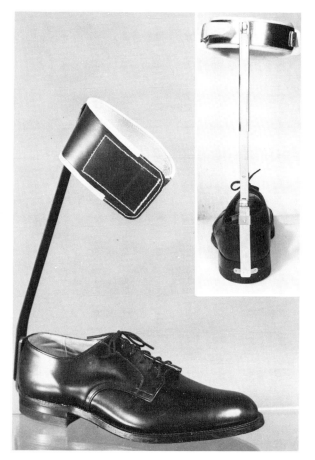

Fig. 10-41

Type: AFO (ankle-foot orthosis)
Name: Rigid orthosis

					Rotation	
	Flex	Ext	Abd	Add	Int	Ext
A-Ankle	(Dorsi) H	(Plantar) H				
F-Foot { Subtalar					(Inver) H	(Ever) H
F-Foot { Midtarsal	H	H				

Biomechanical purpose: To restrict all motion at ankle and in foot.

Material and design: Molded plastic or leather orthosis to extend on calf and to metatarsophalangeal joints to distribute pressure.

Fabrication: Requires plaster cast model of foot and leg.

Special consideration: Immobilizes foot and ankle in position provided by cast. Heel and sole of shoe are usually modified to provide roll-over action. Rigidity depends on type of plastic used and full encasement of foot and leg.

REFERENCE

Simons, B. C., Jebsen, R. H., and Wildman, L. E.: Plastic short leg brace fabrication, Orthot. Prosthet. **21**:215-218, Sept. 1967.

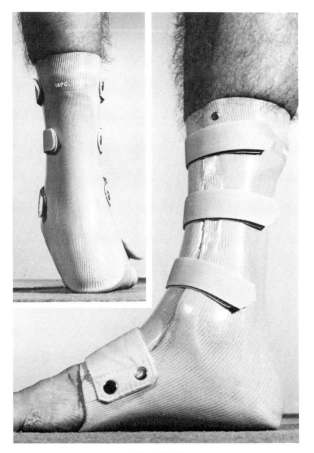

Fig. 10-42

Type: AFO (ankle-foot orthosis)
Name: Flexible plastic shell orthosis

					Rotation	
	Flex	Ext	Abd	Add	Int	Ext
A-Ankle	(Dorsi) A	(Plantar) R				
F-Foot Subtalar					R	R

Biomechanical purpose: To provide dorsiflexion assistance during swing phase while providing various degrees of mediolateral stability depending on lateral or medial trim.

Material and design: Flexible plastic.

Fabrication: Over plaster cast. Some models are available commercially in several sizes and design modifications.

Special consideration: Normally uses Velcro closure (Fig. 10-43, *A*). Trim can be varied to modify flexibility as noted in the posterior views (Fig. 10-43, *B* and *C*). Needs a larger size shoe, but shoes can be interchangeable.

REFERENCES

Engen, T. J.: Research developments of lower extremity orthotic systems for patients with various functional deficits, Houston, 1971, Texas Institute for Rehabilitation and Research.

Engen, T. J.: Instructional manual for fabrication and fitting of a below knee corrugated polypropylene orthosis, Houston, 1971, Texas Institute for Rehabilitation and Research.

Rubin, G., and Dixon, M.: The modern ankle-foot orthoses (AFOs), Bull. Prosthet. Res. **10-19:**20-41, Spring 1973.

Yates, G.: A method for the provision of lightweight aesthetic orthopaedic appliances, Orthopaedics 1(2):153-162, 1968.

A   B   C

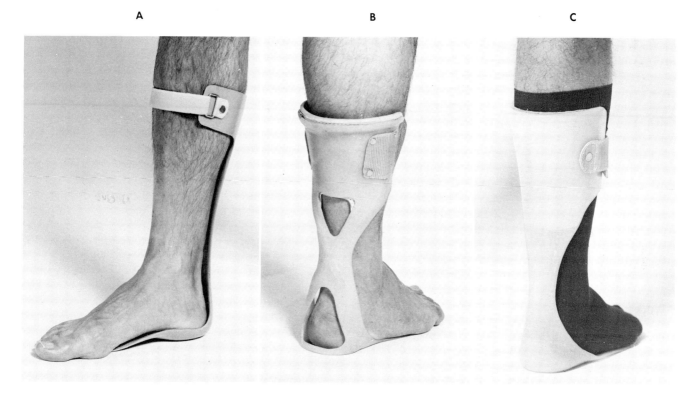

Fig. 10-43

Type: AFO (ankle-foot orthosis)

Name: Molded spiral orthosis (Institute of Rehabilitation Medicine)

					Rotation	
	Flex	Ext	Abd	Add	Int	Ext
A-Ankle	(Dorsi) A/R	(Plantar) A/R				
F-Foot Subtalar					S or R	S or R

Biomechanical purpose: To provide dorsiflexion assistance during swing phase and some plantar flexion assistance at push-off while the shoe insert portion provides moderate mediolateral stability.

Material and design: Plexidure; Nyloplex thermoplastic, polypropylene.

Fabrication: Requires plaster cast model of foot and leg over which hot forming of thermoplastic is performed. Proper trimming and fit are critical.

Special consideration: Shoes are interchangeable with same heel height but may need larger size.

REFERENCE

Lehneis, H. R.: New developments in lower limb orthotics through bioengineering, Arch. Phys. Med. Rehab. **53**(7): 303-310, July 1972.

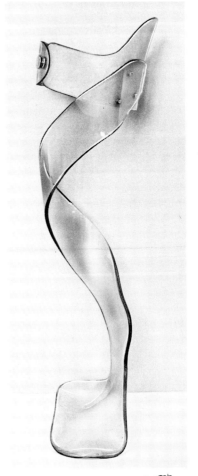

Fig. 10-44

Front of right

Type: AFO (ankle-foot orthosis)

Name: PTB weight-bearing orthosis (Veteran's Administration Prosthetics Center)

					Rotation		Axial Load
	Flex	Ext	Abd	Add	Int	Ext	
A-Ankle	(Dorsi) S_V	(Plantar) S_V					H
F-Foot Subtalar					(Inver) H	(Ever) H	H

Biomechanical purpose: To partially unweight leg with ankle motion control as desired by choice of orthotic ankle joint and by setting of stop, maximum of mediolateral stability is provided.

Material and design: Plastic laminate (PTB) socket with metal uprights, metal ankle joints, and metal shoe attachment. Socket may be lined.

Fabrication: Requires plaster cast model of leg for socket lamination and for fitting prefabricated uprights. Uprights can be made adjustable to vary unloading. Shoes are modified for stirrup attachment and for roll-over action, usually through use of a soft heel and rocker bar.

Special consideration: The amount of leg unloading varies considerably depending on soft-tissue tolerance and motion at ankle joint.

REFERENCE

McIlmurray, W. J., and Greenbaum, W.: A below-knee weight-bearing brace, Orthop. Prosthet. Appliance J. **12**(2):81-82, June 1958.

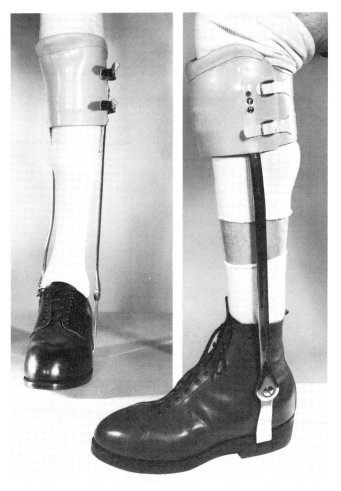

Fig. 10-45

Type: KO (knee orthosis)
Name: Molded plastic orthosis (Institute of Rehabilitation Medicine; Nitschke)

					Rotation	
	Flex	Ext	Abd	Add	Int	Ext
K-Knee	F	S	H	H	S	S

Biomechanical purpose: To prevent hyperextension of the knee joint while providing mediolateral stability.
Material and design: Plastic laminate (polyester-nylon stockinet) or thermoplastic.
Fabrication: Requires cast model of leg-knee-thigh area, which is used for laminating or forming thermoplastic orthoses.

Special consideration: Requires careful fitting; Institute of Rehabilitation Medicine design (Fig. 10-46, *A*) donned and removed over foot and leg. Nitschke model (Fig. 10-46, *B*) uses bivalved design. Good cosmesis, since orthosis is contoured to leg, but does protrude anteriorly when patient is sitting.

REFERENCES

Lehneis, H. R.: New developments in lower-limb orthotics through bioengineering, Arch. Phys. Med. Rehab. **53**(7): 303-310, July 1972.
Nitschke, R. O., and Marschall, D.: The PTS knee brace, Orthot. Prosthet. **22**(3):46-51, Sept. 1968.

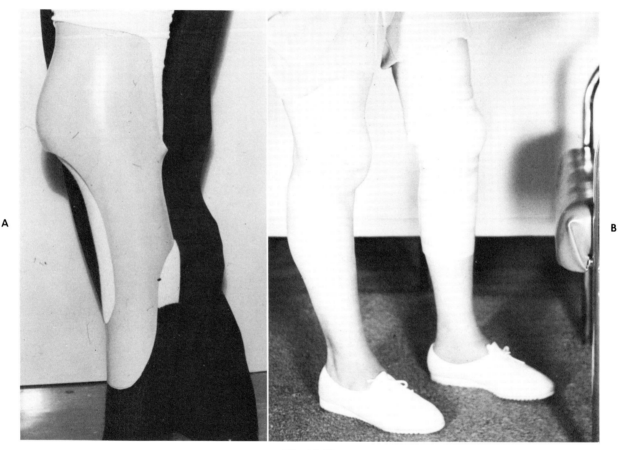

Fig. 10-46

Type: KO (knee orthosis)

Name: Rigid three-point pressure orthosis (Swedish knee cage)

	Flex	Ext	Abd	Add
K-Knee	F	S	H	H

Biomechanical purpose: To prevent mild hyperextension yet provide good mediolateral stability.

Material and design: Prefabricated in metal with soft posterior pad. Thigh and calf straps are heavy elastic.

Fabrication: Commercially available in prefabricated form. Fitting requires very minor adjustments.

Special consideration: Cosmesis is poor, mediolateral dimension is bulky and orthosis protrudes slightly when sitting.

REFERENCE

The Swedish knee cage, Artif. Limbs **12**(2):54-57, Autumn 1968.

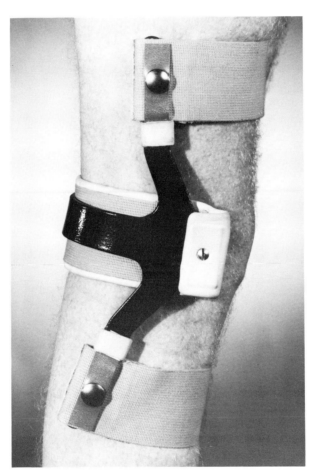

Fig. 10-47

Type: KO (knee orthosis)
Name: Double anterior loop knee orthosis (Lenox Hill orthosis)

					Rotation	
	Flex	Ext	Abd	Add	Int	Ext
K-Knee	F	F	H	H	H	H

Biomechanical purpose: To allow full knee flexion and yet provide some mediolateral and rotatory stability.

Material and design: Metal, gum rubber, and fabric straps.

Fabrication: Requires cast model of leg-knee-thigh for fabrication.

Special consideration: Used generally during competitive sports activity only. Generally not used for day-long knee support.

REFERENCE

The Lenox Hill Derotation Brace, a descriptive brochure on its use published by Lenox Hill Brace Shop, Inc., 100 East 77 Street, New York, New York 10021.

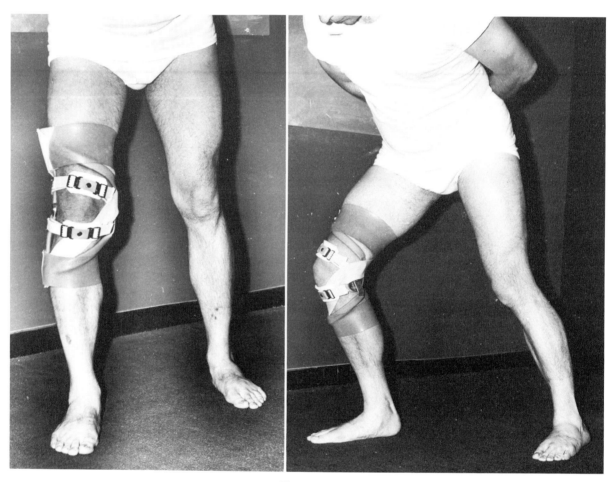

Fig. 10-48

Type: KO (knee orthosis)
Name: Hinged knee cage

					Rotation	
	Flex	Ext	Abd	Add	Int	Ext
K-Knee	S$_L$	S$_L$	H	H	R	R

Biomechanical purpose: To provide mediolateral stabilization. Control of flexion or extension depends on stop or lock used at knee joint.

Material and design: Bands may be plastic, leather, or fabric. Hinged uprights may be plastic or metal (Fig. 10-49, *A*). In Fig. 10-49, *B*, note the screw locking orthosis in extension.

Fabrication: Plastic type requires cast model of leg-knee-thigh area. Orthosis also available commercially.

Special consideration: None.

REFERENCES

Dixon, M. A., and Palumbo, R. L.: Polypropylene knee orthosis with latex suprapatellar strap suspension, Orthot. Prosthet. **29**(3):29-31, Sept. 1975.

American Academy of Orthopaedic Surgeons: Orthopaedic appliances atlas. Vol. 1. Braces, splints, shoe alterations, Ann Arbor, Mich., 1952, J. W. Edwards.

A   B

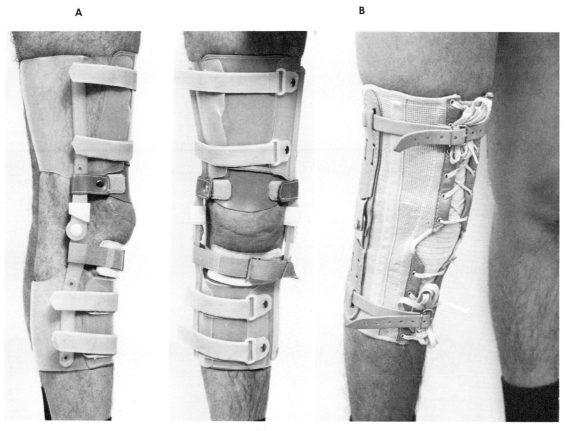

Fig. 10-49

Type: KO (knee orthosis)
Name: Knee extension cage (Rancho Los Amigos)

					Rotation	
	Flex	Ext	Abd	Add	Int	Ext
K-Knee	R	R	R	R	H	H

Biomechanical purpose: To provide adjustable extension of knee joint to reduce knee flexion contractures. May provide stabilization of knee for ambulation.

Material and design: Leather, Velcro straps, felt or plastic padding, and aluminum bars.

Fabrication: Requires tracing and leg-thigh measurements, bending of bars, attachment of cuffs that pivot (with padding), and kneecap. Dial locks, elastic turnbuckle, and straps can be used to modify function.

Special consideration: Used as a temporary orthosis to reduce knee flexion contractures. Effective use requires long lever arm.

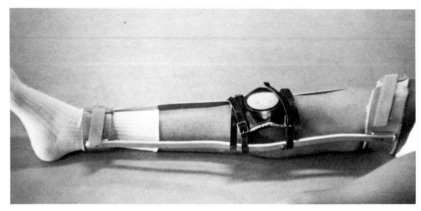

Fig. 10-50

Type: KAFO (knee-ankle-foot orthosis)
Name: Long leg double bar orthosis

	Flex	Ext	Abd	Add	Rotation Int	Rotation Ext
K-Knee	F/S∨	F/S∨	H	H	H	H
L-Leg						
A-Ankle	(Dorsi) A/F/S	(Plantar) F/R/S				
F-Foot Subtalar					(Inver) H	(Ever) H

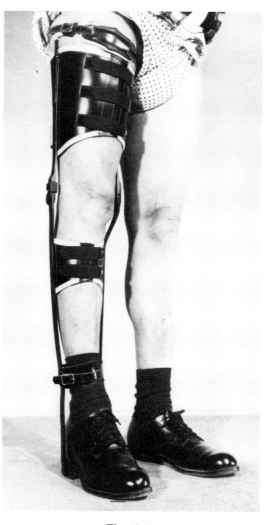

Biomechanical purpose: To provide flexion and extension and mediolateral stabilization of the knee. Orthosis also allows free, limited, or stop action at the ankle joint. It may also provide free or locked knee motion.

Material and design: Metal uprights, bands, joints, and shoe attachment with leather and fabric accessories. Most parts are prefabricated.

Fabrication: Requires tracing of entire lower limb. Alignment of knee and ankle joints critical in relation to anatomic joints in both frontal, sagittal, and coronal planes.

Special consideration: Heel tunnel calipers provide easier shoe change but displacement of ankle axis. Knee flexion deformities may require special knee joints, special alignment of uprights, and a wide calf and thigh band.

REFERENCES

American Academy of Orthopaedic Surgeons: Orthopaedic appliances atlas. Vol. 1. Brace, splints, shoe alterations, Ann Arbor, Mich., 1952, J. W. Edwards.

Lehneis, H. R.: Final report: Bioengineering design and development of lower extremity orthotic devices, Institute of Rehabilitation Medicine, New York University Medical Center, Oct. 1972.

Fig. 10-51

Type: KAFO (knee-ankle-foot orthosis)
Name: Double bar, knee lock, hip stabilizing orthosis
(Craig Rehabilitation Hospital)

					Rotation	
	Flex	Ext	Abd	Add	Int	Ext
K-Knee	S$_L$	S$_L$	H	H	H	H
L-Leg						
A-Ankle	(Dorsi) S$_V$	(Plantar) S$_V$				
F-Foot Subtalar					(Inver) H	(Ever) H

Biomechanical purpose: To provide knee and ankle stabilization and allow passive hip stabilization by ankle alignment in dorsiflexion.

Material and design: Metal uprights, bands, joints, stirrup and shoe attachment. Ankle joint has adjustable stops (A-3-1).

Fabrication: Requires tracing of entire lower limb.

Special consideration: Knee joint is posteriorly offset to facilitate locking and to reduce clothing wear. A bail lock may be used for easier knee-joint unlocking. The shoes are stabilized by double bar stirrup and long shank. Uses heel cushion to provide some simulated plantar flexion at heel strike.

REFERENCES

Hahn, H. R.: Lower extremity bracing in paraplegics with usage follow up, Paraplegia 8(3):147-153, Nov. 1970.

Scott, B. A.: Engineering principles and fabrication techniques for the Scott-Craig long-leg brace for paraplegics, Orthot. Prosthet. 25:14-19, Dec. 1971.

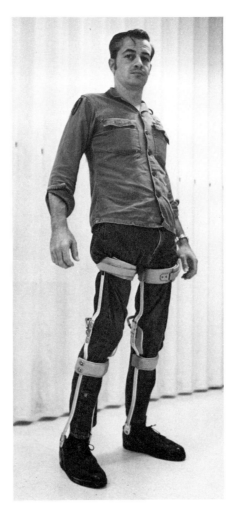

Fig. 10-52

Type: KAFO (knee-ankle-foot orthosis)
Name: Quadrilateral brim, weight-bearing orthosis

					Rotation		Axial Load
	Flex	Ext	Abd	Add	Int	Ext	
T-Thigh							H
K-Knee	S$_L$	S$_L$	H	H	H	H	H
L-Leg							H
A-Ankle	(Dorsi) S$_V$	(Plantar) S$_V$					H
F-Foot Subtalar					(Inver) H	(Ever) H	H

Biomechanical purpose: To partially unload thigh and lower limb with pelvic belt and locked knee and ankle joint.

Material and design: Molded plastic above-knee socket, metal uprights, bands, joints and shoe attachment with leather and fabric accessories.

Fabrication: Quadrilateral brim may be prefabricated or made over plaster-cast model of thigh. Uprights may be made adjustable for unloading. Uses shoe modifications, soft heel, and rocker bar to simulate ankle motion.

Special consideration: Unloading effect only occurs with locked knee and ankle.

REFERENCE

Russek, A., and Eschen, F.: Ischial weight bearing brace with quadrilateral wood top—preliminary report, Orthop. Prosthet. Appliance J. **12**(3):31-35, Sept. 1958.

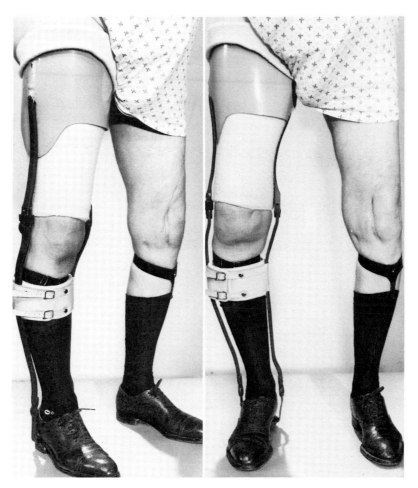

Fig. 10-53

Type: KAFO (knee-ankle-foot orthosis)
Name: Single-bar, knee lock orthosis (Nitschke)

	Flex	Ext	Abd	Add	Rotation Int	Rotation Ext
K-Knee	S$_L$	S$_L$	H$_V$	H$_V$		
L-Leg						
A-Ankle	(Dorsi) A	(Plantar) R				
F-Foot Subtalar					(Inver) H$_V$	(Ever) H$_V$

Biomechanical purpose: To provide flexion and extension and mediolateral stabilization at the knee, using three-point force system. Ankle joint can be varied to meet patient's need.

Material and design: Single metal upright, metal bands and joints with leather and plastic accessories. Molded plastic or leather thigh and pretibial cuffs.

Fabrication: Requires tracing of entire lower limb and a cast model for shaping of thigh and calf band.

Special consideration: Uprights may be attached to shoe insert to provide subtalar control and shoe exchange.

REFERENCE

Nitschke, R. O.: A single-bar above-knee orthosis, Orthot. Prosthet. **25**:4-20-25, Dec. 1971.

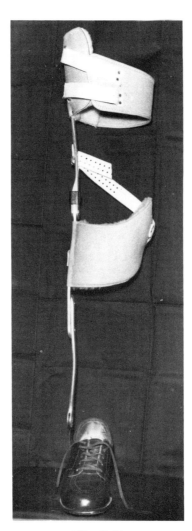

Fig. 10-54

Type: KAFO (knee-ankle-foot orthosis)
Name: Hip abduction orthosis (Ontario Crippled Children's Center)

					Rotation	
	Flex	Ext	Abd	Add	Int	Ext
H-Hip	H$_V$	H$_V$	H	H	H	H
T-Thigh						
K-Knee	F	F	H	H		
L-Leg						
A-Ankle	(Dorsi) H$_V$	(Plantar) H$_V$				
F-Foot Subtalar					(Inver) H	(Ever) H

Biomechanical purpose: To stabilize hip joints bilaterally at 45 degrees of abduction and 15 degrees of internal rotation, to maintain femoral heads in acetabulums.

Material and design: Metal structure and joints; leather or plastic thigh cuffs (Fig. 10-55, *A*).
Fabrication: Assembled from kit of prefabricated parts to match measurements taken from patient.
Special consideration: Orthosis is jointed (Fig. 10-55, *B*) to allow knee flexion for ambulation (Fig. 10-55, *C*) and sitting while maintaining 45-degree hip abduction. Ankle and subtalar joints are stabilized and supported in neutral position by alignment and high-top shoes. Thigh supports essential to avoid genu valgum.

REFERENCE

Bobechko, W. P., McLaurin, C. A., and Motloch, W. M.: Toronto orthosis for Legg-Perthes Disease, Artif. Limbs **12**(2): 36-41, Autumn 1968.

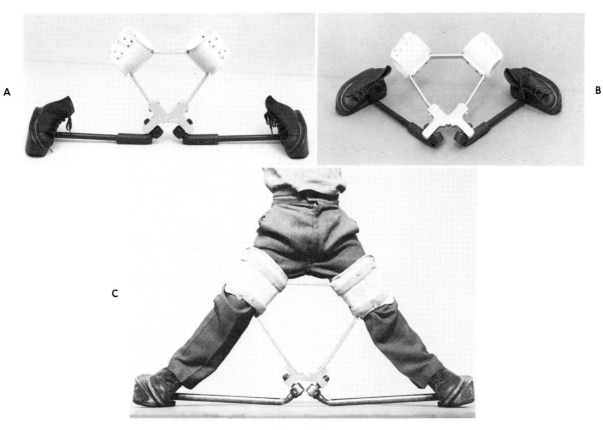

Fig. 10-55

Type: KAFO (knee-ankle-foot orthosis)

Name: Molded plastic orthosis (Institute of Rehabilitation Medicine—Fig. 10-56, *A*—and Veteran's Administration Prosthetic Center [VAPC]—Fig. 10-56, *B*)

	Flex	Ext	Abd	Add	Rotation Int	Rotation Ext
K-Knee	F	S$_V$	H	H	H*	H*
L-Leg						
A-Ankle	(Dorsi) H	(Plantar) H				
F-Foot Subtalar					(Inver) H	(Ever) H

*In VAPC variant

Biomechanical purpose: To allow free knee motion during swing phase and knee extension. Stability during stance by fixed ankle plantar flexion. Hyperextension of the knee prevented by high anterior thigh wall.

Material and design: Molded plastic. Metal knee joints may be used in VAPC variant.

Fabrication: Requires full cast model of the lower limb for molding of orthosis. The VAPC variant requires the metal uprights to be shaped and aligned over cast before lamination.

Special consideration: Length discrepancy must be accommodated because of plantar-flexed ankle. Cosmesis of this orthosis is good since it is contoured. The one-piece design (Fig. 10-56, *A*) will protrude slightly when sitting; use of joints (Fig. 10-56, *B*) overcomes this problem.

REFERENCES

Lehneis, H. R.: New concepts in lower extremity orthotics, Med. Clin. N. Am. **53**(3):585-592, May 1969.

Lehneis, H. R.: Final report: Bioengineering design and development of lower extremity orthotic devices, Institute of Rehabilitation Medicine, New York University Medical Center, Oct. 1972.

Lehneis, H. R.: New developments in lower-limb orthotics through bioengineering, Arch. Phys. Med. Rehab. **53**(7): 303-310, July 1972.

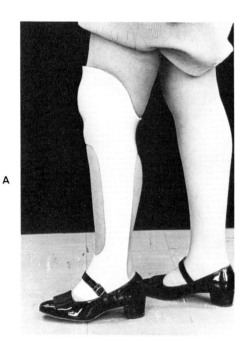
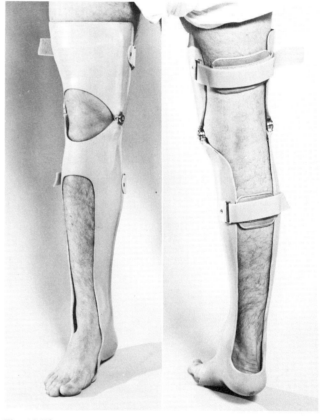

Fig. 10-56

Type: KAFO (knee-ankle-foot orthosis)
Name: Molded plastic hinged orthosis (VAPC)

					Rotation	
	Flex	Ext	Abd	Add	Int	Ext
K-Knee	F	Sv	H	H	H	H
L-Leg						
A-Ankle	(Dorsi) A	(Plantar) R				
F-Foot Subtalar					(Inver) R	(Ever) R

Biomechanical purpose: To control hyperextension knee, to provide dorsiflexion assistance with amount of ankle control varied by trim of shell.

Material and design: All plastic except joint, bolts, and rivets. Several designs are possible using either polypropylene (Fig. 10-57) or a plastic composite (Fig. 10-56, *B*). Fig. 10-56, *B,* also contains a regular metal joint whereas Fig. 10-57 uses a joint with only the pivot pin made of metal.

Fabrication: Requires full cast model of the lower limb for molding of thigh and leg-foot segments and for shaping plastic uprights.

Special consideration: Shoe insert permits shoe interchangeability although shoe may have to be larger. Improved cosmesis and light weight are achieved in this design, but at the expense of stability and durability.

REFERENCE
Rubin, G., and Palumbo, R. L.: A polypropylene knee-ankle orthosis, Int. Soc. Prosthet. Orthot. Bull. **8:**8, Oct. 1973.

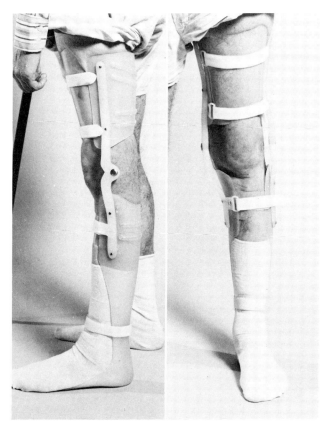

Fig. 10-57

Type: KAFO (knee-ankle-foot orthosis)
Name: Trilateral socket hip abduction orthosis

	Flex	Ext	Abd	Add	Rotation		Axial Load
					Int	Ext	
H-Hip	F	F	F	R	A	R	H V
T-Thigh							H V
K-Knee	S L	S L	S	S	S	S	H V
L-Leg							H V
A-Ankle	(Dorsi) F	(Plantar) F					

Biomechanical purpose: Ischial weight-bearing socket for reducing axial load on hip joint, designed to hold hip in position of abduction and internal rotation providing concentric coverage of femoral head. Weight bearing occurs through medial upright from ischium to walking heel of orthosis.

Material and design: Plastic laminate quadrilateral brim with lateral wall extended superiorly over trochanter and cut out inferiorly to permit abduction of thigh. Stainless steel single medial upright with drop-ring knee lock, and growth adjustments above and below knee joint. Slide guide extension with spring maintains alignment of foot and ankle through stirrup attached to shoe. Opposite shoe requires a build up 3 inches at heel and 2½ inches at sole.

Fabrication: Socket made over positive mold of proximal thigh. Modifications of mold similar to that for above-knee quadrilateral socket. Ischial shelf formed so as to be horizontal when thigh is in 30° of abduction.

Special consideration: Rubber walking heel on stainless steel plate wedged posterolaterally to enhance internal rotation. Elastic strap from toe of shoe to walking heel extension may be used to increase internal rotation. Bilateral orthoses may be used in bilateral cases or in unilateral cases to increase degree of abduction.

REFERENCE

Tachdjian, M. O., and Jovett, L. O.: Trilateral socket hip abduction orthosis for the treatment of Legg-Perthes disease, Orthot. Prosthet. **22**(2):49-62, June 1968.

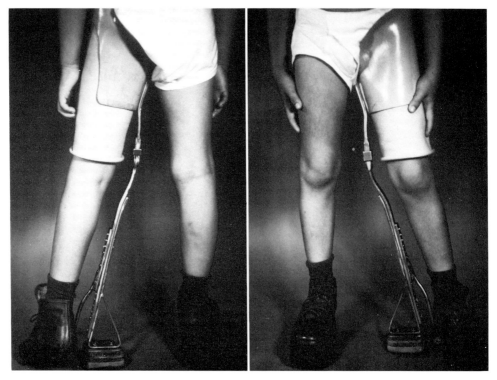

Fig. 10-58

Type: KAFO (knee-ankle-foot orthosis)
Name: Hip abduction orthosis (Newington Ambulatory abduction brace)

					Rotation	
	Flex	Ext	Abd	Add	Int	Ext
H-Hip	H ∨	H ∨	H	H	H	H
T-Thigh						
K-Knee	H	H	H	H	H 15°	
L-Leg						
A-Ankle	(Dorsi) H ∨	(Plantar) H ∨				
F-Foot Subtalar					(Inver) H	(Ever) H

Biomechanical purpose: To stabilize the hip joints bilaterally at 45° abduction and 20° internal rotation, to maintain femoral heads centered in acetabulums.

Material and design: Aluminum 2024 (duraluminum) adjustable frame structure, thigh cuffs, foot plates with neolite soles. Steel ankle- and foot-support brackets. Molded plastic knee-support shells.

Fabrication: Assembled from kit of prefabricated parts to match measurements taken from patient.

Special consideration: Free abduction of hips is prerequisite for use. Plastic knee stabilizing shells maintain knee in 10° of flexion to assist rotation control and avoid locking of knees in full extension. Lofstrand crutches used fore and aft for walking.

REFERENCE

Curtis, B. H., Gunther, S. F., Gossling, H. R., and Paul, S. W.: Treatment for Legg-Perthes disease with the Newington ambulatory abduction brace, J. Bone Joint Surg. **56-A:** 1135-1146, Sept. 1974.

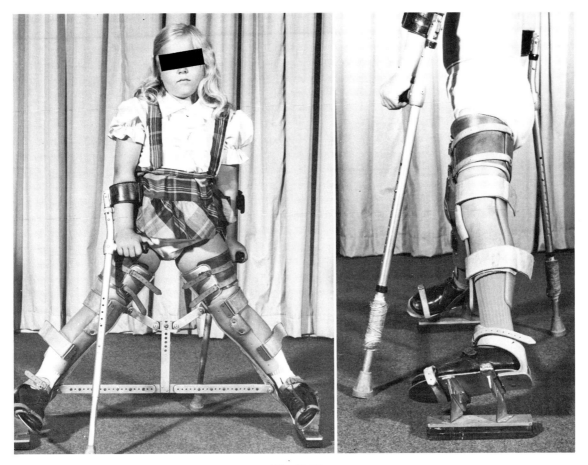

Fig. 10-59

Type: HO (hip orthosis)

Name: Hip control orthosis (Rancho Los Amigos)

					Rotation	
	Flex	Ext	Abd	Add	Int	Ext
H-Hip	F	F	F	S∨	R	R

Biomechanical purpose: To limit abduction at the hip while permitting free flexion and extension of hip.

Material and design: Waist belt and thigh cuff of metal reinforced with padded plastic or leather. Upright is aluminum with double axis joint and variable stop to limit abduction.

Fabrication: Requires tracing of pelvic-thigh region, waist and thigh measurements, and bending of upper segment to conform to waist-hip contour.

Special consideration: None.

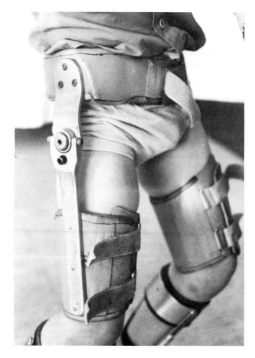

Fig. 10-60

Type: HKAFO (hip-knee-ankle-foot orthosis)
Name: Double bar orthosis (conventional)

					Rotation	
	Flex	Ext	Abd	Add	Int	Ext
H-Hip	F/S	F/S	H	H	H	H
T-Thigh						
K-Knee	S$_L$	S$_L$	H	H	H	H
L-Leg						
A-Ankle	F/S/H	F/S/H				
F-Foot Subtalar					(Inver) H	(Ever) H

Biomechanical purpose: To provide selective hip-joint control with provision for stabilization of knee and ankle as needed.

Material and design: Metal uprights, bands, joints, and shoe attachments; leather and fabric accessories. Most parts are prefabricated. Pelvic attachment can be pelvic band, spinal orthosis, or molded pelvic shell.

Fabrication: Requires tracing of entire lower limb and portion of pelvic area. Shaping of uprights and alignment of joints is done on tracing or on cast model of pelvis when molded shell is used.

Special consideration: This amount of orthotic control is rarely called for.

REFERENCE

American Academy of Orthopaedic Surgeons: Orthopaedic appliances atlas. Vol. 1. Braces, splints, shoe alterations, Ann Arbor, Mich. 1952, J. W. Edwards.

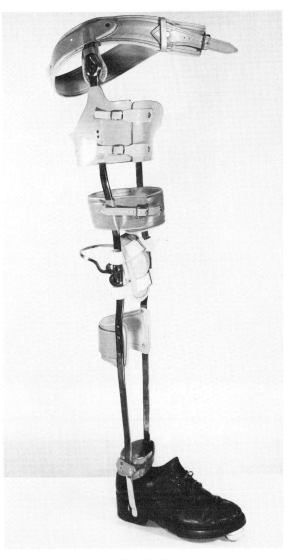

Fig. 10-61

Type: HKAFO (hip-knee-ankle-foot orthosis)
Name: Twister orthosis

					Rotation	
	Flex	Ext	Abd	Add	Int	Ext
H-Hip	F	F	F	F	A or R	R or A
T-Thigh						
K-Knee	F	F	F	F	A or R	R or A
L-Leg						
A-Ankle	(Dorsi) F	(Plantar) F				
F-Foot Subtalar					A or R	R or A

Biomechanical purpose: To provide twisting moment around long axis of limb to assist in external-internal rotation of hip, knee, ankle, or foot.

Material and design: Prefabricated metal-spring cable system.

Fabrication: Requires proper length and attachment to shoe and waist belt.

Special consideration: May cause rotation laxity of knee joint and produce permanent external tibial torsional deformity.

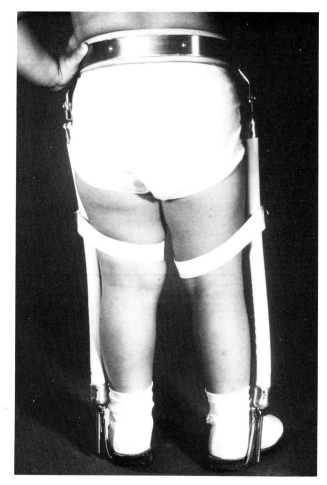

Fig. 10-62

Type: HKAFO (hip-knee-ankle-foot orthosis)
Name: Standing orthosis for children (OCCC standing orthosis)

					Rotation	
	Flex	Ext	Abd	Add	Int	Ext
H-Hip	H	H	H	H	H	H
T-Thigh						
K-Knee	H	H	H	H	H	H
L-Leg						
A-Ankle	(Dorsi) H	(Plantar) H				
F-Foot Subtalar					(Inver) H	(Ever) H

Biomechanical purpose: To stabilize all joints in neutral position for standing. Swing-through or pivoting gait allowed.

Material and design: Prefabricated metal parts with fabric accessories.

Fabrication: Assembly of commercially available parts from a kit with appropriate length adjustments of uprights.

Special consideration: Requires high-top shoes for adequate foot support.

REFERENCE

Motloch, W.: New items for the spina bifida program, Inter-Clinic Information Bull. vol. 10, July 1970.

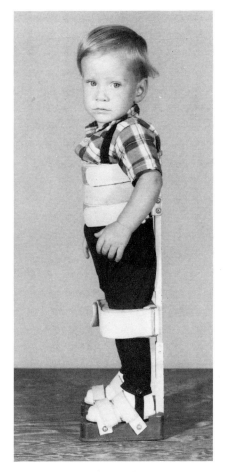

Fig. 10-63

Type: HKAFO (hip-knee-ankle-foot orthosis)
Name: Standing/sitting orthosis for children (OCCC parapodium)

					Rotation	
	Flex	Ext	Abd	Add	Int	Ext
H-Hip	S L	S L	H	H	H	H
T-Thigh						
K-Knee	S L	S L	H	H	H	H
L-Leg						
A-Ankle	(Dorsi) H	(Plantar) H				
F-Foot Subtalar					(Inver) H	(Ever) H

Biomechanical purpose: To stabilize all joints in neutral position for standing, yet allow unlocking for sitting.

Material and design: Prefabricated metal parts with fabric accessories.

Fabrication: Assembly of commercially available parts from a kit used, with appropriate length adjustments of upright.

Special consideration: The ankle and subtalar joints are stabilized in neutral position for standing and sitting by the use of high-top shoes.

REFERENCE

Motloch, W.: The parapodium: An orthotic device for neuro-muscular disorders, Artif. Limbs **15**(2):36-47, Autumn 1971.

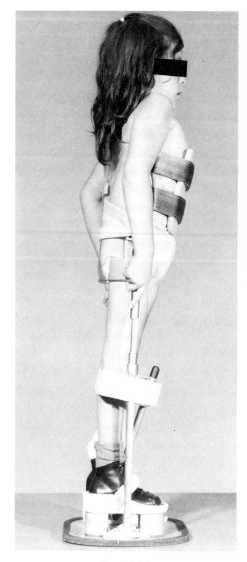

Fig. 10-64

CHAPTER 11

Prescription principles

JAMES M. CARY, M.D.
RALPH LUSSKIN, M.D.
ROBERT G. THOMPSON, M.D.

The adequate prescription of a lower limb orthosis for a patient has four important requisites:

1. Identification of the primary basic purpose for which the orthosis is to be prescribed
2. Definition and understanding of the biomechanical deficits present in the patient
3. Appreciation of the comparative attributes of available orthotic systems
4. Reevaluation of the patient after application of the prescribed orthosis to ensure its effectiveness and its correct use

THE ORTHOTIC TEAM

The treatment of the amputee has been improved by the use of a multidisciplinary, or team approach, to his problem. The patient with biomechanical limb defects who might be aided by the prescription of an adequate orthosis, and who often presents a more complex problem than does the amputee, should benefit even more from this approach to treatment. The amputee generally requires consideration of one or, at the most, two alternative prosthetic devices, whereas the patient who needs an orthosis may present a multiplicity of deficits, and several different possible approaches to treatment.

The first member of such an orthotic team should be a physician with an active interest in the field of rehabilitation. However, he should also have a knowledge and an understanding of effective surgical approaches to the treatment of biomechanical deficiencies. If avenues of surgical reconstruction are denied the patient, whether it be through nonoperative prejudice, lack of awareness, or failure to understand the principles of effective reconstruction, optimum function will not be obtained through orthotic application alone. Conversely, the surgeon who uses as his sole indication for multiple surgical procedures the desire to "get rid of braces" may deny his patient the optimum function and durability that may be attained by a combination of judicious surgical reconstruction and orthotic control. A specialized knowledge of the field of orthotics is needed by the physician to aid his clinical judgment.

The second member of the team is the orthotist. Certification by the American Board of Certification in Orthotics indicates that he has had adequate training in the field of orthotics and has successfully passed an examination by his peers attesting to his ability and skill. He should, in addition, by continued communication with the other members of his team acquire an understanding and an experience with clinical problems, in the solution of which he is asked to participate.

The physical therapist is the third member of the team. The therapist provides help in identifying functional problems and orthotic needs, teaches the patient the proper use of his orthosis, and provides an evaluation of the adequacy of the orthotic device.

Just as amputation clinic teams have multiplied across the country, it is hoped that with new emphasis and interest in orthotics, so too will orthotic clinic teams eventually be available. The complexity of biomechanical problems in the disabled patient makes it advisable to bring these several disciplines together in order to provide an adequate solution. The emphasis should be on scheduled meetings of the orthotic team so that the prescription and resulting appliance represents a consensus.

Occasionally it may not be possible for the group to meet as a team. The patient may be evaluated first by a physician or by the physical therapist who then arrives at a written orthotic prescription for the patient's problems. The *biomechanical matrix* can serve as a useful tool for transmitting this data to the orthotist. A skilled and experienced orthotist might find this the only prescription requirement. He would, however, discuss his orthosis concept with the physician, so that a final design can be established.

In other circumstances a detailed written prescription listing specific components, design, and alignment requirements may be necessary. The orthotist must appreciate the goal or purpose of the orthotic treatment program, and he must be aware of the specific problems in the individual patient. After fabrication of the orthosis the patient and his appliance should then be evaluated by the therapist, physician, and orthotist for its effectiveness and for instruction of the patient in its proper use.

ANALYSIS OF PATIENT PROBLEMS

To obtain a satisfactory evaluation of an individual requiring lower-limb orthotic assistance in order to crawl, stand, or walk, one needs to evaluate systematically the patient's problems. The use of a *technical analysis form,* similar to that illustrated in this volume, will provide the examiner with a standardized approach to the patient's deficits. The form indicates the data to be collected for adequate evaluation of the biomechanical deficiencies present in the foot, knee, ankle, and hip. The patient is examined at rest, standing, and then ambulating. This ambulation may be on an independent basis, or with aids such as cane,

crutches, or walker. When these evaluations are completed, certain biomechanical deficiencies are identified.

The biomechanical deficits are independent of the diagnosis or specific disease state present. Similar defects may be occasioned by conditions that could be quite diverse from an etiologic standpoint. Injuries to the musculoskeletal system, infection of bones or joints, paralysis, either flaccid or spastic, joint diseases, or congenital deformities, are differing causes, yet several may present similar biomechanical deficits. The new approach to orthotic prescription is based primarily, not on the disease, but on the biomechanical deficit present. The character of the underlying disease, nevertheless, must be taken into account in the evaluation because of its prognostic implication or the need for special approaches.

During an evaluation of any patient one needs to be aware that orthotic assistance may be but one part of the treatment program. Judicious surgery may eliminate the need for an orthosis entirely, or it may permit proper or better use of a corrective or supportive device. Physical therapy for joint range of motion, muscle strengthening, and orthotic-use training are usually necessary for optimum orthosis function.

PRIMARY PURPOSE OF ORTHOTIC PRESCRIPTION

We have stated that it is important to identify the primary purpose for which the appliance is to be used. It will be found that the function of a lower-limb orthosis will, in this respect, fall under one or more of three major headings.
1. Prevention of deformity
2. Protection of a weakened or painful musculoskeletal segment
3. Improvement of function

There are certain very specialized applications that may serve a fourth function, that of correction of deformity. For example, the well-known Denis Browne splint may be used in the active correction of the clubfoot. The Milwaukee brace is often used in the corrective treatment of scoliosis. These applications are generally used as a part of a comprehensive active treatment program. Most of these special applications are covered elsewhere in this volume and need not be considered in this chapter.

In prescribing and designing the lower-limb orthosis, the members of the orthotic team, physician, orthotist, and therapist will be wise to keep the primary purpose in mind. The patient and his family must be educated and frequently reminded of the purpose for which the orthosis is prescribed, designed, and worn. All too often, an orthosis applied for the prevention of deformity may be discarded because the patient may walk better without it. The parents may have lost sight of the primary purpose of the appliance, and effective treatment may be interrupted. As an example, a well-controlled hemophilic arthropathy of the knee may be subjected to repeated trauma, hemarthrosis, and recurrence of contracture because the orthosis, prescribed primarily for protection, was not worn because it did not seem to improve the function of the limb.

Prevention of deformity in the child

Prevention of deformity is the most common application in childhood. The indication and the rationale for orthotic use for this purpose is based on two major principles of children's orthopaedics.

1. In paralytic disease in the growing child, it is the active unopposed, or weakly opposed, muscle that causes progressive deformity.

2. In the growing child, skeletal parts demonstrate, with time and growth, "biologic plasticity" in response to forces, normal or abnormal, imposed on them, which thereby produce limb deformity.

To these principles must be added a limitation, of which the orthotic team must be aware. Though in many instances an effective orthosis may be helpful in preventing the effects of muscle imbalance on the biologically plastic skeleton, rarely, if ever, can the orthosis correct a *fixed* deformity that is already present. In these instances preliminary correction, often with serial plaster casts, or in some cases by surgical procedures, is necessary to correct the fixed deformity so that the orthosis may then maintain the desired position.

In prescribing effective orthotic treatment for paralytic muscle imbalance in the lower limb, one needs to keep the principles cited in mind. A normal muscle adapts in length to skeletal growth by repeated full extensile excursion. An effective orthotic prescription will control the active, inadequately opposed, muscle groups expected to create deformity. It will identify the deformity anticipated and, in its application, will allow adequate extensile excursion of the muscle but will prevent (by blocking motion) its excessive contraction. Only if this effect can be accomplished will

undesirable myostatic contracture and failure of physiologic lengthening of the active muscle be prevented.

Again, a limitation in this application must be noted. Certain paralytic deformities have been identified as extremely difficult or impossible to control in their more severe forms by orthotic methods alone. The planovalgus foot, for example, with completely flaccid posterior tibial and toe flexor muscles, with strong dorsiflexors and evertor muscles, with or without triceps surae strength, is notoriously difficult to control. The eventual foot deformity may, at full growth, be difficult to correct even with surgery. The severe calcaneocavus foot, as a second example, with completely flail plantar flexor and strong dorsiflexor muscles is also a poor candidate for orthotic control alone. In these special instances surgical readjustment of the severe muscle imbalance may be necessary to allow orthotic control a chance of preventing irretrievable deformity through growth.

Note that the principles involved in paralytic disease are also pertinent to other conditions. The corrected talipes equinovarus foot deformity may indeed show satisfactory initial correction. If the child's gait is carefully observed, one will, in many instances, see that the peroneal muscles do not function in gait and that only the plantar flexor and invertor muscles of the foot are active. Only when growth catches up with the peroneal muscles, which have been placed in relaxed insufficiency by the correction of the foot, can the foot be maintained in muscular balance. This presents an indication for bracing that utilizes the principle of the unopposed active muscle for the prevention of deformity.

Since this preventive application is used for the most part in children, the consideration of durability of the orthotic appliance may have to preempt emphasis on lightness and cosmetic design. The conventional metal orthoses will usually be found more durable for the hard usage that the child gives them. While he wears the orthosis, the child will be growing, so that some provision for length and size adjustment must be made, and careful supervision to maintain fit and effectiveness is mandatory.

It should be reemphasized that the patient and his parents must be educated in the purpose for which the orthosis is prescribed so that they will be willing to maintain usage without interruption.

The success of orthotic management for prevention of deformity depends on full patient cooperation and understanding of its use.

The patient and his parents can generally be assured that the use of the orthosis is, in most cases, temporary through the growth period. Often, surgical joint stabilization and muscle transfer at the conclusion of growth may allow the patient to discard the appliance altogether, but he and his parents must understand that satisfactory surgical correction is often dependent on minimizing the degree of deformity remaining at full growth.

If an orthosis is needed as a permanent adjunct at full skeletal growth, the appropriate appliance can be prescribed and designed.

Biologic plasticity of the growing skeleton is not influenced by muscle imbalance alone. The forces generated by gravity and joint reaction may indeed be of importance in the creation of, or the accentuation of, deformities of the growing skeleton. An example here might be a severe grade of genu valgum (knock-knee) in which the weight-bearing line passes lateral to the joint and abnormal pressure is borne by the lateral condyles of tibia and femur. The musculature protecting against valgus strain at the knee may have decompensated, and the medial capsule and collateral ligament of the knee joint may be subjected to strong tension at each step. In this instance biologic plasticity and the Hueter-Volkmann epiphyseal pressure rule would indicate that progressive deformity might be inevitable. Orthotic protection to prevent this accentuation may be indicated, not to correct the already-present genu valgum, but to prevent its increase until such time that surgical correction could be considered.

A special instance of control of biologic plasticity may be seen in the orthotic treatment of Legg-Perthes disease. If the damaged, but still growing, capital femoral epiphysis is subjected to a concentration of pressure at the acetabular margin, which occurs with normal walking or even with crutch walking, a pronounced deformity may occur, in which the growing femoral head loses its sphericity. This abnormal femoral head contour may cause future significant limitation of motion and degenerative joint disease.

Petrie originally described a method of ambulation, using plaster casts lined by a broomstick crossbar, in which the hips were maintained in abduction.[9] The method had the disadvantage that range-of-motion exercises for hips and knees were precluded, and distortion in shape of the femoral condyles at the knee by continued localized pressure may be produced.

This method has been modified by orthotic application in hip abduction KAFOs such as the Toronto Legg-Perthes orthosis[2] and the Newington Children's Hospital ambulatory abduction orthosis.[3] A regular standardized exercise program is used in conjunction with these orthoses. Problems at the knee are reduced by either free knee motion, in the case of the Toronto KAFO, or by a limited range of knee motion from an initial position of 15 degrees in the Newington appliance.

These orthoses are bilateral applications, even when only one hip is involved. Containment of the femoral head within the acetabulum is obtained by abduction to 40 to 45 degrees and moderate (approximately 20 degrees) internal rotation of the limbs. A prerequisite is free abduction movement of the affected hip. To obtain this free motion, preliminary limb traction is usually necessary to relieve synovitis and muscle spasm and to allow comfortable use of the orthosis.

The rationale for prescription of these orthosis is the prevention of femoral head subluxation by concentric positioning of the femoral head in the acetabulum, the redirection of gravitational forces of weight bearing toward the center of the acetabulum, the increase of contact area for pressure reception by the entire growing femoral head, and the relief of hip joint pressure from high reaction forces generated by the abductor muscles.

Unilateral applications for Legg-Perthes disease of the hip, such as the ischial weight-bearing, patten-bottom orthosis, previously used to attempt weight relief, have been largely discarded as ineffective. A modification of the abduction principle, however, is occasionally employed as a unilateral KAFO in the trilateral-socket, hip-abduction orthosis.[10]

Prevention of deformity in the adult

Certain applications for prevention of deformity are used in adults, as in a peripheral nerve lesion that is expected to recover. Once again, it is the prevention of myostatic contracture in the active unopposed musculature for which the orthosis is prescribed. In this instance the orthosis must be designed to prevent the muscle contracture. As such it may not be the same design as might be prescribed for a purely functional brace to maintain joint position or stability without the effect of a strong muscle tending to produce fixed deformity. If the patient understands that this is a temporary application, awaiting restoration of muscle balance, he will be more willing to accept an appliance that may be heavier, or more cumbersome, than the functional ideal.

Protection of weakened or painful motor skeletal part

This application of orthotic prescription is common to both adults and children. Its most obvious use is in fracture orthotics, covered in detail elsewhere in this volume.

There are however many other examples of this usage. The minimizing of pain, repeated trauma, and symptomatic synovitis in arthritic joints is a notable instance. That function may be improved and that deformity may also be prevented are issues peripheral to the primary purpose, however, for unless the joint is adequately and firmly protected these secondary functions will not be achieved. The type of design utilized may, again, be quite different from that used specifically to improve function in the painless or asymptomatic joint. Temporary relief of symptoms should not be an indication for discarding the orthosis, since its protective function in an arthritic joint or hemophilic arthrosis is, in fact, prophylactic. Only if the patient understands the purpose for which the brace is prescribed will it be effective in its protective function. At times in the adult, intermittent use of an orthosis may have considerable value. It may offer relief of pain in an inflamed joint or prevent deformity from muscle spasm.

Improvement of function

Improvement of function is one of the primary reasons for orthotic prescription and is the most common reason in the adult. This application of an orthosis to improve function is likely to be permanent. Usage of an orthosis for this reason requires that one carefully evaluate the patient, to be sure that an appliance will, in fact, improve his function and correct the biomechanical deficiencies without adding other problems that may outweigh the advantages expected. These are the most difficult and challenging orthoses to prescribe and to design.[8]

The basic needs of the patient with biomechanical lower limb deficits are those of comfort, significant improvement of function, cosmesis, and ease of application. If an orthosis is uncomfortable, fails to significantly improve function, or is not reasonably cosmetic, he will sooner or later discard it. This is true no matter how long he may train with the appliance. Even if these requirements are met, the resulting orthotic device must also be reasonably cosmetic or he will choose not to wear it. Whether the patient dons and doffs his orthosis independently, or requires assistance, the process must be easily accomplished. If this is difficult, the added effort may produce frustration and the device may be abandoned. All these basic needs should be in balance for the patient to be adequately served by his orthosis.

An orthosis used to improve function may do so by stabilization of an unstable limb segment or segments. Its biomechanical function may be to stop or limit undesired motions or to assist desired or needed motions. It may improve function by providing support in standing that may be an aid in motivation for rehabilitation.

Orthotic contraindications

Particularly in the patient in which orthotic prescription is considered for improvement of function, contraindications must be noted in the evaluation. These may include a lack of motivation or initiative to promote rehabilitation. If he has no innate drive to improve his function, he will rarely use the orthosis even though it may be prescribed and fabricated.

Patients with medical problems that deprive them of sufficient strength or endurance to utilize the orthosis effectively or with severe degrees of muscle weakness may find the use of an orthosis too great an effort for practical use. In some instances the orthosis is not an aid, but rather has become an anchor preventing rehabilitative efforts. A patient with quadriplegia lacking musculature of the trunk and abdomen and who lacks sufficient strength in the upper limbs to utilize crutches or walker does not benefit from application of lower limb orthoses.

Evaluation—foot and ankle

In evaluating the patient's needs for a functional orthosis it is generally advisable for one to examine the lower limb in orderly sequence, noting all biomechanical deficits. Foot deformity and function is evaluated during the sequential phases of gait.

There are a number of defects that may be noted during the stance phase. At heel strike the patient may exhibit a quick plantar flexion, commonly referred to as "foot slap." This is caused by weakness or flaccid paralysis of the dorsiflexor muscles of the foot and ankle. If this is an isolated defect, it may be improved by the use of one of several available lightweight AFOs (ankle-foot orthoses). These may be a molded plastic shell or a double rod AFO that is fabricated either of spring steel wire or of epoxy-fiberglass. The use of an AFO for this problem requires, however, knee stability and a nearly normal range of motion at the ankle joint. By selection of proper trim lines on the medial and lateral sides, an AFO (flexible plastic shell) can provide either considerable, or only moderate resistance, to plantar flexion. If the patient has adequate mediolateral stability in the ankle and subtalar joint, an AFO (VAPC shoe clasp) that clips to the back of the shoe counter is a feasible prescription.

If flaccidity of the ankle control muscles includes both anterior and posterior groups in addition to mediolateral instability, consideration might be given to the AFO, molded spiral.[8] Experience with this orthosis, however, has shown that breakage occurs with relative frequency and, because of its patchy contact with the surface of the leg, is contraindicated in situations where leg edema is a problem; in addition, this orthosis has proved inadequate when major triceps surae weakness is present.

If there is serious mediolateral instability of the ankle with flaccidity of the triceps surae muscle as well as of the anterior leg musculature, the AFO (double upright orthosis) with anterior and posterior ankle stop and dorsiflexion assist is indicated.

As the patient progresses to midstance, a number of other foot deformities may become apparent. Valgus or varus deformity of the foot or a fixed plantar flexion deformity of the ankle may appear, or a forefoot adduction deformity may be seen. It is in this phase of gait that the influence of a shortened leg segment may be noted. This is visible as a dropping of the pelvis on the involved side at midstance.

Flexible deformities confined to the foot, as in passively correctable valgus or varus, may be aided by means of an FO (molded shoe insert) to provide static support. The FO shoe insert may also provide a protective function in treating the pain of arthritis of the midtarsal joints by providing support and limiting motion of the painful structures.

A fixed varus or valgus deformity cannot be corrected by means of a foot orthosis, but shoe accommodation to the deformity, as with a heel lift, sole wedge, or arch support, may be of functional value in improving gait stability. Where fixed deformity is severe, consideration should be given to surgical correction.

Moderate variations in limb length may be aided by sole or heel lifts, as outlined in the chapter on shoe modifications. In certain instances where shorter limb length assists overall function, such as in hip-abductor weakness or instability, the advantageous discrepancy in limb length should not be corrected. This is also true where a rigid or locked knee orthosis is to be worn.

As the patient is observed during push-off, inadequate plantar flexion function, as seen with weakness of the triceps surae muscles may be observed. This might be aided by the use of an AFO with a dorsiflexion stop to stabilize the ankle joint.

In the swing phase of gait one may observe that the patient has inadequate dorsiflexion of the foot and ankle. To avoid stubbing the toe, he may elevate the pelvis, demonstrate steppage, or may circumduct the limb. If this deformity is flexible, function can be helped by one of the several types of AFO previously described. Where the ankle equinus deformity is fixed, surgical correction should be considered.

A function of the musculature of the leg during swing phase is to preposition the foot for weight acceptance in stance. Unbalanced activity of either inversion or eversion muscles during swing phase can carry over into the weight acceptance phase of gait. Orthoses (AFOs) may be used to preposition the foot for properly balanced weight acceptance. The type of orthosis may be varied depending on the amount of control of foot inversion or eversion required. The AFO (plastic shell) with adequate medial and lateral buttresses may be quite satisfactory for a mild deformity. Where the active deformity is quite pronounced, however, and the antagonist muscle is strong, the stability of an AFO (orthosis with double upright) attached to an FO (UCB shoe insert) or to a sole plate, with the use of a sturdy shoe may be required.[6] Varus or valgus correction straps are effective only in swing phase to control flexible foot varus or valgus. These must attach to the shoe at the point of insertion of the upper into the sole and not into the heel or along the side of the shoe. Where deformity is resistant to orthotic control, with poor position of the foot within the shoe, surgical correction is indicated.

If the patient's disability presents as significant pain centered in the ankle or subtalar joint attributable to degenerative or traumatic arthritis, protective use of an AFO (PTB weight-bearing orthosis) to provide partial unweighting of the painful area could be a nonoperative method of treatment. Ideally, ankle or subtalar surgery could be considered, but in some instances the surgical approach may not be feasible.

Knee evaluation

Deformities and deficiencies at the level of the knee joint may also be noted during the various phases of gait. On observing the knee as the patient moves from heel strike to midstance, one may detect knee hyperextension (recurvatum). On the other hand, there may be persistent flexion or valgus or varus knee instability. At midstance, with full loading, the patient may report knee pain, particularly if he exhibits a limitation of complete knee extension.

Hyperextension of the knee joint at midstance may be secondary to quadriceps paralysis when it is associated with soleus weakness. Genu recurvatum may also be produced by a fixed or spastic equinus deformity of the foot and ankle. If the knee hyperextension is associated with this latter deformity, it will be necessary either to provide a heel lift to neutralize the effect of ankle position or to correct the deformity surgically, before orthotic control of the knee dysfunction can be expected.

It is generally considered difficult to prevent or minimize a hyperextension deformity of greater than 10 to 15 degrees by the use of a light molded plastic KO (knee orthosis). Flexible mild hyperextension knee defects, however, can also be aided by an AFO constructed to provide a fixed dorsiflexion attitude of the foot and ankle. The use of fixed dorsiflexion at the ankle provides a function similar to the alignment of the PTB (below-knee prosthesis), which allows a quick roll-over at heel strike to prevent knee hyperextension. This mechanism requires an intact quadriceps muscle. When quadriceps muscle weakness is present, a KAFO with knee lock is indicated.[5]

Patients with mild flexible knee valgus or varus, not exceeding 10 to 15 degrees on weight

bearing, may derive benefit from the use of the molded plastic knee orthosis, or from the use of a rigid three-point pressure KO (Swedish knee cage). In the patient with knee valgus or varus of more than 15 degrees, as might occur with a neurotrophic joint, a more rigid orthosis would be indicated. This may require a KAFO (single or double upright orthosis with a free knee and with flexion and extension). This prescription, of course, requires normal body control of flexion and extension at the knee. If, in addition to a severe valgus or varus deformity, there is recurvatum, it would be necessary to have either an extension stop at zero degrees, or, where muscle control is inadequate, a knee lock of either the bail or crop-lock type. The function of the KAFO (double upright) used in the treatment of severe valgus or varus secondary to a neuropathic knee joint may be improved by a plastic pretibial shell fabricated with a high medial wall.[7]

The patient who exhibits a soft-tissue knee-flexion contracture that does not appear rigidly fixed might benefit from a KAFO with a "dial" knee lock, which can accommodate temporarily flexed attitude at the knee. As the knee flexion contracture is decreased by treatment the "dial" lock can be adjusted to the improvement in extension. This component provides stabilization of a flexed knee in the stance phase and allows the patient to ambulate. Mild knee-flexion instability can be aided by an AFO with dorsiflexion stop at the ankle.

For protection of relaxed medial and lateral ligaments of the knee, stabilization, on a short-term basis, may be accomplished by means of a KO (double anterior-loop knee orthosis, or Lennox Hill orthosis). This requires good muscle function. It is generally used only during active competitive sports. It is not an orthosis used for day-long support of the knee.

A patient disabled by pain in the knee secondary to hypertrophic arthritis, and in whom surgical correction is not feasible, might be benefited by the use of a KAFO designed with a quadrilateral-brim partial weight-bearing section.

Hip joint

Biomechanical defects of the hip present major difficulties to effective orthotic design. Such intrinsic femoral deformities as coxa valga, femoral neck anteversion, and shallow acetabulums may contribute to hip joint subluxation and may eventually produce a dislocation. No orthosis can prevent this complication. The deformations are generated by intrinsic muscle and joint forces of a magnitude that will prevail over external appliances. In the presence of muscle forces tending to produce dislocation, one must observe carefully for early migration of the femoral head. Surgical correction of uncontrollable hip adduction is necessary. Surgical correction to realign muscle forces should be considered when a dislocation is imminent.

Flaccid paralysis

The more proximal the functional deficit in neuromuscular disease, the more devastating is its effect on ambulation. Stabilization of the hip for ambulation is a complex problem and orthotic substitution is difficult.

Before orthotic prescription is undertaken, the physician must understand certain substitution mechanisms, partial solutions that the body may achieve without external support. These substitutions appear as "lurches," or sudden deviations of the center of gravity of the body during the gait cycle that are used when normal stabilizing muscle forces are absent, reduced, or insufficient.

The gluteus maximus lurch consists of hip hyperextension during stance phase. The center of gravity is moved behind the hip joint axis allowing the anterior iliofemoral ligaments to stabilize the hip joint. Anything that interferes with this gluteus maximus lurch will add to the functional and energy demands of walking.

The gluteus medius lurch consists of a shift of the trunk toward the ipsilateral side and over the leg during stance. This limp reduces the demand on the hip abductor muscles, and brings the center of gravity over the stance foot. Interference with this mechanism complicates the patient's gait.

Pelvic and trunk control orthoses may block these substitutions used by the patient to achieve balance in walking. Orthoses that stabilize the hip with a lock, therefore, may have some proximal control of pelvis or trunk, but rarely actually improve functional ambulation.

A hip-flexion contracture adds greatly to the energy requirement of walking. In addition, when associated with hip extensor weakness, it may block a gluteus maximus lurch. The effect of an iliotibial band contracture should also be recognized. This produces abduction of the hip as it is fully extended (Ober test). Its effect on the gait

cycle is to force the patient to maintain the hip in some flexion during stance lest the foot deviate laterally from the line of progression. When such a contracture is present with hip extensor weakness (gluteus maximus and hamstrings) once again, the gluteus maximus lurch necessary to balance may be impaired, and ambulation may be prevented altogether.

These fixed flexion and abduction contractures of the hip must usually be eliminated surgically prior to the use of an orthosis if function in gait is to be improved.

For the most part the proximal control of a KAFO (long leg orthosis) can be achieved by a contoured upper thigh band (gluteal seat) or by a quadrilateral socket. Where obesity causes excessive lateral shift of the orthosis during stance, a pelvic belt may be a useful addition.

Uncontrolled rotation of the entire limb during swing, "windmilling" or "flailing," may be a problem in complete hip-muscle paralysis. This may be managed by a hip-joint control with 1 degree of freedom in the direction of flexion-extension attached to a pelvic belt.

Stabilizing the hip for ambulation in the face of total paralysis, however, is most difficult and often leads to treatment failure.

Complete hip-joint paralysis and lack of hip stabilization is seen in certain lower motor neuron diseases (poliomyelitis, myelodysplasia, and spinal cord injury). In these conditions there may be, in addition to the hip weakness, problems of intrinsic trunk stabilization and pelvic control. Where the trunk and pelvis must be rigidly controlled or stabilized by spinal orthoses, considerable modification of the gait cycle is needed to permit forward progression. The entire body weight may have to be propelled forward in a swing-to, or swing-through, manner, by the muscular effort of the upper limbs and shoulder girdle. With the body further weighted by bilateral leg and body orthoses, the energy required for this is considerable. Usually, adult patients without adequate trunk and pelvic control will not achieve an effective community ambulatory status.

Spastic paralysis

In certain spastic states, trunk stabilization by the hip abductor musculature may be blocked by overactivity of the adductors. The swinging limb may cross behind the stance limb. This can be troublesome in the child who is thus unable to walk but seems to have the potential for bipedal gait.

A HKAFO designed to maintain hip motion in the sagittal plane or line of progression, has been used in these situations. Rigid knee control, however, seriously impairs the patient's ability to take a step. The preferable approach combines an HO with an AFO. The hip is permitted to move in flexion and extension so that the center of gravity may be placed over the foot despite the associated hip, knee, or ankle deformities. Proximal pelvic control is usually simplified by orthosis application to both legs, allowing the stance thigh, instead of the pelvis or trunk, to control the direction of motion of the swing limb. The double limb orthosis uses pelvic bands, which do not fix the pelvis or trunk, to connect the limb appliances. The trunk may move to either side or into as much flexion or extension as is needed to maintain balance. Reinforced orthotic joints are required for this type of firm control. Locks may be added to this system, but this necessitates a drag-to gait. Their practicality is questionable as a functional application is primarily intended for assistance in the development of standing balance.

If the hip-adduction contracture is mild, but internal rotation of the leg is a problem, a HKAFO (hip twister with pelvic band attached to an AFO) may provide some degree of control of internal rotation about the hip. The patient with significant adductor spasm, however, is not well controlled by this orthosis. Either the necessary corrective pressure applied is not tolerated and skin breakdown results or breakage of the orthosis at the hip joint is likely to occur. Excessive external tibial torsion may also result from prolonged use of this device.

Combined deficiencies

The patient who presents himself for evaluation and prescription may not always reveal isolated problems such as those noted for foot, ankle, knee, or hip, but may, in fact, present instability or weakness in all these critical areas. An example might be the paraplegic with a thoracic or lumbar spine lesion. It is generally considered that a patient with a spinal cord deficit at or above the ninth thoracic level will have limited ambulation as an adult even with bilateral HKAFOs. The patient may be able to stand by hyperextension stabilization of his hip joints, with effective orthotic support (KAFO) of the knee and foot. Ambulation with crutches, however, at this level of lesion will be a swing-to or swing-through gait and will depend on the strength of the upper limbs. Those patients who have injuries below the level of the fourth lumbar nerve root may ambulate quite satisfactorily with AFOs that provide foot and ankle stability.[4]

Another design biomechanically related to this application of bilateral orthoses is the parapodium. The concept is interesting in that it discards the traditional anatomic configuration of bracing in favor of pure function. Intended for improvement of function in children, this appliance is basically a standing frame that supports the patient at the level of the hips, knees, and foot-ankle joints and enables him to obtain an upright position with minimum muscular effort. Biomechanically efficient alignment of the lower-limb joints is achieved by adjustment of a system of padded restraints and clamps. The device permits the patient to sit by unlocking the hip and knee joint hinges. This device may enable children to ambulate with, and in a few cases without, crutches.

The principal problem that had been anticipated in employing this device for adults was that of providing sufficient stability. The ratio of the height of the patient's center of gravity from the floor to the area of the base of support in an adult is far higher than in the small child. The adult device requires greater structural rigidity, heavier hip and knee locks, and variations in the padding around the pelvic area. The device may also be equipped with pivoting caster wheels enabling the patient to "walk" by pivoting his body around a longitudinal axis.

TRAINING THE PATIENT IN USE OF FUNCTIONAL ORTHOSIS

Particularly in those appliances intended for improvement of function it is important to recognize that instruction and training in the effective use of the orthosis is a vital part of the program. The opportunity to check fitting and alignment in dynamic testing by the therapist is an important phase in evaluation of the orthosis at delivery.

SUMMARY

In prescribing an orthosis for a patient, one needs to identify the purpose for which the orthosis is to be used. This purpose must be understood by physician, orthotist, therapist, and even more importantly the patient and his family. Orthoses are prescribed for prevention of deformity, protection of a weakened or painful musculoskeletal part, or the improvement of function. Particularly in this last application a complete understanding and definition of the biomechanical deficits present in the patient, and an appreciation of the comparative attributes of available orthotic systems is most important. The limitations, as well as the virtues, of orthotic management, especially in prescriptions for functional improvement, must be appreciated. Reevaluation of the patient after application of the prescribed orthosis is essential to ensure its effectiveness and fit. Training in its correct use is an integral part of orthotic treatment.

REFERENCES

1. Badger, B. M.: An evaluation of the grease-gun (Alamite) cable twister in children with torsional lower limb deformities; bracing of children with paraplegia resulting from spina bifida and cerebral palsy. Report of Workshop sponsored by the Committee on Prosthetics Research and Development, University of Virginia, October 24, 1969.

2. Bobechko, W. P., McLaurin, C. A., and Motloch, W. M.: The Toronto orthosis for Legg-Perthes' disease, Artif. Limbs 12:36-41, Autumn 1968.

3. Curtis, B. H., Gunther, S. F., Gossling, H. R., and Paul, S. W.: Treatment of Legg-Perthes' disease with the Newington ambulatory abduction brace, J. Bone Joint Surg. 56A(6):1135-1146, Sept. 1974.

4. Edberg, E.: Bracing for patients with traumatic paraplegia, Phys. Ther. 47(9):818-823, Sept. 1967.

5. Heizer, D.: Bracing designs for knee joint instability, Phys. Ther. 47(9):859-863, Sept. 1967.

6. Henderson, W. H., and Campbell, J. W.: UC-BL shoe insert: Casting and fabrication, Bull. Prosthet. Res. 11: 215-235, Spring 1969.

7. Lehmann, J. F., and Warren, C. G.: Ischial and patellar tendon weight-bearing braces, function, design, adjustment and training, Bull. Prosthet. Res. 19:6-19, Spring 1973.

8. Meyer, Paul R., Jr.: Lower limb orthotics, Clin. Orthoped. Related Res. 102:58-71, July/Aug. 1974.

9. Petrie, J. G., and Bitenc, I.: The abduction weight-bearing treatment in Legg-Perthes' disease, J. Bone Joint Surg. 53B:54-62, 1971.

10. Tachdjian, M. O., and Jouett, L. D.: Trilateral socket hip abduction orthoses for the treatment of Legg-Perthes' disease, J. Bone Joint Surg. 50A(6):1272-1273, Sept. 1968.

CHAPTER 12

Fracture orthoses

AUGUSTO SARMIENTO,* M.D.
WILLIAM F. SINCLAIR, C.P.O.

Orthoses of various types have been used in the treatment of fractures of the axial skeleton for many years. Such appliances immobilize in varying degrees the injured parts while the reparative process takes place. The concept of using orthotic devices in the management of acute fractures of the appendicular skeleton is, however, relatively new. Traditional orthopaedic practice has called for rest of the fractured bone and immobilization of the joints adjacent to the fracture.

Throughout the years, sporadic attempts to achieve uneventful fracture healing without immobilization of the adjacent joints have had short-lived popularity. Open reduction and internal fixation of fractures, popular during the past 50 years, has helped to perpetuate the concept that rigid immobilization in the fractures of the long bones is highly desirable in achieving osteosynthesis.

Smith[19] from Philadelphia published in 1855 a brief report of his experiences with the use of orthoses that he called prostheses in the treatment of nonunions of femoral shaft fractures. He used the orthotic applicances as a permanent means of stabilization in preference to ablation surgery. In so doing he discovered that in some instances spontaneous union took place some time after the patients resumed weight-bearing ambulation. His work remained unrecognized until recently after the publication of reports suggesting orthotic management of acute fractures.

In the spring of 1963, the idea was first conceived that acute fractures of the tibia could be successfully treated by means of a below-the-knee cast molded like a patellar tendon-bearing prosthesis. This technique permitted freedom of motion at the knee joint and early weight-bearing ambulation without increased shortening of the limb or interference with fracture healing.[13] Successful experiences with this functional shortleg cast led to the development of an orthosis that would permit freedom of motion of ankle and knee joints and weight-bearing ambulation within a relatively short time after the initial injury.[14] Similar methods were developed of treatment for fractures of the femoral shaft. An above-knee orthosis that allowed the patient with a fractured femur to ambulate within a few weeks after the initial injury with freedom of motion of all joints was designed.[18] These experiences were later extended to the management of upper limb fractures.[15]

The work of other investigators during the past decade with various types of orthotic devices, principally for the treatment of femoral shaft fractures, has resulted in wide acceptance of fracture-bracing techniques.[2-4,7-11] This chapter discusses in detail those techniques developed and practiced at the University of Miami School of

*Department of Orthopaedics and Rehabilitation, University of Miami School of Medicine, Miami, Florida.

Medicine.[18] The techniques and experiences of others have been published in the orthopaedic literature.

RATIONALE AND OBJECTIVES

There is considerable evidence in clinical practice suggesting that rigid immobilization of fractures of long bones is not a prerequisite for fracture healing. The uniform and consistent rapid healing of rib fractures in the presence of constant motion is one example. The uneventful healing of clavicular fractures treated with slings; humeral fractures treated with "hanging casts"; femoral fractures with skin or skeletal traction give further credence to the fact that healing can take place in the presence of motion at the fracture site and without immobilization of the adjacent joints. Such observations strongly suggest that some motion at the fracture site, rather than being detrimental to fracture healing, may even favorably enhance osteogenesis. The abundant callus often seen in fractures of long bones suffered by patients with spastic neurologic conditions and those in patients actively ambulatory further supports the value of activity in the osseous reparative process. It is possible that function of the injured limb after a short period of rest after the initial injury creates a healthy physiologic environment conducive to uninterrupted union.[13,14,16]

Trauma severe enough to produce a fracture necessarily causes soft-tissue damage, which is clinically manifested by pain and swelling in varying degrees. These two factors preclude the immediate mobilization and active movement of joints adjacent to the fracture. Pain and swelling subside as early healing of the injured tissues takes place. It is during this time that rest is indicated and desirable.

Up to the present time, orthotic techniques for various long bone fractures have been introduced after a period of initial immobilization either in conventional casts or by traction. Attempts to brace fractures immediately after the onset of disability have often resulted in pain and poor acceptance of the method by the patients.

Even though early bracing techniques for lower and upper-limb fractures were carried out with plaster of paris and other investigators have reported experiences with similar types of orthoses, at the University of Miami, plaster of paris has been almost completely abandoned in favor of orthoplast (Johnson & Johnson). This material, a synthetic rubber, is cosmetically acceptable, lightweight, durable, and easy to apply.[14-17]

Contrary to the popular fear that freedom of motion or weight bearing or both would result in loss of reduction of the fractures and increased shortening of the limb, experience has demonstrated that the shortening experienced by the limb at the time of the initial injury remains essentially unchanged.[1,5,14] The alignment of the fractured fragments, if satisfactory, can usually be maintained except in certain fractures, particularly those of the proximal third of the femur.[17] Laboratory investigations have strongly suggested that the maintenance of length is primarily determined by the containment of the fluid-rich soft-tissue mass of the injured limb within the rigid walls of the orthosis. This creates a hydraulic system of an incompressible nature that precludes major shift changes of the osseous structures.[8,11,12,14] The role played by the interosseous membrane in the case of tibiofibular and radioulnar fractures, the firm fibrous muscular attachments, and the elastic nature of the musculature probably assist the orthotic devices in maintaining reduction of the fractured fragments.[6,12,15]

TIBIAL FRACTURES

The fractured tibia was the first long bone treated by means of orthotic devices. The concept of bracing of this bone came as a result of experiences with below-the-knee amputees managed with patellar tendon–bearing prostheses.

The original below-the-knee functional cast used for fractures of the tibia was constructed like a PTB prosthesis, and specialists assumed for some time that such a cast could, by the firm molding over the proximal tibia and popliteal space, the triangular shape of the proximal portion of the cast, and the lateral extensions over the condyles, successfully prevent shortening of the fractured fragments and maintain adequate rotational stability. However, it soon became apparent that the patellar tendon was not a major participant in the distribution of weight-bearing pressures. The orthosis is still indented lightly in this area as a means of reducing the anteroposterior diameter. The patellar tendon fails to perform as a weight-bearing surface because unlike the patellar tendon–bearing prosthesis, the proximal fragment of the tibia cannot be flexed and still permit erect weight-bearing ambulation.[13,18]

Experiences with this cast demonstrated that the shortening accepted at the time of the application of the below-the-knee cast was usually maintained and that rotational deformities did not develop within the cast.[13]

Acceptance of angulation however at the fracture site at the time of its application can result in increased and undesirable deformities.

Early ambulation after acute fractures of the tibia has proved to be advantageous and has resulted in a significant reduction in the number of complications, such as nonunions frequently encountered from nonfunctional, nonambulatory methods of treatment.[1,5,13,14] It appears that most patients with fractures of the tibia treated with functional orthoses should first have their fractures immobilized in conventional above-knee casts applied with the knee in extension and encouraged to ambulate as early as possible. Most patients with closed fractures and without associated injuries are capable of beginning partial weight bearing in such casts within the first few days after the injury.[1,5] After approximately 2 weeks the long leg cast can be replaced with a below-knee functional plaster cast at which time mobilization of the knee and progressively unsupported weight-bearing ambulation can begin. After that time the patients ambulate with the below-knee functional cast for approximately 2 more weeks. Three to 4 weeks after the fracture, an orthosis can be applied usually without encountering complications.

Attempts to apply an orthotic device that permits motion not only of the knee but of the ankle joint as well too soon after the initial injury may result in the development of uncomfortable swelling of the foot and ankle and pain at the fracture site.[14] To provide the maximum amount of comfort to the greatest number of people, it is best to maintain an orderly transition from the long leg cast to the short leg cast and finally into the brace.

However, patients with fractures of the tibia resulting from injuries with relatively minor soft-tissue damage may be candidates for by-passing the short leg cast stage. Regardless of the way that patients are managed, immediate full weight-bearing ambulation is neither possible nor recommended. All patients should be encouraged to ambulate with the aid of crutches bearing only partial weight on the injured leg. They should gradually increase the amount of weight with anticipation that most of them should be capable of ambulating without external support about the fourth postinjury week.

Open fractures require that the therapeutic regimen be altered according to the severity of the injury. Fractures associated with pronounced soft-tissue damage and swelling may not be ready for transfer to the below-knee functional orthosis for several weeks. Fractures with significant shortening at the time of the initial injury that require mechanical restoration of length by means of metallic pins, above and below the fracture, may not tolerate early weight-bearing activity. In such cases it is also best to postpone freedom of motion of the knee for longer periods of time. Note, however, that even in these patients experiences have indicated that early introduction of function into the injured limb favorably influences the reparative process.[1,2,13,14]

Orthotic system

The orthotic device is simply an extension of the below-knee functional cast, which eliminates the foot and ankle portion of the latter. The orthosis can be made of plaster of paris. The results to be obtained with this material can be expected to be comparable to those from Orthoplast material. The advantages of the Orthoplast material, however, seem to outweigh those of plaster of paris.[14,16,17] The coolness of the material, its lighter weight, its durability, and its ease of application are definite advantages. The orthotic ankle joints can be made of metal or plastic; however, the application of metallic joints such as the flexible cable joints require a greater degree of expertise. Prolonged use may result in breakage of the appliance. Polypropylene plastic inserts that consist of a foot piece and flexible plastic hinges are easier to apply, are cosmetically more acceptable, and have a life-span sufficiently long to last the entire period of immobilization of the fracture in the brace.

The primary purpose of the plastic insert is to prevent the orthosis from sliding down on the leg and to avoid rotational deformities when the shoe is removed during recumbency and cleansing of the foot. The vertical loading transferred through the uprights is only minimal.[12]

Fabrication

The application of the Orthoplast orthosis is carried out preferably with the patient sitting on a high table with his hip, knee, and ankle joints at

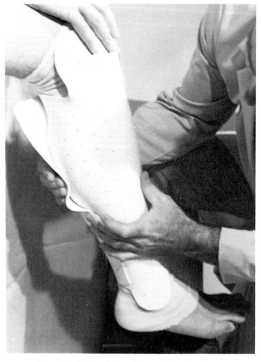

Fig. 12-1. Applying heated Orthoplast.

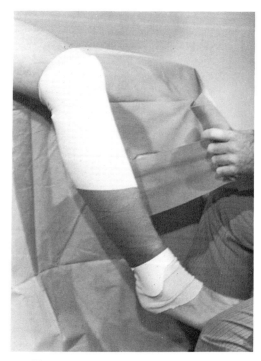

Fig. 12-2. Application of elastic bandage.

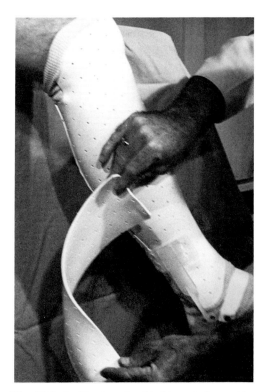

Fig. 12-3. Application of ankle hinge to leg portion.

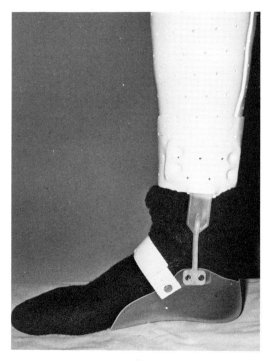

Fig. 12-4. Detail of ankle joint and footplate.

90 degrees. In this manner the operator is in a better position to observe the vertical and rotational alignment of the leg. The prefabricated sheet of Orthoplast is dipped in a hydrocollator with water heated to 190° F. for approximately 1 minute. The soft, malleable Orthoplast is wrapped over the leg, which has been previously covered with a double layer of stockinet that extends from midfoot to just above the knee (Fig. 12-1). The self-adhesive property of the Orthoplast is enhanced by moistening the overlapping surfaces with a non-toxic organic solvent. After overlapping of the surfaces of the Orthoplast, an elastic bandage soaked in cold water is firmly wrapped from just above the ankle to above the knee (Fig. 12-2). This facilitates an even compression of the Orthoplast material and assists the operator in contouring manually around the various bony and soft tissue prominences of the fractured limb. Minor changes in the alignment of the bone are carried out at this time. No anesthetic has been required in over 500 acute fractures treated in this manner. During the 3 to 4 minutes required for the hardening of the Orthoplast the operator firmly contours the medial flare of the tibia and compresses the proximal portion of the leg posteriorly. As contouring is completed and

before the Orthoplast becomes rigid, the knee is extended to approximately 45 degrees. Upon completion of the brace the patient should be able to fully flex and extend the knee. The application of the supracondylar portion with the knee in flexion would make it impossible for the patient to fully extend the knee upon resumption of ambulation, since the anterior wall of the plastic material, extending over the patella, would impinge against the distal thigh. The Orthoplast is trimmed with a sharp knife or scissors so that it has a high anterior wall and a posterior wall opposite the level of the tibia tubercle.

The orthosis extends distally over the malleoli of the tibia and fibula but allows flexion and extension of the ankle by virtue of its higher trimming anteriorly and posteriorly.

The flexible plastic foot insert is applied snugly against the heel. The lateral and medical uprights are fastened against the underlying Orthoplast with a small strip of heated Orthoplast (Figs. 12-3 and 12-4).

The patient's shoe is applied if swelling of the ankle is not present (Fig. 12-5). When swelling is present, it is preferable to apply either a tennis shoe or soft shoe of similar construction. The poste-

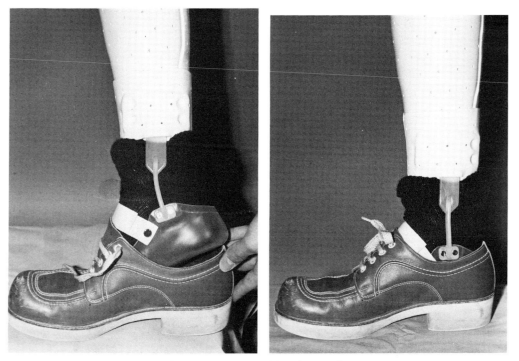

Fig. 12-5. Insertion of footplate in shoe.

rior wall must be cut low enough to permit full flexion of the knee without impingement on the hamstring tendons (Fig. 12-6).

Fractures close to the ankle joint and particularly those with pronounced soft-tissue trauma should have an elastic stockinet used routinely. The elastic sock should only extend to the ankle joint, overlapping the distal end of the orthosis and should not extend the entire length of the leg. The patient should be able to remove the stocking for cleansing purposes.

Fractures of the proximal tibia and particularly those extending into the joint are best treated with a brace made with a thigh corset in order to obtain greater stability[8,9,14,17] (Fig. 12-7 to 12-9). These fractures need to be followed closely because of their ready tendency to develop angulatory deformities when subjected to weight-bearing stresses. These complications are more common with fractures involving the medial plateau and are influenced by the conditions of the fibular neck.

Management

Patients begin ambulation immediately after the application of the orthosis bearing partial weight on the limb to a degree dictated by symp-

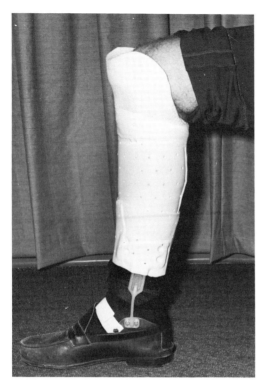

Fig. 12-6. Completed orthosis.

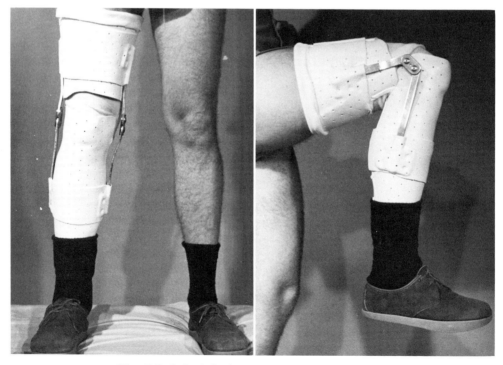

Fig. 12-7. Orthosis for fractures of proximal tibial area.

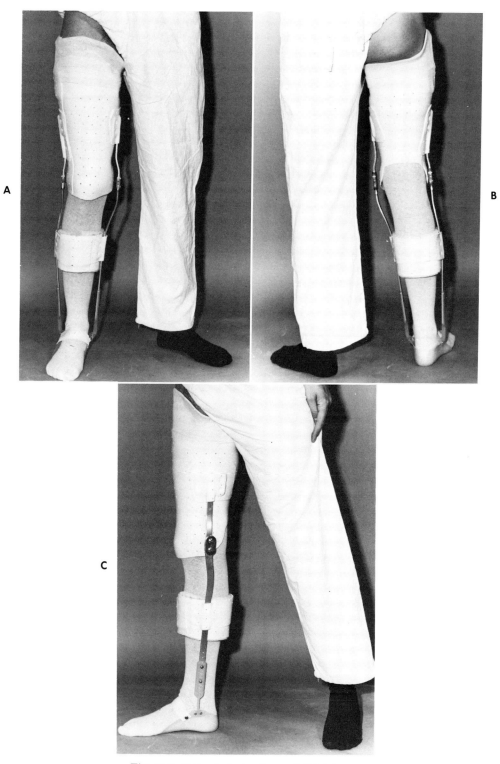

Fig. 12-8. Orthosis for fractures of distal femur.

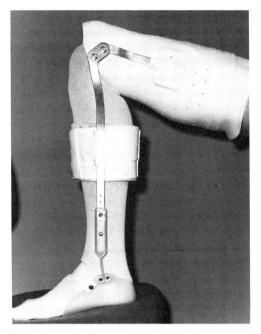

Fig. 12-9. Knee flexion available with orthosis for femur fractures.

toms. The complete freedom of motion of the ankle and knee joints appears to facilitate the physiologic contraction of the musculature, which probably enhances the rapid disappearance of the swelling. In the event that swelling is present at the ankle joint or its development is anticipated, an elastic stocking is prescribed to extend from the toes to overlap the distal end of the orthosis. The patients are instructed to remove their shoes at night and during recumbency. This does not result in rotatory deformities because of the accurate contour of the lateral walls of the plastic insert over the heel.

Usually the orthosis is not removed until radiologic and clinical evidence of fracture healing has been established. It appears that the continued use of the limb and the creation of a physiologic environment results in a more rapid consolidation of the fracture. Oftentimes it is possible to split the Orthoplast material posteriorly to make its occasional removal possible. This is done only after sufficient stability has developed at the fracture site or in cases where infected or granulating soft-tissue defects are accompanied by serous or purulent drainage, which would otherwise macerate the skin. The split Orthoplast orthosis is fastened with Velcro straps in a conventional manner.

The recognition of malalignment of the frag-

ments after application of the orthosis must be corrected by removing it and applying a new one. Wedging the Orthoplast after hardening of the material is possible, but the risk of burning of the skin with the heat gun may be too great. It is also possible to split the orthosis, carry out the corrective manipulation and then reapply the orthosis, which has been softened with a heat gun.

Experience has shown that the shortening accepted at the time of application of the ankle-foot orthosis remains unchanged throughout the entire healing process.[14,17]

The amount of shortening experienced in most closed fractures of the tibia generally does not exceed ¼ inch. In open fractures the initial shortening may be and usually is greater.[13,14]

Upon removal of the orthosis there is usually no need for physical therapy or other treatments to restore motion of the joints, since patients have been able to use them soon after the initial injury.

FEMORAL FRACTURE

As in the case of fractures of the tibia, first efforts to apply orthotic devices for fractures of the femur were inspired by prostheses worn by above-knee amputees.[18] It soon became evident that attempts to obtain ischial weight bearing were unnecessary. The stability of the bony structures is primarily provided by the firm and snug contact between the walls of the orthosis and the soft tissues of the thigh.

Intramedullary nailing remains perhaps the method of choice in the treatment of transverse fractures of the middle third of the femur. Other devices such as single or double plates and nail plates have been used successfully in many instances. There are fractures of the femoral shaft, however, which for various reasons are best not treated surgically. Open fractures with possible contamination and greatly comminuted and oblique fractures may not lend themselves readily to internal fixation. It is in these cases that fracture bracing has a place.

Unlike the rather consistent and satisfactory results obtained with bracing of fractures of the tibia, femoral bracing has been associated with a greater degree of difficulty in its implementation. It appears that ambulation of patients with femoral-shaft fractures that immobilized in orthoses particularly if applied prior to the development of adequate intrinsic stability, often causes the development of deformities at the fracture site.

Those complications are more frequently encountered with fractures located above the middle third of the femur. The deformity usually consists of varus angulation that results in shortening of limb and, if severe enough, an unacceptable malalignment.[16,17]

Therefore it is best to align the fractured fragments by means of skeletal traction for a period of time sufficient enough to obtain early intrinsic stability. Intrinsic stability is defined as absence of pain at the fracture site, evidence of early callus formation, and lack of gross motion. Such a status is achieved about the fourth postinjury week in most instances. It is at this time that the orthosis may be applied. To obtain the greatest degree of success with the brace, it is imperative to have the knee mobilized actively and passively during the period of skeletal traction. The musculature of the limb and the condition of this joint should be in the best possible condition to prevent the development of swelling and pain upon the resumption of weight bearing. Patients who fail to mobilize their knee during the period of recumbency and who present themselves to the orthotic laboratory with painful limitation of motion and lack of extension of the knee are prone to experience discomfort for several days or weeks.

Particularly with fractures located in the most distal portion of the femur, swelling and knee infusion is often encountered. Prebracing activity of the knee joint is most desirable in these situations.

As in the case of the fractured tibia it has been found that Orthoplast orthoses are preferable over those made of plaster of paris. Their lighter weight and easy applicability have been desirable features. However plaster of paris orthoses can be used with satisfactory results.[2,4,7,8,10,11]

Fabrication

The Orthoplast orthoses can be applied with the patient in the erect or supine position. Experience has shown, however, that the recumbent position is preferable. Particularly because patients who have been bedridden for several weeks after a major injury do not readily tolerate standing up for the time required for the fabrication of the brace.

An Orthoplast preformed brim is fit snugly over the proximal thigh and held in place with adhesive tape (Fig. 12-8). It is over this brim, which resembles the quadrilateral above-knee pros-

thesis, that the distal portion of the Orthoplast is applied. The surfaces of the material are made to overlap after being moistened with a cleaning fluid such as Carbona in order to enhance the adhesive properties of the Orthoplast. The soft malleable Orthoplast orthosis is wrapped firmly with elastic bandages saturated with cold water in order to expedite its setting process. During this period the thigh is firmly molded and the femoral condyles are contoured. Because of the ready tendency of the fracture to angulate in a varus deformity, a three-point fixation attempt is made. In doing so the orthotist applies manual pressure at the apex of the fracture as he attempts to displace the distal leg in a lateral fashion. Such a maneuver is not indicated in cases where angulatory deformities are not present or expected. The distal portion of the orthosis is constructed in such a manner that the anterior wall extends below the distal pole of the patella (Fig. 12-8, C), laterally covers the condyles of the femur, and posteriorly allows flexion of the knee (Fig. 12-9). Pelvic bands are not used, as they do not provide significant protection against angular deformities.

Upon completion of setting of the first portion of the brace, aluminum uprights that include polycentric knee joints are fastened to the thigh section by a circumferential strip of Orthoplast. A special alignment jig that connects the two uprights at the knee joint is used to ensure proper placement of of the joints during this procedure. An Orthoplast cuff is then placed about the proximal calf, and the uprights are anchored to this cuff by a second strip of Orthoplast to afford stabilization to the distal portion of the orthosis. A polypropylene shoe insert that encompasses the heel of the foot is then attached to the medial and the lateral uprights by screws after proper adjustment has been made for length (Fig. 12-9).

Upon completion of the bracing procedure and after trimming, all joints should be freely movable. Because patients have been immobilized in traction for variable periods of time, it is impossible in most instances to fully range the knee joint. The orthotist should properly trim the orthosis in anticipation of gradual restoration of motion.

The plastic insert that fits over the heel and is held in place by the shoe prevents the orthosis from sliding down during standing. A Velcro strap attached to the insert and passing across the dorsum of the foot helps to prevent the orthosis from sliding down when the shoe is removed at night. Firm molding of the Orthoplast over the distal portion of the femur with compression medially and laterally above the condyles also assists in this regard. Patients with fat or flabby thighs are more prone to experience difficulty in maintaining stability of the orthosis.

Management

Patients are encouraged to ambulate with external support increasing the weight bearing according to the symptom and the nature of the fracture. It is strongly recommended that patients with proximal femoral fractures be kept from bearing full weight on the limb for a longer period of time and that x ray films be obtained at frequent intervals.

The rapid resumption of ambulation frequently leads to the development of swelling around the knee joint. The elastic stocking that has been used underneath the Orthoplast controls excessive swelling. It is the continued use of the joint and the frequent isometric contraction of the musculature that best assists in the elimination of swelling. Recognition of inadequate alignment of the fragments or development of angular deformities require reapplication of the brace after proper manipulation or after further stabilization of the fracture in traction.

SUMMARY

Fracture bracing techniques are still in their infancy. Their efficacy, however, has strongly suggested their permanent place in the armamentarium of the orthopaedist. Greater knowledge and experience, as well as improved technology, should result in broadening of their indications. Bracing is not applicable to all fractures, and therefore a clear understanding of its principles, indications, limitations and expectations is mandatory. Failure to obtain and maintain satisfactory alignment of the braced fracture dictates that if at all possible, an alternate method of treatment be sought. Although bracing does not propose to totally replace other methods of treatment, it appears that its application is highly beneficial in eliminating the danger of complications that might follow surgical osteosynthesis. By virtue of the fact that muscle and joint function is possible within the brace, the physiologic environment created is conducive to bone healing.

REFERENCES

1. Brown, P. W., and Urban, J. G.: Early weight bearing treatment of open fractures of the tibia. An end result study of sixty-three cases, J. Bone Joint Surg. 51A:59, 1969.
2. Burkhalter, W. E.: Experiences with brace-cast for femoral fractures. Presented at workshop sponsored by the Committee on Prosthetic Research and Development of the Division of Engineering, National Research Council, Fitzsimmons General Hospital, Denver, 1971.
3. Connolly, J. F., and King, P.: Closed reduction and early cast-brace ambulation in the treatment of femoral fractures. Part I: An in vivo quantitative analysis of immobilization in skeletal traction and a cast-brace, J. Bone Joint Surg. 55A:1559, 1973.
4. Connolly, J. F., Dehne, E., and La Follette, B.: Closed reduction and early cast-brace ambulation in the treatment of femoral fractures. Part II: Results in 143 fractures, J. Bone Joint Surg. 51A:1581, 1973.
5. Dehne, E., Metz, C. W., Deffer, P. A., and Hall, R. M.: Nonoperative treatment of the fractured tibia by immediate weight-bearing, J. Trauma 2:514, 1961.
6. Latta, L., Zilioli, A., Sinclair, W. F., and Sarmiento, A.: The role of soft tissues in fracture stability. Presented at the Orthopaedic Research Society meeting, 1974, J. Bone Joint Surg. 56A:854, 1974.
7. Moll, J. H.: The cast brace walking treatment for open and closed femoral fractures, Southern Med. J. 66:345, 1973.
8. Mooney, V., Nickel, V., Harvey, J. P., and Snelson, R.: Cast-brace treatment for fractures of the distal part of the femur, J. Bone Joint Surg. 49A:295, 1970.
9. Mooney, V.: Cast bracing, Clin. Orthop. 102:159, 1974.
10. National Academy of Science, National Research Council, Prosthetic Research and Development, Subcommittee on Design and Development: Fracture bracing, April 1968.
11. National Academy of Science, National Research Council, Prosthetic Research and Development: Cast-bracing of fractures, 1971.
12. Posival, R.: A study of the mechanics of below-the-knee functional braces, Masters-thesis, University of Miami School of Engineering, Miami, Florida, 1973.
13. Sarmiento, A.: A functional below-the-knee cast for tibial fractures, J. Bone Joint Surg. 52A:855, 1967.
14. Sarmiento, A.: A functional below-the-knee brace for tibial fractures, J. Bone Joint Surg. 52A:295, 1970.
15. Sarmiento, A., and Cooper, J. S.: A functional method of treatment of forearm fractures presented at the annual meeting of the American Academy of Orthopaedic Surgeons, 1974.
16. Sarmiento, A.: Fracture bracing, Clin. Orthop. 102:502, 1974.
17. Sarmiento, A.: Functional bracing of tibial and femoral shaft fractures, Clin. Orthop. 82:2, 1972.
18. Sarmiento, A., and Sinclair, W. F.: Application of prosthetic-orthotic principles to orthopaedics, Artif. Limbs 2:2, 1967.
19. Smith, H. H.: On the treatment of un-united fracture by means of artificial limbs, Am. J. Med. Sci., Jan. 1855.

PART FOUR

The foot

CHAPTER 13

Biomechanics of the foot

ROGER A. MANN, M.D.

The subject of the biomechanics of the foot and ankle is a complex one. It cannot be considered as a separate entity, rather it is an integral part of the biomechanics of the lower limb. As we walk, the entire lower segment, consisting of the pelvis, femur, tibia, and fibula, undergoes rotation in the transverse plane. This rotation is then transmitted through the ankle joint and then translated through the subtalar joint into the bones of the foot. The foot is a unique structure in that it is flexible during some phases of activity and rigid during others; it is flexible during swing phase and early stance phase and then converts into a rigid lever arm prior to toe-off. The body requires a flexible foot in order to adapt to its external environment, which may be flat, uneven, or sloping, but it needs a rigid structure for push-off. Although the foot has some inherent structural stability, it only attains rigidity as a result of the external rotation of the entire lower segment, which is then transmitted to the foot from the segments above. In this discussion, the mechanics of these changes are described and correlated in order to present a meaningful picture of foot functions.

As stated above, each lower segment of the skeleton (composed of part of the pelvis, femur, tibia, and fibula) rotates in the transverse plane during normal locomotion (Fig. 13-1). The degree of rotation progressively increases in magnitude from the more proximal segments to the more distal ones. During normal walking on level ground, the pelvis rotates an average of 6 degrees, the

femur 13 degrees, and the tibia 18 degrees. The lower limb rotates internally during swing phase and the first 15% of stance phase; the direction is then reversed and external rotation begins, reaching its peak just after toe-off, when internal rotation again occurs. This transverse rotation is passed to the talus through its articulation with the tibia and fibula.

The axis of rotation of the ankle is directly laterally and posteriorly as projected on the transverse plane and laterally and downward as seen on the frontal plane. The axis of the ankle passes just distal to the tip of each malleolus and may be reasonably accurately estimated by placing one finger at the tip of each malleolus. The angle between the axis of the ankle joint and the long axis of the tibia is approximately 80 degrees, with a range of 68 degrees to 88 degress (Fig. 13-2, A). In the transverse plane (Fig. 13-2, B), the ankle axis is externally rotated 20 to 30 degrees with respect to the knee axis (which is perpendicular to the line of progression). The longitudinal axis of the foot (Fig. 13-2, C), which passes between the second and third toe, is internally rotated 6 degrees to the axis of the ankle joint with a range of 2 degrees of internal rotation to 9 degrees of external rotation.

The type of motion that occurs in the ankle joint (Fig. 13-3) is dorsiflexion and plantar flexion. The ankle joint undergoes plantar flexion at the time of initial floor contact (heel strike), which continues until the onset of midstance phase or throughout the first 15% of the walking cycle, and

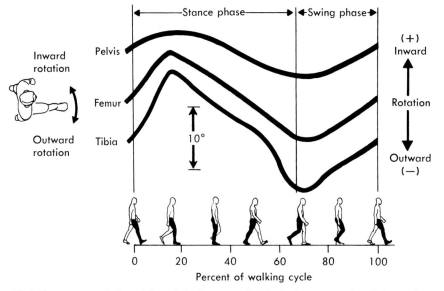

Fig. 13-1. Transverse rotation of the pelvis, femur, and tibia during a normal walking cycle. NOTE: There is inward rotation until foot-flat at 20% of the cycle, after which there is progressive outward rotation until toe-off when inward rotation once again begins.

then progressive dorsiflexion occurs from the time of heel-off until the 40% point of the cycle, when again, plantar flexion begins (Fig. 13-4). During the swing phase, dorsiflexion of the ankle joint takes place until the time of heel strike, when plantar flexion again begins.

The axis of rotation of the subtalar joint is oblique; it passes in the horizontal plane medially to laterally as one proceeds from the distal portion to the proximal portion of the foot. The axis passes at an angle of 23 degrees to the midline of the foot, with a range of 4 to 47 degrees (Fig. 13-5, A). In the horizontal plane, the axis passes at an angle of 41 degrees, with a range of 21 to 69 degrees (Fig. 13-5, B). It becomes apparent when one studies the axis of the subtalar joint that the joint is analogous to an oblique hinge (Fig. 13-6). Thus, when a rotation is imparted to the superior aspect of the talus, it will bring about rotation of the calcaneus in the opposite direction. External rotation of the leg will produce inversion of the calcaneus, and conversely internal rotation of the leg will produce eversion of the calcaneus. As one can readily see, the rotation in the subtalar joint is intimately coupled with the rotation of the lower segment.

The motion that occurs in the subtalar joint (Fig. 13-7) is called "inversion" when the calcaneus is brought toward the midline of the body and "eversion" when the calcaneus is brought away from the midline. The magnitude of inversion during the stance phase of level walking is about 8 degrees in persons with normal feet and about 12 degrees with persons with flatfeet. The degree of eversion that occurs is roughly equal to that of the stated degree of inversion. In normal walking, eversion of the hindfoot takes place throughout the first 15% of stance phase, at which time inversion begins (Fig. 13-8). The motion in the subtalar joint is passed through the talus and calcaneus to the navicular and cuboid bones respectively.

The transverse tarsal joint, which is composed of the talonavicular and the calcaneocuboid joints, is so constructed that any motion in the talus, the calcaneus, or both, will affect its stability. Depending on the position of the hindfoot, two fundamental patterns are seen. When the hindfoot is everted, the axes of the talonavicular and calcaneocuboid joint are parallel to each other, so that relatively free motion can occur about these parallel axis (Fig. 13-9). However, when the hindfoot is inverted, the axes of the talonavicular joint and calcaneocuboid joint are divergent so that some degree of restriction of motion in the joint is present. When the periods of external and internal rotation of the lower limb are correlated with the positions of the hindfoot, the lower limb is found to be in internal rotation at heel strike, causing

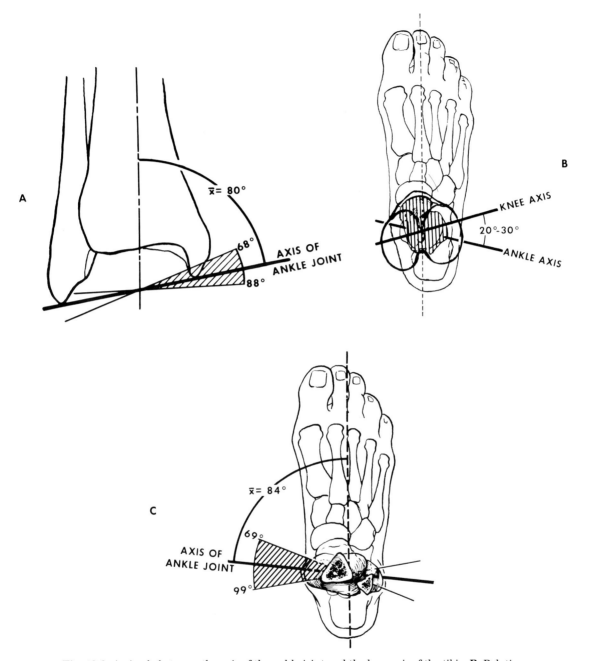

Fig. 13-2. A, Angle between the axis of the ankle joint and the long axis of the tibia. **B,** Relationship of the knee, ankle, and foot axes. **C,** Relationship of the ankle axis to the longitudinal axis of foot.

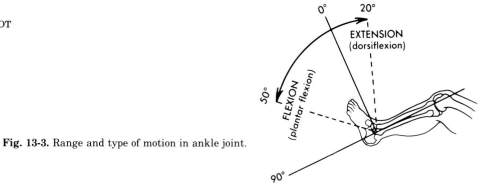

Fig. 13-3. Range and type of motion in ankle joint.

PLANTAR FLEXION-DORSIFLEXION

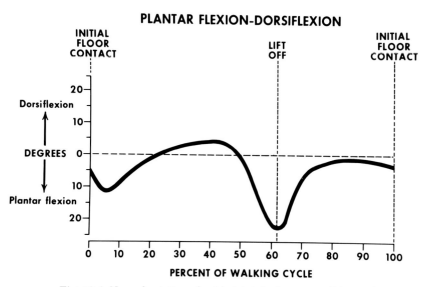

Fig. 13-4. Normal rotation of ankle joint during one walking cycle.

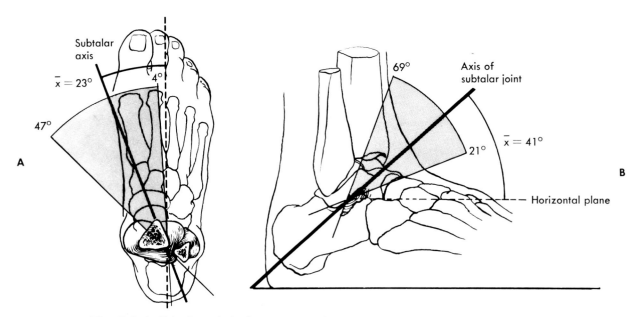

Fig. 13-5. A, Subtalar axis in the transverse plane. **B,** Subtalar axis in the horizontal plane.

eversion of the hindfoot and therefore a relatively flexible longitudinal arch of the foot. As the lower segments start to rotate externally during the stance phase, the hindfoot is inverted and increased stability of the transverse tarsal joint results, producing a more stable ltngitudinal arch of the foot.

One should keep in mind that the navicular articulates with the cuneiforms and the three medial rays. The cuboid articulates with the two lateral rays. So again, external rotation of the leg causes inversion of the heel and consequent elevation of the medial side of the foot and depression of the lateral side. Internal rotation of the leg produces the opposite effect on the foot: eversion of the heel, depression of the medial side of the foot, and

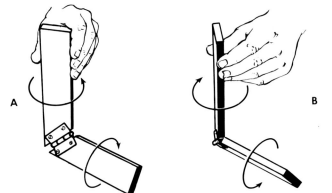

Fig. 13-6. Analogy of subtalar axes to an oblique hinge. **A,** Outward rotation of upper stick results in inward rotation of lower stick. **B,** Inward rotation of upper stick results in outward rotation of lower stick.

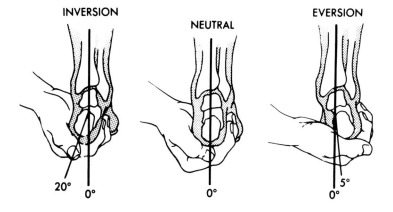

Fig. 13-7. Types of motion in subtalar joint.

Fig. 13-8. Motion in subtalar joint during normal walking cycle. NOTE: There is rapid eversion at the initial floor contact, followed by progressive inversion until lift-off, after which eversion once again occurs. (Adapted from Wright, D. G., Desai, S. M., and Henderson, W. H.: J. Bone Joint Surg. **46A:** 361-382, 1965.)

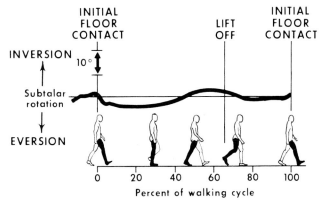

EVERSION   INVERSION

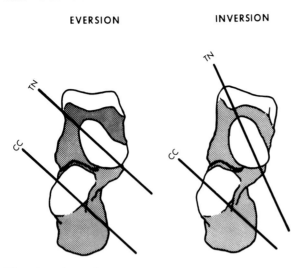

Fig. 13-9. Axes of rotation in the talonavicular, **TN,** and calcaneocuboid, **CC,** joints. When the hindfoot is in eversion, these axes are parallel so that relatively free motion in the transverse tarsal joint is permitted. When the hindfoot is inverted, the axes are divergent; thus there is restriction of motion in the transverse tarsal joint and hence greater stability.

slight elevation of the lateral side of the foot (Fig. 13-10).

The metatarsal break is the name given to the oblique axis that overlies the metatarsophalangeal joints. The axis passes from the head of the second metatarsal, since it is the most distal one, to that of the fifth metatarsal, which is the most proximal (Fig. 13-11). It has been demonstrated that the angle between the metatarsophalangeal break and the long axis of the foot may vary from 50 to 70 degrees.

As one can see, the rotation that occurs in the lower segment acts on the talus. It is the translation of this rotation through the oblique hinge of the subtalar joint that transmits this rotation to the foot. The changing of the axes of the transverse tarsal joint and the changes that occur distal to this joint cause a conversion of the flexible foot into a rigid arch system. If rotation of one of the segments is functioning in an abnormal manner, one can readily see why the entire gait pattern may be altered.

The muscles within the lower segment play a vital role in its function. Only those muscles present below the knee are considered in detail at this time. The extrinsic muscles of the foot or the calf should be viewed in relation to their relative positions about the axes of the ankle and subtalar joints (Fig. 13-12). When one views the muscles in

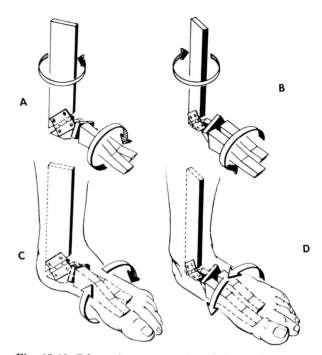

Fig. 13-10. Schematic representation of the mechanism by which rotation of the tibia is transmitted through the subtalar joint into the foot. **A,** Outward rotation of the upper stick results in inward rotation of the lower stick, so that as seen in **C** outward rotation of the tibia will cause inward rotation of the calcaneus and subsequent elevation of the medial border of the foot and depression of the lateral border of the foot. **B,** Inward rotation of the upper stick results in outward rotation of the lower stick, so that as seen in **D** inward rotation of the tibia will cause outward rotation of the calcaneus with depression of the medial side of the border of the foot and elevation of the lateral border of the foot.

this manner, one can appreciate the function of the muscle and also can gain knowledge about the length of the lever arm through which the muscle acts. The more distant the location of a muscle from the axis of rotation (Fig. 13-13), the greater is the leverage exerted by that muscle; conversely, the closer the muscle to the axis of rotation, the lesser is the leverage exerted by that muscle. With this in mind, it becomes obvious that the muscles posterior to the ankle axis are the plantar flexors whereas those anterior to the ankle axis are the dorsiflexors. Those muscles medial to the subtalar axis are invertors, whereas those lateral to the subtalar axis are evertors (Fig. 13-14). Furthermore, it becomes clear that those posterior to the ankle axis and medial to the subtalar axes are plantar flexors and invertors, whereas those muscles anterior to the ankle axis and medial to the subtalar axes are dorsiflexors and invertors. When

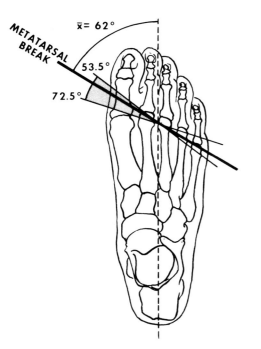

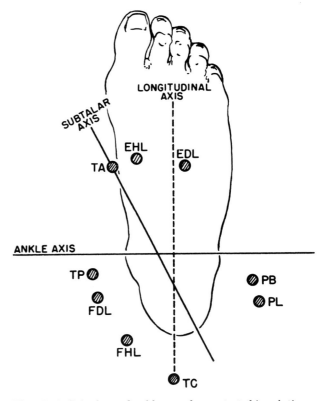

Fig. 13-11. Metatarsal break in relation to longitudinal axes of foot.

Fig. 13-12. Subtalar and ankle axes demonstrated in relation to extrinsic muscles. **EDL,** Extensor digitorum longus. **EHL,** Extensor hallucis longus. **FDL,** Flexor digitorum longus. **FHL,** Flexor hallucis longus. **PB,** Peroneal brevis. **PL,** Peroneus longus. **TA,** Tibialis anticus. **TC,** Tendocalcaneus. **TP,** Tibialis posterior (see text for explanation).

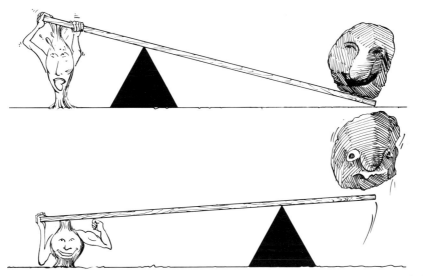

Fig. 13-13. Upper diagram demonstrates that the closer a muscle is to the axis of rotation, the less leverage it has to effect rotation about the axis. Lower diagram demonstrates that a muscle far from the axis of rotation has a longer lever arm and hence the greater moment it can exert across the axis.

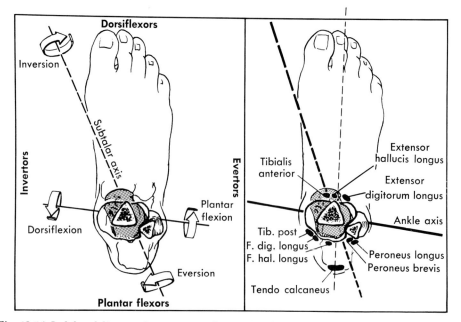

Fig. 13-14. Left-hand diagram demonstrates the rotation that occurs about the subtalar and ankle axes. Right-hand drawing demonstrates the relationship of the various muscles about the subtalar and ankle axes.

one deals with patients with a specific motor loss, and if one keeps a diagram such as this in mind, the type of deformity that would probably result can rather easily be predicted.

The activity of the anterior compartment (or the dorsiflexors) basically occurs during swing and early stance phase (Fig. 13-15). These muscles help the body clear the foot during swing phase and then gently place the foot on the ground after initial floor contact (heel strike). Once the foot is on the ground, they probably help pull the body forward over the fixed foot. The calf group generally functions during the midstance and terminal-stance phases until toe-off.

The intrinsic muscles of the foot (those arising from and inserted within the foot itself) as a group are noted to be active from the middle of midstance phase until toe-off in a normal individual. In a person with flatfoot, those muscles demonstrate a longer period of activity.

Now that we have a generalized idea of the overall function of the lower limb, let us focus our attention upon the mechanisms that stabilize the foot itself and are not directly related to the aforementioned angular rotations of the lower limb. The plantar aponeurosis arises from the inferior tubercle of the calcaneus and passes forward, dividing into bands (Fig. 13-16). These bands

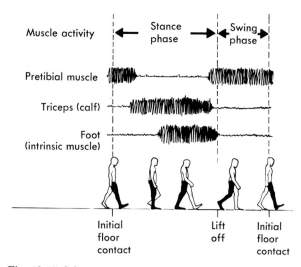

Fig. 13-15. Schematic phasic activity of the leg and foot muscles during normal gait.

circle the flexor tendons and then are inserted along the joint capsule into the base of each proximal phalanx. The combination of plantar aponeurosis and metatarsophalangeal joint capsule is known as the plantar pad. The plantar aponeurosis has essentially a fixed origin and insertion. As the metatarsophalangeal joints are brought into an extended position, beginning after midstance (heel-off) and lasting until toe-off, the

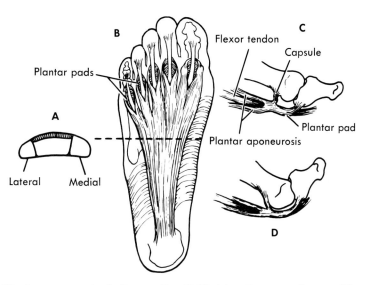

Fig. 13-16. Plantar aponeurosis. **A,** Cross section. **B,** Division of aponeurosis around flexor tendons. **C,** Components of plantar pad and its insertion into base of proximal phalanx. **D,** Toes in extension with plantar pad drawn over metatarsal head.

plantar aponeurosis is wrapped around the metatarsal head and a relative shortening of the plantar aponeurosis ensues. By this mechanism, the metatarsal head is stabilized and the arch of the foot is raised without any muscular action per se. This mechanisms has been likened to a windlass and is most effective for the great toe and least effective for the small toe.

The talonavicular joint consists of a convex talar head and a concave navicular surface (Fig. 13-17). This configuration forms a joint that is shaped like an elliptical paraboloid. When increasing force is exerted across it during heel rise and toe-off, it becomes mechanically stable.

After having discussed individually the main mechanisms of the foot and ankle, let us now walk a step and integrate the events as they occur during the walking cycle.

Initial floor contact (heel strike) will be our starting point (Fig. 13-18). The lower segment is undergoing rapid internal rotation until foot-flat has been achieved at 15% of the cycle. The heel is in an everted position and the forefoot has remained flexible as it is adapting to the ground. The pretibial muscles are active throughout the first 15% of the stance phase. There is no activity in the intrinsic muscles. At approximately the 15% point the midstance phase begins. The direction of rotation of the lower segment is reversed; external rotation of the lower segment and inver-

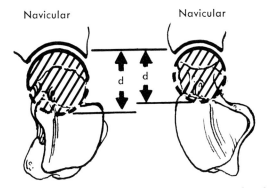

Fig. 13-17. Relationship of head of talus to navicular, left superior view and right lateral view, showing differing diameters of head of talus.

sion of the hindfoot begin. The intrinsic muscles in persons with flatfoot become active, but no activity is present in a person with normal feet until at the 30% of the cycle. From the beginning of inversion of the hindfoot until the time of toe-off, there is progressive stabilization of the transverse tarsal joint and the longitudinal arch. The posterior calf muscles have likewise become active during the midstance phase and will remain active until toe-off.

As the foot is loaded, the convex head of the talus is firmly seated in the concave navicular. The plantar aponeurosis exerts its force on the arch as the body weight passes over the foot, and

WALKING CYCLE

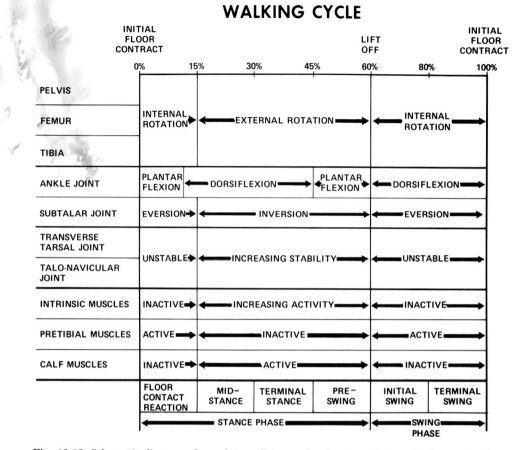

Fig. 13-18. Schematic diagram of complete walking cycle, showing rotations that occur in the various segments and joints as well as the activity in the foot and leg musculature.

the toes are brought into extension. Just prior to toe-off, the lower segment has reached maximum external rotation and the hindfoot is in a position of maximum inversion. The axes of the transverse tarsal joint are divergent, the talar head is firmly seated in the navicular, intrinsic muscle activity has reached its peak, and the activity in the musculature of the posterior calf is at its maximum. All these mechanisms have one common result: stabilization of the longitudinal arch of the foot at the time of lift-off. As soon as lift-off starts, internal rotation of the lower segment begins with associated eversion of the foot. The eversion of the hindfoot unlocks the transverse tarsal joint and in turn the longitudinal arch of the foot. No activity is present in either the intrinsic muscles of the foot or in the posterior muscles of the calf. The foot

once again has become a relatively flexible structure. The internal rotation of the lower segment continues during the swing phase and does not reverse itself until the foot-flat has been achieved at 15% of the new walking cycle.

The most important factor in constructing an orthosis is the proper alignment of the axis of the ankle joint in order to assure freedom of movement. It is important to keep in mind that the ankle-axis alignment of the orthoses is based on a line connecting the inferior tip of each malleolus and that this line transverses both the frontal and transverse planes. The degree of toeing out, as it reflects the relationship between the longitudinal axis of the foot and the ankle axis, also has to be taken into consideration in the overall alignment of a short-leg orthosis.

CHAPTER 14

Shoes and shoe modifications

MELVIN H. JAHSS, M.D.

The commercial shoe is the standard means of protecting and supporting the normal foot in both childhood and adulthood. Orthopaedic surgery may often be necessary to correct deformities of the foot and ankle and relieve painful or anesthetic areas (callus, exostosis, ulcer, hammertoes, and bunion) from abnormal pressure, with and without shoe wear, particularly with weight-bearing conditions. These conditions may also be aided by transfer of weight-bearing stresses or by accommodation of shoes to the deformities. The shoe may also aid in immobilizing painful stiff toes (hallux rigidus) or unstable (ankle) joints. Shoe corrections may be used to equalize leg length and foot discrepancies.

Various conservative methods are thus available to relieve painful or deformed feet. They include the appropriate use of various types of commercial and "orthopaedic" shoes, shoe corrections, foot or arch supports, and pads. These corrective measures, often used in combinations, should be based upon sound biomechanical principles, with each foot being judged individually. To evaluate and prescribe shoes and shoe modifications, one needs to be familiar with anatomy, terminology, and the manufacture of shoes and their component parts.

SHOE LEATHERS—MANUFACTURE

Shoe leathers are made from the skin or hides of animals. Common animal sources are goats, sheep, calves, horses, and cattle. The skins are processed to leather by tanning. Briefly, skins are limed and heated to remove hair and excess fat; the lime is neutralized and the actual tanning carried out by acid, either vegetable (oak) or mineral (potassium bichromate). This process of tanning condenses the skin and denatures the albumin, so that the finished leather will not decompose. The leather is then finished by drying and is oiled, split, stained, and finally polished.

Types of shoe leathers

Leather may be anatomically divided into three types: (1) *grain side* (top grain, outer surface), which is strong, water resistant, and takes a good polish; (2) *split grain,* split from the central portion, more porous, and usually used as side leather; (3) *flesh side,* which is buffed and used as suede, or may be varnished to use as patent leather.

Sole leather is made from dried oak-tanned cattle hides, is dense but somewhat flexible, and is usually about ¼ inch in thickness.

COMPONENT PARTS OF A SHOE
(Figs. 14-1 and 14-2)

The upper portion of a shoe includes the toe box, vamp and lace stay, tongue, throat, quarter, and counter covered by the wall. The construction of the vamp and lace stay determines the two basic shoe styles, Blucher and Bal (Fig. 14-3).

The sole consists of an insole, which has a sock lining (the thin piece of leather covering the in-

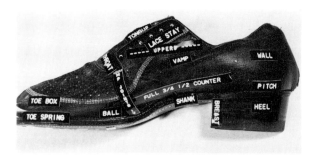

Fig. 14-1. Parts of shoe.

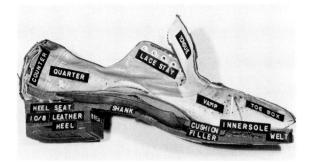

Fig. 14-2. Parts of shoe, sagittal section.

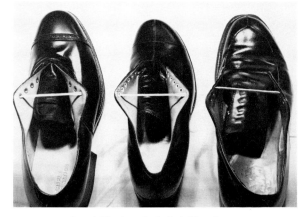

Fig. 14-3. Bal and Blucher. *Left,* Bal. Note lace stays, tongue, and vamp sewn together at the throat. *Middle,* Modified Blucher. Lace stays are not sewn to throat, but there is a seam at the throat where the tongue is stiched to the vamp. *Right,* Tongue is continuous with the vamp and there is no seam at the throat.

sole). Metatarsal pads are placed under this lining and cemented to the insole. Arch supports are usually placed over the sock linings.

A part of the sole is also called the filler, consisting of cork or felt, filling the space between the insole and outsole. It adds resilience and permits some molding of the insole by the foot.

The remaining part of the sole is referred to as the outsole and consists of the welt, a strip of leather that joins the insole and outsole providing a smooth seamless inside to the shoe but allowing it to be readily opened for the insertion of sole wedges, and the ball, the area of the sole on which the metatarsal heads rest with weight bearing. The ball is the widest part of the sole. Metatarsal bars and Denver heels are placed on the outer soles just proximal to the ball to transfer weight bearing posterior and off the metatarsal heads.

The shank portion of sole, between heel and ball, usually includes metal that extends under the heel to stabilize the forefoot. Wide shanks give extra stability for pes planus and unstable subtalar joints. Shanks are completely filled and are flush with ground surface in Space Shoes.

The swing portion of the sole refers to the curvature of the outer edge of the shoe. Abnormal feet, such as splay, metatarsus primus varus, and metatarsus quintus valgus, are better fitted with a greater swing or outer sole edge curvature.

The remaining portion of the sole is the toe spring, the degree of dorsal curvature of sole distal to the ball. Usually this is ½ inch (measured from the floor to top of sole). Toe spring allows for a smooth rocker effect for push-off and lessens creasing of the shoe uppers. This principle is used for sole elevations and rockers, with distal tapering to counteract rigidity of such thickened soles. In effect this rocker sole contour of toe spring provides a smoother gait for patients with ankylosed ankle joints.

The heel portion of the shoe consists of the pad, seat, or rand; the lift, or rubber heel; and the breast, or anterior surface of heel. The higher the heel height, the greater is the downward pitch of the foot (equinus) with increasing forward thrust against the metatarsal heads. Shoe corrections, metatarsal pads, and long arch supports are ineffective when used within commercial high-heel, high-pitched shoes with narrow heels and narrow shanks (Fig. 14-4). With a high-pitched heel, the foot is unstable in a forward direction. Elevation of sole may lessen the effect of pitch of the heels,

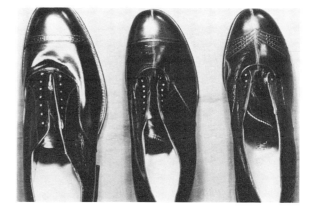

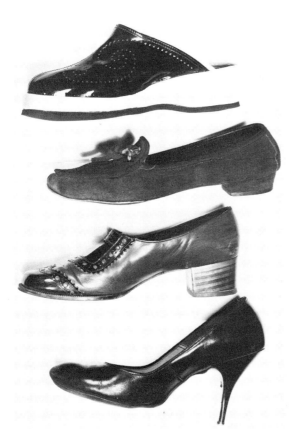

Fig. 14-5. Shoe styles. *Left to right,* Commercial shoe, straight last shoe, and bunion last shoe.

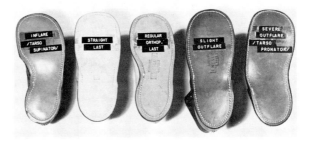

Fig. 14-6. Children's shoe styles from strong inflare to severe outflare. *Viewed from sole, left to right,* Tarsosupinator, straight last, standard orthopaedic last, slight outflare, and tarsopronator.

Fig. 14-4. Women's heel styles and pitch. *Top to bottom,* Platform wedge shoe, suede shoe with low broad heel, Cuban heel, and spike heel.

as in platform shoes. At heel strike, the posterior margin of heel is unstable unless the posterior edge of the heel is curved.

SHOE LASTS AND SIZES

A shoe last is a wood, plastic, or metal form or mold over which a shoe is constructed. A last provides the general shape and construction and conformity of the shoe with regard to deviations from its longitudinal axis (Figs. 14-5 and 14-6). The inner border of sole and upper is in a straight line distally to the medial end of shank or instep in a straight last shoe. This line curves laterally or outward with an outflare shoe. Specific orthopaedic lasts are available for specific deformities, such as the bunion last, which swings medially to accommodate the deformity and then outwardly to accommodate the fifth metatarsal head.

Shoes are measured by width (letters) and length (numerals). For each width (A to B) there is a ¼-inch differential in girth and $1/12$- to $1/24$-inch differential in length. For each one-half size

larger or longer (7 to 7½) there is $1/6$-inch increase in length and ⅛-inch increase in girth of shoe.

SHOE PRESCRIPTION AND FITTING

When called upon to treat foot deformities by conservative means, the orthopaedic surgeon should order the proper shoe and shoe corrections in detail by written prescription, thus maintaining a record for subsequent reference. Shoe corrections or foot supports, if needed, should be prescribed at the same time that the shoe is recommended, since their added bulk within the shoe often requires a wider and long shoe. Shoes and shoe modification prescriptions should probably be made preoperatively rather than postoperatively when there may be residual swelling. A prescribed shoe and shoe modifications should be subject to check by the orthopaedic surgeon. Proper shoe fit should be determined under weight-bearing conditions, the upper should not wrinkle with flexion of the foot, the foot should not bulge the welt. The toe ends should be within

½ inch of the end of the toe box. In the adult, custom-made "space" shoe, the toes should be ¼ inch from the end of the toe box. In children's shoes sufficient room for growth must be included to allow ¾ inch between the end of the child's toe to the end of the toe box. Children may outgrow a shoe within 3 to 4 months. There should be no excess looseness of upper lacing. Relative snug grip of counter about heel is important. Transverse creases develop across the vamp of the shoe with metatarsal head step-off.

PRINCIPLES OF SHOE CORRECTIONS
Children's shoes

Shoes and shoe corrections or modifications are prescribed to apply weight-bearing force against flexible deformities, or rigid deformities, previously corrected by plaster casts or surgical procedures. A corrected clubfoot may be maintained, after plaster or surgical procedure, by outflare shoe. Flexible forefoot varus may be actively treated by primary prescription of an outflare shoe. In the adult such deformities may have become fixed and will *not correct* with prescription of such a corrective shoe, but rather it will require a shoe conforming to the deformity.

The magnitude of correction must be in proportion to severity of deformity, age and tolerance by the child. In the young child, $1/16$- to $1/8$-inch heel or sole wedge is the maximum tolerated, whereas in older children wedges to $3/16$ inch are tolerated and may be prescribed.

Time-lapse studies of young children reveal that the efficiency of shoe corrections may be minimized because a greater proportion of time may occur when they are sitting, kneeling, and lying down, so that benefits of corrections are not utilized.

Finally it should be recognized that the efficiency of many childhood shoe corrections has yet to be proved by long-term control studies, much less by any objective scientific quantitative data. Similarly, there is sparse scientific knowledge of what constitutes the ideal shoe for weight bearing on varied surfaces, for both children and adults with normal feet.

Adults' shoes

Active shoe corrections are generally not functional in adults, instead the foot should be passively stabilized as well as possible in weight bearing plantigrade position. Deformities are usually relatively fixed, and so the floor, by means of the shoe, must be brought up to the foot. Attempts at active correction may only increase symptoms of malfoot weight bearing. When arthritic and rigid joints are present, active correction may only increase stress, strain and pain.

Excess pressure may exist between the foot and upper (bunions, dorsal corns) and between the foot and shoe sole (plantar calluses) and between adjacent toes (soft corns). Shields may be necessary over such prominent deformities to minimize pressure.

Shoes may be modified to minimize excessive weight bearing against deformities such as plantar calluses or local skin change from plantar warts, ulcers, and scars. Shoe pressure and friction must be minimized over any projecting deformity, such as hammertoes.

Areas of decreased weight bearing must be provided with increased weight-bearing support on uninvolved areas of the foot to unload excessive weight-bearing conditions (cavus foot with plantar calluses over prominent metatarsal heads). A simple clinical method indicating this type of shoe adjustment may be determined by the thickness of the plantar skin. Unloaded forefoot plantar skin is usually relatively thin, whereas excessive plantar skin loading provides callusing. This clinical expression of plantar skin represents an actual clinical determination of weight-bearing stresses on the plantar aspect of the foot and may be more accurate than the more sophisticated techniques such as pedograms, pressure transducers,[3] pressure-sensitive dye capsules,[5] or glass mirror reflections of distribution of weight bearing.

Redistribution of weight bearing from areas of excess pressure to areas normally not weight bearing can mechanically be accomplished by foot appliances such as full-length foot or arch supports, or transverse metatarsal arch support, so that proper fitting fills the so-called metatarsal arch or the longitudinal arch, or both, transmitting part of the body weight to normally non-weight bearing surfaces.

In more advanced cases "wells" or depressions must be added to the foot support, with the wells lined with soft resilient shock-absorbing material such as sponge rubber or polyurethane foam.

Arthritic painful joints usually require increased shoe stability to limit motion with weight bearing. A disease ankle joint may be relieved by a high toe shoe. Painful hallux rigidus may be relieved by lengthening the shank or adding rigidity to the sole of the shoe.

Extra or increased stability may be further obtained mechanically by increasing the base of support and altering the axis of heel strike (Ashley heel). Forefoot stability is increased by shoe flanges (outer sole corrections). Subtalar stability is increased by long heel counters or rigid foot supports, and wide shanks. Heel stability is improved with long wide heels, or heel flanges. Ankle joint stability may be increased with high-top shoes with or without extra strength or stiffening. A mild paretic foot drop maybe controlled with a high-top shoe.

Finally, avoid a shoe correction that may aggravate coexisting malfunction condition or cause an additional deformity problem. Inner heel wedge for arch support may only aggravate internal tibial torsion deformity.

CHILDREN'S SHOES AND SHOE CORRECTIONS
Children's commercial shoes

The bootee is soft knit material, used only for warmth and skin protection. The prewalker shoe is made of soft leather, again largely only for skin protection. An infant's walking shoe is usually a high top with firm leather and spring low heel made by adding an extra layer of leather from shank to posterior edge of heel, approximately ¼ inch in height. By age two a low shoe is sufficient with a stable ankle. Generally, a child's shoe is essentially one with a straight last and wide square toe box. Sneakers or tennis shoes of adequate fit are acceptable for the normal foot. The concept of a firm "orthopaedic" shoe to support the foot for maintenance and development of a normal longitudinal arch has not been proved to everyone's satisfaction.

Children's orthopaedic shoes and shoe corrections

Shoe wedges (Fig. 14-7) are flat triangular pieces of leather that are positioned between the inner and outer sole, within heel or sole, occasionally within the shank. The exposed outer margin is the maximum wedge width tapering to paper thinness and covering 50% of the heel or sole. Such corrective modifications are used to aid in derotating the forefoot or heel with flexible deformities. An outer sole wedge will aid in derotating a flexible forefoot varus to valgus. As a secondary

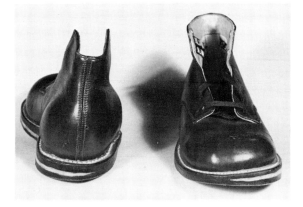

Fig. 14-7. Shoe wedges. Heel and sole wedges are outlined in white.

effect, shoe wedges exert a dynamic force to pivot the heel or forefoot during the gait cycle. Secondarily, wedges exert biomechanical corrective influence upon tibial torsion. However, if metatarsus varus is associated with a valgus heel, a corrective inner heel wedge will dynamically accentuate the associated metatarsus varus and internal tibial torsion if present. On the other hand an outer sole wedge may dynamically accentuate a valgus heel. Derotating or pronating the forefoot may be accomplished with a cuboid or lateral sole wedge. A reverse Thomas heel will rotate the heel toward valgus.

Children's orthopaedic shoes and lasts may incorporate built-in specific heel and shoe wedges as well as straight outflare lasts. A long medial counter extends into the vamp for longer wear. In general, children's orthopaedic shoes include concepts of passive correction with modified lasts and built-in wedges.

Specific types of children's orthopaedic shoes and lasts (Figs. 14-8 and 14-9)

1. The clubfoot prewalker, high-top, open-toe shoe with strong outflare at the level of the tarsometatarsal joints may have a strap and buckle passing anterior to ankle to maintain the heel within the shoe because of common associated underdeveloped heels. This type of shoe is commonly used with connecting intershoe bars and straps.

2. The metatarsus varus–last shoe has a slight outflare of forepart with lateral shoe wedge and long medial counter.

3. The clubfoot shoe has a maximum outflare last with an extralong medial counter, a lateral sole shank, and a heel wedge, used for maintain-

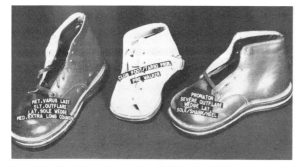

Fig. 14-8. Specific orthopaedic children's clubfoot shoes. *Left to right,* Metatarsus varus last, clubfoot, and tarsopronator lasts.

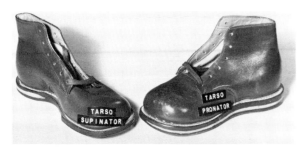

Fig. 14-9. Specific orthopaedic children's shoes. *Left,* Tarso-supinator. *Right,* Tarsopronator.

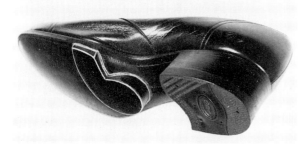

Fig. 14-10. Hauser comma bar and Thomas heel.

ing corrected clubfeet in older-age ambulatory children.

4. The flatfoot shoe, for ambulatory children with flexible pes planovalgus deformity, consists of moderate forefoot inflare with slight supination of foreportion of shoe, incorporating a long medial counter and ⅛-inch inner heel wedge.

5. Children's corrective shoes are also manufactured with inflare, straight last, and varied degrees of outflares (Fig. 14-6). This type of shoe may be prescribed if no special individual correction is necessary.

6. In infancy, a congenital calcaneovalgus foot rapidly responds to straight-last shoes with re-

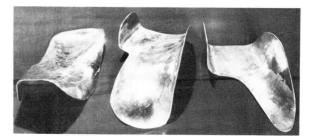

Fig. 14-11. Rigid arch supports, Whitman style.

verse use of inner shoe bar. The tarsal supinator shoe (Fig. 14-9) may be used for young children. For older children, fabricated corrective shoes are available with full medial counter and Thomas heels with inner heel wedge to ³/₁₆ inch, and rubber scaphoid supports are available for nonspecific individual prescription. Specific additional corrective forces may be added, such as a Hauser bar (Fig. 14-10). This appliance is shaped to avoid dorsal displacement, particularly of the fifth metatarsal head.

7. Insert arch supports may also be used. The longitudinal arch and transverse metatarsal arch may be supported by either semirigid or rigid material. The metal Whitman plate (Fig. 14-11) is a rigid arch support but is rarely indicated for children. The Whitman plate is based upon the concept that the heel valgus is secondary to medial displacement of the talus. The basic mechanical effect of the plate is to provide active inversion of the os calcis with ambulation. The outer flange of the plate grasps the heel to provide this force. To construct the Whitman plate with inversion-rotation force potential, a plaster cast of the foot in inversion on a slanted board is constructed as a model. The semirigid-arch foot support is constructed from leather or plastics (Fig. 14-12).

The U.C.B. insert[12] (Fig. 14-12) is a semirigid plastic laminate shoe insert of recent design development based upon biomechanical concepts and has replaced the metal Whitman plate.

The plantar flexed talus shoe,[14] a recent design development, includes reverse calcaneal heel position, forefoot anterior pitch, and forefoot adduction. A long steel shank maintains the necessary rigidity and, as the foot deformity improves, the degree of correction is increased.

In general, one is unimpressed with the value of special shoe lasts, corrections, and foot supports

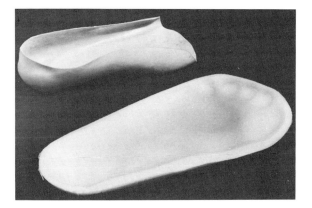

Fig. 14-12. *Top,* U.C.B. laminated plastic shoe insert. *Bottom,* One half inch thick closed-cell polyethylene foam arch support.

as corrective measures for hypermobile flatfoot syndrome, although on occasion such feet are more comfortable with relative rigid support particularly in the adult.

Genu valgum and genu varum. Many authorities suggest medial heel wedges to aid in correcting genu valgum, which is often associated with secondary pes planus. Whitman[18] recommended an outer sole wedge, in addition, to apply a corrective force with associated medial tibial torsion deformity. Dickson and Diveley[7] recommended inner sole and heel wedges for genu varum as well as genu valgum because weight bearing falls generally medially in both the deformities and causes the foot to pronate.

Others prefer inner heel wedge for genu valgum and inner heel wedge with outer sole wedge for genu varum, as inner heel wedge by itself aggravates the toeing-in gait. Not infrequently however, genu varum becomes genu valgum with or without shoe corrections, and the effect of shoe corrections with these childhood deformities is in question.

COMMERCIAL ADULT SHOES AND SHOE MODIFICATIONS

In general, a satisfactory commercial shoe for the normal foot should include a heel no higher than 2 inches, relatively thick leather or rubber sole, and straight last with high wide toe box. Soft suede uppers yield to abnormal bone protuberances or mild toe deformities. A paretic foot will function more effectively with a light, soft shoe for improved antigravity forefoot lift-off and being readily stretchable for minor deformity. Leg-length discrepancy lifts add weight and are less

cosmetically acceptable but more often than not, exact equalization of leg length will not improve the malfunctioning gait.

Inexpensive commercial shoes may be readily modified by mechanical stretching over a last or through the use of a localizing stretcher or a "swan".[13] Acute conditions, such as acute bursitis over hallux valgus deformity may be relieved by cutting out the shoe over the area until the acute reaction subsides.

With toe deformities, particularly hammertoes, a high wide toe box of soft suede is indicated. Split size shoes may be used for unequal foot length. Low heel heights are preferable with toe deformities to lessen the heel pitch angle to prevent compression of toes toward the end of the shoe. Contracted tendon Achilles mechanisms, however, do not tolerate a low heel. For acute conditions of the anterior toes, an open-toed shoe is indicated on a temporary basis. Hallux rigidus symptoms may often be controlled by a thick platform shoe or thick sole.

Commercial shoes of thin leather soles with high heels increase heel pitch and aggravate anterior metatarsalgia. The commercial shoe of choice has soft resilient soles such as thick rubber, ripple, or crepe with low heel height. Metatarsal pads or plantar sole metatarsal bars can be added. A wedge shoe with a filled shank increases the weight-bearing distribution. Application of appliances such as metatarsal bars, however, require relatively thick soles and relatively wide stable shanks. Pathologic conditions such as plantar ulcers and severe calluses may also be relieved by use of wool-lined shoes with or without thick soft rubber or crepe soles and heels with suede uppers for added comfort.

Plantar heel spur syndrome, posterior heel bursae, and irritated os calcis exostosis may be relieved by open heels or removal of the heel counter.

Elasticized vamps are useful for patients with limited knee and hip function as well as those with upper-limb disabilities who are unable to tie a shoelace.

The orthopaedic shoe is constructed for maximum weight-bearing function with comfort and constructed of good leather, relatively thick soles, high wide toe box, and wide stable shanks extending into the heel. The arch is supported by a high vamp and often a long medial counter. Heels are broad, not in excess of 2 inches high, and with low pitch and firm stabilizing heel counter. The last is generally of straight construction. This type of shoe permits the addition of removable or fixed specially constructed foot or arch supports. These shoes come in several styles.

In the Bal (Balmoral) shoe (Fig. 14-3), the upper construction is available in commercial shoes; the tongue, throat, and lace stays are seamed as one unit. This type of upper construction, however, allows less space for the dorsal aspect of the midfoot and therefore is contraindicated for pes cavus and dorsal exostoses.

The Blucher type (Fig. 14-3) of upper shoe manufacture has no seam construction across the dorsum of the midfoot; the tongue piece continues with the uppers. Lace stays are not fixed to the throat; thereby expansion space over the dorsum of the midfoot is permitted.

Specific orthopaedic lasts (Fig. 14-5)

1. The straight last is constructed with a relatively straight inner border and is a standard shoe last for normal feet. Most commercial shoes curve laterally at the level of the base of the hallux, forcing a valgus position. Pointed toe shoes increase this compression toe force both medially and laterally.

2. Bunion last shoes curve medially to provide more space for hallux valgus deformity. Lateral border deviates laterally to provide space for increased prominence of fifth toe base with hallux valgus deformity. This construction is adequate for mild to moderate hallux valgus deformities.

3. Combination last shoes are constructed with a wide forepart and relatively narrow heel widths. Generally, the bunion and combination lasts have wide toe boxes for improved toe spacing.

4. Extra depth shoes have a straight last with high uppers to provide space for foot or arch supports not over ⅜ inch in thickness.

5. Custom-made and -molded ("space") shoes (Figs. 14-13 and 14-14), which are orthopaedic shoes, are hand crafted to fit the foot deformity and include corrective modifications. Molded ("space") shoes are fabricated from individual foot casting, conforming to any deformity present. Shoes of this type provide passive maintenance stability and comfort for severe foot deformities and are not designed for active deformity correction. The molded shoe does not provide space for growth and therefore is not often used for children.

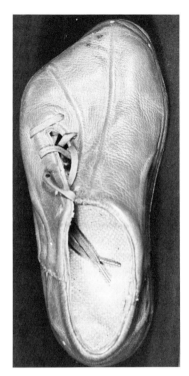

Fig. 14-13. Old style "space" shoe.

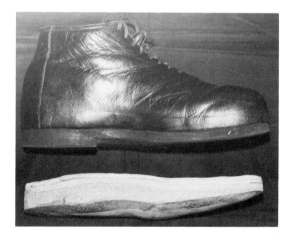

Fig. 14-14. Low boot molded shoe with 1 inch thick rubber adjustable custom full-length arch support.

The molded shoe is fabricated over the positive cast rather than over a wood last. The upper construction is seamless, except for side lacing. The heel and sole are of thick rubber or plastic of similar resiliency and are continuous, since the shank is incorporated. Supplementing the molded shoe with a custom soft foot or arch support adds to passive correction (Fig. 14-15). Stabilizing orthosis may be easily added as indicated.

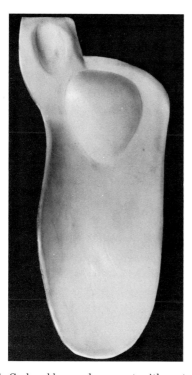

Fig. 14-15. Cork-rubber arch support with metatarsal pad, Morton's extension, and "well" under interphalangeal joint of hallux.

Shoe corrections

Shoe corrections are generally considered internal or external shoe additions—internal by additions to the inner sole, external by additions to the outer sole or heel. Internal additions are generally of soft material, with felt or rubber being more effective, but less tolerated because of space consumption. External corrections include wedges and anterior heels.

Internal shoe corrections. Internal corrections include metatarsal and scaphoid pads fixed by rubber cement to the inner sole and beneath the sock lining, fixed with convexed supporting surface of pads facing the foot. As a temporary measure similar felt pads may be fixed to the foot with adhesive tape (Fig. 14-16). Inside toe corrections include protective metal toe cap and piano felt insertion to protect a hammertoe.

Metatarsal pads are constructed of firm rubber or of plastic material positioned just proximally to the metatarsal heads. These pads principally protect the second, third, and fourth metatarsal heads. Sesamoid (dancers, or "bat") pads are similar to metatarsal pads, but extend proximally to the first metatarsal head. The interior cuboid pad

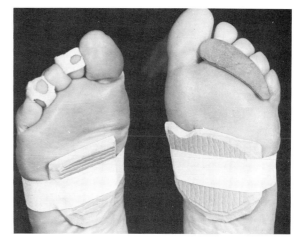

Fig. 14-16. Metatarsal pads and plantar toe shields. Standard metatarsal pad on patient's right and sesamoid pad on patient's left.

is constructed of rubber, positioned beneath the sock lining, under the cuboid bone to derotate the forefoot with flexible forefoot supination deformity.

The longitudinal arch or foot support is constructed of varied thicknesses of moderately firm rubber scaphoids ("cookies"), positioned along the medial border of the insole onto the medial counter. This modification may be built into an orthopaedic shoe, and thus is usually fabricated of firm leather. The addition of ⅛-inch medial heel wedge may add comfort to a high or thick scaphoid.

Interior heel wedges $^1/_{16}$ to ⅛ inch in height (Fig. 14-7) transverse half of the interior heel width. Heel lifts (tapered heel pads) are constructed of moderately firm rubber, ⅛ to $^3/_{16}$ inch in width, tapered anteriorly. Heel elevation of more than ¼ inch should be applied externally. A shoe heel may be narrowed by the addition of felt applied to the medial aspect of the heel wall. An anterior calcaneal bar[1] may be constructed of ½-inch wide foam rubber, ¼ inch in height, positioned transversely anterior of plantar os calcis of spur.

External shoe corrections (Figs. 14-7, 14-17 and 14-18). Shoe wedges are constructed of leather, positioned under the outer sole, usually ⅛ to $^3/_{16}$ inch at wedge width, and may exert corrective force in children. Toe wedges prescribed for adult fixed deformities are not prescribed as corrective forces, but rather are to provide a plantigrade position of the shoe sole. The addition of foot or arch support with wells (depressions) under a

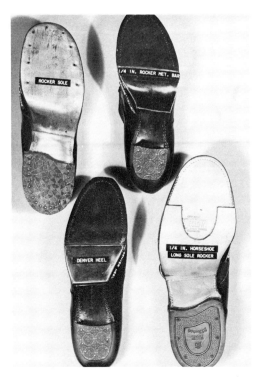

Fig. 14-17. Outside sole corrections. *Top left,* Long sole rocker (rocker sole). *Top right,* One fourth inch rocker metatarsal bar. *Bottom left,* Denver heel. *Bottom right,* Horseshoe long sole rocker.

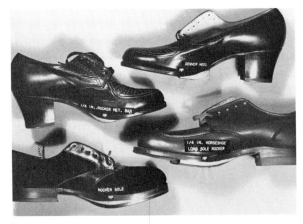

Fig. 14-18. Outside sole corrections. *Upper left,* One fourth inch rocker metatarsal bar. The thickest portion (¼ inch) is at the level of the metacarpophalangeal joints. *Lower left,* Long sole rocker. The leather piece extends to the tip of the sole. *Upper right,* Denver heel that extends to the metacarpophalangeal joints. *Lower right,* horseshoe rocker.

calloused metatarsal head may be necessary with fixed or rigid adult forefoot deformities.

Flanges are medial or lateral extension of sole projecting ¼ inch to provide additional medial or lateral rotary stability to the forefoot.

Metatarsal bars[11] (anterior heels) are constructed of leather or rubber bars fixed transversely onto the outer sole proximal to the metatarsal heads to transfer metatarsal-head weight-bearing pressure posterior to the metatarsal heads.

The Denver heel (Fig. 14-17) is constructed of wide leather metatarsal bars that extend posteriorly to support the distal one-half of metatarsal shafts for added metatarsal distal support.

The Hauser comma bar (Fig. 14-10) is constructed of leather or rubber, comma in shape, and positioned proximally of medial four metatarsal heads with maximum height laterally to pronate the forefoot.

The horseshoe correction (Fig. 14-10) is constructed of leather, horseshoe in shape, and positioned on the outer sole, with distal arms extending to first and fifth metatarsal heads with the central portion positioned proximally of second, third, and fourth heads, applicable to the transmission of excessive midmetatarsal-head weight-bearing deformity. Construction provides a ³⁄₁₆-inch elevation under the first head tapered to ⅛-inch elevation under the fifth head.

The Nutt wedge (medial flared or flagged) is a short wedge constructed of leather positioned posterior to the first metatarsal head. The device prevents medial rotation of hallux and reduces

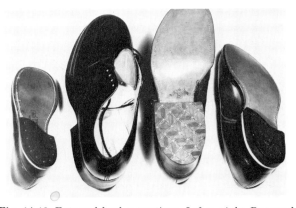

Fig. 14-19. External heel corrections. *Left to right,* Reversed Thomas heel with outer heel wedge; outer sole and heel flange; Ashley heel—note flanges extending wide of shank; Thomas heel with medial heel wedge (left shoe).

medial plantar pressure associated with hallux valgus deformity.

A metatarsal rocker bar (Fig. 14-17) is constructed of leather, positioned transversely distal to metatarsophalangeal joints. The thickest portion of this corrective device is ¼ inch in an attempt to reduce metatarsophalangeal flexion. Rocker function provides smoother plantar roll to toe-off, specifically used with hallux rigidus. Rigidity may be reinforced with a double shoe or long steel shank.

Sole elevation (raises) are prescribed for leg-length discrepancy.

External heel corrections (Fig. 14-19) include Thomas heels constructed with anteromedial heel extension to provide additional support of longitudinal arch. Heel wedges used in adult shoes may be supportive with flexible pes planus, or protective in the presence of tenosynovitis involving the posterior tibial tendon.

Heel flanges (Fig. 14-19) are positioned either medially or laterally ¼ inch to increase plantigrade heel stability. Additional stability may be added with a flanged Thomas heel or application of this heel construction in reverse position.

Tapered heel elevations are limited to ³/₁₆ inch posteriorly and taper to zero thickness at the shoe breast. They are utilized to minimize Achilles tendon tension and decrease weight bearing on the heel.

Heel lifts are prescribed for leg-length discrepancy.

Arch supports

Removable foot or arch supports are preferable to interior shoe modifications in that they are interchangeable from shoe to shoe and may be modified without disturbing the shoe, may incorporate multiple corrections, and may be constructed from several materials. Such orthoses, custom made, may be more accurately and specifically constructed and are preferably to be used with good support orthopaedic type of shoes. By contrast, commercially constructed arch supports are generally comparatively ineffective.

Rigid arch supports (Fig. 14-11). Rigid arch supports were originally developed from the philosophy that "weak" or flat longitudinal arch feet required the addition of firm support and that their constant use would ultimately "mold" a normal longitudinal arch. Rigid metal Whitman plates were originally designed to provide active

inversion force on the heel with weight bearing, particularly for children. Most authors are unimpressed with the prescription of a rigid support as a corrective measure in childhood, being of the opinion that such a support may *occasionally* provide some relief of symptoms associated with flexible adult feet. Whitman supports are constructed of steel from positive casts of the patient's foot, usually extending from the heel area to the metatarsal heads. Corrections may be added to or subtracted from the positive mold. Leather may be added to line metal supports with the exception of the Whitman plate. The Whitman plate (Fig. 14-11) is meant to be rigid, whereas other metal plates or supports may be somewhat flexible, with spring steel. The Shaffer plate is constructed of metal but provides no metatarsal elevation. The Boston arch support is constructed of light metal with an anterior metatarsal elevation and slightly cupped leather-covered heel.

Rigid steel arch supports are most useful as an extension of a leg brace terminating within a shoe to provide maximum foot and ankle stability where indicated.

Semirigid arch supports (Figs. 14-12, 14-15 and 14-20). Semirigid arch supports are constructed from multiple materials—leather, cork, solid plastics, plastic laminates (U.C.B. foot insert), and fiber glass.

Flexible arch supports (Figs. 14-12 and 14-15). Flexible arch supports are constructed from cork,

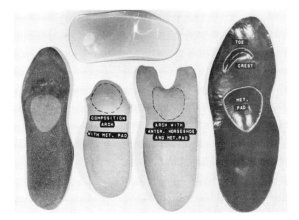

Fig. 14-20. Semirigid arch supports. *Top,* Solid plastic extending to metatarsal heads including flange for arch. *Bottom, left to right,* Full-length leather-lined cork support showing addition of firm rubber metatarsal raise; cork support extending to metatarsal heads and including a metatarsal raise; cork horseshoe support including a metatarsal pad; semirigid support with toe crest and metatarsal pad.

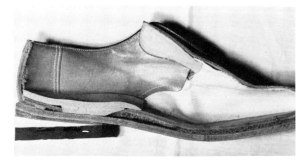

Fig. 14-21. Sagittal section of shoe with Steindler plantar heel spur correction. Note gouged-out heel area filled in with sponge rubber.

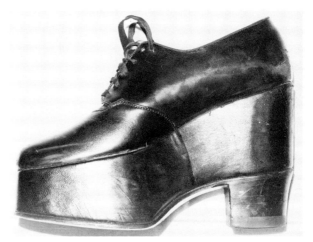

Fig. 14-22. Cork heel and sole raise for leg-length discrepancy.

rubber, soft plastic, or plastic foams. They are therefore softer and more comfortable and may be altered. Rubber is the least acceptable because of heat and compression with weight bearing. Flexible and soft supports are usually covered with thin leather or plastic. Mixtures of rubber and cork, called "rubber butter," may also be used for soft supports. Flexible arch supports are usually constructed as full-length orthoses, thickened where protective weight bearing is indicated. "Wells" (Fig. 14-15) for metatarsal callosities are easily incorporated as are other interior sole and heel corrections. Morton's extension is an elevated extension of arch support anterior to the first metatarsal head to increase weight bearing of this segment of the forefoot.

False toe boxes, toe filler, and inner sole filler are constructed from cork, fixed to an insole support for foot deformities such as toe or forefoot amputations. Fillers constructed in this manner add ambulation stability.

MISCELLANEOUS FOOT-CORRECTIVE DEVICES
Steindler heel spur correction (Fig. 14-21)

The middle one-third longitudinal section of heel interior is removed and the depression defect is filled with a moderately firm sponge rubber. The entire heel surface is then covered with a layer of $3/16$-inch sponge rubber. The exterior heel is elevated with $3/16$-inch tapered wedge and rubber scaphoid is added. The medial shoe counter is lengthened and on occasion $1/8$-inch inner heel wedge is added.

Leg-length discrepancy (Fig. 14-22)

Heel elevation for leg-length discrepancy of less than $1/2$ inch does not require the addition of

outer sole elevation. Elevation of heel greater than $1/2$ inch for leg-length discrepancy requires the addition of outer-sole elevation of approximately 50% of the heel elevation. Outer-sole forefoot shoe elevation should be tapered forward of the ball of the shoe to the toe.

A fixed-foot equinus deformity requires heel elevation for plantigrade foot position, requiring increased heel-to-ball anterior pitch gait, which also requires metatarsal head protection. Upon completion of shoe elevation correction for fixed equinus foot deformity, one must recognize secondary leg-length discrepancy with the foot made plantigrade by shoe correction and must measure the discrepancy with the normal leg (with the patient standing on blocks of predetermined thickness) in order to balance the pelvis. The shoe of the normal leg may require heel and sole lift to balance the deformity.

Minor leg-length discrepancy, less than $1/2$ inch, may be compensated by application of internal heel pads of $1/4$ inch.

Foot-size discrepancy

Discrepancy in foot length may be compensated for by a toe filler in standard commercial shoes. For severe differences, prescribe custom-molded shoes with size differential or matched custom-molded shoes containing toe or partial foot filler.

The anesthetic foot

The anesthetic rigid foot is more likely to break down than the anesthetic flexible foot. Shear and thrust forces applied to the plantar soft tissue of anesthetic foot, particularly with toe-off, are a primary cause for ulceration over plantar bone prominences. To minimize shear and thrust, application of a metatarsal rocker to sole may be prescribed, or one may use a shoe with rigid shank sole, lined with sponge rubber. Space shoe with modifications may be indicated.

Shoe correction in the treatment of the insensitive foot does not depend on rigidity per se, but rather on adequate support in the transference of weight bearing, a soft heel strike, and a smooth roll-off. This principle is therefore no different from those used for the therapy of the foot with normal sensation.

REFERENCES

1. American Academy of Orthopaedic Surgeons: Orthopaedic appliances atlas. Vol. 1. Braces, splints, shoe alterations, Ann Arbor, Mich., 1952, J. W. Edwards.
2. Anderson, A. D.: The shoe and leather lexicon, ed. 15, New York, 1952.
3. Bauman, J. H., and Branch, P. W.: Measurement of pressure between foot and shoe, Lancet **1**:629-632, 1963.
4. Bauman, J. H., Girling, J. P., and Branch, P. W.: Plantar pressure and trophic ulceration. An evaluation of footwear, J. Bone Joint Surg. **45B**:652-673, 1963.
5. Brand, P. W., and Ebner, J. D.: Pressure sensitive devices for denervated hands and feet, J. Bone Joint Surg. **51A**:109-116, 1969.
6. Clawson, D. K., and Seddon, H. J.: The late consequences of sciatic nerve injury, J. Bone Joint Surg. **42B**:213-225, 1960.
7. Dickson, F. D., and Diveley, R. L.: Functional disorders of the foot. ed. 2, Philadelphia, 1944, J. B. Lippincott Co.
8. Gibbard, L. C., editor: Charlesworth's Chiropodical Orthopaedics, ed. 2, London, 1968, Bailliere, Tindall & Cassell.
9. Gross, R. H.: Modern foot therapy. In Lewi, M. J., editor: Modern foot therapy, New York, 1948, R. H. Gross.
10. Jordan, H. H.: Orthopaedic appliances, ed. 2, Springfield, Ill., 1963, Charles C Thomas, Publisher.
11. Lewin, P.: The foot and ankle, ed. 4, Philadelphia, 1959, Lea & Febiger.
12. Mereday, C., Dolan, C. M. E., and Lusskin, R.: Evaluation of the University of California Biomechanics Laboratory shoe insert in "flexible" pes planus, Clin. Orthop. Related Res. **82**:45-58, Philadelphia, 1972, J. B. Lippincott Co.
13. Milgram, J. E.: Office measures for relief of the painful foot. Instructional course lectures, J. Bone Joint Surg. **46A**:1095-1116, 1964.
14. Outland, T., McKeever, G. R., and Glaubitz, A.: Clinical application of the plantarflexed talus shoe. Preliminary report, Orthop. Prosthet. Appliance J. **20**:23-27, 1966.
15. Price, E. W.: Studies on plantar ulceration in leprosy. VI. The management of plantar ulcers, Leprosy Rev. **31**:139-171, 1960.
16. Ross, W. F.: Footwear and the prevention of ulcers in leprosy, Leprosy Rev. **33**:202-206, 1962.
17. Schuster, O. N.: Foot orthopaedics, ed. 2, Albany, 1939, J. B. Lyon Co.
18. Whitman, R.: A treatise on orthopaedic surgery, ed. 8, Philadelphia, 1927, Lea & Febiger, pp. 736-926 and 933.
19. Wickstrom, J., and Williams, R. A.: Shoe corrections and orthopaedic foot supports, Clin. Orthop. Related Res. **70**:30-42, Philadelphia, 1970, J. B. Lippincott Co.

PART FIVE

The spine

CHAPTER 15

Biomechanics of the cervical spine

HENRY LaROCCA, M.D.

The human neck is a cylindrical conduit that supports the head and renders it mobile. It provides avenues of passage for essential connections in the respiratory, gastrointestinal, vascular, and nervous systems and serves as the locus for two vital ductless glands and for the organ of phonation. As such, it is a compact aggregate of numerous critical structures related to the cervical spine, which serves as the major architectural member (Fig. 15-1). The anatomic structures within the neck are segregated into compartments divided by fascial planes for efficient utilization of relatively restricted space. The cervical spine, with its investing musculature, is housed within the vertebral compartment, situated centrally and posteriorly. The contents of this compartment provide points of anchorage and suspension for fascial layers defining all remaining compartments. Though these fascial layers provide stabilization to their contents, they are sufficiently lax to permit motion of the neck as a unit, as well as motion of one compartment relative to another (as exemplified in the act of swallowing).

The cervical spine is a highly mobile structure that functions principally to position the head in space to permit effective adaptation of the organism to his environment. Motion of the neck is therefore inseparably linked with motion of the head, and this linkage is a critical concept in both normal and pathologic states. When the neck muscles contract, their net effect is to move the head to a new position. Further, so long as the

head is free to move, at least part of the cervical spine must move with it.

NORMAL BIOMECHANICS OF CERVICAL SPINE
Generation of motion

The various types of motion that occur in the neck are generated by *muscles,* which may be categorized into four groups: (1) cervicocapital motors, (2) visceral motors, (3) suspensor motors of the first ribs, (4) suspensor motors of the shoulder girdles. Individual muscles in each of these columns are oriented craniocaudally and traverse much of the length of the neck. The *cervicocapital motors* consist of three groups, all of which move the spine *(cervical)* and skull *(capital)* simultaneously in integrated, combined motions. The first of these groups lies extrinsicly to the spine, passing from the shoulder girdle to the skull in peripheral regions of the neck, producing primary motion of the head on the neck. The major members of this group are the sternocleidomastoid muscles. The remaining two groups of cervicocapital motors have origins directly from the spine and insertions onto either the spine or skull and thus are intrinsic to the spine. They occur in right and left pairs, and members of a pair independently act to rotate and tilt the head and neck. One of these groups is located entirely anteriorly and includes the longus muscles (thoracis, cervicis, and capitis). When its members contract in concert, flexion results. The second is located entirely

283

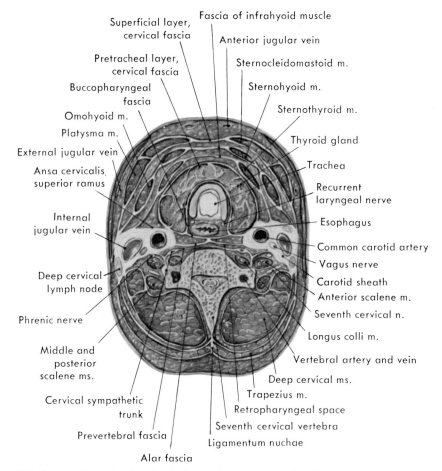

Fig. 15-1. Cross section of neck at level of seventh cervical vertebra illustrating compact aggregation of numerous critical anatomic structures. (From Sobotta, J., and Becher, H.: Atlas der deskriptiven Anatomie des Menschen, Part 1, München, 1957, Urban & Schwarzenberg Verlag.)

posteriorly, comprising the erector spinae and splenius muscles, which produce head and neck extension, often acting in concert. These long cervicocapital motors are supplemented by smaller muscles in the atlantoaxial region, which produce discrete motion of the structures in this special region.

The *visceral motors* of the neck include those muscles associated with the pharynx, larynx, trachea, hyoid bone, and thyroid bone, and thyroid gland. The *suspensor motors of the first ribs* are the scalene muscles, which pass from the spine to cover the domes of the thoracic cavities; thus they have an intimate relationship with great vessels emerging to supply the head and upper limbs. The brachial plexus gains access to the thoracic outlet region by separating the muscle bundles of the scalenes. The *suspensor motors of the shoulder girdle* include the trapezius, rhomboids, and

levator scapulae. These muscles, taking origin from the cervical and thoracic spine, suspend and mobilize the scapula and thereby link neck motion with upper-limb motion.

While the muscles of the neck are generating motion, the ligaments serve as constraints to motion, confining it within physiologic ranges. Thus, as the neck is brought into extension by muscular activity, the anterior longitudinal ligament becomes increasingly taut until finally it prohibits further extension. Similarly, the extremes of flexion are constrained by the posterior ligamentous structures, including the ligamentum nuchae, the interspinous ligaments, and the posterior longitudinal ligament. The ligamentum flavum and the capsules of the zygapophyseal joints also serve as ligamentous constraints in sagittal plane motion but constrain both rotary and tilting motion as well. In the upper cervical

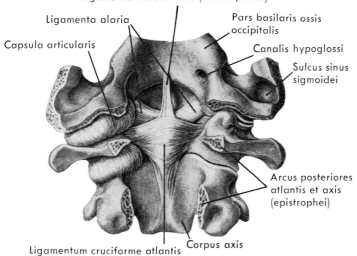

Fig. 15-2. Specialized bony and ligamentous anatomy of atlantoaxial region. (From Sobotta, J., and Becher, H.: Atlas der deskriptiven Anatomie des Menschen, Part 1, München, 1957, Urban & Schwarzenberg Verlag.)

region there are specialized ligaments that contribute to the stability of the occipitoatlantal and atlantoaxial articulations (Fig. 15-2).

Determinants of motion

The potential for motion of the cervical spine arises from the contours, dimensions, and relationships of the vertebrae, whose geometry is a fundamental determinant of both the direction and the extent of possible motion. The seven cervical vertebrae are organized structurally and functionally into two regions: the upper and lower cervical spine. The upper cervical spine includes the atlas and the axis, and the lower cervical spine includes all the remaining cervical vertebrae.

The *atlas* is a ring of bone with two broadened lateral articular masses. The anterior aspect of this ring articulates directly with the odontoid, and the interior extensions from both lateral atlantal masses give rise to the transverse ligament to complete the encirclement of the odontoid. This special construction permits rotation of the atlas about a vertical axis, which is physically represented by the odontoid. The *axis* features the odontoid, a bony prominence directed cranially from its vertebral body, representing what was the embryologic body of the first cervical vertebra. The body of the axis also gives rise to two stout pedicles that partially support the superior facets and then flatten to form the laminae. These join the spinous process, a large and bifid structure.

The special geometry of the atlas and axis therefore determines much of the direction and extent of motion of the head in the sagittal and axial planes.

The lower cervical vertebrae (C3 to C7) are shaped alike, with regional variations in the size of substructures (Fig. 15-3). Each consists of a body, two pedicles, two pairs of facets, two laminae jointing centrally to form a spinous process, and two specialized transverse processes. Contrary to the shape suggested by radiographs, the body is *not* rectangular in either frontal or sagittal section. Instead, the end plates are caudally convex in the frontal plane and cranially convex in the sagittal plane, forming saddle-shaped structures.[14] The superolateral margin of the vertebral body rises to form a ridge, the uncinate process, which articulates with the intervertebral disc and the inferolateral side of the vertebral body above. The pedicles, emerging from the bodies and projecting posteriorly, form the floor of the intervertebral foramen and then support the articular processes. The laminae and spinous processes complete the segmental unit posteriorly. The transverse processes are specialized structures consisting of an anterocostal element (a vestigial rib) and a true transverse element, which join laterally to form a foramen surrounding the vertebral artery. Between the vertebral artery and the transverse element is a trough for the emergence of the spinal nerve. Both the costal and

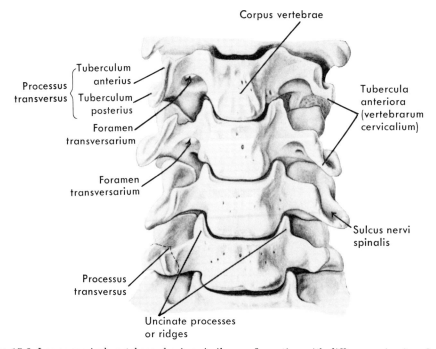

Fig. 15-3. Lower cervical vertebrae sharing similar configuration with differences in size of substructures. (From Sobotta, J., and Becher, H.: Atlas der deskriptiven Anatomie des Menschen, Part 1, München, 1957, Urban & Schwarzenberg Verlag.)

transverse elements terminate in tubercles for muscle attachment.

From the level of the second vertebra downward, each pair of vertebral bodies is connected by an intervertebral disc, composed of two avascular hyaline cartilage end plates, an annulus fibrosus, and a nucleus pulposus. The intervertebral discs are the structures through which intervertebral motion occurs, and they therefore play an important role in the determination of motion capacity. Cervical discs are often tall structures, and the separation between vertebrae that this dimension produces imparts the high degree of mobility noted in the cervical spine.[14]

The vertebral bodies are positioned in series to support the load delivered by the head, and the form assumed by the bodies reflects both weight-bearing and motion-determining functions. The basic structure is a modified cube with upper and lower surfaces broadened to receive and transmit the load. These surfaces are larger than the vertical height of the corresponding vertebral bodies, and thus the width of the body is greater than its height or depth. Hence there is a greater capacity for flexion-extension than for lateral bending, since lateral bending is dampened by the breadth

of the bone present. In addition to being broadened for transmission of the weight of the head, the upper and lower surfaces of the vertebral bodies are shaped into cavities and projections, which determine motion possibilities. The upper surface of the body is concave in the frontal plane and convex in the sagittal plane. The frontal concavity is increased by the cranial projections of the uncinate processes. The lower surface of the body is convex in the frontal plane and concave in the sagittal plane. These structural refinements produce shallow sockets in which one vertebra moves with tilt and rotation against its subjacent neighbor. The secondary uncovertebral articulations (Luschka joints) may guide flexion and extension and may also prohibit lateral displacement of one vertebra on another.

The zygapophyseal joints are also guides to motion, and their configuration and orientation allow considerable freedom. The articular plates are small ovoids that slide freely upon one another. The surfaces of the joints are nearly perpendicular to the sagittal plane and thereby permit considerable horizontal rotation and lateral bending. These surfaces incline obliquely from anteriorly to posteriorly, thus guiding flexion and extension. Since the right and left joints are parallel in orientation to one another, they offer no mechanical locking effects against motion.

In summary, the determinants of the direction and extent of motion reside in the geometry of the vertebral bodies and in the contours and orientations of the intervertebral articulations. The presence of the intervertebral disc adds a special determinant to motion by providing a fulcrum upon which the vertebrae can displace and by containing a nucleus pulposus that is sufficiently mobile to participate in the action. The ligaments, membranes, and capsules invest the spine function passively to provide constraints to motion. When their elastic limits are reached, the tension created causes motion to halt.

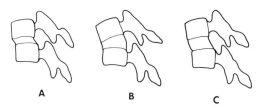

Fig. 15-4. Cervical vertebrae move on their discs with either sliding motion, **A,** tilting motion, **B,** or a combination of both, producing rolling motion, **C.**

Patterns of motion

The motion of the neck observed grossly is the culmination of multiple activities occurring either simultaneously or in series in which muscular contraction initiates positional changes to which vertebral bone and intervertebral soft tissues respond. The unit of activity is intersegmental motion, occurring between two adjacent vertebrae. The combination of multiple intersegmental motions provides the neck with six degrees of freedom: flexion, extension, right and left bending, and right and left rotation. Coupling of motions in the sagittal, frontal, and axial planes allows an almost infinite variety of head and neck positions.

Three distinct types of motion occur: (1) sliding of one vertebra on another, (2) tilting of one vertebra on another, and (3) rotation of one vertebra on another about a vertical axis (Fig. 15-4).[14] *Sliding motion* is seen principally in the sagittal plane as vertebrae displace forward and backward on one another in a linear path during the actions of flexion and extension. In flexion, the vertebrae move forward in a stair-step pattern and return to form a smooth curve as extension progresses (Fig. 15-5).[6,7,20] Sliding in the frontal plane is blocked by the uncovertebral projections. In sliding (and rotational motion) a vertebra displaces on its subjacent nucleus pulposus and continues

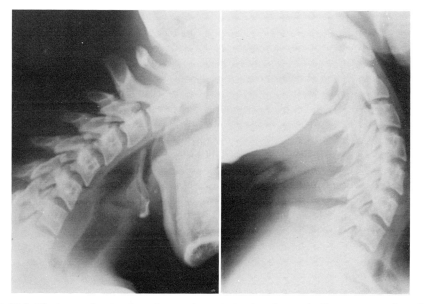

Fig. 15-5. Flexion and extension of normal cervical spine demonstrating no separation of atlas from odontoid, sliding motion at upper segments, rolling motion at middle segments, tilting motion at lower segments, and stair stepping in flexion.

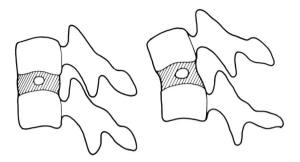

Fig. 15-6. As the vertebra moves on its disc, the nucleus displaces toward convexity of curve thus formed and assumes tapered shape.

to do so until all laxity in the annulus fibrosus is eliminated, at which point the motion must cease.

Tilting motion occurs on both the frontal and the sagittal planes. In the frontal plane, lateral bending of the head causes a tilting of the vertebral body toward the side to which the head displaces. In the sagittal plane, flexion and extension are associated with tilting of the vertebrae on their subjacent neighbors about an axis that runs perpendicular to the direction of motion. In this particular displacement, the vertebrae do not roll smoothly on one another, but instead take a more angular path.[14] In tilting motions, a vertebral body moves along the spherical surface of the nucleus pulposus and thus initially assumes a rolling path of progress. However, the nucleus does not remain stationary[5] but moves in a direction opposite to the path of vertebral motion, and in so doing its configuration begins to taper (Fig. 15-6). Hence the moving vertebra then displaces along a more angular course. When the spine moves into flexion, the nucleus displaces posteriorly with its taper directed anteriorly. With the spine going into extension, the nuclear changes are reversed. Similar configurational changes occur with lateral bending.

Sliding and tilting motions are the two principal patterns demonstrated in flexion and extension of cervical intervertebral units. In those units in which the intervertebral disc is *rectangular* in shape in the sagittal plane, the predominant type of motion is a *sliding* one. In those units in which the disc configuration is that of a *wedge* with the base anterior, the predominant motion of the upper vertebra on the lower is a *tilting* one. As a generalization, sliding motion is the predominant type in upper segments; the central segments demonstrate combinations of both sliding and tilting.[7,14]

Rotation about a vertical axis occurs as the spine and head turn toward right or left. In this motion, the vertebrae turn toward the direction of the head displacement by rotating through the intervertebral disc.[7]

When the neck moves, there are quantitative differences in the degree of participation in the motion exhibited by the upper cervical column as contrasted with the lower. Motion in the upper column, which includes the occipitoatlantal and the atlantoaxial articulations, is the result of the special bony and ligamentous anatomy of the region.[11,12] At the occipitoatlantal joint, motions occurs primarily in the sagittal plane. This joint contributes approximately 30 degrees of sagittal motion as the head moves from the fully extended position to the fully flexed position. At the atlantoaxial joint, the major motion is in the axial plane, permitting rotation of the head to the right and left through 45 degrees in either direction as the atlas pivots about the odontoid. Thus the greatest absolute quantity of head motion normally is provided by the atlantoaxial joint. However, rotation is not the only motion possible at this level and both flexion-extension and lateral bending occur. In flexion, the space between the posterior tubercle of the atlas and the spinous processes of the axis widens and the atlas displaces forward on the axis over an arc of 15 degrees. A maximum of 2 millimeters of separation between the anterior arch of the atlas and the odontoid process occurs with normal flexion. In extension, the atlas tilts 15 degrees posteriorly on the axis and the space between its posterior tubercle and the spinous process of the axis narrows while the anterior arch of the atlas approximates the odontoid. In lateral bending of the head, the atlas displaces laterally on the axis toward the side to which the head deviates.[11,12] However, pure lateral displacement of the axis is prohibited by the anatomy of the area, and this phenomenon can only occur with associated rotation of the atlantoaxial joint. Thus there is an obligatory coupling of the actions of lateral displacement and rotation, producing a definite offset of the articular facets and an asymmetric position of the odontoid. The posterior tubercle of the atlas is displaced away from the direction to which the head deviates. When lateral bending of the head exceeds 30 degrees, the spinous process of the axis also deviates away from the direction of motion, indicating greater quantities of rotation.

An additional type of motion peculiar to the atlantoaxial joint is one described as vertical approximation.[7,12] With rotation of the unit, the atlas rides up and down in a vertical manner on the axis. With this motion there are observable changes in the appearance of the lateral articulations between these two vertebrae. Facets on the side to which the spinous process deviates become superimposed while the facets on the opposite side approach one another to cause the appearance of apophyseal joint narrowing. This telescoping motion of the atlas on the axis with rotation results from the configuration of the surfaces of the facets. Instead of being mated, as is the usual case, both surfaces of the atlantoaxial facets are convex. In the neutral position, the high points of the convexities are opposed, holding the atlas high on the axis. With rotation, the atlas slides downward on the convex slope of the axis. With alternating direction of rotation, the atlas pistons up and down on the axis.

As a result of all of these features, the upper cervical spine contributes large quantities of motion of the head in both the sagittal and axial planes, accounting for approximately 30% of flexion and extension and 50% of head rotation.

The lower cervical spine supplies the remaining mobility that the neck possesses. Its principal directions of motion are in the frontal and sagittal planes, although a significant amount of axial rotation is available as well.[6] Flexion and extension are accomplished as one vertebra slides and tilts on the vertebra below. Since the sagittal curve of the cervical spine is normally lordotic, the vertebrae in the center of this curve have intervertebral discs that are trapezoidal in shape with a greater anterior disc height than posterior. As these central units begin to move, sliding is initiated, but as a body displaces on a moving nucleus pulposus, tilting is added, and the two types of motion resolve into a roll.

In the normal neck, the C2-C3 segment ordinarily has a short and rectangular intervertebral disc and the motion is principally a sliding one in which the body of the second vertebra displaces forward in flexion on the body of the third.[14] The C4-C5 and C5-C6 segments contain the tallest intervertebral discs, and these are wedge shaped. Motion at these segments should therefore be a smooth roll. The C6-C7 segment usually has a tall

disc, which is rectangular (or even trapezoidal with the tallest height posteriorly), and motion here is usually tilt.

Besides determining the type of motion, the intervertebral disc height and configuration also determine the quantity of motion present in a given segment. The most mobile three segments of the lower cervical spine are C4-C5, C5-C6, and C6-C7.[2,14] In general, the amount of excursion into flexion is greater than that into extension for all segments from C2 to C6. At the C6-C7 and C7-T1 segments, extension excursion is somewhat larger than flexion excursion.[2]

Motion in the lower cervical spine involves the participation of all segments.[6] In flexion, a smooth rhythmic sequence occurs as each vertebra displaces forward on its subjacent neighbor. The anterior intervertebral disc heights shorten, and the posterior heights increase. The facets glide forward and the spaces between the spinous processes widen. Slight stair stepping is apparent in the upper segments because of the relatively greater quantities of sliding motion present in these segments. The cervical lordosis is reversed, and the nucleus pulposus in each segment displaces posteriorly with somewhat of an anterior tapering. With extension, all these phenomena reverse, although no stair stepping occurs. Instead, the cervical lordosis is accentuated and the posterior margins of the vertebral bodies form a smooth convex curve as the nuclei displace anteriorly.

In determining whether the motion that occurs is sliding or tilting, there are two quantitative indices that portray the type of motion occurring at each segment in flexion and extension of the cervical spine: the *top angle*[14] and the *instant center of rotation*.[9,16] Lateral radiographs of the spine in flexion and extension are used to compute both.

The top angle[14] demonstrates whether the motion that occurs is principally sliding or tilting. In its computation, one selects a point on the anterior margin of a vertebral body and a second point on the posterior margin. The positions taken by each of these points in flexion and in extension are connected by a line. These two lines that result are then continued in a cranial direction until they cross, and the angle they form is the top angle (Fig. 15-7). The larger the angle, the greater the slide of the vertebral bodies; the smaller the angle, the greater the tilt of the vertebral body. At C2-C3, the normal top angle ap-

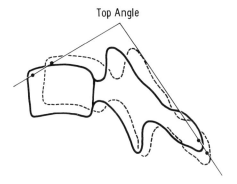

Top Angle

Fig. 15-7. The top angle is computed by identication of one anterior point and one posterior point and then plotting of paths of these points as vertebra moves from flexion into extension. Cranial extension of the lines describing these paths causes them to intersect to form an angle.

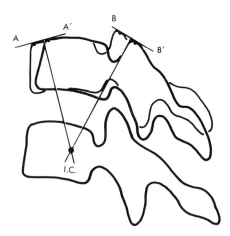

Fig. 15-9. Instant center of motion is computed by identifying paths of one anterior (A to A') and one posterior (B to B') point as they move from flexion into extension. Perpendicular lines are drawn caudally from these paths, and their point of intersection is the instant center about which the vertebra moves. (From Frankel, V.: Whiplash injuries to the neck. In Hirsch, C., and Zotterman, Y., editors: Cervical pain, Oxford, 1972, Pergamon Press.)

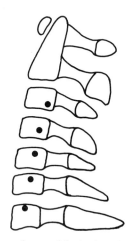

Fig. 15-8. Location of normal instant center of cervical vertebra. (From Penning, L.: Functional pathology of the cervical spine, Amsterdam, 1968, Excerpta Medica Foundation.)

proaches 100 degrees, indicating that there are large amounts of sliding motion as compared with a top angle of 80 degrees at the C7-T1 segment, which moves predominantly by tilting.

The *instant center of rotation*[16] is a point about which a vertebra rotates in the sagittal plane. For each of the cervical vertebrae, the instant center is located within the body of the vertebra below. The center about which the second vertebra rotates is located in the posteroinferior portion of the body of the third vertebra. Progressing down the column, the centers tend to assume a more anterosuperior location in the next lower vertebral body (Fig. 15-8). The center of rotation for the sixth vertebra lies at the level of the upper end plate of the seventh body. If the instant center for a vertebral body is relatively removed from that body

(as in the case of the second cervical vertebra) then motion of the body in question will contain large elements of sliding.[14] If the center is relatively near the vertebra (as in the sixth vertebra) the motion associated is one that is predominantly tilt. In addition to the description of segmental motion provided by the instant center of rotation, this concept also has bearing on the function of the zygapophyseal joints.[9] With normally located centers, the surfaces of these joints glide smoothly on one another in an arc of a circle as the vertebra rotates. If the instant center is displaced, however, then the path of motion taken by the inferior facet of the upper moving vertebra cannot conform to the arc over which the surface is intended to pass. Hence the facet surfaces tend to abut against one another when the instant center has been displaced from its normal position. Because of its clinical significance, a simplified method of computation of the location of the instant center can be utilized by selecting two points on a vertebra and locating the positions of these two points as the spine passes from full flexion to full extension. For each point the position in flexion is connected to the position in extension by a line. Perpendicular bisectors are then dropped caudally from these lines and their point of intersection corresponds to the location of the instant center of rotation (Fig. 15-9).

In addition to sagittal plane motion, the lower cervical column also exhibits motion in both the frontal and the axial planes. Motion in the *frontal* plane is that of right and left lateral bending, and in this motion each vertebra tilts on its subjacent neighbor. A small measure of lateral displacement occurs, but this is severely restricted both by the breadth of the vertebral bodies and by the upward projection of the uncinate processes, which prohibit significant lateral displacement. Hence the act of bending is one mediated primarily through a pattern of intersegmental tilt. Motion in the *axial* plane occurs in the act of right and left turning of the head. In this, the spinous process rotates away from the direction toward which the head is turning, and the tangential orientation of the fibers of the annulus fibrosus permits a spiral motion to take place between the body regions of the intervertebral units. The overall contribution of the lower cervical spine in axial rotation is in the order of 50%, since much of this motion is provided by the upper segments, as described earlier.[6]

In studying the lower cervical spine in frontal and axial plane motions, one uniformly observes a coupling phenomenon (Fig. 15-10). Observation of the lower cervical spine in the laterally deviated position discloses that the vertebrae are axially rotated as well. Observation of the axially rotated lower cervical spine discloses that the vertebrae are also tilted in the frontal plane. These two motions always occur in concert in the normal situation. Frontal and axial plane motions are greater in the more cranial segments (C2 to C4) of the lower cervical spine than in the more caudal ones (C5 to C7).[14]

Special considerations in children

The cervical spine of the child is considerably more mobile than that of the adult, and as a result, intersegmental motion patterns differ from those accepted as normal in the adult without signifying the presence of disease.[4] At the atlantoaxial joint, flexion may be associated with widening between the arch of the atlas and the odontoid in the order of 3 mm. or greater as compared with a 2 mm. maximum accepted in the adult. With extension, the anterior arch of the atlas may come to lie upon the tip of the odontoid in many normal children (Fig. 15-11). At the C2-C3 segment, pseudosubluxation may appear in flexion as the body of the second vertebra displaces forward on the third by a distance of 3 mm. or more. Similar seemingly exces-

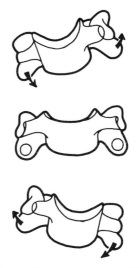

Fig. 15-10. Motions of lateral bending and horizontal rotation demonstrate obligatory coupling of the two. (From Lysell, E.: Motion of the cervical spine, Acta Orthop. Scand., Suppl. no. 123, 1969.)

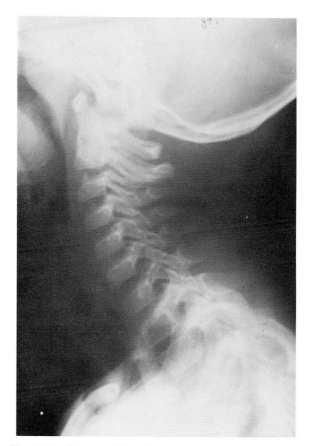

Fig. 15-11. Great mobility of child's neck allows ring of atlas to approach tip of odontoid in extension.

sive excursion of the third vertebra on the fourth is also noted in normal children. The sagittal curve of the spine may also deviate from the expected without indicating a pathologic condition. There may be no lordosis, and in forward flexion the curve may not be uniform with a posteriorly directed convexity, but instead may demonstrate more or less acute angulation at one segment. All of these phenomena are indicative of the immaturity and hypermobility of the juvenile cervical spine.

BIOMECHANICS IN DISORDERS OF THE CERVICAL SPINE

Disorders in the neck alter the biomechanics of the cervical spine when they produce changes in the determinants of motion. Change in the structural soundness of the vertebral bones and articulations, the integrity of the intervertebral disc and ligaments, or the tension and strength of muscles, alone or in combination may lead to functional decompensation of varying degree, from the barely perceptible to the gross. Disorders that involve one segment only may be responsible for derangement at several segments since the units of the cervical spine work in series to produce overall effects. Disorders of a more generalized nature may involve several segments simultaneously and produce derangement throughout the entire cervical spine.

Thus disease and injury in the cervical spine produce biomechanical alterations by changing the anatomic shape of vertebral bone, by altering the normal relationships between vertebral articulations, by interfering with intervertebral disc function, or by attenuating or shortening ligamentous structures. These changes are the common pathways of expression of a pathologic condition and may be produced by all of those varied causes responsible for cervical spine disease. Hence destruction of vertebral bone, whether attributable to infection, neoplasm, or trauma, leads to the same type of functional derangement, since the change in bone architecture is the responsible factor.

Pathologic effects are manifested as changes in the pattern of motion for the spine as a whole or for specific segments thereof. Motion may be abnormally increased or decreased, or the normal type of motion for a given segment may be replaced by motion atypical for that segment. Increased motion arises from disease or injury of ligaments that can no longer constrain the segment to physiologic ranges. Hence, in rheumatoid arthritis of the upper cervical spine, subluxation of the atlas on the axis may result from attenuation of the transverse ligament. Decreased motion, on the other hand, may result from changes that destroy segmental relationships, such as occurs in ankylosing spondylitis or vertebral infection.

When either the quantity or the pattern of motion in a given segment has been altered, the adjacent normal segments are required to accommodate by changing their participation in overall spinal movement.[6,20] Hence, when one segment has been immobilized by disease, the segment above may increase its quantity of motion to substitute for the deficiency that the disease has generated. Conversely, when one segment is rendered unstable, motion of the neck as a whole tends to be concentrated at this level of least resistance, and adjacent segments diminish their participation in overall spinal motion. Further, when a normal pattern at a segment has been changed, some pattern changes in adjacent segments may be provoked.

If disease retards the function of the upper cervical spine, its function must be assumed by the lower cervical spine, to whatever extent this is mechanically possible. Similarly, in extensive disease of the lower cervical spine, compensation for loss of function occurs by increasing the contribution of the occipitoatlantoaxial region to overall neck function.

Paralytic disorders that involve neck musculature specifically lead to difficulties in moving the head or in maintaining it erect.[17] If the cervical muscles are paralyzed, control of the position of the head and neck on the thorax is lost. Lacking sufficient muscle strength, the neck becomes mechanically subject to the weight of the head, which it cannot support. Hence functional decompensation of the spine results. Spastic conditions of muscle also cause functional derangements in the biomechanics of the neck by holding the spine in an abnormal position for excessive lengths of time, ultimately allowing bony changes to develop.

Disorders that cause pain add yet another dimension by triggering protective muscle reflexes that restrict motion.

Congenital anomalies

Congenital anomalies of the soft tissues of the neck, such as muscular torticollis, interfere with normal neck function by introducing abnor-

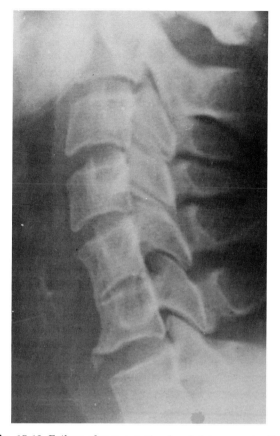

Fig. 15-12. Failure of segmentation has led to concentration of motion at the mobile segment below and has contributed to degeneration of its disc with calcific deposition centrally.

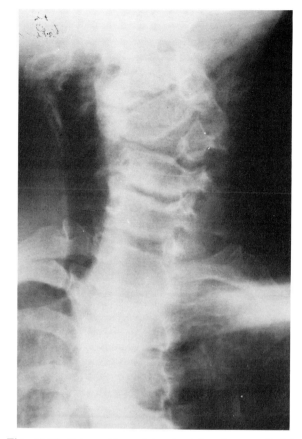

Fig. 15-13. Interposition of hemivertebra has resulted in structural scoliosis.

mal constraints to motion. Thus a contracted sternocleidomastoid muscle tilts the head in one direction and severely limits the ability of the remaining musculature to set the head straight or to tilt it in the opposite direction. If such soft-tissue contractures persist during growth, the spine develops structural changes that tend to perpetuate the restrictions that the original soft-tissue disorder initiated.

Congenital anomalies of the spine have a more immediate and direct effect on spinal biomechanics. In congenital absence of the odontoid, excessive motion at the atlantoaxial region is present, and the atlas subluxates forward on the axis as the neck is flexed. Failures of segmentation remove all motion capacities from the segments so involved and cause the concentration of motion to occur at more normal adjacent segments (Fig. 15-12). Unbalanced hemivertebra of the cervical spine causes an acute scoliosis, which leads to increasing spinal deformity with growth (Fig. 15-13). As the spine deviates in the frontal plane,

axial rotation also occurs so that motion in the lower cervical spine may be virtually eliminated. In this event, all head motion is the result of the continuing function of the atlantoaxial region, which overcompensates. The effect observed clinically is an overall reduction in head and neck motion with specific restrictions against motion toward the convexity of the curve.

Depending on the number, location, and type of congenital anomalies, the spine may be caused to concentrate all its motion at fewer segments than is customary. The ultimate effect of motion concentrations on segments adjacent to immobilized anomalous structures is the hastening of degenerative changes. Hence the effects of the congenital anomalies on cervical spine biomechanics are both immediate and delayed.

Cervical spondylosis

Cervical spondylosis is a degenerative process that begins in the intervertebral disc with progressive alterations in its consistency and there-

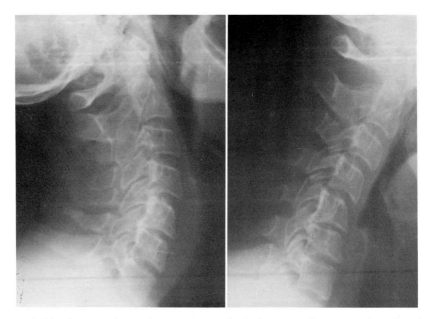

Fig. 15-14. Disc degeneration and narrowing at C5-C6 has caused concentration of motion at C4-C5, which has exhausted its reserve motion capacity and strained ligaments and anulus to permit early subluxation. C4-C5 disc has thus degenerated and pathomechanics has led to zygapophyseal degeneration as well.

fore in its function. As the combined anatomic and functional derangement persists, secondary degenerative phenomena begin to appear about the margins of the vertebral bodies, where spur formation develops. The uncinate processes hypertrophy and intrude on the neural foramina. The alteration in segmental function leads to pathologic motion in the zygapophyseal joints, and these too undergo degenerative arthritic changes with marginal hypertrophy, capsular thickening, and cartilage erosion.

In the early stages of the disorder, the segments affected are those that normally demonstrate the greatest degrees of motion. Hence, the C5-C6 segment is almost invariably the first to undergo the degenerative process.[10,14] The functional derangements that occur in the early stages are the result of the inability of the intervertebral discs to guide the appropriate balance of sliding and tilting motion characteristic of these segments, where normally the sliding and tilting components resolve into a smooth roll with forward flexion. When the intervertebral disc becomes incompetent as a result of changes in its physical consistency, this resolution is no longer possible. Hence either the sliding or tilting phase becomes exaggerated or pronounced. By the substitution of one or the other pattern of motion for the normal rolling motion, excessive stress is placed upon the annulus fibrosus and then upon the anterior and posterior longitudinal ligaments. The deranged motion pattern then becomes increased and perpetuated (Fig. 15-14). The position of the instant center of rotation alters and the zygophyseal joint surfaces abrade one another rather than glide smoothly. Cartilage injury and degeneration follows.[9]

In the intermediate phase of the disorder, the intervertebral disc begins to narrow in its height and the segmental motion begins to diminish. Hypertrophic spur formation occurs as a result of the stresses applied to those regions where the collagen fibers of the anulus fibrosus and the longitudinal ligaments attach to bone.

In the advanced stage of the disease, the vertebral bodies approach one another with little remaining intervertebral disc tissue between. The hypertrophic spurs come into contact with one another, and motion at the segment is eliminated (Fig. 15-15). Because the vertebral bodies tend to approximate one another, the facets of the zygapophyseal joints subluxate into a tilted position. With the altered positions of substructures, and with the presence of hypertrophic excrescences, the tunnels of passage for neurologic and vascular structures become constricted.

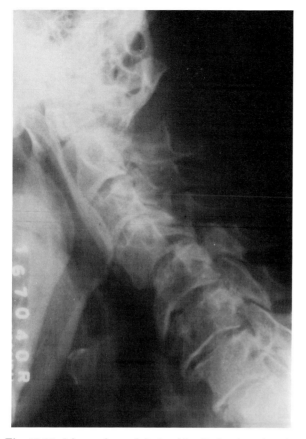

Fig. 15-15. Advanced spondylosis with elimination of motion at segments involved has led to motion concentration at segment above. Application of minor flexion stress then resulted in dislocation of zygapophyseal facets.

Secondary neurologic and vascular disease may supervene.

When one segment is in the early phase of the disease and is demonstrating altered quantities and patterns of motion, it may be a weak point in the spine and may elicit concentration of motion. As the disease advances into an intermediate phase and motion begins to diminish, the adjacent segment may be recruited to compensate by increasing its motion. Initially, this adjacent segment utilizes a reserve quantity of motion, but the continued requirement to do so may hasten the onset of degenerative changes as a result of the added wear imposed.[13] Hence a second segment may develop spondylosis as well. Whether a third segment will be added depends in part on the normal motion capacities inherent in this third segment. Should these be large as the result of a tall intervertebral disc, then the possibility for continuing spondylotic development is present.

However, if these capacities for motion are small because the disc is short and rectangular, only small additions of compensatory motion are possible and the disc may be, in a sense, protected from abuse. In this event, the requirement for dispersal of motion is distributed throughout the spine rather than concentrated at another segment. The process of extension of any mechanical cause of cervical spondylosis to multiple segments is restricted therefore to those units with the largest inherent motion capacities.

If only one segment progresses to the advanced stage of the disease and has its motion eliminated, there will be little by way of observable restriction in motion in the neck (unless observation is done during an episode of muscle spasm). If three segments progress to the advanced stage of the disease, there is sufficient compensatory ability in the remaining cervical spine, particularly in the upper regions, to continue to permit ranges of motion indistinguishable from normal in the clinical examination. Gross loss of neck motion secondary to cervical spondylosis is uncommon, except in the elderly or until the seventh decade.

Trauma

Injury to the normal cervical spine produces changes in its biomechanics if it causes ligamentous attenuation or disruption, fracture, dislocation, bone deformity, or intervertebral disc disruption. In the upper cervical spine, fracture of the ring of the atlas leads to little biomechanical derangement once the injury has healed. Fracture of the odontoid, however, leads to pronounced derangement in cervical spine function both acutely and chronically if the fracture fails to unite.[3] The separation of the odontoid from the body of the C2 allows for excessive excursion of the atlas on the axis with varying degrees of subluxation on every motion of the head-neck unit. The instability produced by the initial displacement of the odontoid from the body of the axis seems to contribute to the subsequent failure of union, which is common in this injury. Chronic subluxating motion at this level leads to neck pain and, in some cases, to gradual neurologic compromise. The hangman's fracture of the pedicles of the axis is a totally unstable injury that separates the upper segments from the lower. Healing of bone is required to restore stability.

Injury to the lower cervical spine produces a variety of anatomic alterations with their attendant functional changes.[18] Flexion forces applied to the head will cause the sudden application of enormous loads to the cervical vertebrae, leading to their mechanical failure. If the spine is in flexion along with the head, the vertebrae are driven toward one another and compression fracture may result. Since all of the energy is dissipated at the time of fracture, the resultant deformed vertebral unit is frequently stable. However, if the flexion force causes the neck to be displaced forward, the posterior ligamentous structures stretch and the zygapophyseal joints begin to subluxate. If the energy is dissipated at this point, the segment may demonstrate some measure of instability, but healing can occur. If the force continues to be applied to the point of interspinous ligament rupture and the zygapophyseal joint capsules tear, the upper vertebra of a segment may move forward sufficiently to rupture the posterior longitudinal ligament and the posterior fibers of the annulus fibrosus. Facet-joint subluxation may then appear. By the time of clinical presentation, spontaneous reduction of the subluxation may have occurred so that the precise nature of the lesion may not be immediately apparent. Unless accurate diagnosis is made and prompt and adequate management begun, the segment is likely to remain permanently unstable.

If the flexion force continues to the point that the facets actually dislocate, the unit becomes locked, and no further segmental motion can occur unless the dislocation is reduced (Fig. 15-16). Depending on the amount of associated disruption of the intervertebral disc occurring with the facet dislocation, there will be some measure of segmental instability as a result of the soft-tissue disruption that fails to heal after reduction. The quality of the scar tissue formed may not be adequate to prevent chronic instability. Although the precise morbid anatomy of flexion injuries is quite variable depending on the position of the head and neck at the time of force application, the end result may include fracture, subluxation or dislocation, and ligamentous and intervertebral disc disruption. Both residual deformity and soft-tissue incompetency may lead to chronic segmental instability and result in a traumatic spondylosis by virtue of persisting functional derangement.

Extension injuries occur either as a result of *acceleration*[15,19] of the head on the neck or as the result of *direct contact*[18] between the extended

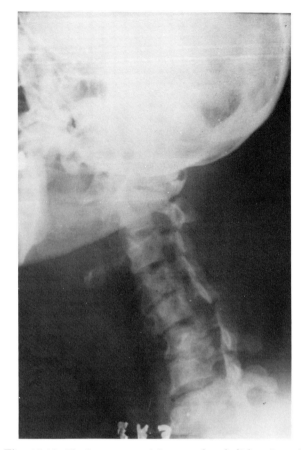

Fig. 15-16. Flexion contact injury produced dislocation of zygapophyseal facets at C5-C6.

head and a surface that delivers a force. In acceleration injuries, if the head is thrust backward with sufficient violence, the anterior longitudinal ligament may rupture and the anterior soft-tissue structures of the neck may be stretched beyond their elastic tolerance. Various degrees of intramuscular and intrafascial hemorrhage may result, but healing of an injury that extends only this far usually results in no chronic derangement. However, if the anterior ligament rupture extends into the upper fibers of the anulus fibrosus, the upper vertebra of the segment may continue to extend backward, and tearing of the intervertebral disc away from the vertebral end plate may result. Even though the proper anatomic relationships may be restored after energy dissipation, the intervertebral discs remains permanently avulsed from the vertebral body and healing is poor. Chronic segmental instability then follows, with excessive excursion and abnormal motion patterns.

When extension injuries result from direct force to the head, the mechanisms of anterior soft-tissue disruption occur as with acceleration injury, but the spine in addition receives vertical loading, which is delivered to the posterior elements. Multiple fractures of laminae and pedicle may result and lead to a total loss of all segmental stability from disruption of both anterior soft tissue and posterior bone.[8] Such an injury is almost inevitably associated with a degree of permanent functional segmental derangement. If the driving force continues, the upper vertebra in the injured segment may actually be driven forward and dislocate anteriorly. Full understanding of the mechanism of injury is mandatory for accurate diagnosis and adequate management.

Neoplasm and infection

The functional derangements produced by neoplasm and infection of the spine are similar to one another, since both disease processes lead to similar alterations in the anatomy of the spine, that is, destruction of vertebral bone and intervertebral disc. The quantity and location of tissue destruction determines whether the units can continue to move on one another in normal patterns. As destruction advances, the vertebral bodies tend to approach one another and motion in the involved segments becomes eliminated (Fig. 15-17). In an infectious process, the end result may be a spontaneous arthrodesis of the segment with permanent elimination of motion. The ultimate outcome in neoplastic processes depends entirely on the nature of the neoplasm and on the altered natural history induced by treatment.

Inflammatory arthritides

Inflammatory arthritides in the cervical spine tend to involve several segments and may be active in both the upper and lower columns. Rheumatoid arthritis leads to a proliferative synovitis in all of the diarthrodial joints in the cervical spine, and the chronic synovitis produces joint destruction, capsular and ligamentous attenuation and rupture, and joint subluxation and dislocation. Affection of the synovial component of the atlantoaxial joint leads to attentuation of the transverse ligament and atlantoaxial subluxation. After the proliferative phase of the disease subsides, a degenerative arthritis of the joints remains with varying effects. Some joints may develop chronic subluxation of a dynamic nature,

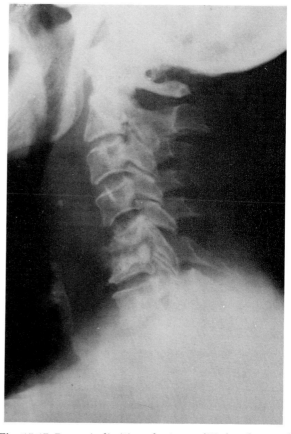

Fig. 15-17. Pyogenic discitis and osteomyelitis has destroyed and deformed C5-C6 and has caused concentration of motion at segment above.

whereas others may ankylose. Rheumatoid arthritis is thus likely to produce a mixed pattern of functional derangement throughout the cervical spine.

Ankylosing spondylitis leads to progressive elimination of the zygapophyseal joints of the lower cervical spine and to ossification of the longitudinal ligaments. The ultimate effect is total spinal rigidity because of the elimination of all articulations. Should the upper column be spared, some residual head motion will be possible.

Surgical alterations in cervical spine mechanics

Surgical procedures performed on the cervical spine are done either to remove offending structures or to eliminate undesired motion. Laminectomy, if performed unilaterally, is generally not associated with sufficient loss of spinal stability to cause functional difficulties. However, more extensive laminectomy, in which the spinous pro-

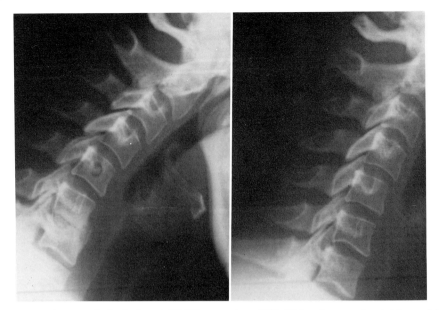

Fig. 15-18. After interbody fusion at C6-C7, excursion of C5-C6 has increased notably, and this may quicken pace of disc degeneration at C5-C6.

cesses, interspinous ligaments, and laminar bone are removed, takes away significant posterior stability. Subsequent to such surgery, the vertebral segments lack posterior constraints and become hypermobile. In so doing, they tend to subluxate forward. Further, the load of the head causes a gradual increase in the cervical lordosis.[1] The increased lordosis and the hypermobility can lead to profound functional derangement of the spine and inadequate support for the head.

Arthrodesis of the spine eliminates motion of the segments included. If these segments are in the most mobile region of the lower cervical spine, the adjacent segments[20] compensate for the loss of motion by increasing their excursion (Fig. 15-18). If these neighboring segments have insufficient motion capacities, they are subject to increased rates of wear and degenerative processes may be hastened.

Arthrodesis in the upper cervical spine is generally accomplished through a posterior approach. With atlantoaxial subluxation, arthrodesis is generally confined to the posterior elements of the atlas and axis. By fusing these two bones, the rotation provided by the odontoid mechanism is eliminated, and all residual head turning must be accomplished at lower spine levels. The amount of loss of head rotation is generally appreciable clinically. If the arthrodesis must be extended to the occiput, then all of the upper column motion is eliminated and appreciable reductions in sagittal plane motion as well as axial plane motion will be clinically apparent.

REFERENCES

1. Bailey, R. W.: Observations of cervical intervertebral-disc lesions in fractures and dislocations, J. Bone Joint Surg. **45A:**461-470, 1963.
2. Bhalla, S. K., and Simmons, E. H.: Normal ranges of intervertebral joint motion of the cervical spine, Can. J. Surg. **12:**181-187, 1969.
3. Blockley, N. J., and Purser, D. W.: Fractures of the odontoid process of the axis, J. Bone Joint Surg. **38B:**794-817, 1956.
4. Cattell, H. S., and Filtzer, D. L.: Pseudosubluxation and other normal variations in the cervical spine in children, Bone Joint Surg. **47A:**1295-1309, 1965.
5. Exner, G.: Die Halswirbelsäule. Pathologie und Klinik, Stuttgart, 1954, Georg Thieme Verlag KG.
6. Fielding, J. W.: Normal and selected abnormal motion of the cervical spine from the second cervical vertebra to the seventh cervical vertebra based on cineroentgenography, J. Bone Joint Surg. **46A:**1779-1781, 1964.
7. Fielding, J. W.: Cineroentgenography of the normal and cervical spine, J. Bone Joint Surg. **39A:**1280-1288, 1957.
8. Forsyth, H. F.: Extension injuries of the cervical spine, J. Bone Joint Surg. **46A:**1792-1797, 1964.
9. Frankel, V.: Whiplash injuries to the neck. In Hirsch, C., and Zotterman, Y., editors: Cervical pain, Oxford, 1972, Pergamon Press, Ltd., pp. 97-112.
10. Friedenberg, Z. B., and Miller, W. T.: Degenerative disc disease of the cervical spine, J. Bone Joint Surg. **45A:**1171-1178, 1963.
11. Hohl, M.: Normal motions in the upper portions of the cervical spine, J. Bone Joint Surg. **46A:**1777-1779, 1964.

12. Hohl, M., and Baker, H. R.: The atlantoaxial joint, J. Bone Joint Surg. **46A:**1739-1752, 1964.

13. Jones, M. D.: Cineradiographic studies of degenerative disease of the cervical spine, J. Can. Assoc. Radiol. **12:** 52-55, 1961.

14. Lysell, E.: Motion of the cervical spine, Acta Orthop. Scan. Suppl. No. 123, 1969.

15. Macnab, I.: Acceleration injuries of the cervical spine, J. Bone Joint Surg. **46A:**1797-1799, 1964.

16. Penning, L.: Functional pathology of the cervical spine, Amsterdam, 1968, Excerpta Medical Foundation.

17. Perry, J., Nickel, V. L., and Garrett, A. L.: Capital fascial transplants adjunct to spine fusion in flaccid neck paralysis, Clin. Orthop. **24:**128-136, 1962.

18. Whitley, J. E., and Forsyth, H. F.: The classification of cervical spine injuries, Am. J. Roentgenol. Radium Ther. Nucl. Med. **83:**633-644, 1960.

19. Wickstrom, J., Rodriguez, R., and Martinez, J.: Experimental production of acceleration injuries of the head and neck, in accident pathology, Washington, 1968, U.S. Government Printing Office, pp. 185-189.

20. Woesner, M. D., and Mitts, M. G.: The evaluation of cervical spine motion below C2, Am. J. Roentgenol. Radium Ther. Nucl. Med. **115:**148-154, 1972.

CHAPTER 16

Biomechanics of the thoracic spine

MARIA T. COTCH, M.D.

NORMAL BIOMECHANICS

Twelve superimposed vertebral units comprise the thoracic portion of the spinal column; together they serve to anchor the rib cage. As is true of the rest of the column, the thoracic spine functions to protect the spinal cord, redirect applied mechanical loads, and provide muscular attachments. Thus trunk balance is effectively maintained above the pelvis. A series of specialized ligaments and intervertebral discs bind each segment to its subjacent one. The back muscles, which are arranged both longitudinally and obliquely, further stabilize the thoracic spine and provide intersegmental motion. In its midportion, the thoracic spine consists of homogeneous units that display similar behaviour. Its extreme cephalad and caudal portions conform more to the mechanics displayed by the cervical or lumbar regions respectively, and therefore are considered transitional in nature.

Vertebral bodies in the thoracic region have a diameter slightly greater in the sagittal plane than in the frontal plane and appear heart shaped (Fig. 16-1). The mass of each thoracic vertebra increases with caudal progress as each supports a successively greater superincumbent load. The vertebral foramen, formed by the junction of the bodies and posterior elements, is circular and has a cross-sectional area significantly smaller than

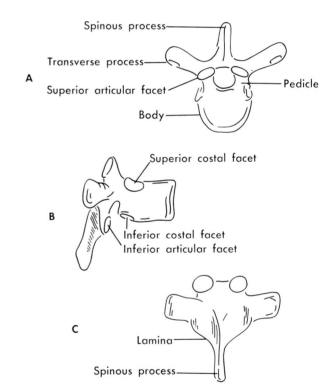

Fig. 16-1. Anatomy of representative thoracic vertebra, from above, **A;** the side, **B;** and the back, **C.**

300

in either the cervical or lumbar regions. This provides for little room between the thoracic spinal cord and its bony vertebral encasement.

Thoracic spine configuration

Each vertebral region contributes to a natural or physiologic curvature of the spinal column. The thoracic spine presents posteriorly directed sagittal curvature that is osseous in nature. This contrasts with the cervical and lumbar areas where the physiologic curves result from variations in disc height. The thoracic discs, however, are uniform, whereas there is a disparity in height between the anterior and posterior portions of each thoracic vertebra. For example, T7 may be normally wedged up to 5 degrees. A total posterior thoracic convexity up to 40 degrees is considered normal. Physiologic variations relate to the degree of lumbar lordosis and pelvic inclination. Natural kyphotic alignment subjects the anterior bodies and discs to compressive stresses, and the posterior arches and ligaments to tractive ones. Although essentially undetectable, a slight right convex asymmetry also exists in the frontal plane. It is purported to be a consequence of continual thoracic aortic pulsation.

Supportive soft tissues

Thoracic discs are uniform in height and comprise approximately one fifth of thoracic spine length. They permit motion and act like shock absorbers between adjoining vertebrae. In the thoracic spine, isolated from the rib cage, maximal flexibility occurs in the midthoracic region, T3 to T7.[7] Here the supporting structures are relatively tall with smaller cross-sectional areas. Composite discal structure is the same throughout the spine, consisting of nucleus pulposus, anulus fibrosus and cartilaginous end plates.

The nucleus pulposus is composed of an incompressible gel-like material. It functions to redistribute spinal loads sustained during daily activities. Discography reveals nuclear displacement with motion. During lateral bending, for example, the nucleus pulposus migrates to the convex side of the disc space. Its symmetric central position is resumed with the return to erect position.

The anulus fibrosus encases the nucleus and attaches to the cartilaginous end plates. Closely packed layers of fibrous rings form this portion of disc and furnish its mechanical strength. Strong annulus fibers are arranged in a specialized intersecting fashion to resist pure horizontal motion between segments. Mechanical failure from degeneration or extreme loading is most likely to occur in the posteriolateral area. For the thoracic region, however, failure is an uncommon event.

The cartilaginous end plates are the most sensitive portions of the disc structure. Experimentally, compressive loads first cause mechanical failure of this discal component before any deformation is noted in the osseous spine. In fresh cadaver specimens end plates fractured at static compressive loads averaging 290 kilograms. Integrity of the vertebral bodies (T12) was maintained until average loads of 750 kg. were reached.[5]

Ligamentous structures also contribute to the stability and mechanical behavior of the thoracic spine. Anterior and posterior longitudinal ligaments are thickest in the thoracic region. The anterior ligament is firmly bound to each vertebral body, but none of its fibers are interwoven with disc complexes. The posterior ligament on the other hand widens at each disc level and is firmly interwoven with discal fibers (Fig. 16-2). In addition to stabilizing the column, these ligaments modify flexion and extension ranges in the thoracic spine.

The ligamenta flava are also biomechanically important. They connect the laminae of adjacent vertebrae. These strong ligaments, composed

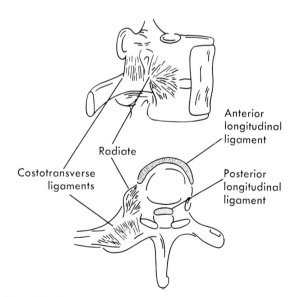

Fig. 16-2. Intervertebral and costovertebral ligaments of thoracic spine.

primarily of elastic material, limit excessive forward flexion of the spine and also assist the return to full upright position. Elastic properties of these ligaments, however, are age dependent. Less flexibility is provided in the elderly.

Rib articulations

The ribs are mechanically significant articulations of the thoracic spine. These 12 pairs of thin arc-shaped bones form a protective cavity for the heart, lungs, and great vessels. They also provide attachment for muscles concerned with respiration posture and arm function. Cartilaginous junctions fix the ribs to the sternum. Characterized as true ribs, the first seven attach to the sternum by individual cartilages. The eighth, ninth, and tenth ribs have a common junction with the sternum and are called "false." The final two ribs, terms "floating," simply end in the trunk musculature.

Ribs and vertebrae are united at two locations. The radiate ligament anchors each rib head to two adjacent vertebral bodies and the disc between them. This occurs at the superior and inferior costal demifacets located at the junction of the vertebral body and posterior arch. Costotransverse ligaments join the rib tubercle and corresponding vertebral transverse process. To accommodate this articulation, each long transverse process is capped by a costal facet (Fig. 16-1).

Since the rib cage actually encloses the thoracic spine, any external stabilizing force must be indirectly applied through the ribs. Because of their size and configuration, the ribs are more plastic than are the vertebral bodies.[23] As such, they readily yield to applied forces. Mechanically, therefore, the ribs are limited as lever arms to transmit corrective forces to the thoracic spine. Rib shape will be altered before any corrective effect is noted on a rigid spine.

Respiratory mechanics

Normal respiration requires the well-coordinated action of the diaphragm and chest wall. The dome-shaped diaphragm is the major muscle involved in quiet breathing. As it contracts, the diaphragm descends, compressing abdominal contents downward. This expands chest volume longitudinally, thus permitting lung expansion. The tidal volume exchange for quiet breathing involves minimal movement of the chest wall.

Periodic sighing is also an important phase of quiet respiration. About six times each hour, one reflexly inspires a volume of air approximately three times that of tidal exchange. Sighing prevents areas of lung, not active with each regular respiration, from totally collapsing. Chest-wall motion is an essential part of this sigh reflex. Contraction of the chest-wall muscles draws the ribs upward and forward, thereby increasing the volume of the thoracic cavity.

The intercostals and levatores costarum are muscles primarily concerned with respiratory rib motion. The external intercostals extend from the rib tubercles to the costochondral junctions. Their muscle fibers pass obliquely forward and downward from the rib above the rib below. Electromyographic studies demonstrate activity during the inspiratory phase of the respiratory cycle. The internal intercostals, thinner than the external system, extend from the anterior portion of the intercostal space to the rib angle. Their fibers pass downward and backward. Electrical activity of the internal intercostals primarily occurs during expiration. The levatores costarum are also assumed to contribute to lifting the ribs during inspiration. Their phasic activity has not yet been confirmed by electromyograph studies.[2]

If sighing is prevented either by binding the thorax or maintaining a uniform inspiratory volume with a respirator, symptoms of breathlessness readily occur. Continued restriction of thoracic movement causes a decrease in arterial oxygen. This is caused by blood flowing through areas of unexpanded lung. Taking a few deep breaths expands collapsed areas and soon brings relief.

Hence any orthoses that encompass the thorax, especially casts, may interfere with the sigh reflex. Fixed thoracic spine deformity similarly restricts thoracic expansion.

Thoracic spine motion

Because of the anatomically restrictive structure of the rib cage, the thoracic spine has long been regarded as the least mobile portion of the spine. Various ranges of motion have been ascribed to this region, depending on the materials employed and the sophistication of measurement. For example, intravital determinations often do not agree with cadaver results. Even the quality of the cadaver specimen must be considered. Embalming chemicals significantly reduce the flexibility of soft tissues, therefore embalmed

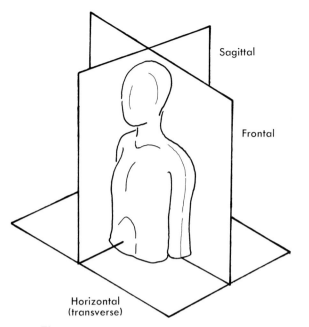

Fig. 16-3. Representation of anatomic planes.

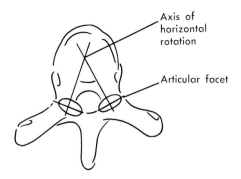

Fig. 16-4. Orientation of articular facets and axis of horizontal rotation typical of thoracic vertebra.

specimens yield data at variance with fresh ones.

Types of motion. Vertebral motion takes place in the discs and posterior joints. The thoracic spine can move through a physiologic range in each anatomic plane—rotation in the transverse plane, flexion-extension in the sagittal plane, and lateral bending in the frontal plane (Fig. 16-3). Limits to excessive intersegmental motion are offered by (1) orientation of articular facets, (2) size and shape of spinous processes, and (3) flexibility of ligament and discs. Since these factors vary in each vertebral region, column motion is modified accordingly.

Horizontal rotation is most closely related to articular facet configuration. For the typical thoracic vertebrae, these flat structures, while situated oblique to each plane, are fairly horizontal and lie along an arc of a circle. This alignment permits greatest freedom of movement in the transverse plane. Perpendiculars constructed from the facet surfaces intersect at the axis of horizontal rotation (Fig. 16-4). In the thoracic spine, this axis lies well within the anterior vertebral body. Beginning at T9 or T10, however, the facets become more sagittally aligned and rotation is reduced. The axis of rotation also recedes to a more posterior position in this transitional area.

The range of thoracic rotation (T1 through T12) totals 70 degrees, as determined in an intravital study.[7] It was also noted that during ambu-lation the trunk above T7 rotates in the same direction as the shoulders, whereas below T7, it rotates with the pelvis in the opposite direction. Thus it is virtually impossible for any orthotic device to totally immobilize the midthoracic spine.

Greater freedom for flexion and extension is present in the lower thoracic region. Long oblique spinous processes and more oblique articular facets restrain this motion in the upper and midthoracic spine. Distal to T8 or T9, the spinous processes are shorter and more horizontal. Articular facets also assume a more sagittal orientation. Both anatomic features permit greater sagittal plane motion. A total range of thoracic flexion-extension is 35 degrees. Approximately one third of this total represents the range of extension.

The range of lateral bending is approximately the same at each thoracic level and totals 50 degrees. Disc and ligament flexibility, rather than bony vertebral hindrance, limits the range of lateral bending in the thoracic spine.

Physiologic lateral bending is accompanied by a small degree of trunk rotation. In this mechanical coupling of motion, thoracic vertebral bodies rotate into the concavity of formed curvature. Bending to the left is accompanied by rotation of the trunk to the left. Similarly, with bending to the right, the trunk rotates to the right. Biomechanical analyses of fresh cadaver spines likewise confirm this coupling pattern. In the upper thoracic spine, level T2, a definite pattern of vertebral body rotation into the concavity of lateral curvature emerged.[30] Neither a consistent nor significant pattern was evident in the middle or lower levels, however, with T5 and T11 as points of investigation.

In pathologic lateral curves of scoliosis there

Horizontal rotation

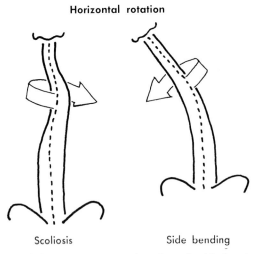

Scoliosis   Side bending

Fig. 16-5. Schematic representation of vertebral body rotation in scoliosis and in normal side bending.

is also a component of rotation, but in the opposite direction. Vertebral bodies involved are rotated into the convexity of the formed curvature (Fig. 16-5). Thus rotational deformities in scoliosis cannot be simply attributed to a physiologic mechanical phenomenon.

Muscular control

Interactions of the back muscles provide motion and stabilization for the thoracic spine. Clinical evaluation is quite difficult, however, because of their limited accessibility for individual palpation. As the back muscles extend upward from the pelvis, they decrease in size. In the middle and upper thoracic regions, total back muscle mass is only one half to one fourth that of the lumbar region.[4]

The larger, more superficial muscle complex is collectively known as the erector spinae. Muscle fibers are longitudinally directed and span multiple vertebral level in three distinct columns (Fig. 16-6). Iliocostalis dorsi, the laterally positioned muscle column, has no direct vertebral attachment. Fibers arise from the angles of the lower six ribs and insert on the angles of the upper six ribs. Its cross-sectional area averages 1 square centimeter. Longissimus dorsi, the intermediate column, is the largest component of the erector spinae group. Unilateral cross-sectional area for this muscle approximates 2.5 square centimeters. Both the vertebral column and the ribs receive fibers from the longissimus. The majority of fibers pass to the transverse processes of each vertebra, but

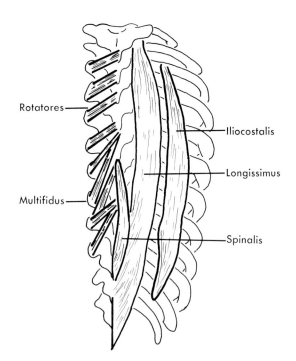

Fig. 16-6. Components of erector spinae muscles.

additional slips insert on the ribs between their tubercles and angles. Spinalis dorsi is the smallest column (cross section nearly 1 square centimeter) and most centrally placed. Its fibers arise and insert into the spinous processes at each vertebral level.

Deep to the erector spinae complex are the two shorter, more obliquely arranged muscle groups. The multifidi span an average of four vertebral levels. Their fibers take origin from the transverse processes and insert onto spinous processes. The smaller rotatores have similar origins and insertions, but span only one vertebral level.

Electromyograph (EMG) recordings demonstrate the patterns of back-muscle interaction required for physiologic vertebral motion. In maintaining an erect posture, all back muscles are active. The longissimus and rotatores continuously discharge, while the iliocostalis and multifidi are recruited when swaying is grossly observed. Bilateral activity of the erector spinae and shorter oblique muscles is also recorded during flexion-extension and lateral bending. During the middle and final phases of the body's returning to erect posture, however, minimal muscle activity is noted. The elasticity of the supportive ligaments, then, is presumed responsible for this antigravity action. Note also that as the trunk becomes erect little force is required to maintain posture. Rotation of the trunk to one side involves activity of the erector spinae of the same side and the multifidi and rotatores on the opposite side. Ipsilateral erector spinae activity may indeed represent primary rotatory participation, or a trunk-stabilizing mechanism. To date, this function has not been resolved.[19]

It is also important to note that the back muscles display phasic activity during ambulation. With heel strike, activity occurs in the erector spinae, multifidi, and rotatores of the opposite side.[29] Combined extensor muscle action prevents extreme forward flexion of the trunk during forward acceleration. The short rotatores contribute to the observed counterrotation of the pelvis and shoulders during ambulation.

Spinal supports alter this electrical periodicity of trunk muscles. EMG recordings decline in the iliocostalis and longissimus when such supports are worn.[28] With fast walking, the back muscles increase their activity. Abdominal muscle activity lessens when spinal supports are worn. If the devices encompass the midthorax, intercostal recordings are likewise reduced.[20]

Trunk support

During the course of maintaining an upright balanced posture, the spine is subject to innumerable combinations of deforming forces, which include compression, tension, shearing, and twisting. The elements that provide vertebral column stability are the trunk muscles and supportive ligaments. The fresh thoracolumbar spine, with its ligamentous system intact, but devoid of all musculature, can support a compressive load of only 2 kg. before collapsing.[14] Combined weight of the head, neck, upper limbs, and trunk to T12 comprises 32% of total body weight. For the average 70 kg. person, this superincumbent weight totals 22.6 kg. Thus, the primary support of the trunk must be furnished by the trunk musculature.

The thoracic cavity also plays a role in trunk support. To aid in reducing spinal loads, the thoracic cavity acts like a rigid walled cylinder filled with air. This action can reduce theoretical spinal loads up to 50%.[20] Spinal orthoses perform a similar function. They fix the trunk and aid in unloading the spine. When these devices are worn, activity of the trunk muscles lessens, so that it is desirable to incorporate a program of muscle-strengthening exercises with any orthotic program.[18]

PATHOMECHANICS

The spine may be likened to a modified flexible rod—a series of osseous (rigid) elements and intervertebral soft tissues (elastic). Spine pathomechanics then may be related to similar factors that influence column behavior. Both systems can support certain compressive loads and maintain equilibrium. Once subjected to a maximum or critical load, the spine, just as the rod, will fail by bending. Buckling occurs and deformation becomes permanent.

Critical load

Euler expressed the mechanical behavior of a column under a buckling load in the following formula[15]:

$$\text{Critical load} = \frac{\text{Column length} \times TT^2}{\substack{\text{Flexibility} \\ \text{factor}} \times \substack{\text{End support} \\ \text{factor}}}$$

Although it was originally expressed quantitatively for a uniform material, it can serve as a quantitative relationship for the analysis of the pathomechanics of the spine.

End support. When all variables but the mode of column-end fixation are constant, four categories of stabilization can be identified. Greater freedom of motion permitted at each column end reduces the column's critical load.

In the normal spine, the pelvis serves as a horizontal fixed base, while spinal ligaments and trunk musculature provide concentric spine alignment above the pelvis. Cervical and shoulder girdle muscles and righting reflexes serve to fix the column's top. With both base and top fixed, maximal column stability is established. Under these circumstances superincumbent body weight is less than the column's critical load and spine deformation does not occur with gravitational stress.

Clinically when spine deformation occurs with no abnormality in end-fixation control, the pattern stimulates that of idiopathic scoliosis.

With its base fixed, and the top totally unrestrained and allowed to deviate in any manner, the critical load is diminished 16-fold. Lucas[14] has demonstrated this behavior in the ligamentous thoracolumbar spine. Here the thoracolumbar spine of adult length with fixed pelvic stabilization can support only 2.2 kg. before buckling. This critical load approximates one sixteenth of superincumbent body weight. Clinically this condition may be compared to the unconscious patient or one with totally paralyzed spinal musculature.

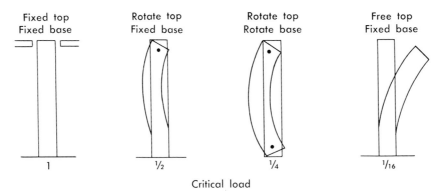

Fixed top	Rotate top	Rotate top	Free top
Fixed base	Fixed base	Rotate base	Fixed base

1       $\frac{1}{2}$ $\frac{1}{4}$ $\frac{1}{16}$

Critical load

Fig. 16-7. End support situations.

When each column end is free to rotate but not to deviate laterally, the spine can support a greater critical load (Fig. 16-7). Still, superincumbent body weight cannot be maintained by the column with an unstable base. Here spine deformities present with pronounced pelvic obliquity typified by the patient with muscular dystrophy.

With the column base remaining fixed but the top allowed only to rotate and not deviate laterally, greater stability is imparted to the flexible column. The critical load however remains less than the superincumbent body weight; so spine deformities will develop. Clinically these circumstances would compare to the partial loss of control of upper spinal musculature.

A spinal orthosis can function to provide maximal restraint for the unstable spine ends. This permits improved support of body weight.

Column length. Length is the factor that most influences the critical load of the spine. Any increase in length makes the spinal column more susceptible to deforming loads. Buckling will occur, unless each increment of column length can be balanced by added ligmentous stability and increased muscle strength.

Study of the skeletal system has forwarded the concept of normal growth patterns and the factors influencing them. The rate of spinal growth is not a constant process. A juvenile or midgrowth spurt occurs between 6 and 8 years of age. A more pronounced growth spurt of adolescence occurs between 13 and 15 years.

These periods of rapid gain in spinal column length coincide with the greatest incidence of idiopathic spinal deformities. In established deformities, regardless of etiology, these growth spurts correlate with the most rapid deterioration of spinal alignment. In the natural history of spinal deformity, cessation of growth does not fully halt progression. Curvature does increase, but at a minimal rate, about 1 degree per year.

Congenitally malformed vertebrae provide an inadequate support mechanism for the spine. Continued growth produces asymmetric lengthening of the vertebral column. Spinal ligaments and muscles cannot compensate for this bony column instability. As a result spinal deformity is progressive.

Experimentally, unilateral arrest of vertebral growth can be accomplished by either excising or stapling vertebral growth plates,[21] or cauterizing and wiring a number of vertebral laminae.[25] These procedures affect only a limited portion of the growing column. As the remainder lengthens, these tethered areas fail to grow. Excessive exposure to irradiation can also damage the vertebral growth plates and cause nonuniform spinal growth.[9] Progressive deformity results because there are defective bony components in the column.

Vertebral growth also responds to pressure. According to Wolff's law, bone adapts its architecture as a response to mechanically applied stresses and strains. In the case of scoliosis, the vertebral bodies change configuration and become wedge shaped. The lesser heights are noted on the concave side of the curve. This bone remodeling is believed to result from the unequal application of forces on the bone as it grows.

An alternate theory for wedge deformation of the vertebra is the Heuter-Volkmann law. It suggests that intermittent compressive and tractive stresses applied to the growing bone lead to areas of retarded and expanded bone growth. Theoretical pressures acting upon the concave side of the vertebrae in scoliosis are several times the superincumbent body weight.[1] This would support the belief that constant and excessive pressure does retard bone growth.

In idiopathic scoliosis, pathologic examination of the involved vertebrae reveals no inherent defect in bone composition. Rather, the bone changes represent an adaptation in ossification caused by external pressure.[4]

Flexibility. The area within the spine that yields under load may be the bone, ligaments, or muscles. The response may be abrupt as with trauma or gradual when the repetitious demands of trauma or of daily life cannot be met. Spinal flexibility is inversely related to stability.

Bone. Erosion of the vertebrae by infection or tumor produces inadequate bone support to maintain spinal alignment. In some generalized metabolic disorders, as rickets, bone strength is lessened, making the vertebrae incapable of providing the needed stability for trunk support. Malalignments ensue.

Ligamentous support. Restraint to column failure is imparted by thick, strong ligaments and intervertebral discs with a large cross-sectional area. Any portion of the column gains greater freedom of motion by virtue of longer ligaments or thicker discs having a smaller cross-sectional area. With greater freedom of motion, the column fails under a smaller load. In the isolated ligamentous spine, the area of greatest flexibility lies in the midthoracic region, levels T3 to T7.[14] Pathologic curvatures, especially the idiopathic variety, most commonly develop at this site. Hence, whatever the inciting factors may be, progressive deformation is enhanced by the increased flexibility.

Integrity of both the spinal ligaments and ribs is mechanically important in providing vertebral column support.[11] Spinal deformity with vertebral rotation and wedging occur in experimental animals when (1) ribs are resected in the region of the neck and tubercle, (2) ligaments of the rib head are sectioned, or (3) both the internal and external intercostal muscles are resected. The operative side is convex to the resultant deformation in each instance. Bodies of the involved vertebrae rotate into the convexity of the curvature. Intervertebral discs are also deformed. The nucleus is displaced to the convex side, similar to that of the idiopathic curve.

Thoracoplasty procedures involve similar surgical resections. Ribs lateral to their tubercles are removed in the affected hemithorax. In some instances, the corresponding transverse process as well as rib head and neck are resected. Spinal deformation does appear subsequent to thoracoplasty.[13,26] These deformities develop even when spinal growth is complete. More than half the curves are present 1 week postoperatively. The remainder develop during the first 6 months to 1 year after surgery. Progression is slight beyond this time. This appears to be primarily wound guarding, since the deformity is preventable with early postural management.

When the operative procedure involves removal of the transverse processes and proximal ribs, a greater incidence of spinal deformity occurs. Larger curves result when greater numbers of ribs are resected. These resultant curves develop convex to the operative side. Vertebral bodies involved in the deformity rotate into the convexity of the curve.

It is possible to consider the lateral curvature and rotational deformities occurring after thoracoplasty in terms of altered spinal stability. Disruption of the costovertebral ligaments, as well as removal of the proximal ribs and transverse processes decrease the ligamentous support of the spine. Loss of the natural muscle insertions for the longissimus and iliocostales reduces the supportive capabilities of the spinal musculature. Both factors produce a segmental increase in spinal flexibility and thereby hasten column failure.

In certain metabolic derangements, such as Marfan's syndrome, abnormalities in biochemical composition alter the flexibility of spinal ligaments and discs. These defective elements are unable to satisfactorily support body weight. As a result, column failure occurs.

Disc deformation has been documented in idiopathic scoliosis. In radiographic tracings of typical curves, discs, as well as vertebral bodies, are wedge shaped.[16] Curve tracings after a period of orthotic treatment reveal persistent disc wedging, while the vertebral bodies regain a more natural configuration. When deformed to this extent, the normal ability of the disc to equally transmit compressive loads may well be altered. No conclusive data exist, however,

Muscular support. Since the isolated ligamentous spine can support only 2 kg. before buckling, the major portion of trunk stability is provided by balanced trunk musculature. Abnormalities of these muscles are clearly relevent to spinal column failure. If muscle support is severely unbalanced or totally lacking, spine deformation occurs.

Resections of the back muscles in rats and mice produce abnormal spinal curvatures.[27] These curves are small, however, and readily correctable. Immature animals simply immobilized in a position of lateral flexion by means of plaster casts also develop scoliosis.[10] Some curves produced in this manner progress once the plaster has been removed. Thus muscle contracture as well as muscle ablation affect normal spinal alignment. Muscle denervation at a number of levels can also produce abnormal spinal curvatures. Deformities result from motor nerve damage, spinal cord injury, or partial cerebral damage.

In poliomyelitis, for example, only the anterior horn cells of the motor nerves are affected. Muscle paralysis results, but sensation remains intact. Abnormal spinal growth and structural deformity commonly develop. The most important determinants are specific patterns of muscle paralysis and the stage of spinal maturity.

In the fully grown spine, paralytic deformity is limited by the available range of intervertebral motion. For lateral flexion, this approximates 40 degrees. The immature spine however not only collapses to this extent once trunk muscles are symmetrically paralyzed, but also continues to deform. A long, mobile C-shaped curve is characteristic of paralytic deformity. Without a means to stabilize the ill-supported growing spine, the progressing curvature becomes fixed.

Patterns of motor weakness correlate with regional paralytic deformation. In the thoracic spine, unilateral intercostal weakness significantly influences the development of lateral deformity.[6,8] These affected muscles are located on the convexity of the paralytic curvature. A greater extent of unilateral muscle paralysis results in more severe spinal deformity. Isolated upper-limb paralysis has no particular influence upon spinal growth. Paralytic curvature develops only when trunk muscles are involved. Limb weakness is merely coincidental.[8]

In spinal cord injury, the modulating effects of the higher neural centers are lost, because cerebrospinal pathways are disrupted. As a result, sensory and motor control below the level of injury is absent. Only primitive spinal motor reflex arcs remain intact. High spinal cord injuries cause paralytic deformities in the immature spine. These long C-shaped curves often include pelvic obliquity. Degenerative neuropathies or myopathies may also lead to inadequate muscular support of the trunk. Under these conditions, similar paralytic spinal deformities result.

Not all neuromuscular disorders produce muscular inactivity, however. In cerebral palsy or brain injury, for example, muscle tone is increased and overactive primitive reflexes predominate. Asymmetric spastic muscle tone alters the normally balanced support of the trunk, pulling it to the stronger side. Structural deformation of the growing spine is likely to ensue. Spinal stabilization either by orthotic or surgical means is difficult in these cases, because spastic phenomena are involuntary and are often provoked by simple postural changes.

Experimentally, immature animals deprived only of proprioceptive or balance input to the spinal muscles develop abnormal curvatures.[17] This information is carried by the dorsal nerve roots. If these structures are sectioned in growing animals, scoliosis will develop. Severity of curvature correlates to the number of dorsal roots resected. Curves develop convexly to the operative side. In the clinical situation, segmental spinal proprioception is difficult to ascertain. Its importance to developmental spinal deformities has yet to be elucidated.

Vertebral rotation

Computer analogs of the spine can simulate characteristic patterns of scoliotic deformity.[24] Only spatial alterations between specific anatomic sites in the region of the transverse processes yield typical patterns of spinal deformation, lateral deviation, and convex vertebral body rotation. Most mild curves involve movements well within the physiologic range of intersegmental motion. In a proposed mechanical model of the spine, characteristic deformation was produced by a restraining force developed in the region of the dorsal ribs and transverse processes.[12]

The observed pattern of convex vertebral body rotation in scoliosis remains an enigma. Physiologic coupling of lateral bending and horizontal rotation is not the explanation. Normally, bending to one side is accompanied by trunk rotation to the same side. In idiopathic scoliosis, however, the trunk rotates to the contralateral side. At the present time, no accepted biomechanical explanation exists for the vertebral rotation in scoliosis. Investigative efforts are continuing.

Secondary factors in spinal deformation

Regardless of etiology, progressive failure of the spine follows a similar chronologic course. Persistent asymmetric spinal loading with respect to gravity occurs. This leads to unbalanced soft-tissue tension. Supportive structures shorten and contractures form. Finally, disc and vertebral deformation becomes irreversible.

Once deformity has developed in the spine, constant gravitational effects provoke its worsening. As long as the spine remains in a horizontal position, the effect of gravity is minimized. Once upright posture is resumed, however, deformity will relapse and worsen. The body weight above the curvature contributes a major portion of the deforming forces acting upon the curve. As curvature progresses, the compressive deforming component of the superincumbent body weight increases with the degree of deformity.

Abnormal curvature distorts the natural head and shoulder alignment over the pelvis. Hanging over the pelvis on one side, the upper trunk mass hastens further mechanical failure. In essence then, one primary objective of spinal orthotics is to reestablish the normal balance between thorax and pelvis.

Vertebral column deformation also alters the effective mechanics of the longitudinal and oblique back muscles. Normal lines of action for these muscles deviate and asymmetric tensions are developed. With continued curve progression, these muscles may actually contribute to active deforming forces rather than function as major column stabilizers[3] (Fig. 16-8).

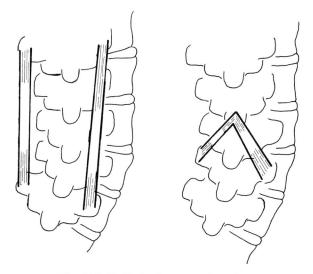

Fig. 16-8. Scoliosis alters muscle action.

Spinal stabilization

In stabilization and correction of spinal deformities, two basic methods of control are employed: (1) longitudinal traction or distraction and (2) counteractive horizontal forces—three-point pressure sytem. Any external orthosis, then, will be limited by the areas over which corrective forces can be applied, and the by tolerance of the underlying tissues to withstand correction while not endangering their viability.

Early in progressive spinal deformities, changes in vertebral alignment remain within the normal range of intersegmental motion patterns, and supporting structures are still flexible. Thus a greater portion of the deforming forces can be overcome and result in an improved vertebral alignment. Once the pathologic curvature exceeds the normal limits of vertebral motion, however, posterior joints and supportive ligaments and discs become distorted and contracted. Then, greater corrective forces must be externally applied to overcome structural deformity. As the deformity progresses, the successful use of external orthoses becomes increasingly limited.

Respiratory pathomechanics

Progressive thoracic spine deformity adversely affects respiratory mechanics. Combinations of lateral curvature and rotation distort the natural shape and spatial relationships of the ribs. Concave to the deformity, ribs are more horizontal in position and are crowded together. Ribs on the convex side are less crowded, but their downward slope is accentuated; therefore that lung space is narrowed. Rotation of the involved vertebrae into the convexity of the curve causes the convex ribs to protrude at their angles, while those on the concave side become more prominent anteriorly.

Chest-wall motion during respiration is also diminished. As thoracic spine and rib deformities progress, chest-wall muscles, which normally provide chest expansion, lose their effective mechanical advantage. Contraction no longer lifts the ribs upward and outward. Further restraint to rib motion is caused by the contracture of soft tissues that accompanies spinal deformity. As a result, there is a decrease in lung expansion and loss of an adequate sighing mechanism. These changes produce restrictive lung disease.

Respiratory symptoms of fatigue and shortness of breath are more severe in the paralytic type of thoracic spine deformity. In these patients the effects of a deformed thorax are compounded by weakened or paralyzed chest muscles and diaphragm. In idiopathic scoliosis, diaphragm excursion is present and contributes to respiratory control even when the chest wall is severely deformed.

Respiratory function in idiopathic scoliosis noticeably begins to fall short of predicted norms when curvature ranges from 55 to 65 degrees.[22] Patients with curves below this range demonstrate minimal respiratory restriction. Vital lung capacity in these patients is slightly decreased, and exercise elicits a greater than normal fall of arterial oxygen. Beyond 65 degrees, both the total lung capacity and vital capacity are significantly reduced. When deformity progresses beyond 90 degrees, almost two thirds of the vital capacity and one half the total lung capacity are lost.[31] In the more severe deformities studies demonstrate increased shunting of the pulmonary blood flow.

Adult scoliotics are prone to repeated bouts of respiratory infections and pulmonary insufficiency. Their already compromised pulmonary function is easily subject to decompensation. Respiratory failure and chronic failure of the right side of the heart lead to an early demise. Realizing these long-term cardiopulmonary effects of spinal curvature, those involved in treating spinal deformities must consider not only the spine, but the respiratory system as well. Early spinal stabilization efforts are necessary to reduce the incidence of pulmonary failure when these patients reach adulthood.

Altered respiratory mechanics must also be kept in mind when orthoses are fitted for spinal deformities. Such devices will hamper any effective respiratory reserve if they rigidly encompass the thorax or abdomen. Available rib motion will be inhibited, and the piston action of the diaphragm will be reduced by tight abdominal components.

REFERENCES

1. Arkin, A. M., and Katz, J. F.: The effects of pressures on epiphyseal growth, J. Bone Joint Surg. 38A:1056, 1956.
2. Campbell, E. J., and Davis, J. N.: The respiratory muscles, mechanics and neural control, London, 1969, Lloyd-Luke (Medical Books), Ltd.
3. Comeaux, L. J.: Some alterations in the biomechanics of the spine in idiopathic scoliosis, Orthopaedic Seminars 5:93-100, 1972, University of Southern California, Department of Orthopaedic Surgery, LAC-USC Medical Center, Rancho Los Amigos Hospital, Downey, California.
4. Enneking, N. F., and Harrington, P.: Pathologic changes in scoliosis, J. Bone Joint Surg. 57A:165, 1969.
5. Evans, F. G.: Some basic aspects of biomechanics of the spine, Arch. Phys. Med. 214:226, 1970.
6. Garrett, A., Perry, J., and Nickel, V.: Paralytic scoliosis, Clin. Orthop. 21:117, 1961.
7. Gregersen, G. G., and Lucas, D. B.: An in vivo study of the axial rotation of the human thoraco-lumbar spine, J. Bone Joint Surg. 49A:247, 1967.
8. James, J. I. P.: Paralytic scoliosis, J. Bone Joint Surg. 38B:660, 1956.
9. Katzmann, H., and Waugh, T. R.: Skeletal changes following irradiation of childhood tumors, J. Bone Joint Surg. 51A:825, 1969.
10. Langenskiold, A.: Growth disturbances of muscle: A possible factor in pathogenesis of scoliosis. In Zorab, P. A., editor: Scoliosis and growth, Edinburgh, 1970, Churchill Livingstone.
11. Langenskiold, A., and Michelsson, J. E.: Progressive experimental scoliosis in the rabbit, J. Bone Joint Surg. 43B:116, 1961.
12. Lindahl, O., and Raeder, E.: Mechanical analysis of forces involved in idiopathic scoliosis, Acta Orthop. Scand. 32:27, 1962.
13. Loynes, R. D.: Scoliosis after thoracoplasty, J. Bone Joint Surg. 54B:484, 1972.
14. Lucas, D. B.: Mechanics of the spine, Bull. Hosp. Joint Dis. 30:115, 1970.
15. Lucas, D. B., and Bressler, B.: Stability of the ligamentous spine, Report No. 40, Biomechanics Laboratory, University of California, San Francisco, January 1961.
16. MacEwen, G. D.: Factors affecting the growth of vertebral bodies and intervertebral discs. In Zorab, P. A., editor: Scoliosis and growth, Edinburgh, 1970, Churchill Livingstone.
17. MacEwen, G. D.: Experimental scoliosis. In Zorab, P. A., editor: Proceedings of a second Symposium on Scoliosis: Causation, London 1967, Edinburgh, 1968, Churchill Livingstone.
18. Morris, J. M., and Lucas, D. B.: Biomechanics of spinal bracing, Ariz. Med. 21:170, April 1964.
19. Morris, J. M., Benner, G., and Lucas, D. B.: Electromyographic study of the intrinsic muscles of the back in man, J. Anat. 96:509, 1962.
20. Morris, J. M., Lucas, D. B., and Bressler, B.: Role of the trunk in stability of the spine, J. Bone Joint Surg. 43A:327, 1961.
21. Nachlas, I. W., and Borden, J. N.: Experimental scoliosis: The role of the epiphysis, Surg. Gynecol. Obstet. 90:672, 1950.
22. Riseborough, E. J., and Shannon, D. C.: The effects of scoliosis on pulmonary function. In Keim, H., editor: Second annual post-graduate course on management and care of the scoliosis patient, New York Orthopaedic Hospital, Presbyterian Medical Center, New York, Warsaw, Ind., 1970, Zimmer.
23. Roberts, S., and Chen, P. H.: Global characteristics of typical human ribs, J. Biomech. 5:191, 1972.
24. Schultz, A. B., LaRocca, H., Galante, J., and Andriacchi, T. P.: A study of geometrical relationships in scoliotic spines, J. Biomech. 5:370, 1972.
25. Somerville, E. W.: Rotational lordosis: The development

of the single curve, J. Bone Joint Surg. **34B**:421, 1952.

26. Stauffer, S., and Mankin, H. J.: Scoliosis after thoracoplasty, J. Bone Joint Surg. **48A**:339, 1966.

27. Swartzmann, J. R., and Mills, M.: Experimental production of scoliosis in rats and mice, J. Bone Joint Surg. **27**:59, 1959.

28. Waters, R. L., and Morris, J. M.: Effects of spinal supports on the electrical activity of muscles of the trunk, J. Bone Joint Surg. **52A**:51, 1970.

29. Waters, R. L., and Morris, J. M.: Electrical activity of muscles of the trunk during walking, J. Anat. **111**:191, 1972.

30. White, A. A.: Analysis of the mechanics of the thoracic spine. An experimental study of autopsy material. Acta Orthop. Scand. Suppl. 127, 1969.

31. Zorab, P. A.: Respiratory function in scoliosis, In Zorab, P. A., editor: Scoliosis, Springfield, Ill., 1969, Charles C Thomas, Publisher.

CHAPTER 17

Biomechanics of the lumbosacral spine

JAMES M. MORRIS, M.D.
KEITH L. MARKOLF, Ph.D.

Section I

The normal spine

The spinal column possesses a number of unique features that make it distinctive in an engineering sense. First and most obvious, it is not a homogeneous structure but is instead composed of relatively rigid units (vertebrae) interspaced with highly deformable discs arranged within a complex of guiding and restraining facet joints. This combination of strength and flexibility is a workable compromise that affords maximal protection for the spinal cord and nerves with minimal restriction of mobility. Second, the spine is not straight, but rather curved to adapt to our upright posture, a feature that allows the column to more efficiently damp vertical shocks such as those imposed by running or jumping. If the spine were straight, these shocks would be transmitted along the axis of the spine and truly be a jolting experience for the head. The curvature of the column allows it to bend as well as compress. The third major feature of the spine is its variation in size and geometry. The spine is not only tapered, but the variation in the geometry of the vertebrae and facets places definite restrictions on which motions are allowed and which are not.

The spinal column serves as a sustaining rod for the maintenance of the upright position of the body and as such is subjected to many forces of different types (such as compression, shearing, tension, bending, and twisting). The spinal column possesses an *intrinsic* as well as an *extrinsic* stability. The former is caused by the interplay of disc ligamentous forces, whereas the latter is related to muscle support, especially of the abdomen and thoracic cage.

GROSS ANATOMY OF SPINE

The bones of the spinal column consist of 24 presacral vertebrae, the sacrum, and the coccyx. The presacral segments increase in size from the first cervical to the fifth lumbar vertebra. The sacral and coccygeal segments decrease from the first sacral segment caudally. Each typical presacral vertebra is composed of four parts (Fig. 17-1): (1) the body, which is primarily for transmission of forces; (2) the lamina and pedicles, which (with the body) enclose the spinal canal; (3) the spinous and transverse processes for attachments of muscles and ligaments; and (4) the posterior articular processes, or facets, which guide and limit motion between adjacent vertebrae.

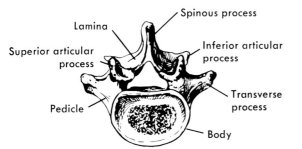

Fig. 17-1. Fifth lumbar vertebra. (From Morris, J. M.: Biomechanics of the spine, Arch. Surg. **107:**418-423, Sept. 1973.)

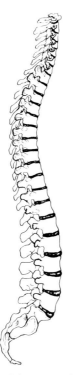

Fig. 17-2. Lateral view of the spine, showing the four typical curves.

At the time of birth, the infant's spine has only one long curve, which extends over its entire length and is convex dorsally. It is generally assumed that when the infant raises his head, the cervical lordosis develops, and that as he assumes the upright position, the lumbar lordosis results. Completion of these curves gives the spine its adult shape of four typical curves in the sagittal plane (Fig. 17-2).

The vertebrae articulate by means of three joints: the intervertebral disc anteriorly (between the vertebral bodies) and two articulations posteriorly between the facets, which are of the gliding type and which possess true synovial joint cavities. In the posterior intervertebral joints, the inferior articular facets of the vertebra above usually overlie the superior facets of the vertebra below.

A series of ligaments placed under tension by an expanding intradiscal force firmly bind the vertebral segments together. These ligaments include (1) a longitudinal system that binds all the vertebrae together into a mechanical unit (that is, anterior and posterior longitudinal ligaments, supraspinous ligament) and (2) a longitudinal system that secures one segment to another (that is, interspinous, intertransverse, and iliolumbar ligaments and ligamentum flavum). This arrangement accounts for the relative stability of the spine when dissected free of musculature.

STRUCTURE AND COMPOSITION OF INTERVERTEBRAL DISC

The intervertebral disc, which provides for spinal flexibility, is generally considered to be composed of three parts: the nucleus pulposus, which occupies the central 50% to 60% of the cross-sectional area of the disc; the surrounding anulus fibrosus; and the two cartilaginous plates that separate the disc from the vertebra above and below. Embryologic and certain functional studies, however, indicate that these plates are better considered portions of the vertebral body.

The nucleus pulposus is an oval gelatinous mass that occupies the central portion of the disc, nearer the posterior than the anterior border of the anulus fibrosus. The nucleus consists of chondrocyte-like cell bodies dispersed within an intercellular matrix consisting of a fairly dense network of poorly differentiated collagen fibrils, which are covered by a polysaccharide-protein complex. The polysaccharide is chondroitin sulfate. Because of its polar (—OH) groups, the nucleus has a great capacity to imbibe and bind water (depending on age, it contains from 88% to 69% water by weight). These components of the intercellular matrix form a three-dimensional lattice gel system.

The anulus fibrosus is formed of layers of collagenous tissue and fibrocartilage (inner portion) and is firmly anchored to the vertebra. The fibers within these layers are directed obliquely between the vertebrae, and successive layers have fibers that are perpendicular to those of the neighboring layer, an orientation that gives the disc its elasticity. The layers are firmly bound by an intercellular cement-like substance. The anterior and lateral portions of the anulus are approximately twice as thick as the posterior portion. Here the layers are narrower and fewer in number, and the fibers appear to be oriented in a direction more parallel to those of the adjacent layer. There is also less binding substance. These conditions, no doubt, contribute to the propensity of a disc to herniate posteriorly. Fibers of the innermost layers of the anulus pass into the nucleus and blend with its intercellular matrix. There is therefore no distinct demarcation of anulus and nucleus.

BIOMECHANICS OF INTERVERTEBRAL JOINT

The intervertebral joint complex is a three-dimensional junction and as such has six possible degrees of freedom: three in rotation and three in translation. Because of the anatomy of the joint, certain motions are allowed more readily than others. Compression, lateral bending, anteroposterior bending, and torsion occur most readily, whereas tension and anteroposterior and lateral shear are seen to a lesser extent in the normal joint (Markolf[14]).

The response of the intervertebral joint to forces and bending moments is of fundamental importance to an understanding of the biomechanics of the spine. The deformations and rotations that occur in the joint are related in a most interesting way, because of the anatomic configuration of the joints, to the forces and moments that produce them. The load-deformation behavior of the intervertebral joint will be examined for the most significant modes of deformation.

AXIAL COMPRESSION

Experimental studies on cadaver spines have shown the posterior facets to play a relatively minor role in withstanding pure compressive force (Hirsch and Nachemson[7]).

The structure responsible for withstanding compressive forces is the intervertebral disc, which is remarkably well suited for this task since it is capable of sustaining enormous forces without loss of mechanical function. It is so strong, in fact, that laboratory tests on cadaver discs have failed to crush them irreversibly before failure of the vertebral bodies. The so-called weak link of the disc-vertebra complex is the end plate, the

cartilaginous barrier between the porous cancellous bone and the highly liquid-gel nucleus. As a disc is compressed, the first structure to fail is the end plate, usually by one or more cracks, which allow escape of nuclear material into the spongiosa. This occurs at a compressive force of 453.6 to 635 kg. (1000 to 1400 pounds) for healthy lumbar discs from young persons and at lower loads for degenerated specimens. If the compression is increased beyond this point, the next structure to fail is the vertebral body itself—this failure may be catastrophic, with complete loss of structural integrity. The force required to crush a vertebra can range from 589.7 to 1088.6 kg. (1300 to 2400 pounds) for healthy lumbar specimens. The most remarkable point here is the fact that irreversible damage to the disc cannot be produced by compression alone, and an intact intervertebral disc specimen has never been experimentally herniated.

Of equal importance to the failure load of the disc is the response of the disc to lower loads. The information of most interest is the load deflection curve for pure compression. The curve for the disc (Fig. 17-3) is unique in that it does not show a steady increase in deflection proportionate to increasing force, which would be indicated by a straight line, but rather shows stiffening behavior, the stiffness being the slope or rate of increase of load with deformation measured in units of kilograms per millimeter (pounds per inch). The tangent or slope of the curve increases as the curve bends upward—indicating stiffening of the disc as a result of loading. Most engineering materials have a curve that tends to flatten out or "soften" for high loads; thus the disc is truly unique as a compressive unit. Another very interesting feature of the load-deflection curve is its dependence upon loading rate. The disc becomes "stiffer," the faster it is loaded. The most rapid loading rates tested approximate conditions present during high-speed ejection from jet aircraft.

Another interesting phenomenon exhibited by the disc under constant compressive force is its tendency to compress with time. The term used to describe this behavior is *creep,* and it commonly occurs in metals at very high temperatures. The disc, however, will creep at room temperature. The rate of creep increases as the force level increases (Fig. 17-4). This long-term compressive deformation of the disc is probably responsible for the change in height of an individual noticed be-

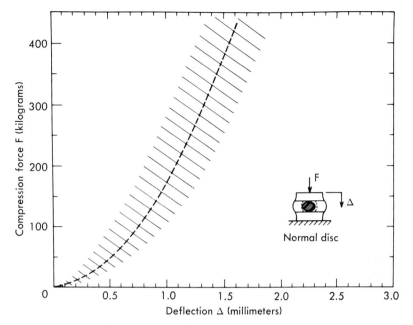

Fig. 17-3. An average force-deflection curve for compression of 24 normal discs. Range of variation is indicated by the shaded area.

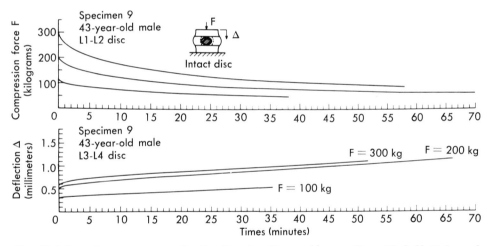

Fig. 17-4. Long-term creep curve for the disc of a 43-year-old man. (From Markolf, K. L., and Morris, J. M.: The structural components of the intervertebral disc; a study of their contributions to the ability of the disc to withstand compressive forces. J. Bone Joint Surg. **56A:**675-687, June 1974.)

tween morning and evening. The origin of this creep behavior is probably fluid transfer into and out of the disc since, as mentioned above, the nucleus is hydrophilic. Also shown in (Fig. 17-4) are *load relaxation* curves, which show the decrease of load as a function of time for a constant deformation. Like creep, load relaxation is a phenomenon observed in viscoelastic materials.

Because of its unique gel nucleus center structure, the disc (in vitro), when small radial tears are present in the anulus, exhibits a remarkable "self-sealing" behavior characterized by a return to normal compressive behavior. In this instance the load-deformation curves (Fig. 17-5) show that the first time the disc is compressed, nuclear material is extruded through the opening, as evidenced by visual observation and loud popping sounds. The

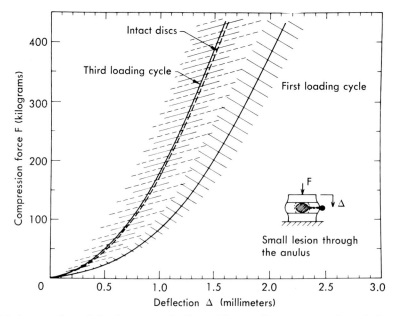

Fig. 17-5. Average force-deflection curves for discs with a small passage cut through the postero-lateral wall of the anulus, repeated loading. Ranges of variation are indicated by the shaded areas. (From Markolf, K. L., and Morris, J. M.: The structural components of the intervertebral disc; a study of their contributions to the ability of the disc to withstand compressive forces, J. Bone Joint Surg. **56A:**675-687, June 1974.)

load-deflection curve is also much "softer," indicating that the disc is more compressible than normal for a given load. If the load is removed and the disc is again loaded in precisely the same manner, the disc becomes stiffer; by the third loading cycle the lesion has sealed and normal compressive behavior is restored. It should be noted, however, that because of loss of nuclear material, the sealed disc is now slightly less in height even though it has a normal load-deflection curve (Markolf and Morris[7]).

Further insight into the properties of the components of the disc is provided by the results of yet another load-deflection test—this time on an autopsy specimen that consists only of the anulus, with the nucleus, end plates, and supporting bone above the end plates having been removed (Fig. 17-6). This preparation excludes any possibility of self-contained pressure generation within the nucleus. The first time the disc is compressed, a very "soft" curve is revealed, indicating that the anulus has been compressed to a new configuration. The remarkable thing is that after the anulus has stabilized to a new, more compressed configuration and the loading cycle is repeated, the third cycle of the load-deflection curve has nearly approached that for a normal disc. This would indicate that

the anulus alone is strong enough, as a structure on its own, to carry the compressive force of the disc in a normal fashion (in vitro). The role of the nucleus is probably, therefore, one of load distribution more than direct load-carrying (Markolf and Morris).

The expansile intradiscal pressure created by nucleus imbibition pressure serves to maintain normal ligament tension and normal facet alignment. A disc composed of solid material would provide no mechanism for resisting tension of the binding ligaments, and thus stability would not be assured. The self-contained pressure system of the disc also acts as an efficient energy absorber. The process of end-plate rupture may be likened to a safety fuse that dissipates energy before the vertebral bone itself is fractured. Since it appears that the nucleus plays a lesser role in load carrying, it is perhaps not too surprising how well patients with disc protrusions or discectomies are able to do after discectomy. The ability to sustain load is probably intact but with the sacrifice of some loss of joint stability and a reduction of disc height.

BENDING OF THE JOINT

The next most common motions of the joint are those of bending, namely, flexion, extension, and

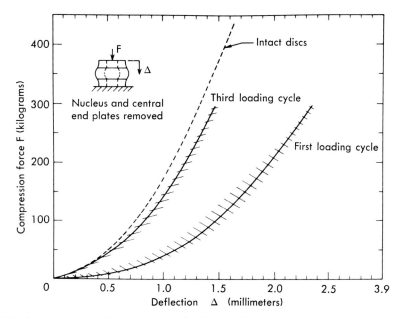

Fig. 17-6. Average force-deflection curves for discs with the anulus only remaining, repeated loading. Ranges of variation are indicated by the shaded areas. (From Markolf, K. L., and Morris, J. M.: The structural components of the intervertebral disc; a study of their contribution to the ability of the disc to withstand compressive forces, J. Bone Joint Surg. **56A:**675-687, June 1974.)

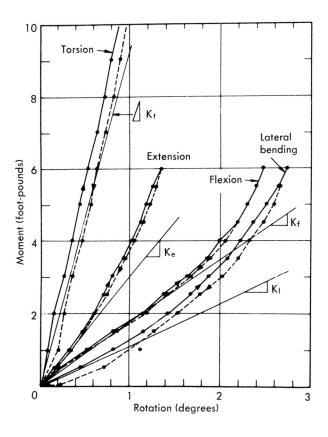

Fig. 17-7. Moment-rotation curves for a typical disc, the one between the twelfth thoracic and first lumbar vertebrae, showing the relative initial stiffness for lateral bending, K_l; flexion, K_f; extension, K_e; and torsion, K_t. *Solid lines,* Loading cycles. *Broken lines,* Unloading cycles. (1 foot-pound = 0.138 kg.-meter.) (From Markolf, K. L.: Deformation of the thoraco-lumbar intervertebral joints in response to external loads: A biomechanical study using autopsy material, J. Bone Joint Surg. **54A:**511-533, April 1972.)

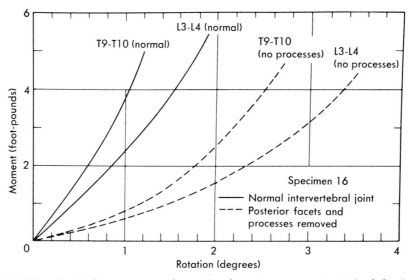

Fig. 17-8. Effect of articular processes and posterior elements on moment-rotation behavior of a thoracic and a lumbar intervertebral joint in extension. (1 foot-pound = 0.138 kg.-meter.) (From Markolf, K. L.: Deformation of the thoracolumbar intervertebral joints in response to external loads: A biomechanical study using autopsy material, J. Bone Joint Surg. **54A**:511-533, April 1972.)

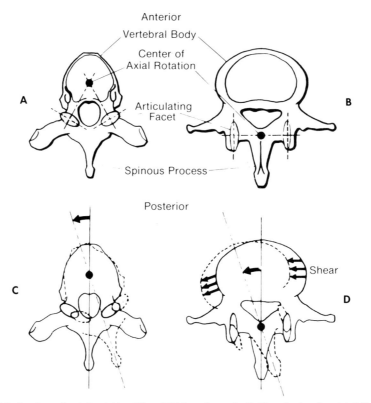

Fig. 17-9. Mechanism of axial rotation (**C** and **D**) in a thoracic (left) and a lumbar (right) vertebra. (From Gregersen, G. G., and Lucas, D. B.: An *in vivo* study of the axial rotation of the human thoracolumbar spine, J. Bone Joint Surg. **49A**:247-262, March 1967.)

lateral bending. To characterize the mechanics of these motions, a curve similar to that of force versus deflection for axial compression is used. For bending movements, the motion observed is rotation, measured in degrees, and the force acting to produce this rotation is called moment. A moment is a force applied in such a way as to produce rotation about a fixed point; the value of the moment is force times the distance of the lever arm, and it is measured in units called newtonmeters or foot-pounds. The curve of a moment-rotation test is similar to that of a force-deflection test (Fig. 17-7).

The moment-rotation response of an in vitro intervertebral joint (thoracic and lumbar) with and without the posterior facets presents a non-linear curve with increasing stiffness just as was observed for the force-deflection curves. Again, this behavior is characteristic of collagenous biologic materials. The importance of the posterior facets for bending varies with the motion. For lateral bending the facets have a minimal effect on the bending behavior. In flexion the curves vary slightly but are essentially the same. For extension (Fig. 17-8), however, the facets have a definite stiffening influence since for both the lumbar and thoracic discs the stiffness for a normal joint with posterior structures intact is about three times that for a joint with the facets removed. This stiffening effect by the facets is probably attributable to facet-joint compression and impingement upon one another as the joint is extended, with resulting resistance to further rotation. The presence of the facets provides a safety feature for the bending motions of the intervertebral joint, particularly for the motion of extension, because extreme extension could cause pinching of nerve branches exiting posteriorly from the spinal canal.

The existing data relate to low loads and small rotations. Bending data for high moment level and rates of loading are not yet available. It is expected that the bending response for diseased joints will differ significantly from the data for normal joints.

TORSION OF INTERVERTEBRAL JOINT

Torsion of the intervertebral joint about its long (spinal) axis (rotation) is a complex motion and is greatly dependent on structural features of the posterior facets. The mechanics of torsion in the thoracic and lumbar joints differs significantly because of differences in facet orientation (Fig.

17-9). In the thoracic spine the center of torsional rotation lies within the nucleus and the disc is subjected to rotation forces. For a lumbar joint, however, the center of axial rotation lies posterior to the disc nearer the facet joints, and the disc is thus subject to transitional shearing forces. As was the case for bending, the response to a moment is stiffening in character. Before and after removal of the posterior facets (by sawing across the neural arch) two normal joints were tested for torsion (Fig. 17-10). The thoracic joint showed little change in torsional (moment-rotation) behavior before and after facet removal. This was to be expected since the facet articulating surfaces for thoracic joints are more horizontal in orientation and thus present little resistance to torsion. Conversely, the lumbar facets project downward with nearly vertical surfaces, thus providing direct in-

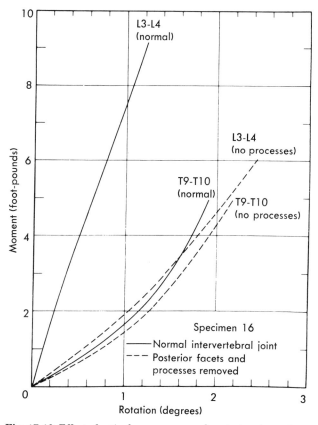

Fig. 17-10. Effect of articular processes and posterior elements on moment-rotation behavior of a thoracic and a lumbar intervertebral joint in torsion. (1 foot-pound = 0.138 kg.-meter.) (From Markolf, K. L.: Deformation of the thoracolumbar intervertebral joints in response to external loads: A biomechanical study using autopsy material, J. Bone Joint Surg. **54A:**511-533, April 1972.)

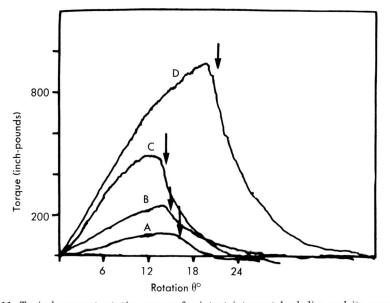

Fig. 17-11. Typical moment-rotation curves for intact intervertebral disc and its components loaded to failure. **A,** Intact joints between articular processes with capsule of contralateral articular process removed. **B,** Ruptured isolated disc. **C,** Intact (normal) isolated disc. **D,** Intact intervertebral joint with a normal discogram. (1 inch-pound = 0.0115 kg.-meter.) (From Farfan, H. F., Cosette, J. W., Robertson, G. H., Wells, R. V., and Kraus, H.: The effects of torsion on the lumbar intervertebral joints: The role of torsion in the production of disc degeneration, J. Bone Joint Surg. **52A:**468-497, April 1970.)

terference with one another to resist torsional motions, and presence of the facets results in stiffening. Torsional tests by Farfan indicate an average failure torque of 881×10^6 dyne-centimeters, or 8.99 kilogram-meters. He estimates that the disc provides 40% to 50% of the torsional stiffness, with the remainder provided by the posterior facet capsules. When torsion was applied to the point of failure (Fig. 17-11), it was found that intervertebral joints with degenerated discs were, as would be expected, weaker than normal specimens.

LIGAMENTOUS SPINE

The isolated spinal column, devoid of musculature, demonstrates an intrinsic stability. As we have seen, the self-contained balance of forces of internal pressure within the nucleus acting against the external binding tension of the ligaments results in a stable unit. This stability is minimal, however, as far as the entire column is concerned, for although the ligamentous spine is capable of standing erect on its own without external support, a compressive force of only 2 kg. (4½ pounds) applied at the top is enough to buckle the column laterally (Fig. 17-12).

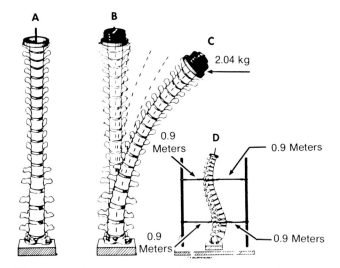

Fig. 17-12. Adult thoracolumbar ligamentous spine, fixed at base and free at top, under vertical loading, and restrained at midthoracic and midlumbar levels in anteroposterior plane. **A,** Before loading. **B,** During loading. **C,** Stability failure occurring under 2.04 kg. load. **D,** Lateral view showing anteroposterior restraints. (Courtesy D. B. Lucas and B. Bresler.)

Although the spinal column is nonuniform in size, the bending and compression stiffnesses are nearly constant throughout the thoracolumbar spine. This result is a curious balance between the counteracting effects of disc height versus cross-sectional area. A large disc area acts to provide increased stiffness, whereas increased disc height favors greater flexibility. The spine is so proportioned that the disc height increases as the disc area increases. This provides constancy in bending and compressive stiffness, an unusual circumstance for a tapered column.

Torsional stiffness, however, is not uniform since the lower lumbar joints are far stiffer than the thoracic joints. This discontinuity between lumbar and thoracic torsional stiffness presents a potential inherent weakness within the column for torsional injury. The upper thoracic vertebrae (the tenth vertebra and above) articulate with the rib cage in such a manner that resistance to torsional motion is increased; the thoracic vertebrae may be visualized as a rigid unit bound together by the rib cage. Since the lumbar vertebrae possess an inherently high torsional stiffness, they may also be considered as a stiff structural unit. This leaves the discs between the tenth and twelfth thoracic vertebrae as the intermediate elastic elements. When sudden torsional moments are applied, such as those that might be developed within the column during a fall or during acceleration, these intermediate discs would be likely to absorb a great deal of energy since rotations would be greatest at these levels. Thus it appears that the lowest thoracic discs are the most prone to injuries involving torsion.

AXIAL ROTATION OF SPINE AS A WHOLE

Gregersen and Lucas studied axial rotation of the erect spine in vivo while the trunk was rotated from side to side. Steinmann pins were inserted into spinous processes under local anesthesia and angular displacement between various vertebral levels was measured by special transducers designed to measure only rotation. They concluded from studying rotation of the trunk from side to side that approximately 74° of rotation occurred between the first and twelfth thoracic vertebrae. The average cumulative rotation from the sacrum to the first thoracic vertebra was 102 degrees (Fig. 17-13).

Measurements obtained during walking in-

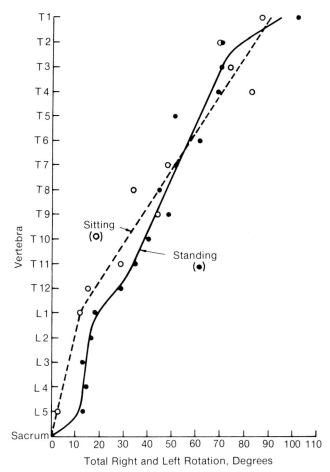

Fig. 17-13. Maximum total axial rotation of thoracolumbar spine in standing and sitting positions, pelvis immobilized. (From Gregersen, G. G., and Lucas, D. B.: An *in vivo* study of the axial rotation of the human thoracolumbar spine, J. Bone Joint Surg. **49A:**247-262, March 1967.)

dicated the following:
1. The pelvis and lumbar spine rotate as a functional unit.
2. In the lower thoracic spine, rotation diminishes gradually up to the seventh thoracic vertebra.
3. The seventh thoracic vertebra represents the area of transition from vertebral rotation in the direction of the pelvis to rotation in the opposite direction—that of the shoulder girdle (Fig. 17-14).
4. The amount of rotation in the upper thoracic spine increases gradually from the seventh to the first thoracic vertebra.

Axial rotation at the lumbosacral level in vivo was measured by Lumsden and Morris using a specially designed transducer. Approximately 6

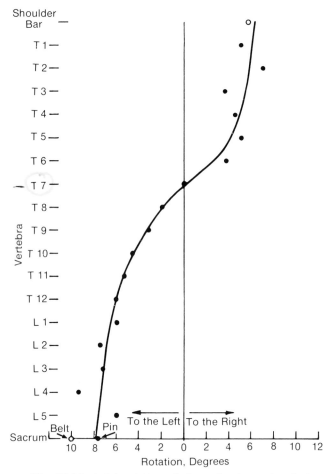

Fig. 17-14. Axial rotation of thoracolumbar spine during locomotion. Left heel strike to right heel strike, 4.38 km. per hour. *Solid circles,* Values for readings from pins. *Open circles,* Readings from belt. (From Gregersen, G. G., and Lucas, D. B.: An *in vivo* study of the axial rotation of the human thoracolumbar spine, J. Bone Joint Surg. **49A:**247-262, March 1967.)

degrees of rotation were found to occur at the lumbosacral joint during maximal rotation when the subject was either standing or straddling a bicycle seat with his pelvis fixed. Approximately 1.5 degrees of rotation occurred during normal walking. Rotation at the lumbosacral joint was not measurably affected by asymmetrically oriented lumbosacral facets. It was always associated with flexion of the fifth lumbar vertebra on the sacrum.

SPINE STABILITY

The combined intrinsic and extrinsic support of the spinal column enables it to withstand the great forces to which it may be subjected. At the same time, the number of articulations and interposed intervertebral discs allow the column to act

as a modified elastic rod. Intrinsic stability is the result of the expansile pressure within the discs, which tends to push the vertebral bodies apart, and the resistance provided by the ligaments, which tends to force the bodies together. This combination produces a very stable arrangement between adjacent vertebral bodies.

One can calculate from a static diagram that when an individual bends forward to lift a heavy weight, a large force is generated at the lumbosacral junction (Fig. 17-15). This force results largely from the contraction of the erector spinae muscles acting through a very short lever arm. The ratio of the anterior to the posterior lever arm is approximately 10 to 1. Therefore, if a weight of 90.7 kg. (200 pounds) is lifted, there is, theoretically at least, a force of 907.2 kg. (2000 pounds) at the lumbosacral level. However, a number of biomechanical experiments have been carried out to determine the strength of the discs and vertebral bodies, and it has been demonstrated that such great forces (907.2 kg.) cannot be tolerated. By placing two vertebral bodies with their intervening discs in a materials-testing compression machine or by subjecting them to sudden dynamic forces, investigators have obtained considerable information.

Compression tests have shown that the disc behaves as an elastic body only up to a maximal total pressure of 635 kg. (1400 pounds) (in specimens from young adults). In specimens from older persons, the elastic limit is approximately 158.8 kg. (350 pounds). Beyond this amount the disc is rapidly deformed by very little additional pressure.

Compression forces have been imposed up to the point of failure of a particular segment of the spine being studied. This failure is characterized by an audible crack followed by leakage of sanguineous fluid from one of the vertebrae (usually the superior) through the vascular foramen, and occasionally at some point along the attachment of the peripheral fibers of the anulus to the vertebral bodies. The evidence of failure is often difficult to visualize either upon gross examination or roentgenographically. It may consist of compression of a few spicules of bone, cracks in the end plate, or sometimes collapse of the plate. It has been shown that this failure occurs in specimens from young persons at a compressive load of 453.6 to 771.1 kg. (1000 to 1700 pounds). When specimens from older persons were studied, the

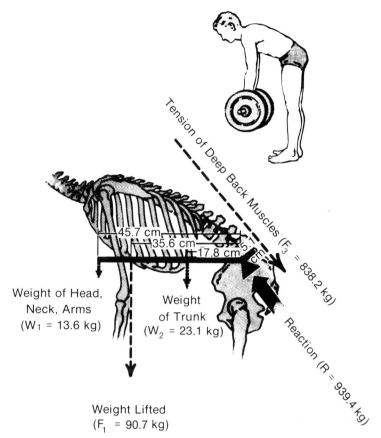

Fig. 17-15. Force on lower lumbar part of spine, with role of trunk omitted. (From Morris, J. M., Lucas, D. B., and Bresler, B.: Role of the trunk in stability of the spine, J. Bone Joint Surg. **43A**:327-351, April 1961.)

critical load was much less, even as little as 136.1 kg. (300 pounds).

It is noteworthy that when the anulus is intact its elastic limits cannot be exceeded without vertebral fracture. The end plate is most susceptible to fracture as a result of the forces exerted on the spine, and this structure generally gives way first. It is most likely to fracture centrally when the disc is normal and when the resistance of the vertebral body is greater than the pressure generated in the nucleus. This type of end-plate failure might explain the origin of the so-called Schmorl's nodes in young persons. Peripheral plate fractures or fissures across the end plate occur when various degrees of disc degeneration are present and thus lead to an abnormal distribution of forces across the disc space.

The vertebral body itself is the next most susceptible portion of the segment under study and usually collapses before herniation of the nucleus occurs through the anulus. Even when well-developed defects of the anulus are present, end-plate or vertebral fractures are more likely to occur than would disc herniation. (It is to be emphasized that the above values are not in vivo measurements.)

Investigations of injuries sustained by catapult ejections of jet pilots with an acceleration of 20 g (gravities), or less than 907.2 kg. (2000 pounds), demonstrated that vertebral compression fractures occurred in 27% of the cases.

It has also been shown experimentally in dogs that a single violet trauma will cause fracture of the vertebra more often than disc herniation will. This would agree well with the opinion that trauma per se seldom causes disc herniation. Organic as well as inorganic materials generally are able to withstand stresses during a short period more readily than stresses exerted for longer periods of time. It has been shown that an approximately equal number of end-plate fractures occurred when a static force of approxi-

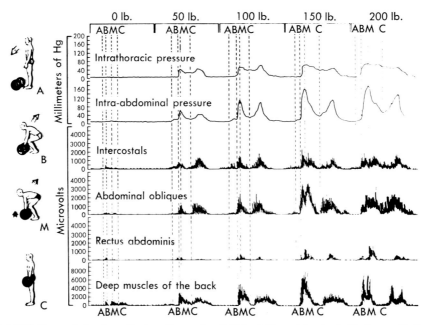

Fig. 17-16. Dynamic loading of spine. (1 pound = 0.45 kg.) (From Morris, J. M., Lucas, D. B., and Bresler, B.: Role of the trunk in stability of the spine, J. Bone Joint Surg. **43A:**327-351, April 1961.)

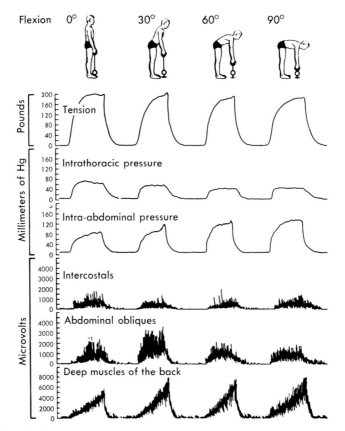

Fig. 17-17. Static loading of spine. (1 pound = 0.45 kg.) (From Morris, J. M., Lucas, D. B., and Bresler, B.: Role of the trunk in stability of the spine, J. Bone Joint Surg. **43A:**327-351, April 1961.)

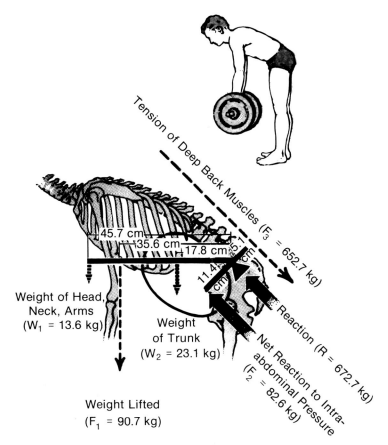

Fig. 17-18. Force on lower lumbar part of spine, with role of trunk included. (From Morris, J. M., Lucas, D. B., and Bresler, B.: Role of the trunk in stability of the spine, J. Bone Joint Surg. **43A:** 327-351, April 1961.)

mately 589.7 kg. (1300 pounds) was exerted as when dynamic stresses of 1179.3 kg. (2600 pounds) were applied. (This is apparently related to the viscoelastic properties of the involved structures.)

How, then, can the spine support the apparent loads to which it is subjected? One explanation for the ability of the spine to withstand such forces is to consider it as a segmental elastic column, supported by the paraspinal muscles and attached to the sides of and within two chambers, the abdominal and thoracic cavities, which are separated by the diaphragm. The first cavity is filled with a combination of solids and liquids, while the second is filled largely with air. The action of the trunk musculature converts these chambers into semirigid-walled cylinders of air and semisolids capable of transmitting forces generated in loading the spine and thereby relieving the spine itself.

This hypothesis was studied, and it was possible to show that, during the act of lifting, the action of the intercostal muscles and the muscles of the shoulder girdle rendered the thoracic cage quite rigid. An increase in intrathoracic pressure resulted, converting the thoracic cage and the spine into a sturdy unit capable of transmitting large forces. By contraction of the diaphragm and the muscles of the abdominal wall, the abdominal contents were compressed into a semirigid mass, thereby making the abdominal cavity a semirigid cylinder. The force of weights lifted by the arms is thus transmitted to the spinal column by the muscles of the shoulder girdle, principally the trapezius, and then on to the abdominal cylinder and the pelvis, partly through the spinal column and partly through the rigid rib cage and abdomen. The larger the weight lifted or the greater the static loading of the spine (pulling on a strain ring), the greater was the activity of the trunk and chest and abdominal musculature. Also, a concomitant increase in intracavitary pressures resulted (Figs. 17-16 and 17-17). In regard to the effects of the increased cavitary pressures, the calculated force on the lumbosacral disc during the lifting of any load was found to be decreased by 30%, and the load on the lower thoracic portion of the spine was about 50% less than it would have been without support by the trunk. Thus, when 90.7 kg. (200 pounds) is lifted, instead of approximately 907.2 kg. (2000 pounds) of force being transmitted along the spine to the lumbosacral level, only about 680.4 kg. (1500 pounds) is actually transmitted (Fig. 17-18). It is interesting to note that when a tight corset is worn about the abdomen, an increase in the intra-abdominal and intrathoracic pressures resulted from tightening of the corset. At the same time, during the act of lifting, there was a decrease in the activities of the thoracic and abdominal muscles, indicating that the effect of the muscles can be replaced by such an external appliance.

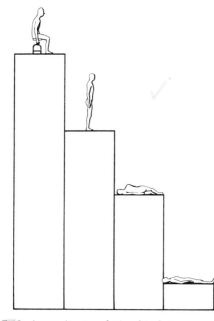

Fig. 17-19. Approximate relationship between position and total pressure on normal third and fourth lumbar discs. Positions shown are sitting, standing, reclining (with tilting), and lying with complete muscle relaxation (in one subject under general anesthesia, with the use of additional muscle relaxants, pressure recorded was similar to that obtained from autopsy specimens). (From Nachemson, A., and Morris, J. M.: *In vivo* measurements of intradiscal pressure: Discometry, a method for the determination of pressure in the lower lumbar discs, J. Bone Joint Surg. **46A:**1077-1092, July 1964.)

In an attempt to confirm the above calculations, intradiscal pressures were measured in vivo by Nachemson and Morris.[20] A needle with a pressure-sensitive polyethylene membrane at its tip was inserted into the disc under study. Intradiscal pressures of 10 to 15 kg./cm. were found in normal discs with subjects in a sitting position. There was approximately 30% less pressure during standing and about 50% less in the reclining position (Fig. 17-19). From these measurements one can determine that the lower lumbar discs of adults have to support total loads of as much as 99.8 to 174.6 kg. (220 to 385 pounds) when the subjects are seated. For the standing position, total loads between 90.7 and 120.2 kg. (200 and 265 pounds) were calculated from the pressure values obtained. The intradiscal pressures were significantly elevated when weights were lifted, especially when associated with forward flexion of the trunk. The figures obtained agreed closely with the theoretical calculations of forces on the spine mentioned above. Nachemson and Elfström[19] have recently extended this study to record intradiscal pressures during a variety of tasks or activities.

Section II

Pathomechanics

The majority of cases of chronic low back pain are related directly or indirectly to intervertebral disc degeneration. It is estimated that almost 90% of the patients with this condition encountered in a general orthopaedic practice or clinic have symptoms as a result of abnormal physiologic aging or degeneration of the intervertebral disc. Therefore, this chapter will deal primarily with physiologic changes in the disc that predispose an individual to acute or chronic low back pain. Certain anatomic variations and static disorders of the spine will be discussed briefly. Unusual causes of back pain such as tumors, infection, and metabolic bone disease will not be considered.

In the past, certain static conditions of the spine or anatomic variations of the lumbosacral region were believed to predispose or give rise to low back pain.

GENERAL CONDITIONS AFFECTING MOBILITY AND STABILITY OF LUMBOSACRAL AREA

The peculiar anatomic makeup of a particular spine may allow for the imposition of static stress upon it, such as the narrow, long back of some women whose lumbar spine is high upon the sacrum. This is frequently associated with flattening of the lumbar spine and poor supporting musculature. Such a back was felt to be quite susceptible to strain even with ordinary activity.

There are conditions remote to the lumbar spine that increase its lordosis and thereby might facilitate production of ligamentous strain. Examples might be old tuberculous gibbus of the dorsal spine, the kyphosis of Scheuermann's disease, congenital hip dislocation, or coxa vara.

Anatomic variations affecting mobility of spine

The attainment of the orthograde position imposes considerable static stress on the lumbosacral junction, which is less equipped to handle it than any other part of the spinal column. Certain anatomic variations from the normal that occur in this region may affect the mobility or stability of the spine. If mobility is resisted or checked, the burden of added mobility may be thrown onto higher levels of the spine. In other cases in which motion is not checked soon enough, strain may fall primarily on the soft tissues of the region. These variations are outlined below.

Abnormally long transverse process of L5. This is seen more commonly in painful backs, though it may be seen in backs without pain. The process may cause pain by impinging on the ilium to lock motion and cause strain at a higher level, or it may cause pain on lateral motion by impingement.

Sacralization. In this condition motion of the spine in any direction is transferred to the L4-L5 disc. However, the articular processes of this junction are directed in the sagital plane, and therefore the freedom of motion found in the lumbosacral joint is absent. Though this articulation usually adjusts to this situation, it may be a cause of stress during rotation.

Tropism. In this condition the articular facets of the lumbosacral junction are asymmetrically arranged. The articulation is directed in the frontal plane on one side and in the sagittal on the other. Here again, the sagittal articulation resists rotatory and lateral movement; this resistance leads to added stress upon the articulations above. Also, Farfan[2] has pointed out that this condition imposes additional shearing stress on the anulus and thereby accelerates degenerative changes.

Anatomic variations affecting stability of spine

Spina bifida. A defect in the arch may encroach upon the ligamentous attachments and thus cause a certain degree of instability.

Spondylolysis and spondylolisthesis. The articular processes may separate as the upper vertebra slips forward on the vertebra below leading to spondylolisthesis. Because of the original defect, spinal stability depends entirely on the ligamentous structures, especially the iliolumbar ligament, which holds L4 and L5 to the ilium. This ligament is frequently not strong enough to prevent forward slipping of L5.

Horizontal sacrum leading to abnormal forward shearing stress at lumbosacral junction. The more nearly this junction approaches a 90-degree angle, the more the force acting on the spine acts as shear. The spine in this condition is particularly susceptible to jars and jolts in that the almost vertical disc is unable to adequately intercept them. In this condition strain is thrown on the sacroiliac ligaments, which must resist the forward rotation of the upper end of the sacrum under the body weight.

The Munkfors report of 1954,[9,10] however, indicated that most of these conditions were not related to a higher incidence of back pain, nor were they indicative of increased susceptibility to back pain. The one exception was spondylolisthesis, which was associated with a high incidence of disc degeneration.

DISC DEGENERATION

As mentioned before, disc degeneration is the basic factor in the production of the majority of cases of low back syndrome. In Friberg's studies,[4] roentgenographic evidence of various degrees of degeneration, such as instability as shown by "rocking" of the upper vertebra on the lower, narrowing of disc space, and osteophyte formation, was found in one half of all the patients examined for complaint of back pain. How many had back pain caused by this degeneration in which changes were not great enough to be seen roentgenographically? Even with a normal roentgenogram, considerable degenerative change may be present.

Physiologic changes in the disc from age or degeneration begin at about 20 years and increase progressively in later life. In the nucleus, the water content decreases with age. At birth it is 88% water, whereas in persons in the seventies it is only 69%. There is progressive fibrosis with increasing cellular degeneration, central fissuring, and cavitation, as well as focal deposition of calcium salts.

The anulus shows swelling of the lamellae with areas of mucinous degeneration between them, which stain dark blue with hematoxylin. These areas give rise to concentric fissures that enlarge and coalesce increasingly with age. The fibrous structure becomes increasingly homogenized or hyalinized and may become fragmented. Radial fissures, most prominent posterolaterally, occur in the lower lumbar discs. These begin centrally and may extend through the anulus, causing bulging. They disturb the function of the disc more than the other changes. Fibrous tissue with vascularization may be seen at the borders of the anulus after trauma and healing. Areas of brown pigmentation may be seen in the region of fissure, presumably from hemosiderin deposits.

The cartilage plates become thinner, cellularity decreases, and cells in various stages of degeneration may be found. Schmorl's nodes occur with increasing frequency, and fibrillation or parallel tears in the cartilage may be seen.

In attempting to explain relatively early degeneration of the disc, several factors must be taken into account. Age changes in the nucleus and the anulus are similar to the changes seen in the aging of other mesenchymal tissues, such as articular cartilage, tendons, and connective tissue itself.

There is no conclusive evidence that heavy physical labor is the direct cause of disc change. There is a similar incidence of disc degeneration in stevedores, lumberjacks, and sedentary workers. If we consider, however, that these changes not only become more frequent as age advances but also are found more often in the lower lumbar discs, we cannot avoid the assumption that mechanical forces play some part in disc degeneration and in the resistance of the anulus to rupture.

Some idea of the effect of mechanical stresses can be obtained from the work of Brown and his group.[1] As noted in the previous chapter, the anulus and nucleus of the disc are better able to withstand compressive or single dynamic forces than is the end plate or the vertebral body. However, in a fatigue test using a disc and adjacent vertebrae, a load of only 6.8 kg. was applied. The superior vertebra was then rapidly flexed on the inferior vertebra by means of a machine with 1100 cycles per minute. After only 1000 cycles,

less than 1 minute, there was an almost complete horizontal tear through the anulus. This demonstrates the susceptibility of the disc to combined loading and bending forces.

Pressure is also a factor to be considered, since the radial fissures are first seen and are most pronounced in the portion of the disc on the concave side of a spinal curve. They occur in the posterior anulus in the lordotic lumbar region and in the anterior anulus in the kyphotic dorsal regions. Lindblom[11] noted that when rats' tails were fixed in a sharply bent position, radial ruptures of the anulus on the concave surface were induced.

The absence of a blood supply to the discs is of importance both in the early onset of degeneration and in the absence of repair once this degeneration has begun. The lack of blood supply leads to changes in oxygen tension and pH, with resultant metabolic changes in the ground substance of the nucleus.

There is also evidence that hereditary factors may play a part. In breeds of dogs in which chondrodystrophic changes develop, such as the dachshund, pekinese, and French bulldog, disc degeneration is much more pronounced than it is in dogs of other breeds.

Thus it would seem that the normal underlying process of degeneration with aging is, in the case of the intervertebral disc, further influenced by lack of blood supply, heredity, and mechanical factors.

All regressive changes begin in the nucleus. No ruptures occur in the anulus unless the nucleus shows appreciable structural changes.

The nucleus has been described as a three-dimensional lattice-gel system composed of interlacing collagen fibers within a protein-polysaccharide matrix, which gives the nucleus its pronounced hydrophilia. The efficient functioning of the disc depends largely on the plasticity of the nucleus, which is, in turn, related to its water-binding capacity.

There are two possible physiochemical bases for this water retention: osmosis and the imbibition pressure exerted by the protein-polysaccharide gel. That osmosis is relatively unimportant is shown by the fact that the nucleus retains an almost constant degree of hydration when placed in fluids of different tonicity. Therefore, it is virtually certain that the hydration of the nucleus is attributable to the imbibition pressure of the gel. It is interesting to note that a gel with a saturation of 1% will have an imbibition pressure of 5000 atmospheres. This is the amount of force necessary to separate the water and the solid phase. This characteristic of gels provides a powerful and adaptable force to meet the functional needs of the disc.

In the process of degeneration or physiologic aging of the nucleus, the high content of chondroitin sulfate A, which is present in the young, is gradually replaced to a degree by keratosulfate and chondroitin sulfate B. Also, the amount of hyaluronic acid decreases. Presumably, this is a result of decreased oxygen tension and pH changes resulting in decreased metabolic activity in the ground substance. The protein cores of the protein-polysaccharide complexes divide and the amount of collagen within the nucleus increases in relation to the amount of mucopolysaccharide. The effect of this is to decrease the viscosity of the nucleus by first decreasing the strength of the water binding within the nucleus and later by decreasing the actual amount of water. In this process the collagen protein seems to occupy a larger number of the polar hydroxyl groups of the polysaccharide, leaving a smaller number available for water binding. Studies by Hendry[6] have shown that the degenerated nucleus is much less hydrophilic than is the normal nucleus. When this degenerate nuclear material is subjected to low pressure, it will lose more water than normal.

The importance of the preceding data relates to the weight-bearing stresses placed on the spinal column. Normally, the stress through the vertebral bodies can be regarded as being resolved into two components: (1) a force transmitted through the nucleus and balanced by its own imbibition pressure, and (2) a residual force transmitted by the anulus.

Hirsch[7,8] has suggested that if the nucleus loses its ability to produce an even distribution of pressure, the anulus is no longer capable of meeting even physiologic demands upon it.

This reduction of the imbibition pressure of the nucleus has three effects:

1. A greater proportion of the total stress will be thrown on the anulus. Nachemson[18] has calculated by means of measuring the intradiscal pressures in normal and degenerated discs that if the nucleus is degenerated, the stress on the anulus is four times greater than in a normal disc. He has also calculated that the weight-bearing capacity of a normal disc is 50% greater than that of a degenerated disc.

2. The character of the stress on the anulus may change from an alternating tension and compression to unrelieved compression. The collagen fibers of the anulus are adapted to withstand tensile forces but degenerate when subjected to continuous compression.

3. Under conditions of prolonged relaxation, the nucleus will imbibe fluid only to be unable to retain it when stress is reapplied. This will cause a sudden loss of fluid and a rapid redistribution of hydrostatic pressure, which cannot be dissipated rapidly through the avascular disc. This forceful expulsion of fluid from the nucleus into existing small fissures and cracks within the anulus tends to enlarge the fissures and separate the lamellae of the anulus. Since the elastic properties of the anulus depend on the oblique sheets of fibers running perpendicular to each other, one can see that separation of these sheets would allow for increased motion of one upon the other and thereby allow more compression and bulging of the anulus. This, in turn, permits increased motion of one vertebra on another and leads to a condition of instability.

Thus degeneration of the nucleus gives rise to effects that, in turn, hasten the degenerative processes occurring within the anulus and pave the way for possible herniation of the degenerated nuclear material.

In the course of events of degeneration, usually within 5 to 6 years, fibrosis of the nucleus and fibrous proliferation in the anulus (partially because of ingrowth of granulation tissue through the fissures) transforms the disc space into a modified fibrous ankylosis between the two vertebrae. At this time there is little danger of herniation, and pain, if it has been present, often disappears. This explains the clinical observation that whereas disc degeneration proceeds on into old age, the peak incidence of herniation and disc disease occurs in the 30- to 50-year age group.

Whether a mechanical derangement of the disc actually occurs may depend on the age and activity of the patient at the time of degeneration, on the speed and extent of collagen deposition in the nucleus, on the relation of anular damage and fibrosis to hydrostatic effect, and on unknown biochemical factors.

It may be that the difference in normal aging and that seen in degenerative disc disease is that the two phases of mucopolysaccharide loss and collagen deposition are out of step in the latter. In normal aging, a slow orderly mucopolysaccharide loss with simultaneous collagen replacement would allow progressive physiologic dehydration to occur without severe damage to the anulus and without the appearance of hydrostatic effects.

It has been shown that degeneration of the disc leads to loss of the intrinsic stability of the spine, which is the result of tension of the binding ligaments opposed by the turgor or imbibition pressure of the nucleus. With the combination of loss of turgor, or desiccation, of the nucleus and the fissuring, lamellar separation, and settling of the anulus, the tension of the spinal ligaments is decidedly decreased. These factors give rise to the condition known as *instability of the spine,* in which an abnormal amount of movement occurs between contiguous vertebrae. In extension the upper vertebra is displaced posteriorly and in flexion it may be displaced forward. Instability is said to exist when the amount of motion exceeds the normal limit of 3 mm. of displacement. This condition is most frequently seen at the L4-L5 disc and next most frequently in the L5-S1 disc. It may be the first sign of disc degeneration detectable roentgenographically. With increasing degeneration, the disc space narrows and bulging of the anulus elevates the periosteum at the edges of the vertebral body. Beneath this elevated periosteum new bone forms, as osteophytes or spurs.

This excessive mobility of the unstable spine may cause pain by the undue stress placed upon the surrounding ligamentous structures.

Narrowing of the disc and instability tend to cause posterior displacement of the center of rotation in the involved segments during flexion and extension. In severe degeneration, the axes of motion may even pass through the posterior articulations. The abnormal motion thus imposed on these posterior joints leads to degenerative changes of various degrees, in the form of fibrillation and pitting of the cartilage, fibrosis, fractures of the articular surfaces, bony impingement of an articular process against the laminae of adjacent vertebrae, or even subluxation.

Pain may arise by motion within the degenerated posterior articulation, capsular stretching, bony impingement, or occasionally entrapment and squeezing of redundant synovia between the articular surfaces. The latter condition is believed to be a basis of some cases of "catching" pain in the back.

Another mechanism of pain production is suggested by Hirsch.[8] He was able to reproduce back pain in patients by injecting saline into the degenerated disc. If procaine was used, pain did not occur. He believes that the pain is attributable to distension of the anulus causing tension in the posterior ligament at its junction with the anulus. It may be that fractures of the end plate of the degenerative disc are sensitive to pain, thus accounting for the rapid action of procaine in relieving this pain. Hirsch has also suggested that pain may arise by irritation of the vascular granulation tissue that grows into anular fissures from the periphery. Nachemson has suggested the possibility of leakage of a chemical irritant resulting from the degenerative process.[18]

In all of these conditions the existing pain is usually the deep type. It is a dull, aching pain that is poorly localized and that may be associated with visceral symptoms. Radiation may occur across the back or down the thigh. This radiation does not correspond with the dermatome distribution of sensory cutaneous nerves in the region, but follows a more or less constant, reproducible sclerotomal pattern characteristic of "deep pain."

Finally, low back pain with or without sciatica may arise from compression of the spinal nerve in the intervertebral foramen. This is most commonly seen in the lower two lumbar nerves and the first sacral nerve. This would, of course, be expected because of the high incidence of disc degeneration at this level. It would also be expected from an anatomic standpoint, since the size of the lumbar intervertebral foramen decreases from above downward while the sizes of the spinal nerves increase. Thus the lower nerves are more susceptible to compression.

This compression may be caused by several conditions such as herniation of nuclear material or bulging of the posterior anulus. However, other factors such as the presence of osteophytes, subluxation of the posterior joints, hypertrophy of the ligamentum flavum seen quite frequently in spinal instability and edema or congestion of a spinal nerve and dural lining are of importance. The fundamental cause of sciatic pain or low back pain in cases of nerve root compression is difficult to elucidate. Certainly, compression does not appear to be the complete answer. With pressure on a nerve, the first fibers to be blocked are the large, myelinated fibers responding to touch, proprioception, and the motor impulses. This is illustrated by the leg "going to sleep" from pressure being placed on the sciatic nerve in sitting. The pain fibers (especially the smaller fibers of deep pain) are affected later.

In sciatica, however, pain is one of the first symptoms. Some mechanism must therefore be assumed to lower the threshold of pain fibers. Perhaps the edema and inflammation of the nerve root found in conditions of compressions and irritation are involved.

REFERENCES

1. Brown, T., Hansen, R. J., and Yorra, A. J.: Some mechanical tests on the lumbosacral spine with particular reference to the intervertebral discs. A preliminary report, J. Bone Joint Surg. 39A:1135-1164, Oct. 1957.
2. Farfan, H. F.: Mechanical disorders of the low back, Philadelphia, 1973, Lea & Febiger.
3. Farfan, H. F., Cossette, J. W., Robertson, G. H., Wells, R. V., and Kraus, H.: The effects of torsion on the lumbar intervertebral joints: The role of torsion in the production of disc degeneration, J. Bone Joint Surg. 52A:468-497, April 1970.
4. Friberg, S., and Hirsch, C.: Anatomical and clinical studies on lumbar disc degeneration, Acta Orthop. Scand. 19:222-242, 1949.
5. Gregersen, G. G., and Lucas, D. B.: An in vivo study of the axial rotation of the human thoracolumbar spine, J. Bone Joint Surg. 49A:247-262, March 1967.
6. Hendry, N. G.: The hydration of the nucleus pulposus and its relation to intervertebral disc derangement, J. Bone Joint Surg. 40B:132-144, Feb. 1958.
7. Hirsch, C., and Nachemson, A.: New observations on the mechanical behavior of lumbar discs, Acta Orthop. Scand. 23:254-283, 1954.
8. Hirsch, C., Ingelmark, B.-E., and Miller, M.: The anatomical basis for low back pain. Studies on the presence of sensory nerve endings in ligamentous, capsular and intervertebral disc structures in the human lumbar spine, Acta Orthop. Scand. 33:1-17, 1963.
9. Hult, L.: Cervical, dorsal and lumbar spinal syndromes: A field investigation of a non-selected material of 1,200 workers in different occupations with special reference to disc degeneration and so-called muscular rheumatism, Acta Orthop. Scand. 17(suppl.):1-102, 1954.
10. Hult, L.: The Munkfors investigation. A study of the frequency and causes of the stiff neck–brachialgia and lumbago-sciatica syndromes, as well as observations on certain signs and symptoms from the dorsal spine and the joints of the extremities in industrial and forest workers, Acta Orthop. Scand. 16(suppl.):1-76, 1954.
11. Lindblom, K.: Intervertebral-disc degeneration considered as a pressure atrophy, J. Bone Joint Surg. 39A: 933-145, July 1957.
12. Lucas, D. B., and Bresler, B.: Stability of the ligamentous spine. Biomechanics Laboratory, University of California, Tech. Rep. 40. San Francisco, Jan. 1961, The Laboratory.
13. Lumsden, R. M., II, and Morris, J. M.: An in vivo study of axial rotation and immobilization at the lumbosacral joint, J. Bone Joint Surg. 50A:1591-1602, Dec. 1968.
14. Markolf, K. L.: Deformation of the thoracolumbar intervertebral joints in response to external loads: A biomechanical study using autopsy material, J. Bone Joint Surg. 54A:511-533, April 1972.
15. Markolf, K. L., and Morris, J. M.: The structural components of the intervertebral disc: A study of their contributions to the ability of the disc to withstand compressive forces, J. Bone Joint Surg. 56A:675-687, June 1974.
16. Morris, J. M.: Biomechanics of the spine, Arch. Surg. 107:418-423, Sept. 1973.
17. Morris, J. M., Lucas, D. B., and Bresler, B.: Role of the trunk in stability of the spine, J. Bone Joint Surg. 43A: 327-351, April 1961.
18. Nachemson, A.: Lumbar intradiscal pressure. Experimental studies on postmortem material, Acta Orthop. Scand. 43(suppl.):9-104, 1960.
19. Nachemson, A., and Elfström, G.: Intravital dynamic pressure measurements in lumbar discs: A study of common movements, maneuvers and exercises, Scand. J. Rehabil. Med. 1(suppl. 1):1-40, 1970.
20. Nachemson, A., and Morris, J. M.: In vivo measurements of intradiscal pressure: Discometry, a method for the determination of pressure in the lower lumbar discs, J. Bone Joint Surg. 46A:1077-1092, July 1964.

CHAPTER 18

Biomechanical analysis of the spine

NEWTON C. McCOLLOUGH, III, M.D.

Of the three major areas of the body under consideration for orthotic application, the spine is perhaps the most difficult to accurately describe in terms of biomechanical analysis. The upper and lower limb, by virtue of the accessibility of their articulations and motors to physical examination lend themselves well to diagrammatic representation on a technical analysis form. The deeply seated joints of the spine with their gross and less well defined motor control units present the clinician with a difficult problem in examination, diagnosis, and identification of biomechanical deficits. Of course, orthotic prescription for the spine can reach no greater level of sophistication than that permitted by the accuracy of identification of biomechanical abnormalities. With these considerations in mind, some method of tabulation or diagrammatic representation of the biomechanical status of the spine is still considered to be highly desirable as a basis for proceeding with a rational orthotic prescription. The method to be described, utilizing the spinal technical analysis form, provides the examiner with a systematic and illustrative means of recording pertinent data upon which the orthotic prescription may be based.

DESCRIPTION OF SPINAL TECHNICAL ANALYSIS FORM

The spinal technical analysis form consists of four pages suitable for inclusion in the patient's

hospital record. The first page (Fig. 18-1) contains spaces for patient data and a summary of major impairments. In general, the impairments noted on this page are those that do not lend themselves well to diagrammatic representation. The second page (Fig. 18-2) contains a legend for symbols to be used in conjunction with the skeletal outline to complete the biomechanical analysis. The third page (Fig. 18-3) contains a skeletal outline of the spinal column and pelvis in the coronal, sagittal, and transverse planes. The fourth page (Fig. 18-4) provides a space for summarizing the functional disability and for identifying treatment objectives. The orthotic recommendation or prescription form is also included on this page for the purpose of indicating the type of motion control desirable at each level of the spine in each plane.

INSTRUCTIONS FOR USE OF SPINAL TECHNICAL ANALYSIS FORM
Major impairments (Fig. 18-1)

Most of this portion of the form is self-explanatory. In general, observations to be recorded here are those that do not lend themselves to diagrammatic illustration on the following page. These observations include structural abnormalities such as the character of bone and disc space involvement; sensory abnormalities; upper and lower limb deficits that may influence spinal alignment and orthotic prescription; balance im-

TECHNICAL ANALYSIS FORM   SPINE   May 1974

Name_____ No._____ Age____ Sex____ Weight_____ Height_____

Diagnosis_____ Occupation_____

Present Orthotic Equipment_____

_____

    Ambulatory☐   Non Ambulatory☐   Wheelchair☐

Standing Balance: Normal☐   Impaired☐   Walking Aid_____

Sitting Position: Stable☐   Unstable☐   Reclined☐   Upright☐

Sitting Tolerance: Normal☐   Limited☐

MAJOR IMPAIRMENTS

A. Structural: No Impairment☐

  1. Bone: Osteoporosis☐   Fracture☐   Level_____

        Other_____

  2. Disc Space: (Describe)_____

  3. Alignment: Scoliosis☐   Kyphosis☐   Lordosis☐

B. Sensory: No Impairment☐

  1. Anesthesia☐   Location_____

  2. Pain☐   Location_____

C. Upper Limb: No Impairment☐

  1. Amputation☐_____

  2. Other_____

D. Lower Limb: No Impairment☐

  1. Limb Shortening: Right☐   Left☐   Amount_____

  2. Hip Contracture☐   Ankylosis☐   Flexion☐   Degree_____

      Adduction☐ Degree_____;   Abduction☐ Degree_____;

      Extension☐ Degree_____

  3. Major Motor Loss☐ Location_____

  4. Sensation: Anesthesia☐ Location_____;

      Hypesthesia☐ Location_____

      Pain☐ Location_____

E. Associated Impairments:_____

_____

Fig. 18-1

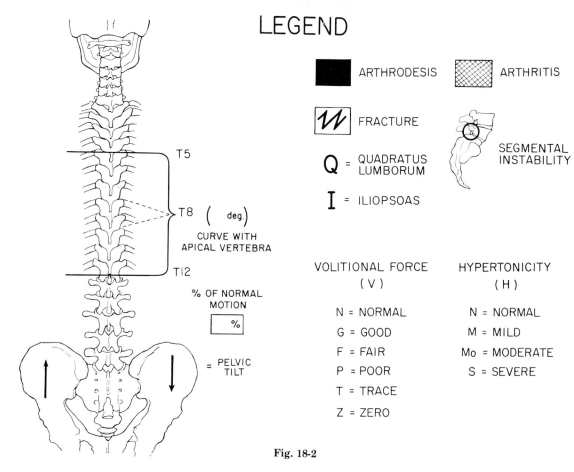

LEGEND

ARTHRODESIS

ARTHRITIS

FRACTURE

Q = QUADRATUS LUMBORUM

I = ILIOPSOAS

SEGMENTAL INSTABILITY

T5

T8 (deg.)

CURVE WITH APICAL VERTEBRA

T12

% OF NORMAL MOTION

%

= PELVIC TILT

VOLITIONAL FORCE (V)

N = NORMAL
G = GOOD
F = FAIR
P = POOR
T = TRACE
Z = ZERO

HYPERTONICITY (H)

N = NORMAL
M = MILD
Mo = MODERATE
S = SEVERE

Fig. 18-2

pairment; and any associated impairments that may have bearing upon selection of treatment.

Legend and spinal diagram
(Figs. 18-2 and 18-3)

On either side of the spinal column in the coronal, sagittal, and transverse plane small rectangular boxes with appended arrows are located at the cervical, thoracic, and lumbar levels for the purposes of indicating range of motion of the spinal segments. Range of motion is recorded within these boxes to indicate the estimated percent of normal motion retained at each level and in each direction. In cases of fixed rotational deformity, such as is present in scoliosis, the estimated degree of rotation at each level is recorded in the appropriate box using the radiologic method described by Nash and Moe.[1] Also located adjacent to the spinal column are small boxes labeled B and H for the purpose of recording muscle strength of the lateral flexors, extensors, and forward flexors of the spine. Since these muscle groups are not

readily distinguishable in their effects upon the thoracic and lumbar spine separately, thoracolumbar motors are graded together. The quadratus lumborum (Q) and iliopsoas (I) are graded separately on each side of the lumbar spine in the coronal plane. Active volitional strength of these muscles is recorded in the box labeled V and hypertonicity, if present, is recorded in the box labeled H at each level according to the scale in the legend.

Curvature of the spine in the coronal or sagittal plane is indicated by drawing transverse lines through the spinal column at the upper and lower limits of the curve. The direction of the curve is indicated by a bracket on the convex side extending between the end vertebrae. The apical vertebra is identified at the center of the bracket as is the magnitude of the curve in degrees and whether it is a primary or secondary curve.

Pelvic tilt is indicated by directional arrows overlying the outline of the pelvis as depicted.

Symbols for arthrodesis, fracture, arthritis, and segmental instability contained in the legend

CORONAL SAGITTAL TRANSVERSE

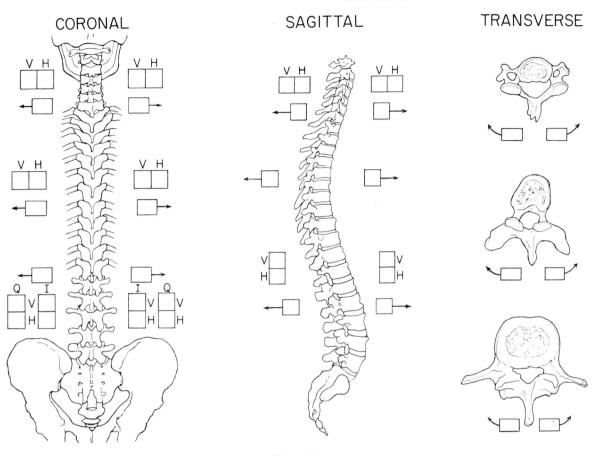

Fig. 18-3

are to be used in an overlay fashion on the diagram to indicate specific areas of involvement.

Summary of functional disability
(Fig. 18-4)

The summary is intended to be a concise analysis of the factors that are significant in producing functional impairment and for which orthotic control is desirable.

Treatment objectives (Fig. 18-4)

The objectives of orthotic treatment are identified by checking the appropriate boxes. There frequently may be more than one objective of treatment.

Orthotic recommendation (Fig. 18-4)

The level of orthotic application is selected on the basis of the information obtained. A full spinal orthosis to include the cervical spine, thoracic spine, lumbar spine and sacrum is identified in the chart as a CTLSO, or cervicothoracolumbosacral

orthosis, whereas a device to control only the lumbar and sacral spine would be designed as an LSO.

For each segment of the spine to be encompassed or controlled by the orthosis, the type of control in each direction of motion in each plane is inserted in the blanks provided, abbreviated according to the key at the bottom of the page. Thus the types of control to be provided, and not the specific components to be used, form the basis of the orthotic recommendation. Under the section concerning remarks more exacting recommendations as to components or special considerations in fabrication can be recorded.

CASE ILLUSTRATIONS
Case 1 (Figs. 18-5 to 18-7)

This 58-year-old female was seen for low back pain, secondary to osteoporosis, compression fractures, and osteoarthritis. Fig. 18-5 provides the basic background information regarding this patient's disability. One may note that she has compression fractures of the eleventh and eighth

Summary of Functional Disability: ______________________

____

____

Treatment Objectives:

Spinal Alignment ☐ Motion Control ☐
Axial Unloading ☐ Other ______________________

____

ORTHOTIC RECOMMENDATION

SPINE		FLEX	EXT	LATERAL FLEXION R	LATERAL FLEXION L	ROTATION R	ROTATION L	AXIAL LOAD
CTLSO	Cervical							
TLSO	Thoracic							
LSO	Lumbar							
	(Lumbo sacral							
SIO	Sacroiliac							

REMARKS:

____

KEY: Use the following symbols to indicate desired control of designated function:

F = FREE - Free motion
A = ASSIST - Application of an external force for the purpose of increasing the range, velocity, or force of a motion.
R = RESIST - Application of an external force for the purpose of decreasing the velocity or force of a motion.
S = STOP - Inclusion of a static unit to deter an undesired motion in one direction.
v = Variable - A unit that can be adjusted without making a structural change.
H = HOLD - Elimination of all motion in prescribed plane: specify position, e.g. in degrees or (+) (-).
L = LOCK - Device includes an optional lock.

____
Signature

____
Date

Fig. 18-4

TECHNICAL ANALYSIS FORM   SPINE   May 1974

Name _Eleanor Mosely_____   No. _89266_ Age _58_ Sex _F_ Weight _138_ Height _5'4"_

Diagnosis _Osteoporosis, Compression Fractures_ Occupation _Housewife_____
        and Osteoarthritis

Present Orthotic Equipment _____Thoracolumbar Corset_____

_____

    Ambulatory ☑   Non Ambulatory ☐   Wheelchair ☐

Standing Balance: Normal ☑   Impaired ☐   Walking Aid _____

Sitting Position: Stable ☑   Unstable ☐   Reclined ☐   Upright ☐

Sitting Tolerance: Normal ☑   Limited ☐

MAJOR IMPAIRMENTS

A. Structural: No Impairment ☐

    1. Bone: Osteoporosis ☑   Fracture ☑   Level _T_{11}, T_8_____

                 Other_____

    2. Disc Space: (Describe) _Narrowing $L_4 - L_5$; $L_5 - S_1$_____
                 _Pseudo spondylolisthesis $L_4 - L_5$_____

    3. Alignment: Scoliosis ☐   Kyphosis ☑   Lordosis ☐

B. Sensory: No Impairment ☐

    1. Anesthesia ☐   Location_____

    2. Pain ☑   Location _Low dorsal ; Low lumbar_____

C. Upper Limb: No Impairment ☑

    1. Amputation ☐ _____

    2. Other_____

D. Lower Limb: No Impairment ☐

    1. Limb Shortening: Right ☐   Left ☐   Amount _____

    2. Hip Contracture ☐   Ankylosis ☐   Flexion ☐   Degree _____

        Adduction ☐   Degree_____ ;   Abduction ☐   Degree_____ ;

        Extension ☐   Degree_____

    3. Major Motor Loss ☐   Location _____

    4. Sensation: Anesthesia ☐   Location_____ ;

        Hypesthesia ☐   Location _____

        Pain ☑   Location _Ⓡ hip and posterior thigh_____

E. Associated Impairments: _None_____

Fig. 18-5

CORONAL　　　　　SAGITTAL　　　　　TRANSVERSE

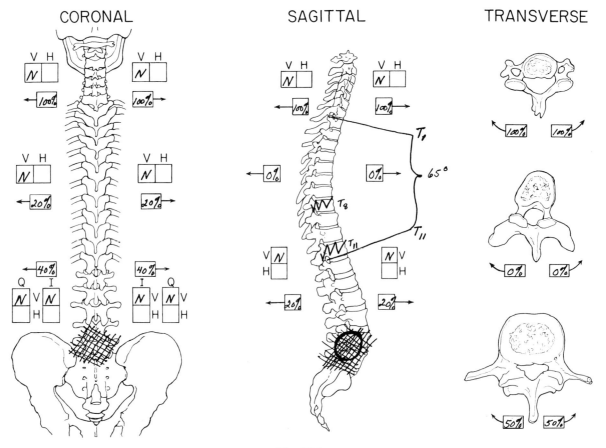

Fig. 18-6

thoracic vertebrae, as well as narrowing of the interspaces between L4 and L5, and L5 and S1. Pseudospondylolisthesis is present at the L4-L5 interval. The patient's pain is primarily in the low dorsal and low lumbar areas and radiates into the right hip and posterior thigh.

Diagrammatic analysis of the spine (Fig. 18-6) gives a more detailed picture of the abnormalities present. In the coronal plane, it is to be noted that there is limitation of lateral flexion in the thoracic area to about 20% of normal, and in the lumbar area, 40% of normal lateral flexion is retained to either side. Muscle strength is designated as being normal throughout the spine, and degenerative arthritis is noted at the low lumbar area involving L4, L5, and S1. In the sagittal plane it is noted that although full range of motion is retained in the cervical spine, there is essentially no remaining motion in flexion and extension in the thoracic area. Only 20% of normal flexion and extension remains in the lumbar spine. Compression fractures are noted at the level of T8 and T11, and a

kyphotic curve is described extending from the first thoracic vertebra to the eleventh thoracic vertebra, measuring 65 degrees. An area of segmental instability secondary to pseudospondylolisthesis is present between L4 and L5, and once again, degenerative arthritis of L4, L5, and S1 is diagrammed. In the transverse plane normal cervical rotation is retained, while rotation in the thoracic area is abolished completely, and 50% of normal rotation remains to either side in the lumbar segment.

In Fig. 18-7, it is noted that the functional disability consists primarily of limited mobility, secondary to pain that is, in turn, secondary to compression fractures, osteoporosis, osteoarthritis, and segmental instability. The objective of orthotic treatment is motion control to reduce or eliminate the existing pain. The orthotic recommendation calls for stopping motion of the spine in all three planes at the thoracic, lumbar, and lumbosacral levels. In addition, reduction of axial load is desirable. The specific orthosis recom-

Summary of Functional Disability: *Mobility Compromised by pain 2° to Compression Fractures, Osteoporosis, Osteoarthritis, and Segmental instability L4-L5*

Treatment Objectives:

Spinal Alignment ☐   Motion Control ☑
Axial Unloading ☐   Other _____

ORTHOTIC RECOMMENDATION

SPINE		FLEX	EXT	LATERAL FLEXION R	L	ROTATION R	L	AXIAL LOAD
CTLSO	Cervical							
TLSO	Thoracic	S	S	S	S	S	S	R
LSO	Lumbar	S	S	S	S	S	S	R
	(Lumbo sacral	S	S	S	S	S	S	R
SIO	Sacroiliac							

REMARKS: *A-P and M-L control thoracolumbo-sacral Orthosis (TLSO) with abdominal corset*

KEY: Use the following symbols to indicate desired control of designated function:

F = FREE - Free motion
A = ASSIST - Application of an external force for the purpose of increasing the range, velocity, or force of a motion.
R = RESIST - Application of an external force for the purpose of decreasing the velocity or force of a motion.
S = STOP - Inclusion of a static unit to deter an undesired motion in one direction.
v = Variable - A unit that can be adjusted without making a structural change.
H = HOLD - Elimination of all motion in prescribed plane: specify position, e.g. in degrees or (+) (–).
L = LOCK - Device includes an optional lock.

Signature
Date 6/17/74

Fig. 18-7

TECHNICAL ANALYSIS FORM   SPINE   May 1974

Name _Karen Cross_   No. _15268_ Age _13_ Sex _F_ Weight _116_ Height _5'6"_

Diagnosis _Idiopathic Scoliosis_   Occupation _Student_

Present Orthotic Equipment _None_

Ambulatory ☑   Non Ambulatory ☐   Wheelchair ☐

Standing Balance: Normal ☑   Impaired ☐   Walking Aid _____

Sitting Position: Stable ☑   Unstable ☐   Reclined ☐   Upright ☐

Sitting Tolerance: Normal ☑   Limited ☐

MAJOR IMPAIRMENTS

A. Structural: No Impairment ☐

    1. Bone: Osteoporosis ☐   Fracture ☐   Level _____

          Other _Early Scheuermann's Disease_ _____

    2. Disc Space: (Describe) _____

    3. Alignment: Scoliosis ☑   Kyphosis ☐   Lordosis ☐

B. Sensory: No Impairment ☑

    1. Anesthesia ☐   Location _____

    2. Pain ☐   Location _____

C. Upper Limb: No Impairment ☑

    1. Amputation ☐ _____

    2. Other _____

D. Lower Limb: No Impairment ☑

    1. Limb Shortening: Right ☐   Left ☐   Amount _____

    2. Hip Contracture ☐   Ankylosis ☐   Flexion ☐   Degree _____

       Adduction ☐   Degree _____ ;   Abduction ☐   Degree _____ ;

       Extension ☐   Degree _____

    3. Major Motor Loss ☐   Location _____

    4. Sensation: Anesthesia ☐   Location _____ ;

       Hypesthesia ☐   Location _____

       Pain ☐   Location _____

E. Associated Impairments: _None_ _____

Fig. 18-8

CORONAL   SAGITTAL   TRANSVERSE

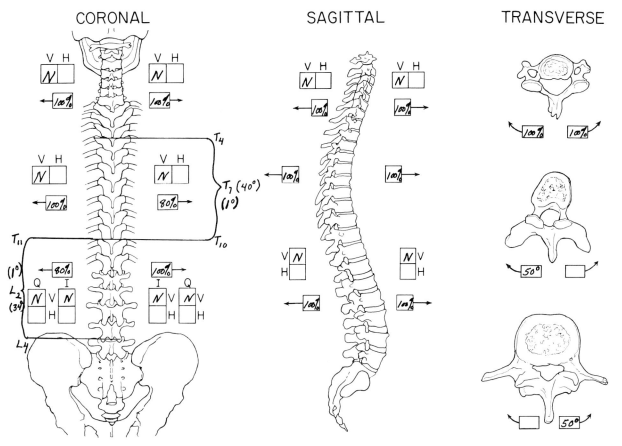

Fig. 18-9

mended to accomplish these biomechanical objectives is a thoracolumbosacral orthosis (TLSO) providing both anteroposterior and mediolateral control, utilizing an abdominal corset.

Case 2 (Figs. 18-8 to 18-10)

This 13-year-old female was seen with the diagnosis of idiopathic scoliosis. Fig. 18-8 indicates the presence of early Scheuermann's disease and the absence of any other major impairments.

Diagrammatic analysis of the spine (Fig. 18-9) details the abnormalities present. In the coronal plane, one may note a primary curve extending from T4 to T10, convex to the right, with the apex at T7 measuring 40 degrees. There is also a lumbar curve, which is also primary, extending from T11 to L4, convex to the left, with the apex at L2 measuring 34 degrees. Right lateral bending is limited to 80% of normal in the thoracic area, and left lateral bending is limited to 80% of normal in the lumbar area. Muscle strength is recorded as normal throughout. In the sagittal plane, a full range

of the cervical, thoracic, and lumbar spine is present in flexion and extension, and the flexors and extensors of the spine are normal in strength. In the transverse plane, one may note that there is a 50-degree fixed rotational deformity to the right in the thoracic area, and a 50-degree fixed rotational deformity to the left in the lumbar area.

In Fig. 18-10, the functional disability is considered to be that of progressive deformity, secondary to idiopathic scoliosis, and the orthotic objectives of treatment are spinal alignment, motion control, and axial unloading. The orthotic recommendation chart indicates that the cervical, thoracic, lumbar, and lumbosacral segments of the spine are to be controlled with an orthotic device. The types of motion control desirable at each level of the spine in each plane of movement are recorded by symbols in the chart. The orthotic device recommended to achieve these biomechanical controls is a Milwaukee brace, utilizing a throat mold, a polypropylene pelvic girdle, a right

Summary of Functional Disability: *Idiopathic Scoliosis with progressive deformity (double primary curve)*

Treatment Objectives:

Spinal Alignment ☑   Motion Control ☑
Axial Unloading ☑   Other _____

ORTHOTIC RECOMMENDATION

SPINE		FLEX	EXT	LATERAL FLEXION		ROTATION		AXIAL LOAD
				R	L	R	L	
CTLSO	Cervical	S	S	S	S	F	F	R
TLSO	Thoracic	S	S	F	S	S	F	R
LSO	Lumbar	H (+)	H (-)	S	F	F	S	R
	(Lumbo sacral)	H (+)	H (-)	H	H	H	H	R
SIO	Sacroiliac							

REMARKS: *Milwaukee Brace*
Throat Mold
Polypropylene pelvic girdle
Ⓡ thoracic pad T₈ ; Ⓛ lumbar pad L₄

KEY: Use the following symbols to indicate desired control of designated function:

F = FREE   – Free motion
A = ASSIST – Application of an external force for the purpose of increasing the range, velocity, or force of a motion.
R = RESIST – Application of an external force for the purpose of decreasing the velocity or force of a motion.
S = STOP   – Inclusion of a static unit to deter an undesired motion in one direction.
v = Variable – A unit that can be adjusted without making a structural change.
H = HOLD   – Elimination of all motion in prescribed plane: specify position, e.g. in degrees or (+) (–).
L = LOCK   – Device includes an optional lock.

_____
Signature
6/27/74
_____
Date

Fig. 18-10

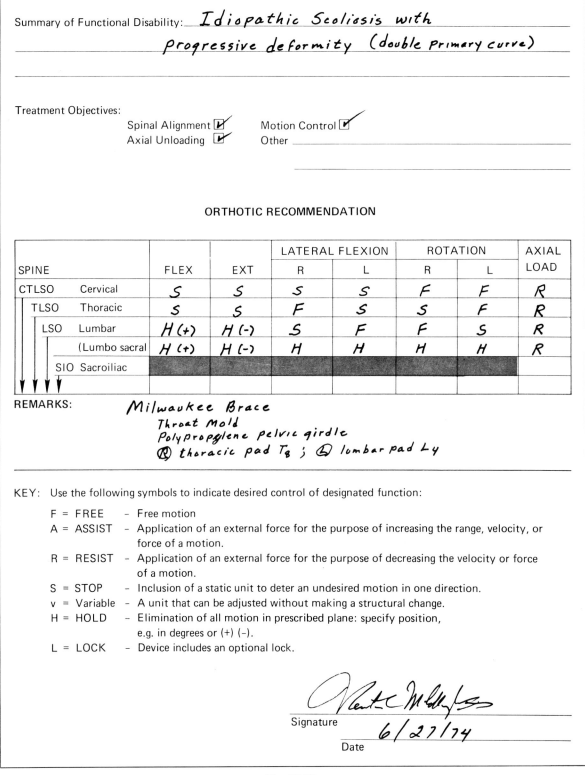

thoracic pad at the level of T8, and a left lumbar pad at the level of T4.

SUMMARY

The initial step in orthotic prescription for the spine must be the identification of abnormal biomechanical factors, for which orthotic control is desirable. The factors to be studied include strength, motion, alignment, and intrinsic disease processes, as they relate to the clinical picture of pain or deformity, or both. Diagrammatic representation of these abnormalities permits one to select better the types of motion control that are most desirable for the individual patient. The orthotic device prescribed thus represents a synthesis of the desired controls at each level of the spine in each plane of movement.

REFERENCE

1. Nash, C. L., and Moe, J. H.: A study of vertebral rotation, J. Bone Joint Surg. **51A**:223-229, 1969.

CHAPTER 19

Orthotic components and systems*

NORMAN BERGER, M.S.
RALPH LUSSKIN, M.D.

The biomechanical consequences of wearing a spinal orthosis are attributable to the fact that the orthosis applies forces to the body. The location, direction, and magnitude of these forces vary with the design of the orthosis, the tightness with which it is worn, and the patient's attempts to move against it.

As a result of force application, virtually all orthotic designs produce three effects:

1. The effectiveness of the abdominal musculature in elevating intracavitary pressure is significantly increased.
2. The ability of the trunk to move is restricted.
3. Skeletal alignment is modified.

In turn, these general effects have many specific physiologic consequences, which are discussed in the following chapter.

Forty or more orthosis designs can be easily identified through perusal of the literature in this field, but it is not possible to determine why components are differentially located and shaped. Rationales either conflict or, more often, do not exist. Additional designs and variations are currently being developed and evaluated.

Despite this proliferation, most physicians use a very small number of different orthoses. A recent survey of the orthopedic community in the United States[4] found that only two designs are widely prescribed in the treatment of low back disorders. These are the Knight and chairback, mentioned by 54% of the responding orthopedists, and the Williams, mentioned by 19%. Though the survey produced a listing of many other orthoses, none of these was mentioned by more than 4.6% of the respondents. It should be noted that the corset was also widely prescribed in the management of low back pain. The quoted figures, however, refer only to preferences among the rigid spinal orthoses.

This chapter presents the components of spinal orthoses and a limited number of orthosis designs composed of the described components. Though the number of designs is small, they form a logical, cumulative system in terms of their biomechanical functions.

COMPONENTS OF SPINAL ORTHOSES

This presentation of spinal components emphasizes their relationship to skeletal and other anatomic landmarks. The purpose of this emphasis is clear. The effectiveness of an orthosis is directly related to the proper fit and alignment of its components, and hence the evaluation of an orthosis requires an understanding of these same principles.

---

*This chapter is based in part on material previously published in the manual *Spinal Orthotics,* printed by New York University Post-Graduate Medical School, Prosthetics and Orthotics, Sept. 1973.

Pelvic band
Alignment and location

1. The lateral ends of the band fall midway between the trochanters and the iliac crests. This position avoids bony prominences and provides an attachment for a pelvic strap that is as low as possible consistent with sitting comfort. This low attachment also helps prevent upward displacement of the brace caused by abdominal protrusion below the abdominal support.

2. The lateral ends of the band extend to the midtrochanteric line to prevent lateral shift of the brace.

3. Posteriorly, the middle section of the band lies above the inferior edge of the sacrum and below the posterosuperior iliac spines. To achieve an efficient distal pressure point, the band should be as low as possible on the sacrum within the limits of comfort and cosmetic acceptability. This section of the band may be tilted slightly, particularly if the sacrum itself is abnormally tilted as in pronounced lordosis. The tilt of the band, however, cannot equal the tilt of the sacrum, since sitting would then be uncomfortable.

4. Just lateral to the sacrum the band dips slightly to increase contact area for lower unit pressures. In these posterolateral sections the band should be as vertical as possible to minimize upward displacement of the brace caused by the buttock bulging below the pelvic band when the patient sits.

Material and dimensions

Aluminum alloy, 2024-T3
Width: 1⅝ inches ± ¼ inch
Thickness: 0.063 to 0.081 inch

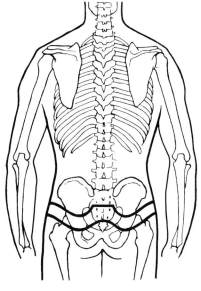

Fig. 19-1. Pelvic band.

Thoracic band

Alignment and location

1. The superior border is at level of T9-T10, approximately 1 inch below the inferior angles of the scapulae. In current practice, thoracic bands are often placed up to 3 inches below the inferior angles, depending on the physician's preference and local custom. The higher band placement recommended here probably results in sightly greater restriction of motion in the lumbar spine and more effective reduction of lordosis.
2. The lateral ends are at the lateral midlines of the rib cage (midaxillary lines).
3. The band is horizontal as worn.

Material and dimensions

Aluminum alloy, 2024-T3
Width: 1⅝ inches ± ¼ inch
Thickness: 0.063 to 0.081 inch

Anterior extensions of thoracic band with subclavicular pads (Cowhorns)

Alignment and location

1. The band extends horizontally forward before curving up around the pectoralis major.
2. The superior border extends to approximately ½ inch below the clavicle when the patient sits.
3. The lateral border extends to a point just medial to the deltopectoral groove so as not to interfere with arm motions.
4. The subclavicular pads are about 2 inches in diameter for the average adult and may be pivotable.
5. To maintain their position, centers of pads are joined by a strap, which may be lowered for cosmetic purposes.

Material and dimensions

Aluminum alloy, 2024-T3
Width: 1⅛ inches ± ¼ inch
Thickness: 0.125 inch

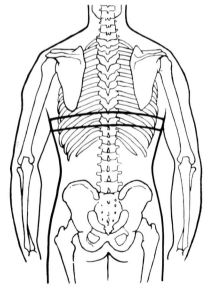

Fig. 19-2. Thoracic band.

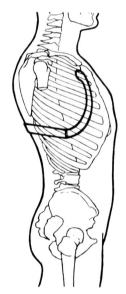

Fig. 19-3. Anterior extensions of thoracic band with subclavicular pads.

Lumbosacral and thoracolumbosacral posterior uprights
Alignment and location

1. The superior ends of lumbosacral uprights are at the superior edge of the thoracic band, 1 inch below the inferior angles of the scapulae. The superior ends of thoracolumbosacral uprights are at the level of the lateral aspects of scapular spines. ✓
2. The inferior ends are at the level of the inferior edge of the pelvic band at its posterior midline.
3. There is spacing of the uprights.
   a. The distance between the medial edges of the uprights is 2 inches ± ½ inch.
   b. The apices of the paraspinal muscle bulges, when palpable, are an excellent guide to spacing of the uprights.
   c. Uprights must avoid contacting bony prominences, particularly the vertebral spines and the posterosuperior iliac spines.

Material and dimensions

Aluminum alloy, 2024-T4
Width: ¾ inch ± ⅛ inch
Thickness: $3/16$ ± $1/16$ inch

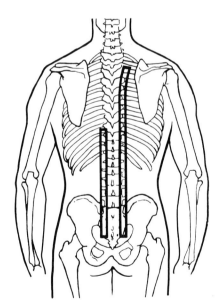

Fig. 19-4. Lumbosacral and thoracolumbosacral uprights.

Lateral uprights
Alignment and location

1. The superior ends are at the superior edge of the thoracic band. ✓
2. The inferior ends are at the inferior edge of the pelvic band. ✓
3. They extend along the lateral midlines of the torso, best approximated by a line from midtrochanter to midaxilla.

Material and dimensions

Aluminum alloy, 2024-T4
Width: ⅝ inch ± ⅛ inch
Thickness: $3/16$ inch ± $1/16$ inch

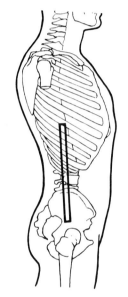

Fig. 19-5. Lateral uprights.

Oblique lateral uprights

Alignment and location

1. The superior ends are pivotably attached to the lateral uprights, approximately 1 inch below the inferior border of the thoracic band. ✓

2. The inferior ends are rigidly attached to the pelvic band at the posterolateral sections of the band.

Allows Flexion

Material and dimensions

Aluminum or stainless steel
Width: ⅝ inch ± ⅛ inch
Thickness: ³/₁₆ inch ± ¹/₁₆ inch

Interscapular band

Alignment and location

1. It extends from 2 inches medial to axillary fold horizontally to the same point on the other side.

2. It crosses the distal third of the scapulae, with inferior edge approximately 1 inch above inferior angles. This location is designed to place the axillary strap attachments slightly above the posterior margin of the axillary fold, which helps prevent upward displacement of the brace. ✓

Material and dimensions

Aluminum alloy, 2024-T3, or stainless steel
Width: 1 inch ± ⅛ inch
Thickness: 0.062 inch in stainless steel to 0.081 inch in aluminum

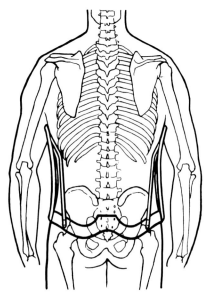

Fig. 19-6. Oblique lateral uprights.

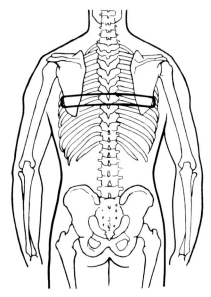

Fig. 19-7. Interscapular band.

Full-front abdominal support

Superior border

½ inch below the xiphoid process. ✓

Inferior border

½ inch above the symphysis pubis, from which point the inferior border roughly parallels the inguinal ligament line.

Lateral borders

It extends to the lateral midlines or to the lateral uprights, except for space required by adjustment straps or laces.

Straps for full-front abdominal support

Pelvic strap

1. It is attached to each end of the pelvic band.
2. It is attached to the apron approximately 1 inch above inferior border.

Waist strap

1. Loop attachments to posterior uprights permit up and down adjustment on the patient (they may also have a fixed attachment to the uprights).
2. It passes between the iliac crests and the rib cage.

Thoracic strap

1. It is attached to each end of the thoracic band or, if no thoracic band, to the posterior uprights.
2. It is attached to the superior border of the apron.

Additional fourth strap

If the patient is tall, an additional fourth strap is used to avoid gapping and wrinkling of abdominal support.

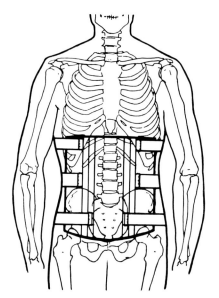

Fig. 19-8. Abdominal support.

SPINAL ORTHOTIC SYSTEMS

Since March 1971, the Task Force on Standardization of Prosthetics-Orthotics Terminology has been attempting to develop a logical nomenclature to enhance communication in this field. The task force has recommended[1] that orthoses be described by the joints they encompass and by analysis of their control of joint motion.

In accord with these recommendations, the four types of orthoses discussed in this chapter are sacroiliac (SIO), lumbosacral (LSO), thoracolumbosacral (TLSO) and cervical orthoses (CO). The orthoses are further described by the letters *F* (free motion) or *S* (stop motion), which denote the degree of motion control. However, *F* does not imply total freedom. Rather, it means a restriction of motion minor enough to be ignored as a function of the orthosis and as a limitation on patient mobility. Also, *S* does not imply complete stoppage or restriction. Rather, it means that the orthosis is designed to *deter* the particular motion.

Probably the majority of patients (perhaps too many patients) are fitted with prefabricated orthoses taken from stock or ordered according to measurements. There are two problems with this approach. First, the orthotic facility must maintain a large and uneconomic inventory to provide rapid service and, second, even with access to large inventories, it is difficult to assure accurately fitted orthoses for the wide variety of figures and body types presented by patients. Custom fabrication and fitting of an orthosis solves these problems and is therefore considered a preferable procedure except where specifically stated otherwise in the following pages. In any case, we wish to stress the importance of proper fitting. The same standards of accuracy should be applied to all orthoses whether custom fitted or prefabricated.

Type: LSO
Name: Lumbosacral flexion-extension control orthosis
(chairback)

			Lateral	Flex	Rotation	
	Flex	Ext	R	L	R	L
Lumbar	S	S	S*	S*	S*	S*
Lumbosacral	S	S	S*	S*	S*	S*

＊ An intermediate degree of motion control, less than S but more than F.

Biomechanical: It provides a three-point pressure system consisting of posteriorly directed forces from the pelvic and thoracic straps and an anteriorly directed force from the posterior uprights in the lumbar area. This system tends to limit trunk flexion occurring in the lumbar spine. A second three-point pressure system, consisting of a posteriorly directed force from the abdominal support and anteriorly directed forces from the pelvic and thoracic bands, tends to limit trunk extension occurring in the lumbar spine and to reduce lordosis. Forces from the abdominal support assist the abdominal musculature to increase intra-abdominal pressure.[2] Lateral trunk motions may be slightly restricted if the pelvic and thoracic bands are sufficiently rigid.

Design and fabrication: Two lumbosacral posterior uprights are attached inferiorly to a pelvic band and superiorly to a thoracic band. A full-front abdominal support is attached to the aluminum frame by means of straps. Measurements and tracings are used as guides in fabrication and final adjustments are made on the patient.[5]

Special considerations:

1. Sufficient clearance should be provided between the posterior uprights and the patient's back so as to allow for reduction of lordosis when the abdominal support is tightened. Additional clearance is needed to permit comfortable sitting.

2. In place of the full-front abdominal support and related straps, a corset may be worn over the orthosis.

3. For patients with pendulous breasts or kyphosis, or whose xiphoid process is considerably lower than the inferior angles of the scapulae, the lateral ends of the thoracic band must be lowered so that the thoracic strap and the top of the abdominal support are ½ inch below the xiphoid level. The center of the thoracic band remains high, 1 inch below the inferior angles of the scapulae.

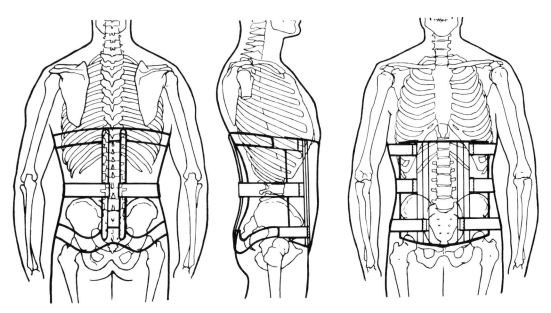

Fig. 19-9. Lumbosacral flexion-extension control orthosis (chairback).

Type: LSO

Name: Lumbosacral flexion-extension and lateral control orthosis (Knight)

	Flex	Ext	Lateral Flex		Rotation	
			R	L	R	L
Lumbar	S	S	S	S	S*	S*
Lumbosacral	S	S	S	S	S*	S*

* An intermediate degree of motion control, less than S but more than F.

Biomechanical: It provides a three-point pressure system consisting of posteriorly directed forces from the pelvic and thoracic straps and an anteriorly directed force from the posterior uprights in the lumbar area. This system tends to limit trunk flexion occurring in the lumbar spine. A second three-point pressure system, consisting of a posteriorly directed force from the abdominal support and anteriorly directed forces from the pelvic and thoracic bands, tends to limit trunk extension occurring in the lumbar spine and to reduce lordosis. Forces from the abdominal support assist the abdominal musculature to increase intra-abdominal pressure. Since the ends of the pelvic and thoracic bands are anchored by the lateral uprights, medially directed forces are applied, which restrict lateral trunk motions.

Design and fabrication: Pelvic and thoracic bands are connected by a pair of lumbosacral posterior uprights and a pair of lateral uprights. A full-front abdominal support or a corset front is attached to the aluminum frame by means of straps or laces. Measurements and tracings are used as guides in fabrication and final adjustments are made on the patient.

Special considerations: The lateral uprights must be fitted carefully as they pass over the iliac crests so as to avoid pressure on these bony prominences.

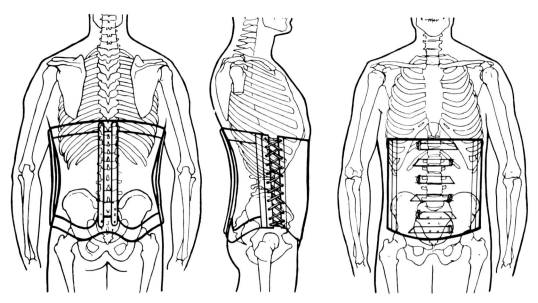

Fig. 19-10. Lumbosacral flexion-extension and lateral control orthosis (Knight).

Type: LSO

Name: Lumbosacral extension and lateral control orthosis (Williams)

			Lateral	Flex	Rotation	
	Flex	Ext	R	L	R	L
Lumbar	F	S	S	S	S*	S*
Lumbosacral	F	S	S	S	S*	S*

* An intermediate degree of motion control, less than S but more than F.

Biomechanical: It provides a three-point pressure system consisting of a posteriorly directed force from the pelvic adjustment strap and anteriorly directed forces from the pelvic and thoracic bands. This pressure system tends to limit trunk extension occurring in the lumbar spine and to reduce lordosis. Forces from the abdominal support assist the abdominal musculature to increase intra-abdominal pressure. The ends of the pelvic and thoracic bands provide medially directed forces that tend to limit lateral trunk motions.

Design and fabrication: Pelvic and thoracic bands are joined by a pair of lateral uprights that are pivotably attached to the thoracic band, but not attached to the pelvic band. The pelvic band is stabilized by a pair of oblique lateral uprights pivotably attached to the lateral uprights and rigidly attached to the pelvic band. An *elastic* abdominal corset is laced to the lateral uprights and a pelvic adjustment strap is provided to tighten the orthosis by pulling the free distal ends of the lateral uprights posteriorly.

Special considerations: For maximum reduction of lordosis, extension control, and abdominal support, a pad may be inserted in the pelvic adjustment strap. The pad fits between the anterosuperior iliac spines and just above the symphysis pubis.

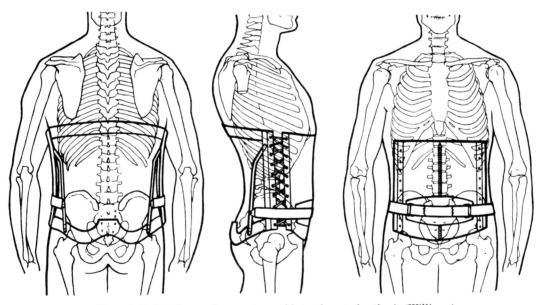

Fig. 19-11. Lumbosacral extension and lateral control orthosis (Williams).

Type: TLSO

Name: Thoracolumbosacral flexion-extension control orthosis (Taylor)

	Flex	Ext	Lateral Flex		Rotation	
			R	L	R	L
Thoracic	S*	S*	F	F	F	F
Lumbar	S*	S*	F	F	F	F
Lumbosacral	**	**	F	F	F	F

* An intermediate degree of motion control, less than S but more than F.
** Compensatory increase in motion.

Biomechanical: It provides a three-point pressure system consisting of posteriorly directed forces from the axillary and pelvic straps and an anteriorly directed force from the posterior uprights in the thoracolumbar area. This system tends to limit trunk flexion occurring in the thoracolumbar and upper lumbar areas. A second three-point pressure system, consisting of a posteriorly directed force from the abdominal support and anteriorly directed forces from the pelvic and interscapular bands and the posterior uprights, tends to limit trunk extension in the thoracolumbar and upper lumbar regions. The flexion-extension restriction causes a compensatory increase in motion at the lumbosacral junction and lower lumbar spine.[3] Forces from the abdominal support assist the abdominal musculature to elevate intra-abdominal pressure.

Design and fabrication: Two thoracolumbosacral posterior uprights are attached inferiorly to a pelvic band. Superiorly, an interscapular band stabilizes the uprights and serves as an attachment for axillary straps. It includes a corset, as illustrated, or a full-front abdominal support and related straps. The axillary straps are attached to the superior ends of the uprights and extend anteriorly over the shoulder and posteriorly under the axilla to pivotable roller loops at the ends of the interscapular band. The straps reverse through the roller loops and run anteriorly to fasten to each other on the chest. The illustrated alternative fastening is by means of webbing buckles at the ends of the interscapular band, thus eliminating the chest strap.

Special considerations:

1. If necessary, comfort may be enhanced by the removal of the axillary straps and substitution of a sternal plate, which eliminates axillary chafing and allows freer arm motion at the expense of increased bulk on the chest.

2. A thoracic band may be added to the orthosis if upward displacement is a troublesome problem. The band also provides a slight tendency to limit rotation and lateral trunk motions.

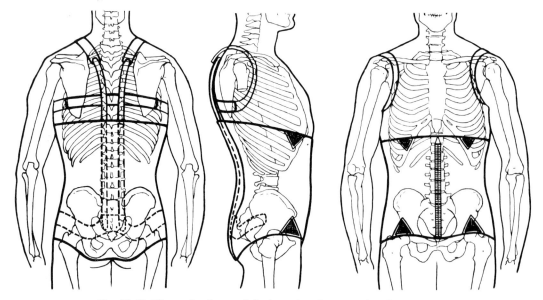

Fig. 19-12. Thoracolumbosacral flexion-extension control orthosis (Taylor).

Type: TLSO

Name: Thoracolumbosacral flexion-extension and lateral control orthosis (Knight-Taylor)

	Flex	Ext	Lateral Flex		Rotation	
			R	L	R	L
Thoracic	S*	S*	S*	S*	F	F
Lumbar	S	S	S	S	S*	S*
Lumbosacral	**	**	S	S	S*	S*

* An intermediate degree of motion control, less than S but more than F.
** Compensatory increase in motion.

Biomechanical: It provides a three-point pressure system consisting of posteriorly directed forces from the axillary straps and the lower portion of the abdominal support and an anteriorly directed force from the posterior uprights in the thoracolumbar area. This system tends to limit trunk flexion occurring in the thoracolumbar and upper lumbar areas. A second three-point pressure system, consisting of a posteriorly directed force from the abdominal support and anteriorly directed forces from the pelvic and interscapular bands and the posterior uprights, tends to limit trunk extension in the thoracolumbar and upper lumbar regions. The flexion-extension restriction causes a compensatory increase in motion at the lumbosacral junction and lower lumbar spine. Forces from the abdominal support assist the abdominal musculature to elevate intra-abdominal pressure. Since the ends of the pelvic and thoracic bands are anchored by lateral uprights, rotation and lateral trunk motions are restricted.

Design and fabrication: Pelvic and thoracic bands are connected by a pair of thoracolumbosacral posterior uprights and a pair of lateral uprights. An interscapular band is fastened to the posterior uprights and serves as an attachment for axillary straps. A corset front is laced to the lateral uprights.

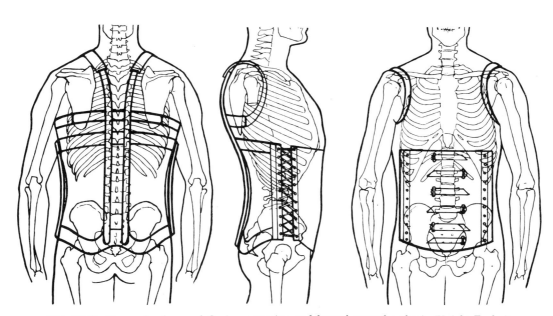

Fig. 19-13. Thoracolumbosacral flexion-extension and lateral control orthosis (Knight-Taylor).

Type: TLSO

Name: Thoracolumbosacral flexion, lateral and rotary control orthosis (cowhorn)

	Flex	Ext	Lateral Flex		Rotation	
			R	L	R	L
Thoracic	S	F	S*	S*	S	S
Lumbar	S	S	S	S	S	S
Lumbosacral	**	S	S	S	S	S

* An intermediate degree of motion control, less than S but more than F.
** Compensatory increase in motion.

Biomechanical: It provides a three-point pressure system consisting of posteriorly directed forces from the subclavicular pads and the abdominal support and an anteriorly directed force from the thoracic band. This system tends to limit trunk flexion occurring in the thoracic and upper lumbar spine. Forces from the abdominal support assist the abdominal musculature to elevate intra-abdominal pressure, and lateral motions are restricted by the stabilized ends of the thoracic and pelvic bands. The lower lumbar and lumbosacral areas display a compensatory increase in flexion but are restricted in extension by a pressure system consisting of anteriorly directed forces from the pelvic and thoracic bands and a posteriorly directed force from the abdominal support. Finally, rotary control is achieved by two force couples: (1) a posteriorly directed force to the pectoral area by the subclavicular pad and an anteriorly directed force to the contralateral dorsal area by the thoracic band, (2) a posteriorly directed force to the pelvis by the lower portion of the corset front on the side opposite to the operative subclavicular pad and an anteriorly directed force to the pelvis by the pelvic band on the same side as the operative subclavicular pad.

Design and fabrication: Pelvic and thoracic bands are connected by a pair of lumbosacral posterior uprights and a pair of lateral uprights. A corset front is laced to the lateral uprights. The thoracic band is extended anteriorly and superiorly, and subclavicular pads are provided.

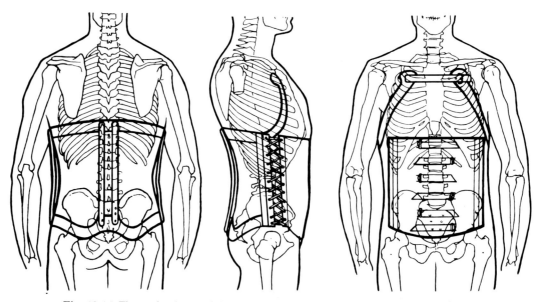

Fig. 19-14. Thoracolumbosacral flexion, lateral, and rotary control orthosis (cowhorn).

Type: TLSO

Name: Thoracolumbosacral flexion control orthosis (Jewett, or anterior hyperextension)

	Flex	Ext	Lateral Flex		Rotation	
			R	L	R	L
Thoracic	S	F	F — S*	F — S*	F — S*	F — S*
Lumbar	S	F	F — S*	F — S*	F — S*	F — S*
Lumbosacral	Insufficient data to specify					

∗ Control of lateral motions and rotation depends on the degree of hyperextension maintained by the orthosis.

Biomechanical: It provides a three-point pressure system consisting of posteriorly directed forces from the sternal pad and the suprapubic pad and an anteriorly directed force from the thoracolumbar pad. This pressure system encourages hyperextension and tends to restrict flexion occurring in the thoracolumbar area. Creation of a hyperextension posture tends to increase lumbar lordosis.

Design and fabrication: This prefabricated orthosis, which is ordered by measurements and adjusted on the patient, consists of an anterior and lateral torso frame to which are attached two lateral pads, a sternal pad, a suprapubic pad, and a posterior thoracolumbar pad. Control of flexion is achieved by the pads only; the frame should not contact the patient. With the patient seated in prescribed posture and the orthosis properly adjusted and aligned, the sternal pad will have its superior border ½ inch inferior to the sternal notch and the suprapubic pad will have its inferior border ½ inch superior to the symphysis pubis.

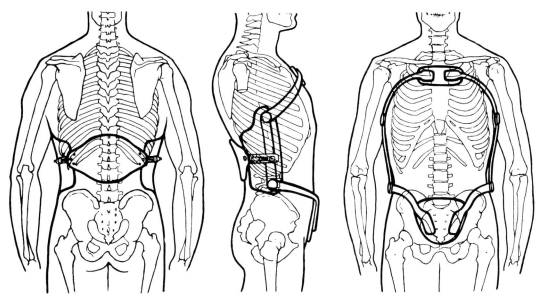

Fig. 19-15. Thoracolumbosacral flexion control orthosis (Jewett or anterior hyperextension).

FLEXIBLE SPINAL ORTHOSES: CORSETS AND BELTS

The previously mentioned survey of the orthopedic community in the United States[4] demonstrated the wide use of flexible orthoses (corsets). As a general preference in the management of low back disorders, 46.6% of the responding orthopedists chose corsets, as compared to 39.0% who preferred rigid orthoses and 14.4% who preferred casts.

Type: Flexible LSO
Name: Lumbosacral corset

	Flex	Ext	Lateral Flex		Rotation	
			R	L	R	L
Lumbar	F — S*	F — S*	F — S*	F — S*	F	F
Lumbosacral	F — S*	F — S*	F — S*	F — S*	F	F

* Degree of motion deterrence is variable and determined by the number, location, and rigidity of vertical stays in the orthosis.

Biomechanical: Anterior and lateral trunk containment assists the abdominal musculature to elevate intracavity pressure. Depending on vertical stays, three-point pressure systems that tend to restrict spinal motions are applied.

Design and fabrication: This orthosis is essentially a cloth garment that wraps around the torso and hips and is adjustable in circumference by means of side, front, or back laces or hooks. Anteriorly, the superior border is ½ inch below the xiphoid process or above the lower ribs, and the inferior border is ½ to 1 inch above the symphysis pubis. Posteriorly, the superior border is 1 inch below the inferior angles of the scapulae, and the inferior border is just below the apex of the gluteal bulge for men and at the gluteal fold for women. The corset is usually a stock garment that should snugly fit all body contours. Wrinkles, failure to maintain position, and discomfort require tucks or alterations for proper fit. If a stock garment cannot be used, a custom corset should be fabricated based upon a pattern derived from careful measurement of the individual patient.

Special considerations: Additions that may be necessary include posterior rigid or semirigid steels, posterior pads or shingles, extra abdominal reinforcements, and a thoracic extension with shoulder straps. Posterior steels should be shaped so as to flatten (not maintain) lumbar lordosis.

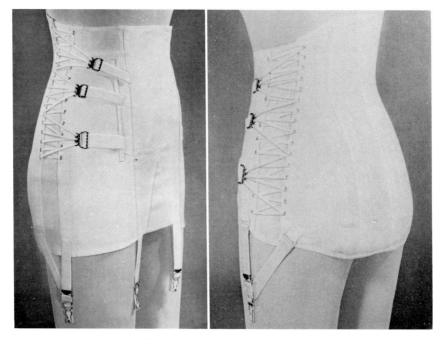

Fig. 19-16. Lumbosacral corset.

Type: Flexible LSO
Name: Lumbosacral belt (high sacroiliac belt)

	Flex	Ext	Lateral Flex		Rotation	
			R	L	R	L
Lumbar	F	F	F	F	F	F
Lumbosacral	F	F	F	F	F	F

Biomechanical: Although not effective in restricting motion, this orthosis does assist in elevating intra-abdominal pressure and may be useful in the obese to support a pendulous abdomen.

Design and fabrication: A cloth garment that wraps around the pelvis and lower abdomen and is adjustable in circumference by means of side, front, or back laces or hooks. Anteriorly and posteriorly, the superior border is at iliac crest level. Anteriorly, the inferior border is ½ to 1 inch above the symphysis pubis, and posteriorly, it extends to the apex of the gluteal bulge. For cosmetic reasons, the superior border may rise to jut above waist level and the inferior border may descend to the gluteal fold, thus reducing bulging. This orthosis is prefabricated and may require tucks or alterations for a comfortable fit.

Special considerations: Additions that may be necessary include posterior rigid or semirigid steels, posterior sacral pads, and extra abdominal reinforcements.

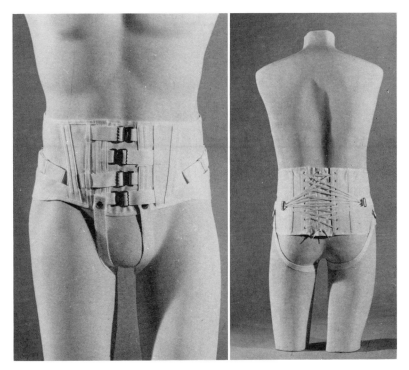

Fig. 19-17. Lumbosacral belt (high sacroiliac belt).

Type: Flexible SIO
Name: Sacroiliac belt

Biomechanical: It partially stabilizes sacroiliac joints and the symphysis pubis.

Design and fabrication: This prefabricated belt (2 to 4 inches wide) encircles the pelvis between the iliac crests and the trochanters.

Special considerations: Used in postpartum and post-traumatic separations of sacroiliac joints and symphysis pubis.

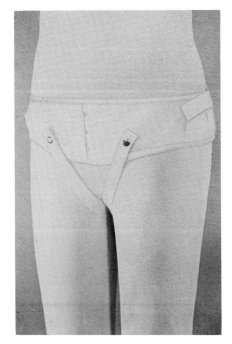

Fig. 19-18. Sacroiliac belt.

CERVICAL ORTHOSES

There are three basic designs of cervical orthoses: orthopedic collars, poster appliances, and custom-molded devices. All these serve as reminders to restrict head and neck motions. In addition, depending on the design and fit of the particular orthosis, they can impose forces to position the head according to prescription (if the muscles are not spastic and the deformity is not rigid); to mechanically limit flexion, extension, rotation, and lateral flexion of the head and cervical spine; and to partially unload the cervical spine by supporting a portion of the weight of the head.

Type: CO

Name: Cervical flexion control orthosis (orthopaedic collar)

	Flex	Ext	Lateral Flex		Rotation		Axial Load
			R	L	R	L	
Cervical	S* or S	F or S*	S*	S*	F	F	F

* An intermediate degree of motion control, less than S but more than F.

Biomechanical: Through sensory feedback, orthopaedic collars serve as a reminder to limit head and neck motions and mechanically restrict flexion of the cervical spine.

Design and fabrication: These are essentially prefabricated devices that wrap around the neck and are adjustable circumferentially. They may also have provision for height adjustment and for single or multiple layers and are of variable softness. Construction materials include sponge, felt, foam (Fig. 19-19, *A*), polyethylene (Fig. 19-19, *B*), and other plastics.

Special considerations: Depending on the padding and contour of both the orthosis and the patient, prefabricated orthopaedic collars may be difficult to fit comfortably. Such problems should be solved by custom fabrication of a collar based on a pattern made for the individual patient.

For maximum control, a chin support (plastic cup) may be added to the hard collar.

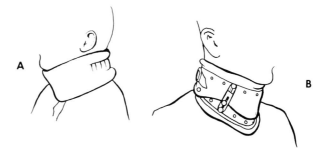

Fig. 19-19. Cervical flexion control orthosis (orthopaedic collar). **A,** Soft collar (foam). **B,** Hard collar (polyethylene).

Type: CO

Name: Cervical flexion-extension control orthosis (poster appliance)

			Lateral	Flex	Rotation		Axial
	Flex	Ext	R	L	R	L	Load
Cervical	S	S	S*	S*	S*	S*	R**

* An intermediate degree of motion control, less than S but more than F.

** Amount of axial load resistance depends on the length of the uprights.

Biomechanical: It applies forces under the chin and occiput to restrict flexion and extension of the head and cervical spine. These forces also tend to limit lateral flexion and rotation. Since the distances between the chin support and sternal plate and between the occipital support and thoracic plate are easily varied, the orthosis can be adjusted to position the head as required and to partially relieve the cervical spine of a portion of the weight of the head.

Design and fabrication: These prefabricated orthoses include an anterior section, consisting of a sternal plate, one or two uprights, and a chin support, and a posterior section, consisting of a thoracic plate, one or two uprights, and an occipital support. Usually, the two sections are connected by flexible straps between the chin and occipital supports and by over-the-shoulder straps between the thoracic and sternal plates. The uprights are adjustable for height, and additional fitting flexibility is obtained by built-in swivel arrangements or by bending of parts. The orthosis is commonly made of aluminum with leather or plastic padding of parts that touch the body.

Special considerations:

1. If, for a variety of reasons, this orthosis cannot be tolerated, the same functions can be provided (though to a lesser degree) by adding chin and occipital supports to a hard orthopedic collar.
2. Control of motion can be increased by adding a rigid attachment between the chin and occipital supports.
3. Thoracic extension can be added to provide increased support and rotary control. However this may impart undesired thoracic movement to the head.

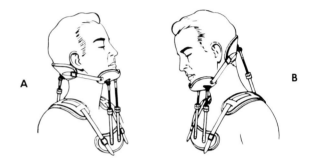

Fig. 19-20. Cervical flexion-extension control orthosis (poster appliance). **A,** Cervical spine in slight extension with head erect. **B,** Cervical spine in flexion with chin depressed.

Type: CO

Name: Cervical flexion-extension, lateral, and rotary control orthosis (custom-molded appliance)

			Lateral	Flex	Rotation		Axial Load
	Flex	Ext	R	L	R	L	
Cervical	S	S	S	S	S	S	R*

* Amount of axial load resistance depends on the length of the uprights of the poster appliance and the fit and padding of the molded appliance.

Biomechanical: It applies forces under and around the chin and occiput to restrict flexion and extension, lateral motions, and rotation of the head and cervical spine. It also positions the head as required and relieves a portion of the weight of the head from the cervical spine.

Design and fabrication: The custom-molded appliance requires a modified positive cast over which leather (reinforced when necessary) or plastic is molded or laminated. The cuirass type extends to the chin and mastoid line, whereas the Minerva type encloses the occiput posteriorly and includes a band around the forehead.

Special considerations: Since the molded appliance involves a difficult fabrication procedure, the same functions can be accomplished (though probably to a lesser degree) by a custom-fitted poster appliance with larger and more intimately contoured chin and occipital supports connected by a rigid bar. For still greater control, a thoracic band attached to the thoracic plate by a rigid upright may be added.

REFERENCES

1. Harris, E. E.: A new orthotics terminology, Orthot. Prosthet. **27**(2):6-19, June 1973.
2. Morris, J. M., Lucas, D., and Bresler, B.: Role of the trunk in stability of the spine, J. Bone Joint Surg. **43A**:327, 1961.
3. Norton, P. L., and Brown, T.: The immobilizing efficiency of back braces, J. Bone Joint Surg. **39A**:111, 1957.
4. Perry, J.: The use of external support in the treatment of low-back pain, J. Bone Joint Surg. **52A**:1440-1442, Oct. 1970.
5. Spinal orthotics, New York University Post-Graduate Medical School, Prosthetics and Orthotics, New York, 1973.

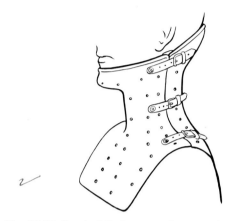

Fig. 19-20. Cervical flexion-extension control orthosis (poster appliance). **A,** Cervical spine in slight extension with head erect. **B,** Cervical spine in flexion with chin depressed.

CHAPTER 20

Prescription principles

RALPH LUSSKIN, M.D.
NORMAN BERGER, M.S.

The proper use of a spinal orthosis requires an understanding of the pathophysiology of the disorder to be treated and an accurate assessment of the effects of the orthosis, both negative and positive. The pathologic condition of many affections of the spine and its supporting mechanisms is obscure, making analysis of the effects of an orthotic device difficult. There is, nevertheless, a rational approach to the application of orthoses that makes full use of our current knowledge of biomechanics.

POSITIVE BIOMECHANICAL EFFECTS

There are three positive effects of spinal orthoses that comprise the physiologic basis for the use of these devices. They are trunk support, motion control, and spinal realignment.

Trunk support

Trunk support is accomplished by two mechanisms: elevations of intracavity pressure and application of a three-point pressure system. The first of these is by far the more important. Enhancement of the thoracoabdominal hydropneumatic support mechanism by anterior, lateral, and posterolateral trunk containment effectively reduces both the functional demand on the spinal extensor musculature and the vertical loading of the thoracic and lumbar spine. Morris[2] documented the role of the orthosis as a substitute for

the abdominal musculature in elevating internal pressure and calculated the consequent reduction in force on the spine. It is also well known that rehabilitative exercise programs directed at the abdominal and gluteal musculature improve trunk stability and alignment and similarly reduce functional demands on the axial musculoskeletal structures, with concomitant reduction of spinal pain in many instances.

Trunk support by mechanical three-point or regional pressure systems is of less importance, for once the trunk is vertical, there is usually little horizontal or vertical loading of the orthosis. In the presence of trunk paralysis, however, the tendency for the trunk to deviate will persist and three-point or multiple-regional pressure will be required to maintain alignment.

Motion control

That gross trunk motion is reduced by both flexible and rigid spinal orthoses is quite evident. However, quantitative analysis of the degree of motion control, particularly intersegmental, by specific orthoses, has been difficult and complete data are not yet available.

There are two mechanisms for the restraint of spinal motion:

1. Mechanical three-point pressure systems, such as those produced by rigid orthoses, stabilize the spine between the end points of the mechanical

364

system. There is some evidence, however, that intersegmental motion may be increased at the ends of the stabilized trunk segments when trunk movement is attempted.[3]

2. Irritative restraint of gross trunk movement is an important effect of all spinal orthoses. The sensation of wearing any of these devices serves as a powerful inhibiting factor and in many situations is the only significant determinant of motion restraint. "Reminder" or "inductive" bracing are terms sometimes used to describe this effect.

Whether irritative or mechanical, restriction of motion is an important goal in diseases of the spinal articulations and intervertebral discs.

It is important to distinguish between motion control and trunk support. In many disorders, if trunk support by thoracoabdominal containment is sufficient to reduce compressive forces on the spinal column and to reduce demands on spinal musculature, joint stabilization need not be required from the orthosis. Within the possibilities permitted by the available braces and corsets, one must seek the minimum restriction required in each instance.

Spinal realignment

Realignment of the spine is accomplished by three-point pressure systems and also by the stimulation of muscle action patterns in withdrawal from an uncomfortable pressure point. Three-point pressure systems are used to produce a shift of gravitational forces from diseased to more normal skeletal components. For example, extension of the trunk produces weight transfer to the posterior elements and away from the vertebral bodies, whereas flexion causes weight transfer to the vertebral bodies and anterior portions of the intervertebral discs, away from the posterior elements.

NEGATIVE EFFECTS

In addition to the foregoing positive results of orthosis application, it is essential to be aware of the following four negative effects of spinal bracing:

1. Muscle atrophy and weakness occur after reduced functional demand. Thoracoabdominal containment and restricted spinal motion reduce the amount of muscular activity required to maintain the erect trunk and reduce total body activity as the patient is psychologically restrained. Although this may often improve symptoms and

induce a recovery phase, it also produces the rapid onset of weakness. The weakness may lead to an early return of symptoms when treatment is discontinued, or make the patient more vulnerable to a recurrence of pain at a later date. The debilitating effect of trunk immobilization, often added to preexisting weakness, may lead to a cycle of pain-treatment-improvement-pain.

Atrophy occurs after prolonged disuse. This implies the structural alterations at a subcellular level that have been shown to develop in atrophying muscle. Mere disuse induces changes in muscle that are indistinguishable from those seen in muscle dystrophies. This problem is easier to prevent than to treat, especially when emotional factors have been added to the structural changes. Many spinal stabilization operations have failed because of these factors, though the skeletal problem was apparently well corrected.

Atrophy should be avoided by maintaining an isometric exercise regimen to the limits of the patient's tolerance while the orthosis is being used, and by the early gradual discontinuation of trunk support as soon as conditions permit.

2. Tightness and contracture occur after immobilization and atrophy. Progressive fibrosis of muscles, fascias, and ligaments are well known sequelae of spinal immobilization. Once developed, this fibrosis may defy intensive treatment. To avoid this, start rehabilitation at the same time that immobilization is instituted, not some months or years later.

3. Psychologic dependence occurs after and enhances physical dependence. Profound emotional disorders often lie beneath the surface of the personality. At times true neurosis develops quickly after injury, and even psychotic patterns may emerge. The laborer is just as vulnerable as the executive and may face more real danger on his return to work. Such problems must be considered at the onset of therapy or they will soon transcend the original disease.

Emotional problems may be enhanced by overtreatment. This means that any treatment modality must be discontinued before it further supports emotional symptom complexes. Early recognition of the problem and termination of nontherapeutic therapy is the best way to avoid trouble. This applies not only to spinal orthotics, but to such modalities as diathermy, ultrasound, massage, and sedatives. Whenever a third party is responsible for the cost of treatment, there is a strong temptation to the patient and provider of therapy to continue the dependency state. The physician must be careful not to become part of the disease.

4. Symptom patterns may be aggravated and undiagnosed disorders may progress. Spinal orthoses, by reducing movement within the confines of their mechanical pressure systems, may cause increased motion at the ends of the restrained segments. If disease is present in this end region, symptoms may be increased. Waters and Morris[4] have demonstrated increased electromyographic activity during ambulation when a spinal orthosis is worn. This is presumed to be attributable to blocking of normal rotations that occur during gait and consequent increased demands on the spinal musculature to stabilize the trunk over the supporting foot. Thus, the orthosis itself may create more difficulty.

The physician must always be aware of the inexact nature of the presumed diagnosis. When symptoms do not respond to a reasonable treatment program, reevaluate the diagnosis.

This discussion of orthosis effects, both positive and negative, should make evident that orthosis application requires the correlation of specific orthotic functions with the demands imposed by each morbid state. The pathophysiology of each patient-disease complex presents its own requirements. If standard formulas are applied to all patients with back disease, the unwanted effects of the treatment may counteract whatever benefits might accrue from therapy.

CLINICAL APPLICATION OF BIOMECHANICAL PRINCIPLES

Based on the foregoing analysis of the physiologic basis for the application of spinal orthoses, we may now apply our knowledge of biomechanical effects of orthotic devices to specific clinical requirements.

First to be considered are the instances where the biomechanical effects of orthotic use may slow recovery. These include some stages of structural-mechanical low-back pain, disc disease, some simple spinal compression fractures, and postsurgical states where posterolateral fusions have been performed. For these conditions, trunk strengthening is a physiologic requirement. To effect trunk strengthening, the orthotic application should be minimized.

In structural-mechanical low-back derange-ments orthotic application should be minimized where there is only low back pain in the absence of physical findings. In these cases, evaluate psychologic evidence and emphasize therapeutic and recreational exercises. Most patients will improve. Keep in mind that when a third party pays, an orthosis may tend to sustain disability.

In stable fractures of vertebral bodies and transverse processes, an early start on an exercise program, especially directed at the abdominal and gluteal musculature, is quite effective, whereas prolonged orthotic support of the trunk is debilitating.

In postfusion patients, orthotic usage has been changing. With the introduction of the posterolateral fusion from the transverse processes to the sacrum, and along the transverse and articular processes in other regions of the spine, many surgeons have discontinued postoperative orthotic stabilization. The vascularity of the graft-recipient bed and broad fusion area often lead to early fusion, which is enhanced rather than suppressed by physiologic demands. Both the trunk musculature and bone grafts seem to do better without external support.

We should now identify the specific orthotic attributes that should be emphasized in the orthotic prescription for various disorders of the spine. The known attributes of various orthoses should be matched with the specific pathologic condition and with patient need. At the same time, any unwanted effects of the trunk orthosis should be avoided insofar as possible, by the proper selection and elimination of unnecessary components.

Trunk support

Trunk support is produced by enhancement of the intracavity hydropneumatic mechanism. Circumferential containment of the flanks and abdomen by corsets or the fabric components of more rigid orthoses is most effective in raising intracavitary pressure. This produces axial deloading while diminishing the demands on muscles and ligaments. Three-point force systems of rigid orthosis can further this effect but at the price of limiting spinal movements.

Mechanical-structural low back pain frequently responds favorably to trunk support.

The causes of low back pain in this condition may be divided into four often interrelated entities: muscle weakness, skeletal instability, degenerative disc disease, and degenerative (osteo)arthritis of the posterior diathrodial (facet) joints. Each of the causes can lead to pain and produce any or all of the others, with resulting accentuation and complication of the disease pattern. Thus muscle weakness enhances instability and encourages disc degeneration. Disc degeneration may produce herniation of the nucleus pulposus and sciatic radiculitis. It may also cause spondylosis or spur formation. Degenerative spondylolisthesis resulting from degenerative disc disease may produce facet-joint arthritis with back pain, but it may also cause sciatica from root compression.[1]

Lumbosacral corsets, which reduce the functional demands on the spinal musculature, are used to permit ambulation and activity in the subacute low back derangement. Discogenic disease with mildly positive sciatic stretch tests, recurrent acute sprains with lumbar pain and restricted mobility, and degenerative joint disease (osteoarthritis) can all benefit from such spinal supports. Not only does the lumbosacral corset produce axial deloading and reduced demand on musculature, which are primary concerns in these low back derangements, but it is virtually mandatory in the obese and elderly; it is more acceptable cosmetically; its effect on trunk movement can be varied by using rigid, semiflexible, or flexible stays; and it is less expensive than the custom-made rigid orthosis.

Trunk support may also be desired after laminectomy. Many patients wear external supports for a 4- to 6-week period. The need for such support increases with the number of vertebral interspaces involved and the preoperative muscular status. Corset containment of the trunk is usually all that is required.

In compression fractures of a lumbar or thoracic vertebral body, uncomplicated by neurologic deficit, axial unloading by thoracoabdominal support is an effective treatment method, as the goal is control of pain rather than control of deformity. When the pain level permits the patient to assume the upright position (7 to 10 days), use of a lumbosacral corset may be needed to control pain. It is not necessary to immobilize the spine, since fracture healing is rapid. A rigid orthosis will not prevent occasional instances of further deformation. The region of the fracture need not be encompassed by the corset.

The transverse-process fracture is essentially a soft-tissue injury and also heals quickly. Trunk support, as in uncomplicated vertebral compression fracture, may be required. Nevertheless, an early start on an exercise program, especially directed at the abdominal and gluteal musculature, can be quite effective in these disorders and may be preferable to orthotic treatment.

Another example of fractures of the spine treated by trunk support is in osteoporosis, which usually presents as a series of more or less acute episodes of back pain. If not produced by metabolic or neoplastic disorders, spontaneous healing brings pain relief.

Though a flexible external support also serves to reduce pain by reducing motion, its main effect is to reduce vertebral body compressive force by its enhancement of thoracoabdominal pressure. By permitting early mobilization of the patient, one may minimize weakness and debility while the acute fracture episode is spontaneously subsiding. The physician must appreciate that muscles rapidly weaken as a result of bed rest, immobility, and external support, leading to further demands on the porotic skeleton.

In osteopenia, therefore, the choice of external support will depend on the severity of the pain and the age of the patient. In the elderly, a flexible lumbosacral corset may be effective and tolerable and need not extend to the upper thorax in most cases even when thoracic spine fractures are present. Younger individuals may require more rigid stays in the corset.

A complication in some of these osteopenic patients is kyphotic deformity. Rigid thoracolumbur orthoses have been used but are rarely tolerated, particularly by the elderly. In any case, the progressive deformity resulting from multiple fracture episodes cannot be prevented by bracing, as the ribs may be fractured by a device that exerts significant pressure on the upper trunk.

Trunk support by three-point or regional pressure systems applied by control orthoses is of lesser importance but may be of some use in paralytic spinal disorders such as poliomyelitis, myelodysplastic states, and dystrophies involving the trunk. However, this is not always the case and a corset may suffice.

In paraplegia, in the absence of pelvic control and balance (hip hikers, abdominal, and erector spinae musculature), the patient will not become a functional walker. In these circumstances, attempts at trunk bracing with high control braces attached to pelvic and leg-control devices will permit ambulation only in an institutional setting. Control devices are expensive, require great rehabilitation efforts, and are usually counterproductive. When there is no pelvic control, a corset will permit the patient to sit in a wheelchair, transfer and engage in activities of daily living, and participate in vocational rehabilitation programs.

Corset containment of the trunk may interfere with respiration if there is diaphragm weakness or paralysis. When accessory respiratory muscles are needed for frog breathing, the abdomen must not be encumbered. Here, special supports on the wheelchair may be used to control and prevent trunk collapse.

In myelodysplastic states, orthotic methods to enhance trunk support may be quite useful. With neurologic deficits, the trunk is to be supported as required, depending on the amount and level of weakness, and the age of the patient. Supports should be related to the development of readiness for sitting, standing, and ambulation. These spinal orthoses are modified for each patient to avoid pressure on a posterior mass or abdominal apparatus (bladder or bowel). When there is a need to control hip rotation, lower-limb orthoses can be anchored to the spinal orthosis. As in paraplegia, potential for ambulation is limited when there is inadequate pelvic control. In adult life, the severely disabled myelodysplastic patient will often abandon complex braces.

The corset therefore should be used in paralytic myelodysplastic states under the following circumstances: (1) if the desired goal is sitting stability only, (2) if, with age, the posterior mass develops tolerance to pressure or is surgically removed, (3) for most adults, as they will discard cumbersome braces, (4) for patients who ambulate using hip hikers, since braces would interfere with trunk movements.

Spinal motion control

Although both the rigid orthosis and corsets limit motion, the rigid orthosis does so to a greater degree, provided that it is properly fitted and includes a large abdominal support. The lumbosacral rigid orthoses reduce segmental motion between L3 and the sacrum with three-point and regional pressure systems that become increasingly loaded as the trunk moves from the resting position.

Thoracolumnar rigid orthoses are effective at their center because of the length of the uprights. However, they induce increased motion at the lumbosacral level and increase the tendency to move the neck.

In low back derangements, rigid orthoses are prescribed when there is incomplete or inadequate relief from a corset and when motion enhances the pain. They are usually reserved for severe, long-term, or deteriorating clinical patterns. As has been stated, they should be used only for limited periods to avoid contracture of the back.

Degenerative spondylolisthesis may lead to degenerative arthritis (osteoarthritis) of the posterior joints. Here motion control is important, especially if there is root compression. A lumbosacral control orthosis is used. Nevertheless, if backache is the only symptom, a corset can reduce axial loading forces without maximum motion control.

Motion control is also useful in the presence of certain tumors of the spine. Spinal supports may be of great benefit as adjuvants to radiotherapy and chemotherapy. The orthosis used for the child is a flexion-extension motion-limiting brace to minimize deformity and restrict motion, whereas for the adult, a corset with rigid stays is often sufficient. In the presence of neurologic deficit or major instability, the situation requires a spinal orthosis that distributes pressure over wide areas and that can be removed from the front or back to facilitate radiation therapy. Here, a split plastic body and/or head-neck support (Minerva or cuirass) with Velcro closures is quite useful.

After spinal fusion in the lumbar area, practices vary widely. It should be realized that not too many years ago all spinal fusions were performed through windows in casts. Later, casts were applied postoperatively for many months, often with recumbency added to the treatment program. More recently, spinal orthoses and earlier ambulation became standard and still more recently, a no-support postoperative regimen has come to be used by many surgeons performing posterolateral fusions.

Nevertheless, postoperative spinal supports are still widely used and the practice is deeply ingrained in many communities. When pure posterior fusions have been performed, lumbosacral flexion-extension and lateral-control orthoses may be indicated to prevent excessive stress from normal physiologic demands and to permit patient transportation without stress to the back. Other factors dictating the use of spinal support are long fusions involving three or more joints and established pseudoarthrosis with pain.

Body casts do not generally provide better immobilization of the lumbar spine, but they do immobilize the patients, are uncomfortable, and tend to produce muscle atrophy and fibrosis.

Motion control is often required in spinal fractures with posterior element involvement. Such injuries include dislocation with pedicle and articular process fractures, concomitant body fractures, and frequently neurologic deficits. Immobilization to permit skeletal healing and spontaneous spine stabilization is likely to be prolonged. Extended bed rest is sometimes acceptable when there is no neurologic deficit, but one is likely to encounter severe morbidity when paraplegia or quadriplegia is present.

If the fracture is stable (compression of body, burst fractures, and dislocation without fractures), the patient can be mobilized without regard for the fusion as flexible segments above and below the injured region will relieve stress. Though many use a lumbosacral or thoracolumbar flexion-extension control brace, a corset with semiflexible stays is usually all that is required.

When an unstable fracture or fracture dislocation is present (rotation fracture dislocation), the situation is more complex. The stability at time of surgery will determine orthotic needs. Internal fixation with plates, wires, or acrylic bridges has been used to give temporary stability while the fusion heals. The more there is internal stabilization, the less the need for rigid external stabilization. The high control braces (thoracolumbar flexion-extension and lateral or thoracolumbar flexion, lateral, and rotary) may be used to permit earlier mobilization of the patient, an important goal of initial therapy, and would be used for long fusions in the absence of internal fixation. The molded plastic body shell can be an excellent tool for motion control in the presence of unstable fractures involving posterior elements.

Motion control is also an important biomechanical requirement for bracing in inflammatory spinal arthritis. This category includes rheumatoid arthritis, Marie-Strumpell ankylosing spondylitis, Still's disease, psoriatic arthritis with spinal involvement, and other similar disorders.

The goals of therapy are relief of pain and prevention of deformity. Any tendency to trunk flexion must be resisted by means of a bed board, sleeping in the prone position, intermittent traction, active extension exercises, and high control orthosis. Here the three-point trunk-control orthosis (thoracolumbar flexion-extension) is useful if the back can be passively brought into extension. Once flexion has occurred, this brace will no longer function properly, and the thoracolumbar flexion, lateral, and rotary orthosis is required to resist flexion. This orthosis uses thoracic band extensions and subclavicular pads for maximum restriction of spinal motion with minimal restriction of chest expansion. Extension exercises and athletics should be encouraged, even when an orthosis is worn, if the hip joints are not involved.

If the disorder is limited to the lumbosacral region, the lumbosacral flexion-extension and lateral control orthosis is used, primarily to control pain. When the cervical spine is involved, an appropriate cervical orthosis is used to control motion and prevent deformity. Atlantoaxial subluxation is a well-documented problem here.

An orthosis may be discontinued once the spine fuses spontaneously and pain and progressive deformity no longer occur. Should there be breakdown of a fused spinal segment, control bracing with or without surgical stabilization will have to be reinstituted.

In general, therefore, spinal motion control is the major functional requirement in arthritis with realignment of secondary importance when some flexibility remains.

Motion control is also a major requirement for the treatment of infectious disorders of the spine (osteomyelitis and tuberculosis). Spinal orthoses are used in conjunction with varied medical and surgical treatments to limit spinal motion, thus controlling pain and permitting healing. The amount of bracing is determined by the spinal level to be immobilized. Control orthoses have largely replaced the large body casts of former years and are used both preoperatively and postoperatively.

Spinal realignment

Spinal realignment demands three-point pressure systems or special orthoses, such as the Milwaukee brace, that influence muscular patterns, leading to the desired trunk positions. Skeletal realignment may transfer weight from diseased segments, and thus pain and inflammation are reduced. It is also used to promote growth in a more normal direction, in the presence of certain developmental disorders.

In certain types of structural lumbosacral derangements, arthropathies of the diarthroidial posterior facet joints play a major role in symptom formation. Degenerative disease (osteoarthritis) of these joints can produce back pain and can lead to narrowing of the spinal canal with root compression as seen as sequelae of degenerative spondylolisthesis. Here, spinal realignment (combined with motion control) may be quite useful in relieving symptoms, for weight can be transferred away from diseased facets to the vertebral bodies. This can be accomplished by the well-fitted lumbosacral flexion-extension and lateral control orthosis of, if less motion restriction is needed, by the lumbosacral extension and lateral control orthosis, both of which reduce lordosis. In the obese and in women it may be necessary to use a corset as an immobilizing and realignment device. Here, four straight, fairly rigid posterior steel stays are used to eliminate lumbar lordosis, since the front of the corset exerts a posteriorly directed force on the trunk.

In compression fractures of the vertebral bodies uncomplicated by neurologic deficit, spinal realignment with hyperextension has been a standard method of treatment in the past. However, these injuries have been the most overtreated of skeletal traumatic disorders. To avoid prolonged disability, treat the patient, not the roentgenogram. Bed rest is used as the primary treatment in the acute stages. When ileus subsides and back pain is tolerable, the patient should be mobilized with as little trunk support as is necessary to control pain. As mentioned earlier, a lumbosacral corset will often suffice. The presence of a concomitant disc injury may demand more rigid immobilization. A large separated body fragment may warrant a hyperextension cast or an orthosis (thoracolumbar flexion) to maintain trunk extension. For the most part, however, surgeons are avoiding the problems of postreduction ileus, abdominal crises, back pain, loss of reduction, and trunk fibrosis and weakness by not performing reductions in these cases. "The less treatment the better the result" is the axiom in this disorder.

External supports can be used to realign the trunk in spondylolisthesis and to improve the effectiveness of the foreshortened musculature in maintaining intracavitary pressure. For these purposes, the lumbosacral extension and lateral control orthosis will establish a three-point pressure system flattening the lumbar lordosis and correcting the tilt of the pelvis.

In some instances of back pain when specific indications are present, trunk support, motion control, and spinal alignment may all be required. Root pain relieved by trunk shift and arthropathies of the posterior facet joints represent two such situations. Here the determination of the specific orthosis to be prescribed requires consideration of the amount of trunk support, the amount and levels of motion control, and the realignment requirements of the spine.

Scoliosis and kyphosis dorsalis juvenalis will be treated in a separate chapter. Spinal realignment is the desired treatment goal in the growing child. Realignment bracing with the Milwaukee brace and intensive exercise programs have been effective in controlling and reversing deformities.

CERVICAL SPINE—SPECIAL ORTHOTIC REQUIREMENTS

The cervical spine is much more flexible than the remainder of the spine, and in addition it supports a 15-pound head. It is subject to injury, degeneration, and inflammatory, paralytic, neoplastic, and infectious disorders. Cervical orthoses function to reduce spinal motion, to realign the cervical spine and cervico-occipital joint, and to somewhat relieve gravitational stress by weight transfer. Hydropneumatic unloading is not possible in the cervical region. Reduction of motion is the main effect of cervical appliances unless weight transfer is specifically built into the device.

The basic cervical orthoses are the simple collars, soft or firm. These function as partial motion restraints, physically blocking movement to only a limited extent. The addition of chin and occipital supports, or the use of appliances with posts, provides more effective restriction of motion and permits a modest amount of weight relief from the spine. When more complete immobility and weight relief are required, the molded plastic cuirass or Minerva types of orthoses are used. The ultimate immobilizing device is skeletal fixation with a halo incorporated in a body cast. This is almost always used as a postsurgical tool.

In each disorder of the cervical spine, a specific requirement will usually predominate, thus permitting matching of the appliance to the patient's needs.

Motion control

Motion control is the primary functional requirement for the orthotic treatment of sprains of the cervical spine. This entity includes flexion, extension, flexion-extension, and lateral sprains. The radiograph is negative for bony injury although preexisting degenerative changes may be present and make the neck more vulnerable to injury. Intervertebral disc injury without herniation occurring in the flexible segments may be a cause for prolonged symptomatology. Pain may be severe and may be referred to the arm, but objective evidence of root compression is rare.

The objectives of therapy are reduction of pain and muscle spasm with resultant increase in cervical mobility. Associated symptoms such as nausea, headache, visual, and vasomotor disturbances usually respond as the neck pain subsides.

In the ambulatory, partially disabled patient, a firm collar by day and soft collar by night serve to reduce neck motion by reminding the patient of his injury and permit healing. The neck must be positioned properly for comfort. Avoid extending a neck that has received a hyperextension injury. Beware of neck injuries where the head has sustained direct impact. Hidden fractures and severe disc injuries may be present.

In more severe circumstances (when disability fails to respond to rest imposed by a simple collar or continually recurs), the rigid cervical appliances, which also reduce gravitational loading, are useful. Here the properly fitted collar with chin and occiput supports or the appliance with posts may be quite effective but should be discarded quickly to prevent atrophy.

Much the same advice can be given for acute torticollis resulting from minor injury or upper respiratory infection.

External supports are not generally indicated for torticollis resulting from rheumatic fever or drugs such as chlorpromazine, nor for adult spastic torticollis (spasmodic torticollis).

Motion control is also useful in degenerative disc disease (cervical spondylosis and spondylitis). This disorder may present as neck pain with restricted mobility, as radicular pain, or with spinal cord involvement. Orthotic restriction of motion often reverses the symptom pattern and permits irritative lesions to become quiescent. The soft night collar and firm day collar make a good combination. The head must be positioned properly for comfort, usually in slight flexion.

Occasionally, weight relief is additionally required for severe pain, but patients in the older age group may find the more restrictive orthoses uncomfortable.

Weight transfer

Weight-transfer orthoses also immobilize the neck, eliminate shear forces on the horizontal spine, and support the head weight when the patient is upright.

Gravitational stress relief may be important in fractures and dislocations of the cervical spine. The orthotic requirements are determined by the stability of the fracture, the state of the nervous system, and the extent and stability of spinal fusion, if performed. Emergency splinting with available materials such as towel rolls should be mentioned. Air collars have been developed and may prove useful for this task.

After initial bed rest and traction, uncomplicated compression fractures or undisplaced posterior element fractures without neurologic deficit may be treated with the patient ambulatory using rigid cervical orthoses that transfer weight, such as an appliance with posts, or hard collar with chin and occiput supports.

When the fracture is unstable, or a dislocation or fracture has been reduced, after an initial program of rest in traction, an immobilizing and weight-transfer orthosis is indicated. The molded plastic jackets are most comfortable. With major instability, the halo device can be mounted on a body cast to unweight and immobilize the cervical spine.

When stability is assured, the simple restrictive collar may be applied to permit gradual resumption of movement and return of muscle function.

After surgical stabilization, external supports are also designed to immobilize and eliminate shear motion and support the head to permit healing. Maximum support is also needed for fusions in the upper cervical and cervico-occipital segments. Posterior and posterolateral fusions create the greatest demands for external support, increasing with the number of levels fused.

In anterior fusion, stability and the length of fusion determine the orthotic needs. One-level locked-interbody fusions after disc excision can be managed with soft or hard simple collars. With multilevel fusions such as long anterior countersunk grafts, relatively complete immobilization and weight transfer are indicated. Therefore, in high cervical, occipitocervical, and long anterior and posterior fusions, use the Minerva jacket appliance created from a mold of the patient, for 3 to 6 months, until fusion is complete. Then progress to a simple collar, which is gradually discarded, with normal activities permitted.

When there is paralysis of the neck musculature, an orthosis can aid in supporting the head and permit the upright position. Support according to the stability of the spine, trying to keep the appliance as simple as possible.

REFERENCES

1. Lusskin, R.: Pain patterns in spondylolisthesis, Clin. Orthop. **40:**125-136, 1965.
2. Morris, J., Lucas, D., and Bressler, B.: Role of the trunk in stability of the spine, J. Bone Joint Surg. **43A**(3): 327-351, April 1961
3. Norton, P., and Brown, T.: The immobilization efficiency of back braces: The effect on the posture and motion of the lumbosacral spine, J. Bone Joint Surg. **39A**(1):111-139, Jan. 1957.
4. Waters, R. L., and Morris, J. M.: Effect of spinal supports on the electrical activity of muscles of the trunk, J. Bone Joint Surg. **52A**(1):51-60, Jan. 1970.

CHAPTER 21

Milwaukee brace principles and fabrication

WALTER P. BLOUNT, M.D.
THOMAS R. BIDWELL, C.P.O.

Introduction to the Milwaukee brace

The Milwaukee brace is a corrective spinal orthosis used in the treatment of scoliosis, lordosis, and kyphosis. It consists of a contoured pelvic girdle attached by three uprights to an occipital pad and throat mold or chin piece. Suspended from the uprights are lumbar and thoracic pads as well as other accessories (shoulder flange, axillary sling, or subclavicular pads).

This device functions to redirect spinal growth by stimulating trunk muscle patterns, while three-point pressure systems play a lesser role.

The description of the components will be found in the discussion on fabrication, whereas the indications and methodology for application will be found in the section on principles of Milwaukee brace treatment. There is also a statement of modifications at the end of this chapter.

The specific term "Milwaukee brace" is used for the orthosis throughout in deference to the wishes of Dr. Walter Blount.

THE EDITORS

Section I

Principles of Milwaukee brace treatment*

WALTER P. BLOUNT, M.D.

The evolution of the Milwaukee brace from 1945 to the present time can be divided conveniently into three periods. Prior to 1950, a crude early model with turnbuckles on the sides, rigid screw fixation of the thoracic pad, and girdles cut out over the anterosuperior spines to prevent pressure sores was used only postoperatively to correct and maintain the improvement of thoracic scolioses. No attempt was made to control curves in the lumbar and cervical regions.

After 1950 the two turnbuckles and four uprights were abandoned and replaced by three extensible uprights, one anteriorly and two posteriorly. By 1960, after 5 years of brace use for nonoperative treatment, we realized that the brace provided more than passive correction. It was shown to maintain the improvement that was

---

*This text is an abstract of the monograph *The Milwaukee brace*, by Walter P. Blount and John H. Moe, Baltimore, 1973, The Williams & Wilkins Company, with many direct quotations. All but two of the illustrations are reproduced from this book by permission of The Williams & Wilkins Company.

accomplished by the movements of the patient during his daily activity or with specific exercises. The uprights were lengthened and the pads advanced 1 cm. at a time to take up slack.

Distraction was still considered important and was obtained by a flat, firm chin pad and a deeply notched occiput support mounted on a heavy neck ring. Pressure on the mandible was considerable and there were some malocclusions and jaw deformities when the brace was first used for nonoperative treatment.

At the end of this decade the increasingly use of the brace in the nonoperative treatment prompted the incorporation of anterior hinges, which had appeared in the Warm Springs model in the late 1950s. This prevented breakage from frequent bending and made it easier to get in and out of the brace without partially dismantling it.

By 1960 the use of the Milwaukee brace plus exercises for the nonoperative treatment of moderate scoliotic curves had become recognized as a successful method. The greatest drawbacks were the conspicuous chin pad and the deranged bite. In the treatment of the latter, the orthodontists were consulted even before the treatment was started and were of considerable help in prevention of deformity.

For many patients a forehead band was provided to alternate with the chin pad at night.[4] This effectively removed the pressure from the mandible while the patient slept.

More significant was the discovery that constant distraction was unnecessary in the correction of deformities that were acceptable for management by nonoperative methods. After the chin pad had been lowered without interference with the maintenance of correction in many scolioses, the throat mold was designed in 1969 (Fig. 21-1). At that time the neck ring was redesigned to be less bulky and to open in the back between the divided occiput pads, which were made smaller and more horizontal. They were fitted under, not behind, the back of the head (Fig. 21-1). The upright element of the throat mold fitted the contours of the neck to maintain the head back over the occiput pads. The tonguelike anterior projection was only a reminder to avoid habitual forward flexion of the neck (Fig. 21-1).

As a result of these many changes the current Milwaukee brace presents a streamlined appearance.[2] It can be worn under ordinary clothing without conspicuous bulging. With a turtleneck

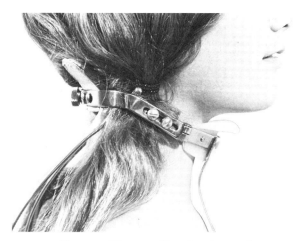

Fig. 21-1. Throat mold and occiput pads.

sweater or a scarf it is nearly invisible. The upright bars conform to the body contours, but they do not embarrass respiration.[4] They are always contoured enough to allow free movement of the torso in the directions that correct deformity. Removal and reapplication of the brace have been simplified so that the patient can perform them himself.

We have continued to use the chin pad, not the throat mold, in the correction of scoliosis for 6 months postoperatively.[4] The forehead band also has remained in the therapeutic armamentarium for those patients who need their chins free for surgery or because they drool.

TREATMENT INDICATIONS

Moderate curves of 30 to 40 degrees are the deformities usually treated nonoperatively today. For these patients the three-point axially directed holding force of the pads is probably more efficient than distraction, which is utilized only intermittently (Fig. 21-2, A).

However, with discontinuation of the chin pad, which had frequently caused bite deformities, 70-degree curves cannot be corrected well. This degree of curve requires mandibular pressure for distraction. Such curves, however, are not generally acceptable for nonoperative treatment.

As the magnitude of the curves increases to 100 degrees or beyond, skeletal traction is desirable and is usually applied with a halo as an accessory to the Milwaukee brace (Fig. 21-2, B).

During nonoperative treatment, the patient continues all physical activities except trampoline, violent gymnastics, and body-contact games. Scoliotic deformities in athletic individuals are

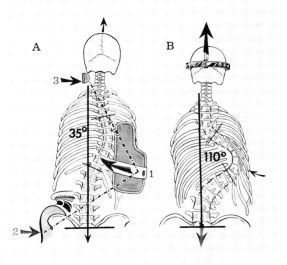

Fig. 21-2. A, Effect of thoracic pad. B, Distraction by halo.

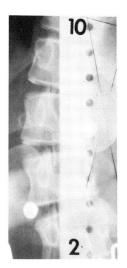

Fig. 21-3. Open vertebral apophyses.

more easily corrected than those in sedentary patients.

All patients must continue with the conditioning program to maintain strength of the abdominal and trunk muscles, which tend to atrophy as the result of the splinting action of the girdle. Several patients who have been referred while wearing braces had improved during their first months in the appliance, only to lose all the initial gain from inactivity. With the adoption of exercise programs, they regained their losses and continued to improve with the nonoperative program.

Better understanding of the principles involved led to further modification of the 1970 model. The carefully molded pelvic girdle was still a basic requirement. It was made of reinforced cowhide lined with soft leather or made of thermoplastic to be worn over an undergarment. The brace was made more streamlined so that it scarcely showed under the clothing. The throat mold could be covered with a scarf or a turtleneck sweater. The top of the girdle was cut low enough and the bars kept far enough from the torso to permit the patient to move freely in the directions that corrected the deformity. Undesirable movements were checked by the pads.

Two principles must not be ignored: (1) The brace must be worn full time until the patient is mature as shown by closure of the vertebral apophyses (Fig. 21-3). (2) Weaning must be gradual (over a period of a year) after the patient

is mature. The brace should then be worn another year or two at night only. A girl who is skeletally 13 will probably have to wear it full time for 5 years. The rapport of the orthopaedic surgeon with the patient and his parents must be adequate to inspire them to carry out this program without faltering.

Occasionally even the most efficient brace treatment may fail to obtain acceptable correction in a seemingly favorable patient. When this is evident after 6 to 8 months of trial, a spine fusion procedure must be carried out without delay. Continuation of nonoperative treatment in this situation will cause dissatisfaction for all concerned.

The indications for nonoperative treatment further depend on a variety of factors, which include the growth potential, size and flexibility of curves, magnitude of the rib hump, curve pattern, back pain, emotional stability, and socioeconomic conditions. A few general guidelines may be helpful. A girl whose skeletal age is 12 or 13, who has a single major curve of 45 degrees or less is suitable for nonoperative treatment. For a boy the timing for the same curve is 2 years older. The younger the child, the greater the curve that may be treated with a Milwaukee brace and exercises. There are intermediary gray zones, however, as shown in (Fig. 21-4). In a child of 7 or 8, a 60-degree curve is not infrequently almost completely corrected and the improvement maintained until maturity. Others with considerable vertebral wedging can be held to an acceptable correction

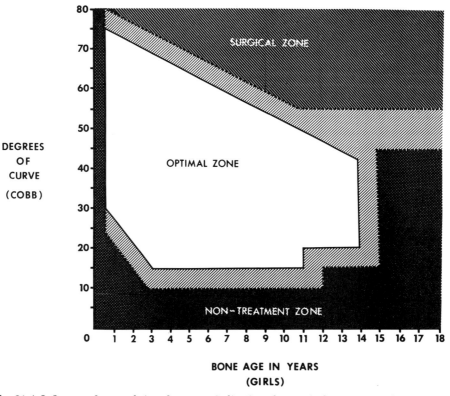

Fig. 21-4. Influence of age and size of curve on indications for surgical or nonoperative treatment of idiopathic scoliosis.

until age 12 or 14 and then fused at that more favorable age.

Girls who have reached the age of 15 are borderline. A 50- or 55-degree curve with considerable rib hump should be operated upon at once without an attempt at brace treatment.[5] In the rare instances in which there is an indication for nonoperative treatment, the brace must be worn full time until maturity and then at night for several years longer if the improvement is to be maintained.

The size of the rib hump and rigidity of the deformity are often more important than the size of the curve. Double curves are better compensated than single ones and may be more suitable for brace treatment.

The essential requisites for brace treatment of scoliosis are a good brace and a cooperative patient and parents. The orthopaedic surgeon must understand brace treatment and be willing to reexamine the patient at intervals of 3 months, take x-ray films as necessary and measure them carefully. A physical therapist should supervise the exercises. The orthotist must be available to adjust the brace to the changing curve pattern, shape, and size of the patient.

If any of these important requirements are missing, the patient with a progressive scoliosis should be referred to another facility or the necessary fusion should be performed promptly.

In a young child, the etiology is of lesser importance. In an older juvenile or adolescent it is most significant. One should not attempt to treat a rapidly progressive paralytic scoliosis with the Milwaukee brace. Other supportive devices are more acceptable.

TECHNIQUE OF BRACE TREATMENT

At the initial visit, the education of parents and patient should begin with reading a brochure about scoliosis and the Milwaukee brace. This should be supplemented, when possible, by conversations with informed members of the nursing, physical therapy, and resident staff. On the first day the patient should be given an outline of the exercises, which are demonstrated for him and a parent.

When a new brace is delivered, it should not be

closely fitted. The neck ring should be left 1 cm. too long and usually the anterior bar one hole too short. The girdle need not be as snugly fitted, as the patient will insist upon having it in a few weeks. The brace may be annoying to the patient but should not be uncomfortable.

The occiput pads should fit well under the back of the head and be low enough to permit the patient to extend the neck almost completely. If the pads are so vertical that they obstruct this movement, they should be bent backward and downward until they present a rounded surface that does not prevent neck extension. The thoracic pad should be tight enough to cause a slight displacement of the chest to the opposite side, but the patient must be able to shift away from it until the pad hangs loose.

If the parents or the patient feel insecure about the program, a few days in the hospital may be desirable when the child first receives his brace. He can then adapt to it and perform exercises under the supervision of a trained staff.

During the first few days in a properly adjusted brace, it may seem too long when the patient sits. He must pull it down or lie down and tilt his pelvis. Any discomfort is usually relieved by recumbency. In repose, muscles relax and the torso elongates while the brace keeps the spine from curving into deformity. The patient will usually soon forget that he is wearing the brace.

BRACE ADJUSTMENTS

A frequent error noted during brace treatment of scoliosis is to have the posterior uprights too long. The patient's complaint is pressure against the throat, and inability to raise the chin from the throat mold. It is a grave mistake to satisfy him by lengthening the neck ring or shortening the anterior bar. Instead, the posterior uprights should be shortened and the neck ring and anterior bar left in their proper position. He will then raise his chin freely and have no discomfort.

After a week the patient should return to have the neck ring shortened, the anterior bar lengthened, the anterior end of the strap to the thoracic pad advanced, and the pelvic girdle tightened. The patient usually does not object to these changes, as the brace will actually be more comfortable after the adjustments.

The pelvic girdle must be low enough in back to maintain the correction of the lumbar lordosis.

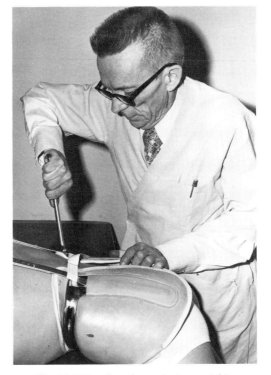

Fig. 21-5. Bending the posterior uprights.

This is the lowest of three pressure points that accomplish this. The other two are the abdominal apron in front and the thoracic pad or upright bars posteriorly. As the patient learns to tilt his pelvis, the girdle may loosen at the lower border posteriorly. This can be remedied by bending the posterior uprights just above the waist[4] (Fig. 21-5).

The pelvic girdle must be cut sufficiently high in front to permit comfortable sitting but must be low enough to support the abdomen. It should reach just to but not over the symphysis pubis while the patient is standing. The patient will soon request that the girdle be made snugger as he finds that it will ride down and press on the lateral surfaces of the crests of the ilia if it is loose. As the subcutaneous fat atrophies during the first 3 months, he will gradually tighten it.

As a result of these alterations in circumference of the pelvis and hips, the posterior edges of the girdle may overlap after a few months. This means that the posterior uprights will converge downward. Neither change is a great disadvantage as long as the fit of the girdle at the waistline is maintained. It is not necessary to remake the girdle in a girl of skeletal age 12 or 13. As her pelvis expands, she may need this additional space and the girdle will again separate in back. Not infrequently there is a weight gain, which does the same thing.

FUNCTION OF PADS

The brace was originally designed to correct a major right thoracic curve. This is still its most frequent function. The L-shaped thoracic pad is attached to a Dacron strap that passes under and around the near posterior upright to a truss stud. The pad is tightened by advancing the anterior end of the strap, which is fastened to an outrigger from the anterior bar. It has the best mechanical advantage of any of the pads used. Its lower rectangular portion should be snug against the ribs at and below the apex of the curve. When double thoracic and lumbar curves are treated, the thoracic pad is shifted one segment higher to avoid exaggerating the lumbar curve. It should be placed one segment lower when there is a structural left upper thoracic curve. With triple curves a smaller pad is used for the middle curve.

With the initial application of this pad, the torso is displaced to the left. If the shift is excessive, the strap is too tight. The patient must be able to move the torso away from the pad. The anterior end of the strap is advanced only to take up slack as the deformity is corrected by the patient's activity. The adjacent upright is bent to uniformily support the entire pad. The upper portion of the pad corrects the rib hump passively, particularly with recumbency. It should overlie the scapula, which moves under it freely.

A double thoracic scoliosis with wedged vertebrae in both curves requires a thoracic pad for the lower curve and a shoulder ring on the opposite side to depress the high first and second ribs and thereby control the upper thoracic curve. In this situation the posterior strap should be fastened high on the ring and then slanted downward 30 or 40 degrees to the opposite upright. To maintain close coaptation of the ring, a second elastic strap is usually fastened to the anterior bar.

The shoulder ring may be used instead of a thoracic pad to prevent excessive increase of the compensatory curve and elevation of the shoulder on the side opposite a thoracolumbar curve that is being corrected by the combination of a lumbar pad and an oval pad. Then the posterior strap is attached halfway down the ring and angulated caudad only 20 degrees from the horizontal.

The shoulder ring has largely replaced the axillary sling because, with excessive displacement of the upper thorax to the left in the correction of a right thoracic curve, there is usually a high left shoulder, which would be accentuated by an axillary sling. In the rare instances in which it is indicated the use of the axillary sling should be withheld until the overhang to the side of the convexity has been completely overcorrected. The routine use of the sling simply to maintain the patient well centered in the brace prevents desirable movement of the thorax.

Since about 1960 lumbar curves have been well corrected by the use of the brace with a lumbar pad. Occasionally, if there is considerable overhang to the left, an oval pad is added to hold against the last three ribs on the same side and increase the compensatory curve in the thoracic region on the opposite side. In a girl with skeletal age 14 or 15, balanced posture is more important than the correction of individual curves. If a rib prominence appears with the thoracic curve, a thoracic pad, or shoulder ring must be added to hold it in check.

Despite the asymmetry of the torso associated with a left lumbar curve, it is imperative that the girdle be symmetric. If the lateral abdominal and quadratus lumborum muscles are extremely tight on the side of the convexity, it may be impossible to mold the negative cast into the waistline on this side. Most of the asymmetry can be corrected on the positive model, which may need to have added plaster in and above the waistline on the concave side. It is a grave error to let the waistline groove be deeper on the right than on the left.

If the symmetry of the girdle is maintained, there is a phenomenon that is difficult for the uninitiated to explain. The patient will be in good balance when out of the brace. As soon as he puts the brace on, he will list to the left. This overhang is caused by pressure of the waistline groove on the quadratus lumborum and lateral abdominals. Before they actually become sore the patient instinctively leans to the left. This relaxes the muscles and takes all the pressure off of them. The patient is not even conscious of this defense mechanism. It can be demonstrated by having the patient stand erect without the brace. First palpate the tense muscles in this position and then have him lean to the left side. The muscles immediately become soft. It is not harmful to allow him to wear the brace and walk with a list as long as he continues to straighten up when the brace is removed. Later, as the muscles stretch out, he

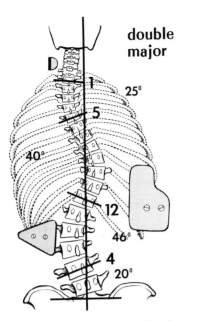

double major

D

1   25°

5

40°

12

46°

4   20°

Fig. 21-6. Correct placement of pads in a double major curve.

will gradually assume the erect position in the brace.

Double major thoracic and lumbar curves are treated with a combination of the thoracic pad raised one segment to avoid exaggeration of the lumbar curve (Fig. 21-6) and the lumbar pad holding against the second and third transverse processes.

When poor posture or round back are associated with scoliosis, the two deformities should be corrected simultaneously by the basic Milwaukee brace plus whatever pads are needed for the lateral curves. Passive improvement of the round back is obtained by bending in the posterior uprights as the patient improves the deformity by active exercises.[4] The orthotist must know how to straighten the anterior displacement of the head, which becomes more apparent as the dorsal rounding is diminished. After this maneuver it is usually necessary for him to increase the pelvic tilt (Fig. 21-5) by bending the lower end of the uprights.

WEANING FROM THE BRACE

The most disastrous error in brace treatment has been premature removal of the brace. Everyone associated with the nonoperative management of scoliosis or round back must understand and make it clear to an adolescent patient at the beginning of treatment that the brace must be worn almost full time until a girl has a skeletal age of 18 and a boy, 20, if the correction is to be maintained. After that the brace should be worn at night for another year or two. The earlier the brace is started, the sooner it may be worn at night only.

In discussing weaning it is important to define the terms accurately. All scoliosis patients should have an initial evaluation of skeletal age according to Greulich and Pyle[6] to aid in establishing a prognosis. During nonoperative treatment the progress of spinal maturation should be followed by clinical and x-ray evaluations. Most conclusive of the positive signs is x-ray evidence of closure of the vertebral-ring apophyses.

Reaching spinal maturity is an indication for testing the stability of the correction by making a standing x-ray film after the patient has been out of the brace for about 3 hours.[3,9] Weaning must not progress faster than the proved stability of the corrected spine. It is important to distinguish clearly between skeletal age, spinal maturity, and stability of correction. Accurate interpretation of these terms will avoid the futile use of the Milwaukee brace or situations in which success is impossible.

The most dramatic permanent cures are those of the juvenile scolioses that may be almost completely corrected.[2] Acceptable lasting improvement can be obtained with moderate idiopathic curves in girls of chronologic age 13 or less, even with some compromise as to the duration of brace treatment. When the brace is first worn at skeletal age 15, flexible curves may be greatly improved and perfect compensation obtained, but, unless a girl adheres to the plan of almost full-time use until 18 and then at night, she will usually lose most of the correction of the curves in the first few years if treatment is prematurely terminated.[3] She will usually retain the compensation that was gained.

Maturity of the spine is sometimes attained before skeletal age 18 in a girl, but usually not before 17. If the curves are well corrected, it is permissible for a patient to occasionally be out of her brace for 3 hours. Before she is allowed 3 hours daily, however, she should have a test of stability of correction. This is accomplished by having an x-ray film made 3 hours after she has been out of her brace. If there is no more than a 3-degree loss as compared with the x-ray film while she was in the brace, then it is safe to allow her 3 hours out of the brace daily. After a few months it may be expedient to give her 6 hours out of the brace daily if divided into two 3-hour intervals with 3 hours in the brace between them. Before her free time is increased to 6 hours at one time, the same test should be repeated after 6 hours out of the brace. This film is compared with the x-ray film after 3 hours out of the brace. There should be no loss of correction. Weaning for at least a year should precede attending school for 9 hours without the brace.

For a year or two before weaning is started, suggest that she will be allowed out of the brace sooner if her muscles are strong enough to maintain the improvement for a period of 3 to 6 hours. This reminder is a great stimulus to exercising. When it fails, the patient must be kept in the brace a longer time. It is better to be too strict, than to be permissive and let the girl out a little too early. This generosity is not appreciated when she loses correction and comes to surgery after 2 or 3 years of brace treatment.

After the patient has been at school for a few months with the brace off 9 hours during every school day, a check-up x-ray film must be made. If there is no loss of correction, the time out can be increased gradually to 12 out and 12 in and eventually to 10 hours in the brace.

Most patients do not object to wearing the brace at night. With this in mind, the orthopaedic surgeon can bargain with a rebellious patient to wear the brace at night for an additional 2 years in exchange for earlier part-time freedom. One should always remind the patient that if he has been out too long and the x-ray film shows an increased deformity, he will have to go back in again. This is not well accepted. It is better to have been miserly with the time so that when the patient asks for more freedom you are safe in giving him an extra hour a day.

The patient's daily activity in the brace improves the deformity. All patients are encouraged to increase rather than diminish their participation in sports, household chores, and yard work. When cooperation can be obtained from the school authorities, we recommend a full program of physical education with the exception of violent gymnastics, trampoline, and contact sports in which the brace would be a hazard to the opponents.

The brace may usually be removed for a hour or more of swimming, which is a most desirable form

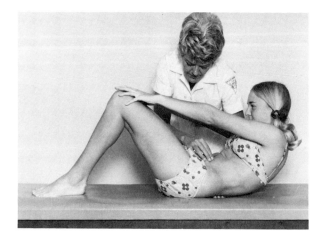

Fig. 21-7. Abdominal strengthening exercises.

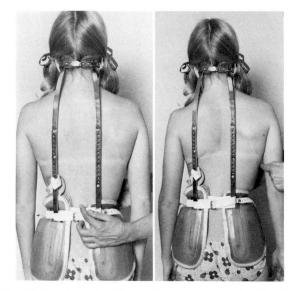

Fig. 21-8. A lateral shift exercise for the patient with a left lumbar curve.

of exercise. Patients may ski in their braces on moderate slopes.

EXERCISE PROGRAM

All patients are given supplementary exercises under the direction of a physical therapist.[4] These exercises are of two types: those designed for abdominal strengthing to counteract the effects of bracing (Fig. 21-7) and lateral shift exercises planned specifically to assist in correcting actively the abnormal curves and rib deformities (Fig. 21-8).

It is true that some good results can be obtained by the intelligent use of a good Milwaukee brace

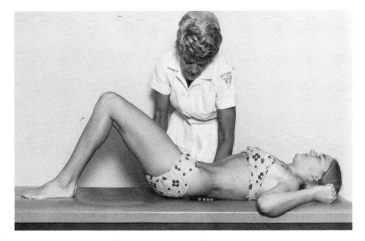

Fig. 21-9. Pelvic tilt exercises.

by an active child without any physical therapy. The improvement however is usually less and is obtained more slowly than with the addition of a relatively simple exercise program. Without exercises, the treatment of a sedentary patient with a Milwaukee brace will generally be unsatisfactory because poor muscle tone will allow deterioration of the deformity in the brace, and collapse of the spine when the brace is removed.

The orthopaedic surgeon or the physical therapist should examine the patient carefully on the first visit for diminished muscle power and contractures. Contracted tensor fasciae latae and iliopsoas muscles cause hip flexion deformities and lumbar lordoses. The pelvis cannot be tilted in the standing position until these tight muscles are stretched out by manipulation, or released surgically.

The release of contractures and an exercise program should be started at once, before the patient is confined to either cast or brace.

The pelvic tilt is learned more easily without the brace. It is basic and is the first movement of all exercises (Fig. 21-9). The routine is modified but continued if a cast is worn and augmented later when the brace is applied.

The first group of exercises maintains and increases the strength of the trunk muscles whose activity is mechanically restricted by the brace. They are performed both in and out of the brace. These exercises prepare the patient to keep his good posture without the abdominal support and holding function of the brace.

The second group of exercises consists of spe-

cific movements designed to diminish the major curve and list, decrease the lordosis, reduce the rib hump, and force out the thoracic valley on the concave side of the major curve. They consist of two routines performed in the brace.[4]

1. Pelvic tilt is followed by deep inspiration and vigorous rounding of the back posteriorly (flexion of the thoracic spine) in an attempt to reach the upright over the thoracic valley. The rib hump impinges on the medial border of the thoracic pad, which is backed up by the other posterior upright. Its motion is effectively arrested while the spine derotates and the valley is filled out. At the same time the thoracic lordosis is reduced.

2. The pelvis is tilted and kept from relapsing into lordosis while the torso is shifted toward the concavity of the major curve. The direction and amount of the list or overhang are determined by dropping a plumb line from the vertebra prominens or occipital protuberance. The shift is primarily to overcorrect the list and secondarily to reduce the major curve.

When these two exercises are repeated in the brace many times a day, the improvement is usually gratifying. After the spinal list is well overcorrected, asymmetric movements should be stopped. A routine check with a plumb line should be made at each visit. When a right overhang from a thoracic curve is inadvertently converted to an excessive left curve, the shifting exercise should be reversed and carried to the right. Rarely, if ever, does one permanently overcorrect an initial curve to an opposite curve.

There is a tendency for some physical therapists to attempt an elaborate exercise program. Do not bore the patient with a complicated routine. Do not remove the brace to facilitate all exercising. The brace is an important adjunct to most of the exercises. Asymmetric exercises without the brace are rarely desirable. Back movements that correct the major curve aggravate the compensatory curves. When asymmetric exercises are performed in the Milwaukee brace, beneficial movements are permitted, whereas unwanted motions are checked before their amplitude is sufficient to produce undesirable effects. As correction progresses, pads must be advanced with upright bars bent in on the side of the convexity and bent out over the expanding thoracic valley and anteriorly. There must be room for deep breathing and exercising.

Excessive fatigue should be avoided. The patient should rest when tired but should resume vigorous activity when rested.

COMPLICATIONS

Over a period of 25 years, there have been two major types of complications with the Milwaukee brace: emotional storms and pressure phenomena. Confirmed rebellion of the patient must be accepted as a contraindication to the use of a brace. An early tearful session is usually only temporary. The late rejection of the brace by a sexually mature but skeletally immature patient will require some compromise or a fusion.

In the early years undesirable skin pressure was a real threat to the success of the method. It has been almost entirely eliminated with the modern girdle, and the use of the throat mold instead of a chin pad.

A well-made plastic girdle fits more closely over bony landmarks than does the molded leather one.[4] Irregularities of its inner surfaces can cause painful blisters and sores. They must be smoothed out with a felt cone. Heating and remolding is necessary to correct the larger troublesome areas. Sores do not occur if the orthotist is skillful in making the negative and preparing the positive. Poorly made girdles can be a vicious cause of painful deep ulcers.

The plastic girdle must be washed on the inside with soap and water everyday. A soft cotton garment should be worn under it.

A few patients have pathologically sensitive skins that break down with pressure under any type of girdle even with the greatest care. They are poor candidates for the Milwaukee brace treatment.

In general, the parents and the patient must be warned against the use of adhesive or moleskin under the girdle. Band-Aids usually cause trouble. Reddened areas or actual breaks in the skin should be protected with Telfa dressings without adhesive edges.

Continuing excessive pressure on the iliac crests means that the brace has been lengthened too much or that the girdle is improperly made or fitted. When the brace is once adjusted, lengthening is usually necessary only once or twice a year as the child grows, but the patient should be seen by the orthopaedist at intervals of 3 months. Correction of a moderate curve may increase the patient's height enough to require elongation of the uprights, but only at the direction of the orthopaedic surgeon. A few zealous parents have overextended the brace repeatedly in their desire for a rapid correction. The only safe rule is to forbid parents ever to lengthen the braces. Occasional exceptions can be made after long acquaintance.

As adolescent fat hips slim down and the circumference of the girdle is diminished progres-

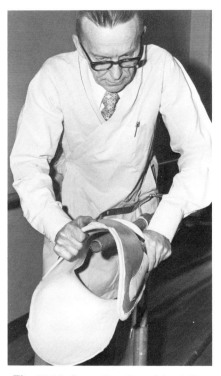

Fig. 21-10. Correcting the pelvic girdle.

sively, there may be overlapping in back and a new cause for pressure. The girdle becomes too narrow from side to side and too wide from front to back. Pressure areas 5 cm. long appear directly laterally at the waist, first on the side opposite the major pad.

With a leather girdle this situation can be remedied easily by bending the Monel Metal bands. The best way is to hold the lateral concavity over a horizontal pipe with the operator's hands equidistant from it on the front and back of the girdle. Forceful pressure against the pipe with simultaneous compression of the girdle from front to back is most effective (Fig. 21-10). The maneuver is then repeated on the other side. The areas of localized lateral pressure disappear immediately. In such a situation a plastic girdle must be replaced.

The best way to avoid troublesome complications is to anticipate them. At each visit the orthopaedic surgeon should inspect the hip regions. There should be symmetric red marks in the waistlines and just medial to the anterosuperior spines but none elsewhere.

Pressure areas over the posterosuperior spines can be relieved by bending the posterior uprights and vertical bands to create some dorsal convexity of the girdle at this point. A plastic girdle can be heated and pushed out over tender bony prominences, but an overlying bar must be bent out at the same time.

The back of the head should be inspected, with the hair carefully held aside. The pressure of the two occiput pads should be equal. They fit under the occiput better when they are bent to incline about 45 degrees from the horizontal.

SUMMARY

The success of brace treatment depends greatly on the rapport between attending physician, patient, and parents. The socioeconomic status of the patient is a most important factor. Emotionally stable, private patients usually do well. In clinics where the control of the patients is poor, brace treatment should not be attempted.

Apparent inexorable progression may actually be attributable to the patient's unrecognized failure to cooperate. However, there are a few idiopathic curves that become worse or fail to improve even when a good patient wears a satisfactory brace faithfully and exercises religiously. This rare variation in the correctability of idiopathic scoliosis cannot be recognized in advance. In a growing child, a trial is justified.

Section II

Fabrication of the Milwaukee brace

WALTER P. BLOUNT, M.D.
THOMAS R. BIDWELL, C.P.O.*

There are certain basic procedures that an orthotist must follow if he is to make a satisfactory Milwaukee brace. He may develop individual variations in preparing the model, molding the girdle and assembling the superstructure, but he will do well at first to follow the techniques that have been developed by trial and error over a period of 28 years.

THE PLASTER MODEL

A plaster model for the pelvic girdle must be prepared for each patient. One can construct the rest of the brace by modifying components that are prefabricated in three or four sizes.

Two layers of stockinet are fitted tightly over the torso from neck to midthighs. A strip of heavy elastic webbing or soft aluminum is run down the back between the layers of stockinet.

The patient stands with the knees slightly bent and the lumbar lordosis flattened (Figs. 21-11 and 21-14). The ischial tuberosities or backs of the thighs are rested against a crossbar that is adjusted to the proper height. The bar may be fastened to a standard prosthetic casting frame,

---

*Milwaukee, Wisconsin.

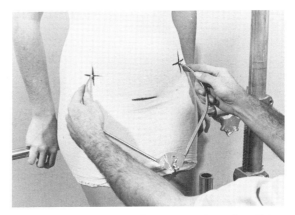

Fig. 21-11. Measurement of anterosuperior spine distance.

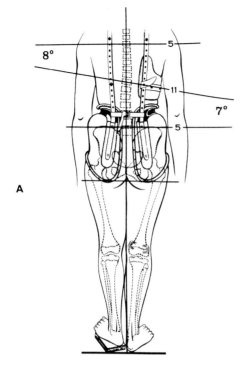

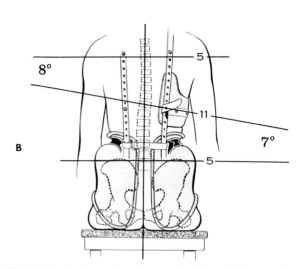

Fig. 21-12. **A,** Correction of a short left leg. **B,** Level pelvis.

the arms should be supported horizontally, and no traction is applied to the head.

A good model for an infant or small child can be made only with deep ketamine sedation or general anesthesia with intubation. The anesthetized patient lies supine on a longitudinal canvas strap of a Risser casting frame. The degree of pelvic tilt can be controlled by varying the amount of tension on the canvas strap and the amount of hip flexion.

If there is inequality of leg length of more than 1 cm., the pelvis must be leveled by a lift under the foot on the short side (Fig. 21-12, *A*). When the patient sits, the pelvis is level and requires a symmetric girdle (Fig. 21-12, *B*). He must wear a lift on the shoe of the short side when ambulatory in the brace.

According to a prepared outline, landmarks are then identified and standard measurements are recorded. The anterosuperior iliac spines, posterosuperior spines, and greater trochanters are located by palpation and marked on the stockinet with an indelible pencil. The distance between the spines is measured with a pelvimeter (Fig. 21-11).

Reference marks are made just above the costal margin and at the top of the symphysis pubis, penciled on the stockinet. With the head in neutral position, measurements are made from the chin to the top of the symphysis and to the reference point near the costal margin (Fig. 21-11). The width of the neck and the anteroposterior distance from the curve of the throat to the occipital protuberance (Fig. 21-13) indicate the size of the neck ring.

Two or three plaster bandages are applied from below the gluteal folds to the scapulae and down again. The bandage is then gathered into a rope at the waist and pulled forward above the iliac crests and downward in front of them (Fig. 21-14), first on the side of the convexity of the lumbar curve, usually the left, and then on the opposite side. The patient steadies himself by holding the horizontal bar or the frame. The pelvic tilt must not be lost. Before the plaster has set, it is molded in the waist and allowed to protrude anteriorly because this abdominal bulge will be removed when the positive is skived (shaved off in layers). Careful preparation of the negative with the bony landmarks accentuated makes it easy to modify the positive accurately.

The reference points at the costal margin and the top of the symphysis are relocated by use of the recorded measurements and marked on the outer surface of the cast (Fig. 21-15). A vertical reference line is drawn while the tape measure

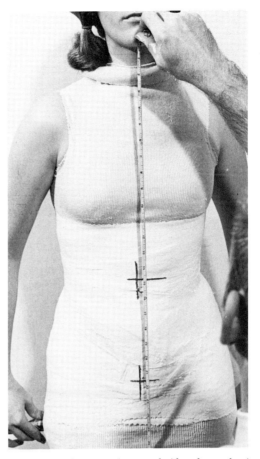

Fig. 21-15. Reference points, xyphoid and symphysis.

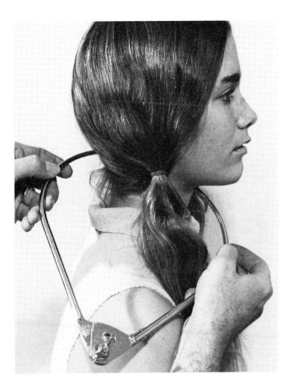

Fig. 21-13. Neck ring measurement.

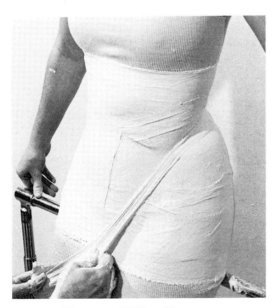

Fig. 21-14. Molding iliac crest.

hangs plumb. This is not the same as the anterior perpendicular midline but will be parallel to it, even if there is a list.

Crosslines are made on the back of the cast to help match the edges later. As soon as the plaster has set, it and the outer layer of stockinet are completely divided down to the protective strip. The cast is sprung open and removed. The inner layer of stockinet remains on the patient. The outer layer is removed from the negative. The original reference marks have been transferred to the inner surface of the plaster. The outside marks for the costal margin and the symphysis can be checked against these by piercing the cast with an awl at these points (Fig. 21-16). The marks on the inner side are then renewed with an indelible pencil so that they will appear on the surface of the positive.

The split negative cast is restored with circular turns of plaster and the bottom is closed. The negative is raised with wedges in front until it stands vertical and is filled with plaster. A metal pipe (Fig. 21-17) with a flattened lower end is inserted as a mandrel before the plaster has set.

After the positive has set, the negative is stripped off. The indelible reference marks are identified and carefully re-marked. The anterior vertical plumb line is extended over the top and bottom of the cast. The mandrel is conveniently held in a pipe vise while the moist plaster positive is skived with a draw knife. The excess plaster is removed anteriorly from the costal margin downward (Fig. 21-18). No matter how bulging the abdomen, the negative is cut back to the depth of the anterior iliac spines.

The anterior vertical midline is drawn perpendicularly to the line between the anterosuperior

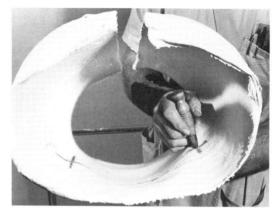

Fig. 21-16. Transfer of reference points to cast.

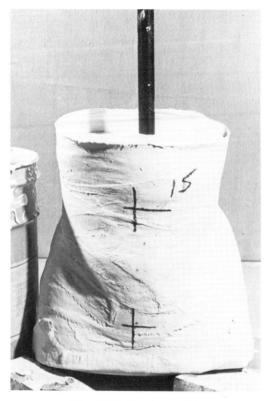

Fig. 21-17. Pouring model.

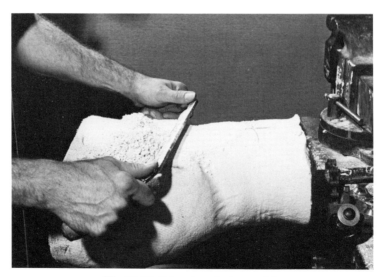

Fig. 21-18. Trimming plaster model.

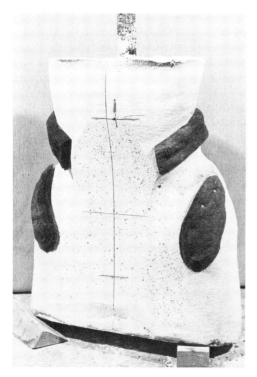

Fig. 21-19. Felt relief pads on the positive.

spines at its midpoint (Fig. 21-19). It is parallel to the plumb line (Fig. 21-17) but not always identical with it. After the plumb line has confirmed the fact that the midline is perpendicular it is discarded.

The waistline is deepened on the shallow side to provide a symmetric purchase on soft tissue over the iliac crests. The groove must not be exaggerated on one side as compared to the other, nor narrow enough to cut into the soft tissues. The grooves are smoothed with a round rasp. The positive is then allowed to dry thoroughly before the leather is applied.

If there is a delay in making their braces, patients with progressive curves should be placed in plaster localizer casts to maintain maximal correction during the waiting period. They may be ambulatory and attend school in their casts.

Preliminary plaster localizer cast correction is often indicated in an obese patient to reduce the waistline and flatten the abdomen, but he must also lose weight by dieting. After a month in a snug cast, a more closely fitted Milwaukee brace can be made.

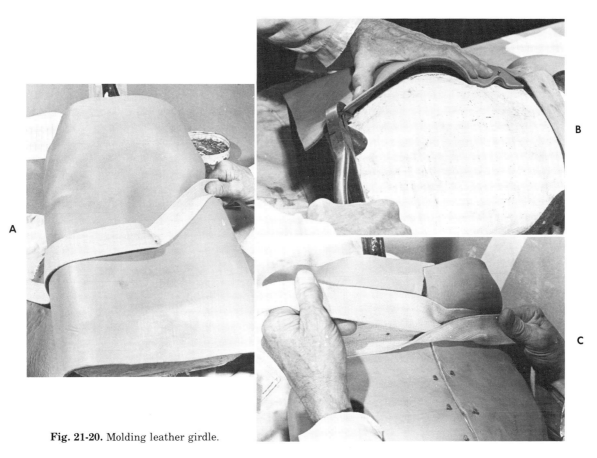

Fig. 21-20. Molding leather girdle.

Preparation of the positive is completed by padding the anterosuperior spines and iliac crests to avoid localized pressure from the completed girdle. Skived felt about 1 cm. thick is nailed over these bony prominences (Fig. 21-19). The modified symmetric positive will now serve as a mold for forming the girdle.

MAKING A LEATHER GIRDLE

Eight- to nine-ounce russet strap leather is thoroughly soaked in water. The cowhide is laid on the model with the thick edge on the side of the concavity of the lumbar curve. Elastic webbing is held with nails in front and drawn upward through the waistline to mold the leather into the grooves (Fig. 21-20, A).

Two diagonal cuts are made in the upper edge of the leather down to the anterior rib margins to allow it to conform as the webbing is pulled backward through the grooves. Wrinkles in the leather at the waist must be entirely eliminated.

Lasting pincers are used to stretch the leather over the buttock prominence (Fig. 21-20, B). The cowhide is secured to the model with nails, and the same procedure is repeated on the opposite side. The ends of the elastic are crossed in back (Fig. 21-20, C), pulled forward in the waistline grooves and drawn downward just medial to the anterosuperior spines. They are secured with nails at the lower margin of the positive.

While still damp, excess leather is removed above the waistline. The edge is then rolled outward and downward on both sides to clear the rib margins and permit active lateral shifting of the torso. The strip of felt above the waist of the positive will hold down the leather. The leather girdle is allowed to dry thoroughly before the elastic straps are removed.

The anterovertical midline and top of the symphysis are identified and marked on the leather (Fig. 21-21). The positive is held vertically in both the frontal and sagittal planes by adjusting two wedges under the front edge. With the aid of a carpenter's square or a triangle, a vertical reference line is drawn downward from one posterosuperior iliac spine (Fig. 21-22). A tape measure is used to record the distance along the waistline groove from the anterior midline to this posterovertical line. The same distance from the anterior midline is measured on the opposite side and another vertical line is drawn. These lines locate

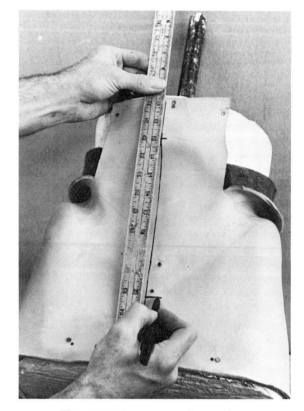

Fig. 21-21. Measuring girdle trim line.

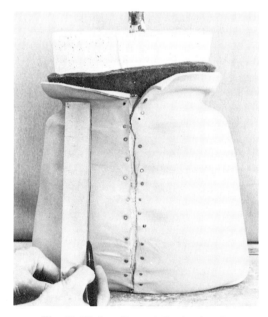

Fig. 21-22. Locating reinforcing band.

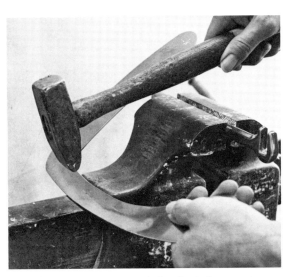

Fig. 21-23. Forming waistband reinforcement.

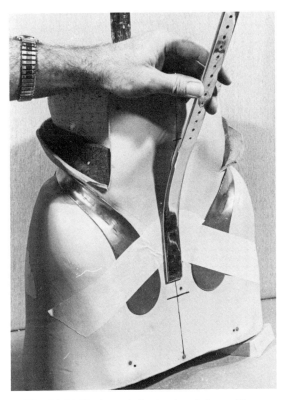

Fig. 21-24. Taping reinforcing bands in position.

the posteromedial segments of the reinforcing bands that are supplied commercially in a prefabricated kit.

The bands provide a firm purchase on the pelvis as a foundation for the superstructure. Each one is cold forged with a flat-peen hammer to form a half tube (Fig. 21-23). It is then turned over and curved to the waistline groove. The band must be a little narrower than the groove. It is fitted by trial positioning. The Monel Metal will need twisting with bending irons.

When the bands fit accurately, they are taped in position (Fig. 21-24) with their posteromedial borders parallel and adjacent to the reference lines. Clearance of 1 cm. in the lumbar region allows for active tilting of the pelvis. The girdle is now ready for the superstructure.

A plastic girdle may be prepared over a similar positive. This technique and the method of installing the superstructure have been published.[4]

FABRICATION OF SUPERSTRUCTURE

The lower anterior bar is held against the front of the girdle and bent as necessary to follow the contour of the abdomen and give support (Fig. 21-27). A reverse bend is made at the rib margin. The anterior bar must have just enough clearance to allow full expansion of the chest.

The lower anterior bar is held against the girdle with the lower end 25 mm. above the level of the symphysis (Fig. 21-25) and the reference point on the chest is marked, and the upper bar is held beside the lower bar and the total length is measured. This length is reduced 25 mm. to allow for the throat mold. The tapped overlapping segments are about one third of the total length. Any excess at either end of either bar is marked for removal with a band saw (Fig. 21-26).

The upper end of the anterior bar is bent in to fit close to the neck and cold forged in its upper 2 cm. (no more) to fit the throat portion of the neck ring (Fig. 21-27). The lower end of the anterior upright is then fastened to the pubic hinge with rivets. The hinge should be on the side of the girdle that requires less stability. With a significant lumbar curve, the hinge is put on the side of the lumbar pad, usually the left.

The anterior bar and neck ring are clamped together. By driving nails into the positive cast, one may attach the hinge to the pelvic bands (Fig. 21-28). With the anterior upright and neck ring in place above the pelvic girdle, the neck ring

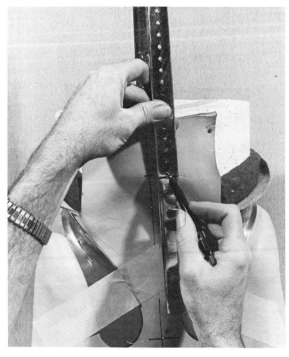

Fig. 21-25. Attachment of anterior bar.

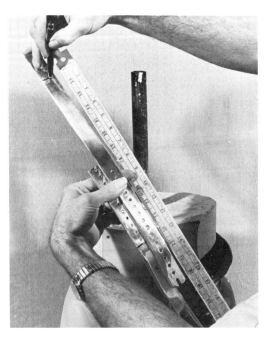

Fig. 21-26. Measurement of bars.

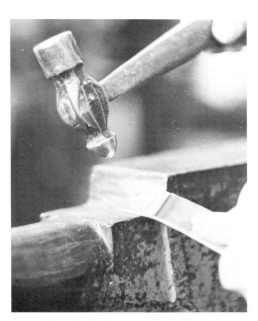

Fig. 21-27. Forming anterior bar.

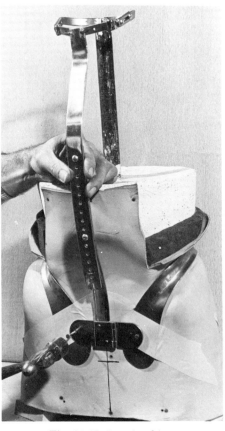

Fig. 21-28. Locating hinge.

should tilt downward anteriorly approximately 20 degrees.

The upper posterior bars are positioned laterally on the back of the neck ring and downward to waist level. Any excess is cut off above the neck ring. They are repositioned and marked 2 cm. below their junction with the neck ring. At this level they are twisted a little to conform to the base of the neck and torso and are bent just enough to clear the body. They are clamped in place on the neck ring and the lower halves of the posterior uprights are held against them. The bottom of the waist groove is marked on the lower bars. They are bent inward here and then outward below and above to conform to the pelvic girdle and the upper posterior bars. They should not protrude excessively above the waist.

The lower posterior uprights are marked approximately 3 cm. below the bend at the waist. Holes are drilled here through uprights and pelvic bands to fasten the uprights to the girdle. In the finished brace, breakage at the screw hole is avoided by fastening a broad, prefabricated bar bridge over each upright at the waistline with two rivets for each bridge but none through the bar (Fig. 21-29). The rivet through the bar is 2 cm. or more below the bar bridge.

The superstructure is now removed from the plaster model. The excess leather is trimmed from the girdle to facilitate the preliminary fitting.

The upper ends of the posterior bars are riveted to the occiput portion of a neck ring of the proper size. The aluminum forms for the occipital pads are screwed in place on the back of the neck ring and temporary foam-rubber pads are glued to them. The throat mold is held in position and holes are drilled to correspond with those in the neck ring. It is then temporarily fastened to the neck ring with rivets.

The upper and lower segments of the anterior bar are joined with screws. The upper and lower parts of the posterior bars are fastened with the clips provided in the kit.

The assembled brace is now ready for a preliminary fitting on the patient. The patient lifts the brace while the girdle is tightened by a strap around the posterior uprights (Fig. 21-30). To accommodate for the built-in pelvic tilt, he may have to lean forward or bend his knees. The brace is inspected for proper fit of the girdle and clearance of the superstructure (Fig. 21-31).

If the posterior uprights are fitted too closely

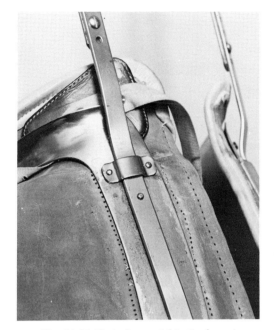

Fig. 21-29. Posterior upright attachment.

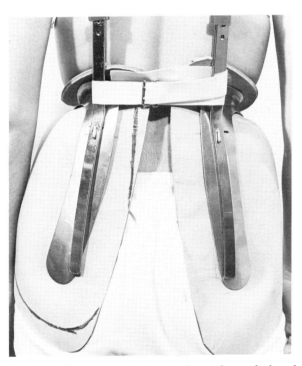

Fig. 21-30. Temporary attachment of uprights and gluteal trim line.

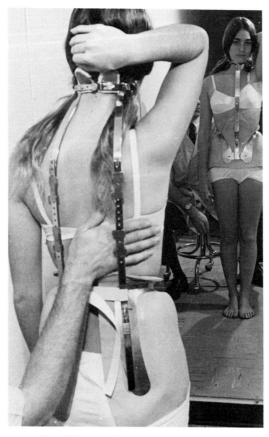

Fig. 21-31. Preliminary fitting of brace.

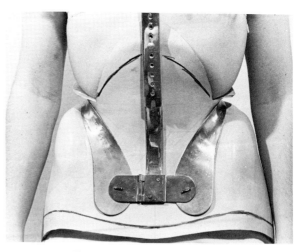

Fig. 21-32. Trim lines of girdle.

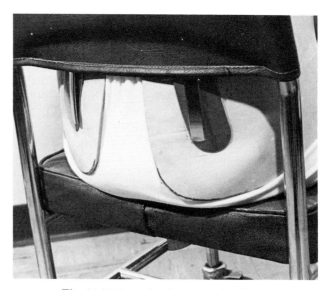

Fig. 21-33. Posterior clearance of girdle.

to the torso, they will restrict respiration and desirable trunk motion. They should be bent outward until they just touch the back on deep inspiration when the thoracic pad is in place. The patient must have room for deep breathing while in the brace.

The throat mold should fit the neck closely but cause no pressure on the mandible. When the chin is raised, the head is supported firmly by the two occiput pads (Fig. 21-31). They must be *under* the back of the head, not behind it.

The location of the top of the symphysis pubis is verified and marked on the leather. Tightening the girdle may have raised the previous mark. The prominences of the greater trochanters are located by palpation. The line is drawn above them and continued in both directions. The lower edge of the girdle is trimmed to this line (Fig. 21-32). The leather must be cut high enough to avoid excessive pressure on the thighs and allow comfortable sitting with good posture.

The abdominal apron should reach just to the ribs. The costal margin is located by palpation

and drawn on the leather. The angle between the apron and the leather at the waist must be below the ribs.

The lower posterior margin is located 25 mm. above the tuberosities of the ischia (Fig. 21-30). The vertical borders of the girdle are marked for trimming to make the edges parallel. The edges should be 5 to 10 cm. apart to allow for loss of weight through the hips. The brace is then removed and the excess leather is cut away along the trim lines.

The brace is reapplied and the patient seated on a stool. The leather is trimmed high enough in the groin to allow sitting without upward dis-

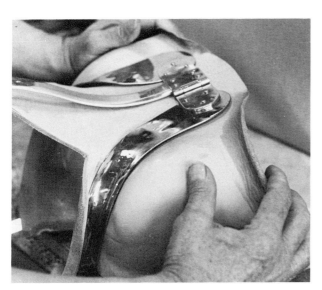

Fig. 21-34. Skiving of pelvic girdle.

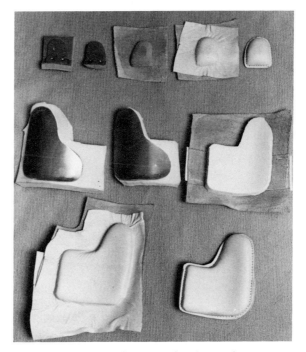

Fig. 21-35. Thoracic and occiput pads.

placement of the brace. The waistline of the girdle must not crowd the ribs. The patient must be able to lean forward without forcing the throat mold uncomfortably high under the chin.

In back, the finished girdle should extend to within less than 3 cm. of the chair (Fig. 21-33). If it is too short, control of the pelvic tilt will be lost.

Alignment of the posterior bars is marked for reattachment to the pelvic bands and leather. The brace is then removed. While it is still assembled, the posterior uprights are welded to the neck ring. If the pelvic bands are too long to permit stitching the lining over the cowhide, the excess is removed.

The lower margin of the leather girdle as far back as the trochanters is skived on the inside to a feather edge. This edge, which is to contact the thighs anteriorly, is moistened with water, flared, and stretched upward for added comfort during hip flexion (Fig. 21-34).

A soft lining leather is centered in the belly portion of the girdle and bonded with rubber cement to the inner surface. Particular care is taken to form the cavities for the iliac crests. The lining leather must be wrinkle free and in total contact with the girdle. It is turned back over the edges of the cowhide and sewed down, except in the groins, where the layers are left unsewed to facilitate later wetting and molding.

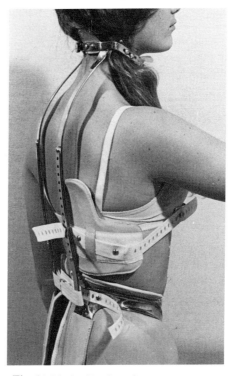

Fig. 21-36. Application of corrective straps.

Firm, not soft, foam rubber is then bonded to the inner surfaces of the prefabricated occipital rests (Fig. 21-35). The rubber is trimmed to the edges of the metal and rounded off in front by sanding. Calf leather is bonded to the outer aluminum surface. The inner surface of the rubber is upholstered with a soft lining. The edges are stitched and the excess leather is trimmed away.

All other pads are backed by more malleable sheet aluminum and upholstered with softer foam rubber in a like manner. The rubber extends 2 cm. in front of the metal of the thoracic pad for added comfort (Fig. 21-35).

Holes are burned at both ends of the Dacron strap for the thoracic pad. The strap is fastened across the center of the rectangular lower portion of the pad with Velcro so that it may be later adjusted to exactly the right angle. To keep the medial border of the pad vertical, the strap usually slants laterally downward on the pad (Fig. 21-36). The position must be checked for each individual chest contour. When the position is satisfactory, the strap is secured permanently with screws or rivets.

FITTING AND ADJUSTMENT

After the brace is polished and assembled, it is ready for the final fitting and adjustment of pads. If there is too much lumbar lordosis, the lower ends of the posterior uprights with the Monel Metal bands can be bent to increase the pelvic tilt. The opposing force is furnished at the waist by a bending iron on the upright (Fig. 21-5).

The lower rectangular portion of the thoracic pad exerts an axially directed holding force against the ribs at and below the apex of their posterior prominence. The pad must not be so snug that the patient cannot shift the torso away from it.

The narrow upper part of the pad corrects the rib hump passively and furnishes a comfortable edge under which the scapula can glide. The medial border should be vertical and fit under the posterior upright, which is bent to give it firm and uniform support. The thoracic pad is held in this position by passing its strap under and around the upright to a truss stud (Fig. 21-36).

To advance the pad, the strap is tightened at the anterior end on the outrigger. The posterior end is not unfastened after it is properly adjusted and may be bound to the upright to keep it from falling off when the brace is removed.

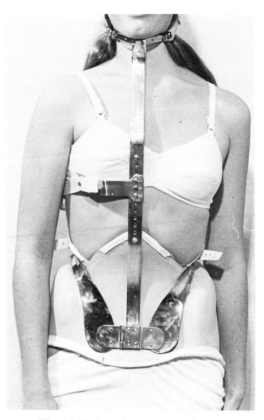

Fig. 21-37. Anterior strap attachment.

The outrigger must be long enough to prevent any pressure on the anterolateral aspect of the chest wall. The lateral end is marked and cut off at the proper length. The expanded medial end is secured to the anterior upright with screws (Fig. 21-37). The outrigger is then bent to the contour of the breast or lower chest wall to permit unimpeded breathing without contact. A truss stud at the lateral end allows adjustment of the tension on the strap.

The lumbar pad must fit laterally to the spinous processes and caudad to the last rib. Its size and thickness are adapted to the position in the girdle and the area of the holding force required. To furnish localized support, it is placed inside the leather girdle and may be fastened in a variety of ways (Fig. 21-38). It may be floated on a Dacron strap, or for a broader holding force it may be placed between the leather and the metal. The lateral end of the strap is then passed under and around the metal band and fastened to a truss stud on the outer surface.

When a plastic girdle is used, the pad must be inside and is fastened to the plastic with Velcro.

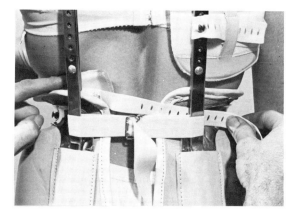

Fig. 21-38. Mounting lumbar pad.

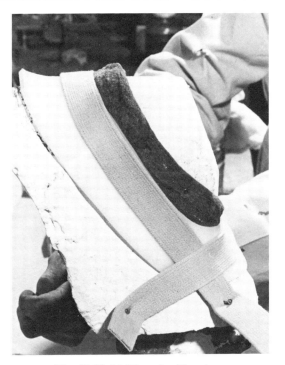

Fig. 21-39. Molding shoulder ring.

Fixation with hinges, metal brackets, or spring steel has proved unsatisfactory; however a rubber block may be inserted between the pad and the upright to increase the holding force. Velcro attachments permit a change of position as the relationships of brace and patient change.

FABRICATION OF SHOULDER RINGS

The shoulder ring is controlled in back by an durable plastic for each patient. It is molded to fit the shoulder and side of the neck. The ideal thermoplastic has not yet been found, but polyethylene has been used because it becomes soft at a temperature of 400° F. and can be formed over a modified positive cast of the shoulder (Fig. 21-39). It is firmly molded by elastic straps, and the edges of the plastic are rolled out, particularly at the angle of the neck. The orthotist's hands must be protected by gloves.

The shoulder ring is controlled in back by an oblique Dacron strap, riveted far enough medially to avoid catching on the posterior upright. The strap that holds down the broad upper surface of the ring supplies a passive corrective force on the shoulder girdle and upper two ribs. When the shoulder is high, this force is increased by raising the attachment of the strap. The location of the strap on the ring controls the direction of the predominant thrust. When it is fastened low, the force is largely medial,[4] and when attached too high, it prevents the shoulder from elevating. When the shoulders are level, the obliquity of the strap is reduced to horizontal by moving the truss stud higher on the opposite upright. The lower transverse segment of the ring then exerts an axially directed holding force on the rib cage.

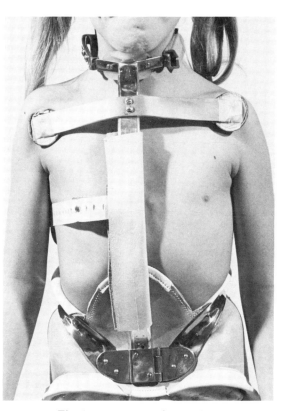

Fig. 21-40. Anterior thoracic bar.

To further secure the ring in position, a second strap may be necessary from the front of the ring to the anterior bar. This is the only place on the brace where it is desirable to interpose elastic to permit free respiration. The more effective posterior strap should contain no rubber.

To correct round shoulders caused by tight pectorals, anterior shoulder pads may be attached to a transverse bar (Fig. 21-40). The bar should be adjustable as to height. The amount of pressure is controlled by bending this bar.

Leather covers on the uprights (Fig. 21-40) protect the clothing and skin to make the brace more comfortable. The edges of the folded leather are fastened like an envelope with Velcro. As the deformity improves, the bars are bent to maintain the holding force.

The child should wear the brace for 20 minutes or more to adjust to it before he is checked by the orthotist, after which it is sent to the orthopaedic surgeon for inspection and patient instruction.

•   •   •

MODIFICATIONS OF MILWAUKEE SCOLIOSIS BRACE

Since the introduction of the Milwaukee brace by Drs. Blount and Schmidt in 1946, several revisions of the orthosis have been suggested although the basic concept has remained virtually unaltered. Clinicians have been aware that to eliminate the irritation along the patient's iliac crest, firm total contact of the pelvic portion of the Milwaukee brace to the pelvic structures is necessary. Perhaps the pelvic girdle could be fashioned better from plastic material than from leather. Experience has shown that a plastic well suited for the pelvic girdle portion of the Milwaukee brace is Orthoplast. This material is easily handled by the orthotist and lends itself quite well to the custom fabrication of a snug-fitting pelvic girdle.[8]

Experience of other orthotists has also indicated that the pelvic portion of the brace could also be prefabricated. A study indicated that with 16 variable sizes of the pelvic girdle, successful fitting of 95% of the scoliotic population could be obtained.[7]

The above modifications of the basic Milwaukee brace concept refer only to the use of different materials for the fabrication of the pelvic girdle. The basic concept of dynamic correction of a scoliosis deformity by the use of this brace remains quite secure.

THE EDITORS

REFERENCES

1. Blount, W. P.: Early recognition and prompt evaluation of spinal deformity, Wisconsin Med. J. **68:**245-249, 1969.
2. Blount, W. P.: Use of the Milwaukee brace, Orthop. Clin. N. Am. **3:**3-16, March 1972, Philadelphia, W. B. Saunders Co.
3. Blount, W. P., and Mellencamp, D. D.: Scoliosis treatment. Skeletal maturity evaluation, Minn. Med. **56:**382-390, May 1973.
4. Blount, W. P., and Moe, J. H.: The Milwaukee brace. Baltimore, 1973, The Williams & Wilkins Co.
5. Blount, W. P., and Mueller, K. H.: Die nicht-operative Behandlung der Skoliose mit dem Milwaukee Korsett, Orthop. Praxis, **8**(6):148, June 1972.
6. Greulich, W. W., and Pyle, S. I.: Radiographic atlas of skeletal development of the hand and wrist, Stanford, 1966, Stanford University Press.
7. Hall, J. E., Miller, M. E., Schuman, W., and Standish, W.: A refined concept in orthotic management of scoliosis, Orthot. Prosthet. **29:**9-16, Dec. 1975.
8. Hall, J. E., and Miller, W.: Prefabrication of Milwaukee braces, J. Bone Joint Surg. **56A**(8):1763, Dec. 1974.
9. The Milwaukee brace: A fabrication manual, Prosthetic-Orthotic Center, Northwestern University Medical School, Chicago, Illinois, 1972, pp. 1-49.
10. Moe, J. H.: Non-operative treatment of idiopathic scoliosis, Clin. Orthop. Related Res. **93:**38, 1973.

CHAPTER 22

Orthotic treatment of kyphotic and lordotic deformities

JOHN H. MOE, M.D.

Kyphotic and lordotic spine deformities present a problem of magnitude similar to scoliosis. Kyphosis, a posterior convexity deformity of the spine must be evaluated in the same manner as scoliosis. Although kyphosis can occur in the cervical and lumbar segments, the thoracic spine is the most common site of kyphotic deformity. The cause of abnormal thoracic kyphosis may be one of the following:

1. Congenital defects of segmentation
2. Abnormal posture, "postural round back" as is found in the relaxed child with prominent abdomen
3. Scheuermann's disease as seen in the adolescent
4. Bone metabolic changes such as osteoporosis
5. Accidental trauma
6. Surgical trauma; laminectomies with excision of facets
7. Infections, including tuberculous
8. Radiation epiphyseal arrest
9. Myelomeningocele

Congenital kyphotic deformities may be recognized early. Developmental kyphotic deformities are most often noted during early adolescent life.

EXAMINATION AND MEASUREMENT

Complete physical and radiologic examinations are essential to determine the best management.

The Cobb method of angular measurement is preferred. A standard method of examination for measurement is recommended—the patient stands with head erect, both arms forward at shoulder level with hands resting on a horizontal bar at shoulder height. With kyphosis deformities, the highest vertebra included in the deformity is determined and a line is drawn parallel to its superior edge. The lowest vertebra involved is likewise marked. Perpendiculars are erected from these lines and at their intersections, and the degree of deformity is determined. Cervical spine lordosis can be measured in a similar way. Lumbar lordosis includes the position of the sacrum, measured by its relative angulation from the lower margin of L5 to the superior margin of the sacrum. When the angle diverges noticeably, the sacrum may approach or even reach a horizontal position in relation to the lumbar spine.

A study at Gillette Childrens Hospital, St. Paul, Minnesota, revealed that the average normal thoracic-spine kyphotic curve is 20 to 35 degrees. Kyphotic angulation beyond 40 degrees in the thoracic spine is considered pathologic.

CLINICAL VARIATIONS

Postural round back deformities of childhood or early adolescence do not alter normal spine flexibility because when the spine is hyperextended, postural curves readily correct and no changes are noted in the vertebral bodies or discs.

397

Persistent vascular channels in the center of apical vertebral bodies may occasionally be present. Their significance is disputable. If these patients cooperate fully and the curve is mild, a well-regulated exercise program will improve posture and help reduce the degree of kyphosis.

Once the measured angulation exceeds 50 degrees in the standing position, there is a strong possibility that the vertebral epiphyseal plates may be compressed sufficiently to retard their growth potential, narrowing anterior body heights and vertebral wedging thus results. Curves of this severity do not respond to simple exercises. Orthoses used in conjunction with a well-regulated exercise program may reduce the degree of kyphosis. Response varies with the degree of pathologic abnormality.

Other postural defects that accompany juvenile kyphosis include increased lumbar lordosis, protuberant abdomen with increased lumbosacral angle and exaggerated pelvic tilt. Often the hamstrings, hip flexors, and pectoral muscles are tight.

Scheuermann's disease is characterized by disturbance of vertebral body growth plates and invagination of the intervertebral disc into vertebral bodies, leading to increased thoracic kyphosis. At the apex of the curve, two or three vertebrae typically exhibit wedging, usually greater than 5 degrees. In the early stages of Scheuermann's disease the amount of wedging and disc protrusion is minimal and the spine remains flexible. Later in adolescence, the spine becomes more rigid, apical wedging increases, and disc invagination further distorts the vertebral body shape. Exercises will help improve posture and strengthen trunk muscles, but orthotic devices should be used until spine growth is complete. Lumbar disc protrusion may be a part of Scheuermann's deformity. If confined to the lumbar area, it need only be treated with low back orthoses. Pain, depending on its severity, usually indicates the need for orthotic protection. Many patients, however, are asymptomatic and do not require any more than periodic evaluation.

LORDOSIS

Lordosis, an anterior concave deformity of the cervical or lumbar spine is evaluated in a similar manner as thoracic kyphosis and scoliosis.

The etiology of abnormal lumbar lordosis may depend on one of the following:

1. A relaxed child with postural round back and prominent abdomen may also have an increased lumbar lordosis.
2. Scheuermann's disease, adolescent round back.
3. Disease of soft tissues such as the Ehlers-Danlos syndrome.
4. Dwarfism, particularly achondroplasia, is characteristically accompanied by extreme lumbar lordosis. The thoracic alignment is unusually flat.
5. Lordosis associated with multiple congenital anomalies. This type of spine is usually rigid and is characterized by multiple failures of segmentation, absence of numbers of growth plates, and difficulty in therapeutic control.
6. After insertion of intradural implants for hydrocephalus.
7. Spondylolisthesis, grade two or greater.
8. Meningomyelocele.
9. Hip-flexion contractures.
10. Lordotic dorsal spine deformity is most frequently seen in adolescent idiopathic scoliosis. Radiologists and many orthopaedic surgeons speak freely of kyphoscoliosis, whereas, in fact, a true lateral x-ray film of a standing spine will show that the thoracic spine is abnormally flattened. This is not related to rotation of the vertebral bodies but is a true flattening, often seen to involve the entire spine.
11. Other conditions such as rheumatoid spondylitis, posttraumatic paraplegia in childhood, compression changes associated with cord tumors, dermatomyositis, arthrogryposis, muscular dystrophies, Werdnig-Hoffman syndrome, and Friedreich's ataxia.

ORTHOTIC MANAGEMENT OF KYPHOTIC AND LORDOTIC DEFORMITIES

An efficient orthotic device for control of kyphotic and lordotic deformities must include the components to correct the associated abnormal postural features accompanying these basic deformities.

The Milwaukee brace, with its well-molded pelvic girdle, specialized uprights, and occipital rests, exerts corrective forces to all spine areas (Fig. 22-1). The forward thrust against the posterior thoracic prominence and lower buttocks is

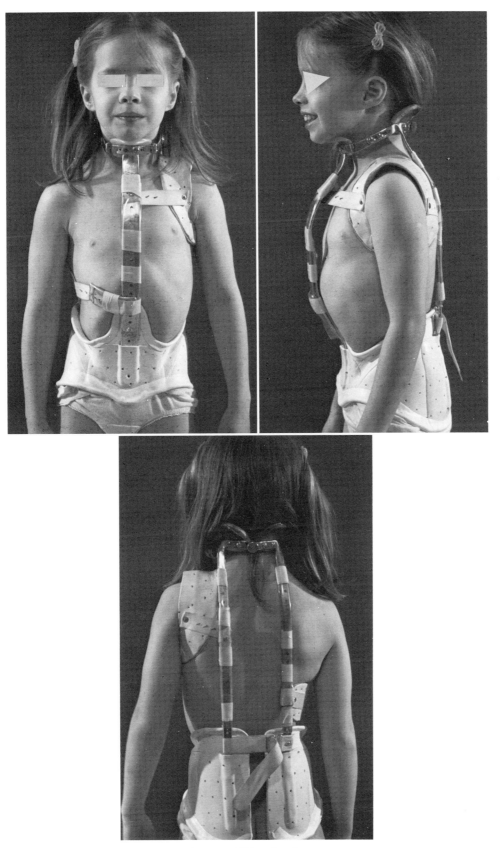

Fig. 22-1. Milwaukee brace.

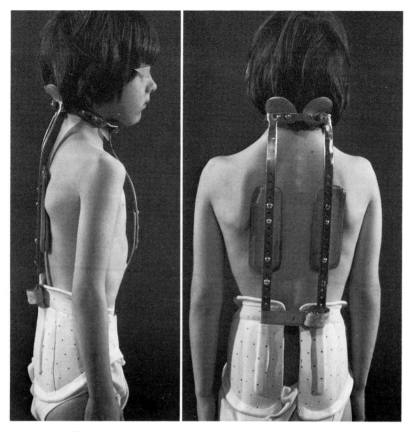

Fig. 22-2. Milwaukee brace with thoracic kyphosis pad.

coupled with counterpressure against the lower abdomen. The head is realigned by forces directed to the anterior neck region. Other three-point pressure systems exert additional corrective forces. In combination they should flatten the lumbar lordosis, reverse the excessive pelvic tilt distally, and at the same time reduce the kyphotic deformity with realignment of the head and neck proximally (Fig. 22-2). The Milwaukee brace may be easily removed for daily bathing and skin care. Exercise is an essential part of abnormal kyphosis and lordosis management and can be performed routinely both in and out of the orthosis.

The Milwaukee brace is preferable in the control of the following:

1. The flexible thoracic kyphotic deformity of Scheuermann's disease responds dramatically. The fixed portion of the deformity can be held and controlled. The abnormal compensatory lumbar lordosis deformity will also decrease.

2. The achondroplasia lumbar lordotic deformity should be corrected and maintained with a Milwaukee brace throughout skeletal growth.

3. The collapsing lumbar lordotic deformity associated with Ehler-Danlos syndrome.

A LSO (extension and lateral control orthosis, Williams) may be prescribed for mild postural kyphosis with no vertebral growth plate change. This orthosis will flatten the lumbar lordotic curve and reverse the pelvic tilt with anterior abdominal pressure. The orthosis conditions the patient to subconsciously extend the thoracic spine and thereby improve postural alignment.

A TLSO (flexion control, Jewett) provides a three-point pressure system and when used with exercise has some influence on postural kyphotic deformities but has limited effectiveness because of lack of postural control of head, neck, and pelvis.

Well-molded plaster body casts or jackets are also used to provide corrective forces for control of kyphotic deformities. These are applied with a pelvic girdle contoured to flatten the lumbar spine. They exert hyperextension force to the thoracic spine region. For maximum effectiveness such a plaster cast should include a cervical collar to fix the head and neck in neutral position.

Clinical experience, however, indicates the superiority of the Milwaukee brace, combined with an exercise program in the treatment of thoracic kyphotic deformities. McAllister and Hardy[2] report that round back deformities are generally improved with a Milwaukee brace. Bradford, Moe, Montalo, and Winter[1] report that kyphotic deformity from Scheuermann's disease treated with a Milwaukee brace and exercise showed an average decrease of thoracic kyphotic deformity from 59 to 35 degrees.

Kyphotic deformities from congenital anomalies accompanied by angular change do not respond to orthoses, rather they require surgical treatment. Neurofibromatosis with acute angular deformity likewise is best treated by surgery. Orthoses are required, however, as long-term protective devices after surgery.

Hip-joint contractures contributing to spine deformities require surgical releases before spine deformity can be effectively improved or controlled with orthoses.

SUMMARY

Dorsal kyphotic and lumbar lordotic deformities that have not become fixed and severe may be controlled by orthoses. If the deformities, however, are severe, orthoses assume a secondary treatment role. The Milwaukee brace provides the maximum control in the treatment of spine deformities of these types.

REFERENCES

1. Bradford, D. S., Moe, J. H., Montalo, F. J., and Winter, R. B.: Scheuermann's kyphosis and round back deformity, results of Milwaukee brace treatments, J. Bone Joint Surg. **56A:**740, 1974.
2. McAllister, D. T., and Hardy, J. H.: Juvenile kyphosis; statistical survey and comparison of methods of treatment, J. Bone Joint Surg. **55A:**1323, 1973.

CHAPTER 23

Treatment of the paralytic spine

WILTON H. BUNCH, M.D., Ph.D.

Frequently it is desirable to support the spine and trunk of a paralyzed child. This seldom, if ever, constitutes definitive treatment but may be of real value in delaying surgery until further growth has been obtained or in improving the function of the paralyzed child.

STANDING DEVICES

The parapodium and its variations constitute a major breakthrough in the care of the paralyzed infant and child. It is designed to provide stability of the ankles, knees, hips, and trunk and permits weight bearing. It allows the otherwise frail and paralyzed child to stand and sit, frees the hands for purposeful activities, and assists in greater socialization. This orthosis is of most value in the child of 12 to 18 months who should, in normal development, be standing, but cannot because of his neurologic disorder. In such an orthosis, the child can proceed with normal intellectual and functional development consistent with the basic defect.

The frame that I use (Fig. 23-1) has the advantage that it can be made from materials found in any orthotic establishment. Placing the child in the frame is simple, since the knee piece swings open anteriorly. Thus children with hip deformities and general lack of mobility can be fit into the frame in a few seconds.

This orthosis is not thought of as a corrective

device for the spine. It will not correct or prevent increase in the curves of scoliosis, lordosis, or kyphosis. It provides lower-limb and spine stability but not spinal correction.

BODY JACKETS

Body jackets and casts of various types have been a popular method of treating the paralytic spine. These are fabricated in many different designs from a wide variety of materials. Unfortunately, these often function only by concealing the curve from patient, parents, and physician. As such, they provide assurance that is totally unwarranted. They can be therapeutic only if replacement is frequent enough to match the changes induced as the child grows.

Effective body jackets utilize two principles. First, they provide pelvic stability and may correct the pelvic obliquity frequently present in children with paralytic scoliosis. This allows the child to sit squarely in the wheelchair with a relatively straight takeoff for the lumbar spine. The second principle utilizes the ribs to support the weight of the trunk on the anterior flare. By utilizing these principles, some very flexible curves may be corrected and held by body jackets (Fig. 23-2).

Like the standing frame, the body jacket should be thought of as providing support for the child to increase his functional activity. If this is

402

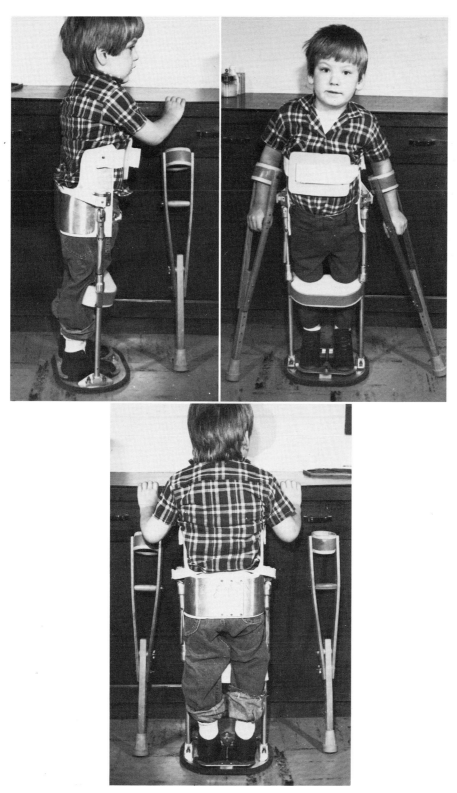

Fig. 23-1. Parapodium.

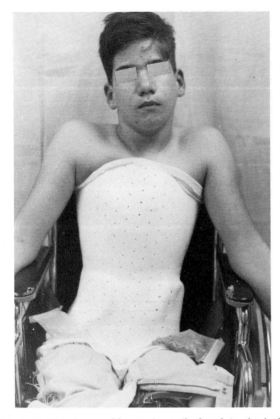

Fig. 23-2. This boy could not sit until placed in the body jacket. Although his flexible scoliosis improved only slightly, his function is greatly improved and he now can attend regular school.

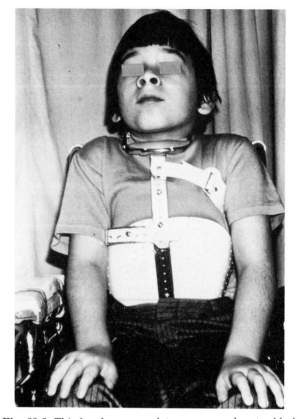

Fig. 23-3. This boy has a complete sensory and motor block at T4, secondary to an astrocytoma. Enlarged pelvic girdle is demonstrated.

the only requirement placed on the orthosis, the body jacket will be successful. Rarely should it be expected to function as a corrective device.

WHEELCHAIR INSERTS

A variety of types of wheelchair inserts have been designed to attempt to support the child with a collapsing spine. These may be as simple as cutouts for intact myelomeningocele sacs, or they may involve multiple lateral supports. These, again, are body supports and are designed only to free the child to use his hands. They may improve the function of the child, but they do not improve his spine.

MILWAUKEE BRACE

If the decision is made to attempt correction of the spine orthotically, the most effective device, because of its adjustability, is the Milwaukee brace. Although it is usually considered an active corrective orthosis in the treatment of idiopathic

scoliosis, it also has excellent passive properties if the design is modified to meet the special needs of the paralyzed child.

Orthotic design

The orthosis for paralytic scoliosis is not radically different from the standard Milwaukee brace as used for idiopathic scoliosis. The pelvic piece is larger and frequently extends up to take some weight from the rib cage. The fit of the pelvic girdle is assessed as carefully as possible, sometimes by use of pressure transducers and thermography. The fit of the girdle is the most critical part of the brace construction (Fig. 23-3).

The thoracic pad is larger than in the standard orthosis and is contoured to fit the rib cage. Since it is impossible for the paralyzed child to "pull away" from this pad as does the patient with idiopathic scoliosis, this pressure must also be monitored. The pad is centered over the ribs leading to the apex of the curve.

Most paralytic curves, fortunately, are lumbar or thoracolumbar. It is difficult to apply corrective pads to high thoracic curves. Neither the axillary sling nor the shoulder ring has worked well. When a high thoracic pad is indicated, we use a modified thoracic pad, shaping it so that the base of the pad is narrow for allowance of higher placement than usual.

No attempt is made to gain distraction by use of a tightly fitted chin rest. The patient should not sag onto the throat mold, since the corrective forces are provided by the trunk pads. Use of a low-placed throat mold eliminates the objection that the patients are left hanging in the brace. The occiput pad is adjusted to provide a low, close fit.

Indications and contraindications

The passive version of the Milwaukee brace is indicated for the child with a paralytic, flexible curve in whom fusion is not desirable. The child may need several brace changes as he outgrows the original while developing trunk height. The brace may be applied even in the absence of skin sensation. Anesthetic skin is not a contraindication.

There are, however, two contraindications to the brace. The first is the obese child, as it is almost impossible to get the desired fit, particularly with anesthetic skin. Orthotic failures have been in this group.

The second contraindication relates to the critical care necessary to monitor the child's anesthetic skin. If the mother cannot provide this type of meticulous fitting schedule supervision, the brace is contraindicated.

Fitting schedule

With anesthetic skin, the brace-fitting schedule is essential. The child should be admitted to a facility with experienced nurses and therapists. The brace is applied for 1 hour and then removed for examination of the skin. If there is no difficulty, it is left off for 4 hours and then reapplied. If the skin tolerates the pressure well, this may be repeated. The child wears the brace no more than 3 of the first 24 hours.

Wearing time is slowly increased by 15 to 30 minutes per day. If skin redness appears, it is allowed to subside before the orthosis is reapplied. Eventually even children with myelomeningocele should be able to tolerate the orthosis 12 to 18 hours a day. The orthosis may be removed at

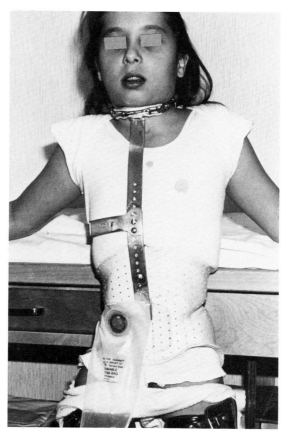

Fig. 23-4. This girl is totally independent although braced from her chin to her toes. She is anesthetic and paralyzed from T9 distally.

night, as gravity is eliminated in the supine position. Frequently they may, in addition, need an hour out of the orthosis in midday.

Ambulation aids

Once spinal stability is provided by the orthosis, some children can ambulate using a swing-through gait and KAFO (knee-ankle-foot orthosis). An example is a girl who is ambulatory despite a total T8-level paraplegia (Fig. 23-4). She is able to balance over the single free joint at the hips and to move at a pace equal to her nonparalyzed classmates.

Most paralyzed children, however, are not this active. For those who need stability at the hips as well, the Milwaukee brace is still a possibility. The pelvic band may be contoured to fit the crest indentation of the Milwaukee brace. Hip locks are adjusted as for any other HKAFO orthosis, and sitting and standing are possible (Fig. 23-5).

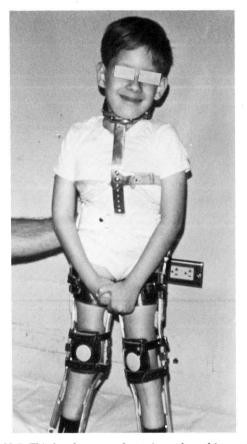

Fig. 23-5. This boy has a myelomeningocele and is paralyzed from T8 distally. Using the braces and pelvic band attached over the Milwaukee brace, he is able to walk short distances with crutches.

SUMMARY

Many types of trunk support are used for children with paralytic spinal deformity. Most of these types make a contribution to the function of the child by stabilizing the trunk and so freeing the upper extremities. Of this group of orthoses, the Milwaukee brace is the most consistent in correcting and holding the scoliosis of the paralytic spine. It should be considered as a temporary, though long-term, expedient to allow spine growth prior to definitive surgical treatment.

CHAPTER 24

Halo traction systems

RONALD L. DeWALD, M.D.

The halo is a method of skeletal skull fixation that provides three-dimensional control of the head. As such it offers the surgeon a way to selectively position the cervical spine in addition to stabilizing it through traction. When combined with appropriate distal counterforces, such as a cast, femoral pins, or pelvic hoop, the halo also provides effective control of the thoracic and lumbar spine and the pelvis.

✳ Indications for halo traction systems are (1) cervical or high thoracic spine instability or deformity, (2) patients with limited respiratory reserve, who could not tolerate localizer casts, (3) severe fixed spinal deformity at any level that requires corrective forces greater than those supplied by conventional external holding devices, and (4) precise fixation for vertebral osteotomy procedures.

HALO APPLICATION

The halo is a metal ring secured to the skull with four pins just below its maximum diameter (Fig. 24-1). Both the halo and the pins are sterilized. Skin preparation includes shaving the hair immediately about the insertion site and then cleansing it thoroughly. Anesthesia may be either local or general. When local anesthesia is used, the periosteum must be infiltrated as thoroughly as the skin. By positioning the halo and making the initial anesthetic insertion through the selected pin channels, the area of infiltration is minimized. This is desirable since small skin wheals lessen the chance of distorting skin-skull rela-

tionships. Puckered skin margins will undergo necrosis unless tension has been relieved. General anesthesia is usually chosen for children because of the need for four separate insertion sites, each with skin and periosteal sensitivity.

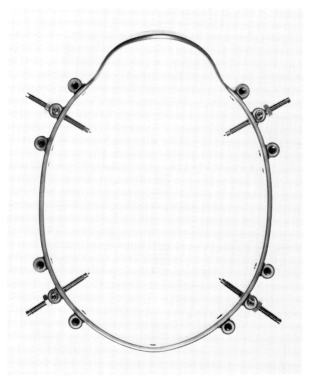

Fig. 24-1. Original cranial halo with skull fixation pins in site. Elevated posterior arc provides an unobstructed access to suboccipital area of spine.

407

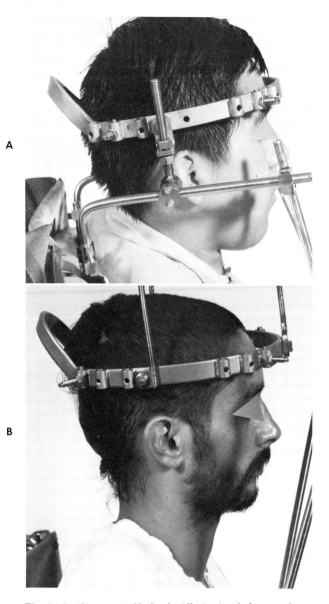

Fig. 24-2. Alignment of halo. A, All pin sites below maximum diameter of skull. B, Common error in placement, posterior pins too high.

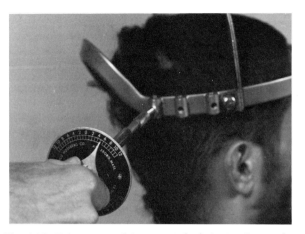

Fig. 24-3. Torque screwdriver control of pin tension used to fix halo to skull.

To ensure that the halo is below the maximum diameter of the skull the front pin holes are centered in the groove at the upper margin of the eyebrows (between the supraciliary ridge and the frontal prominences). Posteriorly the halo is placed about ⅛ inch above the ear. The object is to get the halo as close to the ears as possible and yet certain that it is not touching the pinnae, which are very sensitive to constant pressure (Fig. 24-2). When viewed from above, the halo is aligned to leave slightly more space posteriorly than ante-

riorly. This allows for low-grade edema, which often develops in nonambulatory patients who are more frequently supine than prone.

Anteriorly, the thickest mass of bone is central, under the medial halo channels. Use of this area leaves a very small visible scar, but it also provides the most durable halo fixation. One can avoid all visible scarring by keeping the pin insertions within the hairline through use of the most lateral channels. However, this choice requires penetration of the temporalis muscle and its overlying fascia, a placement that commonly leads to pain during chewing. Also the temporalis bone, being relatively thin, has less holding power. Posteriorly the central channel generally has the best alignment with the skull although the choice is not great in this area.

With the surgeon holding the halo in the appropriate position, an assistant inserts the pins until they just touch the skin. One front pin and the diagonally opposite posterior pin must be tightened simultaneously with fingers to maximum finger tension. Otherwise, the halo will migrate away from the point of insertion with every turn of the pin.

The other pair is then tightened in a similar fashion. Final tension of 6 kg.cm. (5.25 inch-pounds) is achieved with a torque screwdriver (Fig. 24-3). However, if this instrument is not available, one can use a short-handled screwdriver, taking care to apply force only with the fingertips. To minimize the tendency to disturb halo alignment as the pins are tightened, it is best to alternate once or twice between the two pairs of pins, gaining tension in a serial fashion. After

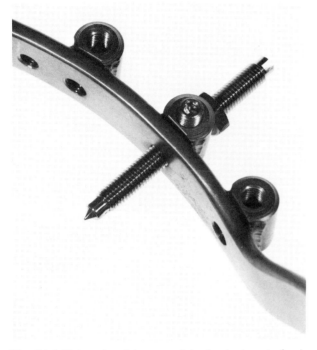

Fig. 24-4. External nut to prevent inadvertent central migration of halo pin with bone erosion.

the desired maximum tension has been obtained in all four pins, they are locked with a nylon-tipped bushing (which catches the threads). Then a nut is fastened tightly against the outside of the halo as a precaution against inadvertent penetration of the skull if the screw works loose (Fig. 24-4). To avoid turning the pin as the nut is tightened, the pin is stabilized with a screwdriver.

To gain firm halo fixation without imminent threat of abrupt or unknowing skull perforation, the threaded pins do not fasten to the skull as ordinary screws, which hold by deep penetration of the basic material. Rather, the pins serve as expanding wedges between the halo and the skull. The sharp pin tip readily catches in the outer surface of the skull (thereby preventing lateral migration). Further penetration is difficult because of its smooth surface and broad bevel. Both the pin and its halo channel have threaded surfaces. With its poor penetration ability, continued twisting of the pin tends to drive (or wedge) the halo away from the skull. Actual displacement is avoided by creating a counterforce with tightening the diagonally opposite pin at the same time. Similar treatment of the other pair of pins gives stability in all planes.

Daily cleansing of pin sites prevents skin and scalp infections. All sites should be swabbed with an antiseptic solution once or twice daily. Additionally, an antibiotic ointment may be applied.

General considerations

Progressive upward migration resulting from bone erosion and consequent eventual loss of contact is avoided by locating the halo below the maximum diameter of the skull. This directs the force into a thick mass of bone rather than against an ever-thinning margin. An occasional patient lacks an enlarged diameter at the midfrontalis level. Then halo fixation tends to be less secure, shortening the period of acceptance.

Maximum fixation tension has been set at 6 kg.cm. (5.25 inch-pounds). Clinical experience suggests this value closely approximates the compression tolerance of living bone. The addition of further force by vigorous head motion or persistent tightening of the pins seems to increase proportionally the rate of erosion by pin loosening. Pins should be tightened only in the presence of serous drainage or patient complaints of 'clicking' sensations. Excessive skin redness indicates pin loosening as well.

Pin replacement

The necessary changing of halo pin sites does not require general anesthesia, even in children. Select an adjacent pin channel and adequately prepare the area. Then infiltrate the skin and periosteum through this pin channel. Insert the pin and very slowly adjust tension to 6 kg.cm. Then remove the offending pin. By following this procedure, three-dimensional head control is continuously maintained. Proximal control would be precarious if the original pin were removed first.

Halo removal

When the halo is to be removed, reverse the application procedure. Be sure to support the head or it will drop when the pins lose hold of the skull and cause pain as they pull on the scalp. Diagonally opposed pins are loosened in sequence. All four pins should be completely disassembled from the halo prior to its removal. Partial pin retraction alone may cause skin injury and pain as the halo is drawn off the head.

Halo complications

Nerve-traction injuries are the major complications of excess traction force applied by means of the halo device. Cranial nerves most frequently involved are those with long pathways prior to exit from the skull. These include the abducens (VI) manifested by internal strabismus. The facial motor (VII) and facial sensory (V) nerves also may be involved. The brachial plexus is particularly threatened by traction when deformity involves the high thoracic spine. Signs of spinal cord neuropraxia are first noted in the lower limbs and in decrease of bladder control because of the layered position of ascending sensorimotor pathways making the sacral tracts most susceptible. Immediate reduction of traction is necessary to avoid permanent neural damage. Thus, neural injury will be avoided if traction is gradually applied and frequent patient observation is performed.

FORMS OF HALO TRACTION

The mode of distal fixation determines the extent of spinal and pelvic control to be provided by the halo-traction system. The halo may be used alone, with the body acting as a counterweight, or distal body fixation may be applied externally or directly attached to the skeleton.

Halo-bed fixation

This halo system provides three-dimensional skull and cervical spine control. Cervical fractures or fracture dislocations are more precisely positioned than is possible with tongs. It is necessary for the rope to fasten to the halo at several symmetrically placed sites, so that tractive forces will be equally distributed to each pin. Usually two U-shaped ropes and a spreader bar work well. This traction system may be used on a regular bed, Stryker frame, or Foster frame.

Halo with distal external fixation

The halo cast and halo orthosis are the two basic systems included in this classification. Each contains a well-molded pelvic portion, which efficiently distributes distractive forces over the iliac crest area.

Halo cast (Fig. 24-5). Rigid spine control is achieved by distraction between the halo and a well-molded body cast. For cervical or upper thoracic immobilization, a body cast must extend to the groin and also contain shoulder straps. Since the primary distractive forces are supported over the iliac crests, it is essential that this area be carefully padded and molded. The halo-cast device also permits greater mobility. Patients are free to

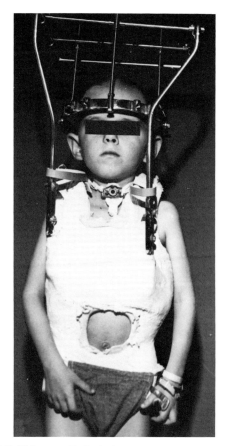

Fig. 24-5. Halo cast. Body jacket countertraction depends on careful molding of cast about pelvis to direct force to soft tissues and not bony prominences. (From Perry, J.: The halo in spinal abnormalities, Orthoped. Clin. N. Am. 3(1):69-80, March 1972.)

ambulate without loss of spinal traction or immobilization.

General considerations. Shoulder straps of the body cast serve an essential purpose for this halo-tractive system. Better than any other cast portion the anterior shoulder areas can support necessary metal attachments for the halo. For this supportive function the body cast must be strongly reinforced. Shoulder strap contour must also permit the full range of shoulder motion present and any gain in trunk height caused by axial traction. As spine curvature is straightened, the trunk accordingly increases in length. Such allowances must be considered when the cast is applied.

The halo cast must be judiciously used for patients with limited respiratory function. Body casts enclose the thorax, thereby further decreasing pulmonary function. Although a large anterior window cut out of the diaphragm area (upper abdomen) serves to reduce cast restriction, not all patients are able to tolerate this device.

Complications of the halo cast are generally related to faulty cast construction. Pressure sores may develop over improperly padded body prominences. Localized pain or a burning sensation is the best indicator of excessive skin pressure, and complaints should be promptly investigated. On occasion single nerve palsies arise from nerve compression at the cast's edges. Adequate trimming will remedy this situation.

Application of body cast. Two unwrinkled layers of stockinet are drawn over the patient's torso to assure a smooth skin and cast interface. To permit optimal trunk alignment before cast application the patient lies supine on a scoliosis-casting table supported only by a wide canvas strap, or paraspinal bars. Care is taken to maintain spinal traction during the entire casting procedure. Proximal fixation is furnished by the halo or chinstraps. Pelvic straps, which provide distal suspension, are adjusted to level the pelvis and define its bony contour. Essentially, their positioning creates a soft-tissue plateau above and medial to the iliac crests.

Next, all bony prominences including the anterior rib margins are well padded with felt or foam rubber. Since the pelvic portion will be quite closely molded, extra effort is made to protect the iliac crests, sacrum, pubis, and greater trochanters. The shoulders should also be free of any cast contact or pressure. All padding is kept in place by a layer of Webril. Only after spinal alignment and protection of bony prominences are assured should any plaster be applied.

First, plaster is evenly rolled about the pelvis in a figure-eight direction over the iliac crests. Splint reinforcements are incorporated over the sacrum and crests as well. Body casting continues by rolling the plaster around the thorax and shoulders. Reinforcements are placed over each shoulder for added strength. A roll of padding is temporarily fastened to the superior shoulder area to allow for increased trunk length resulting from the traction.

Before the plaster sets, it is further smoothed and molded. The hands are firmly swept around and above the iliac crests from behind to define their contour. The inward slope of each ilium is followed, until the flare of the greater trochanter is met. Gentle pressure is also used to smooth over and flatten the lower abdominal area enough to

form a slight indentation superior to the pubis. Similar molding is performed over the sacral area. Once molding is completed and the plaster is set, the patient is removed from the suspension device. An anterior window, in the region of the epigastrium is removed. This "breathing room" permits epigastric expansion during inspiration.

Next all edges of the body cast are sufficiently trimmed with a sharp knife to allow for shoulder motion as well as enough hip flexion for the patient to sit upright. Edges of the stockinet lining are pulled over the cut edges for added smoothness and durability.

Available metal attachments to provide distraction between the halo and body cast are of two designs. Regardless of the system used, all screw-fixation points should be checked daily to assure continued tight fixation.

Overhead frame. A metal frame is horizontally suspended over the halo by two vertical support rods mounted onto the anterior shoulder area of the cast. Three metal traction rods fixed to the halo (one anterior midline and two lateral) are then attached to the overhead metal assembly. The amount of traction provided is regulated by the length of the traction rods between the halo and frame (Fig. 24-6).

Shoulder uprights. This attachment consists of a sturdy rod mounted to a malleable metal-strip base. This is attached to the shoulder piece of the cast so that the metal rod is vertically positioned. Symmetric distraction forces are produced by securing the halo to both lateral uprights (Fig. 24-7).

Halo brace. In this system the well-molded pelvic girdle of the Milwaukee brace serves as the countertractive component. Metal rods, extending from the superstructure to the halo, provide balanced distraction (Fig. 24-8).

Halo-brace design permits adequate inspiratory chest expansion and can be used in patients with borderline respiratory function. Patients are also free to ambulate in this device. The major disadvantage to the halo brace, however, is the lack of rigid spinal immobilization.

Halo-distal skeletal fixation

Included in this category are halo-femoral and halo-pelvic traction. These systems are adapted to control more distal spine deformity and pelvic obliquity. Distraction forces of greater magnitude can be sustained by these systems,

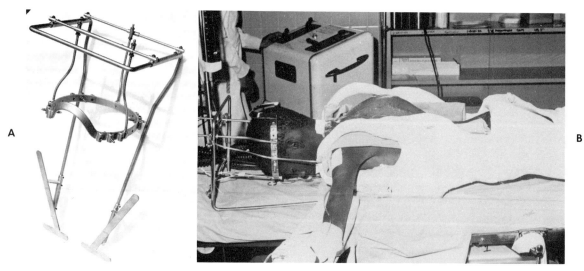

Fig. 24-6. A, Overhead frame and halo that may be attached to brace or cast, or both. **B,** Example of halo with overhead frame attached to cast. (From Ahstrom, J. P., Jr.: Current concepts in orthopaedic surgery, vol. 5, St. Louis, 1973, The C. V. Mosby Co.)

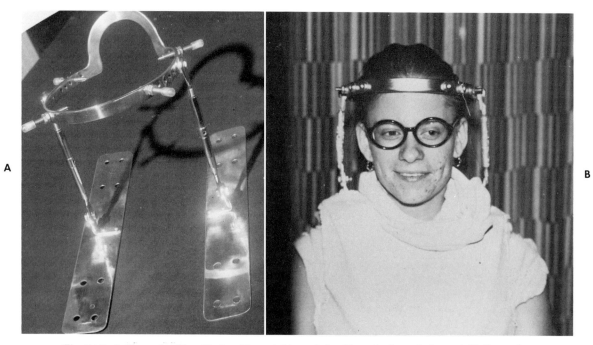

Fig. 24-7. A, Example of head halo with uprights and shoulder attachments for cast. **B,** Example of halo with shoulder attachments.

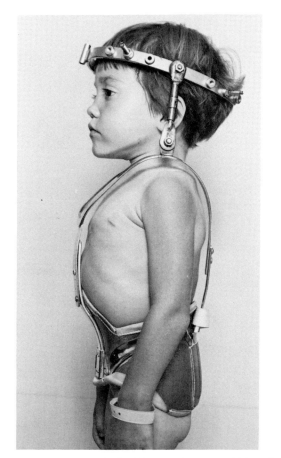

Fig. 24-8. Head halo with shoulder attachments to Milwaukee brace. (From Blount, W. P., and Moe, J. H.: The Milwaukee brace, Baltimore, 1973, The Williams & Wilkins Co.)

since each end is directly fixed to the skeleton. An indication is for traction correction of more severe fixed deformities.

As axial traction reduces skeletal deformity, it also stretches any contracted soft tissues. Traction nerve injuries can be a complication of axial traction. Neuropraxia is most commonly associated with fifth to seventh cranial nerves or the brachial plexus. Spinal cord injury with resulting paraparesis has been reported. By gradually increasing the traction to achieve desired correction and frequent careful checking of the patient, one may avoid catastrophic complication of excessive tension. When any abnormal neural symptoms are noted, traction should promptly be decreased.

Since neither system encloses the thorax, they may be safely used in patients with limited respiratory function.

Halo-femoral traction. This halo traction system is most frequently used to control severe rigid thoracic spinal deformities. Distal skeletal fixation is provided by femoral pins (Fig. 24-9). Weights, suspended from the halo and femoral pins, furnish graduated axial alignment. By suspending a greater portion of weight from the femoral pin on the higher pelvic side, the pelvis is leveled.

Femoral-pin insertion. Femoral pins may be introduced either under general or local anesthesia. In order that each femoral cortex supports equal weight, pins must be transversely directed

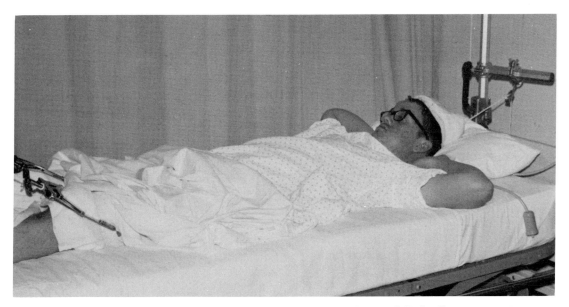

Fig. 24-9. Example of halo and femoral pin distraction. (From Ahstrom, J. P., Jr.: Current concepts in orthopaedic surgery, vol. 5, St. Louis, 1973, The C. V. Mosby Co.)

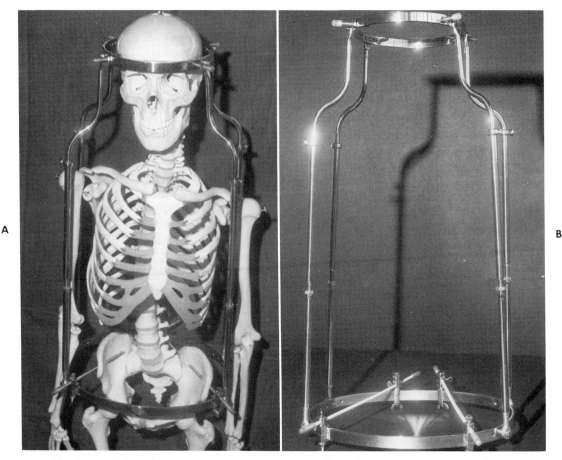

Fig. 24-10. A, Halo-hoop apparatus as applied to a skeleton. **B,** Halo-hoop apparatus. Notice holders for iliac rods and universal joints at ends of four uprights.

through the femoral shaft, in a plane parallel to the knee joint. Care must also be taken to avoid injury to the femoral vessels.

General considerations. Cleansing of pin sites must be a matter of daily routine. Traction ropes and equipment must also be inspected on a regular basis. Maximum total halo-femoral traction should not exceed 25 pounds in either direction. Additional weight does not hasten skeletal correction, but creates a greater likelihood of nerve injury.

Halo-femoral traction exerts axial force though the hip joint in addition to the spinal column. Continuous traction, especially in patients with weakened hip musculature, may lead to hip-joint subluxation. Periodic radiographs of the hips should be reviewed for early detection of this possible complication.

Halo–pelvic hoop. Severe spinal and pelvic malalignments can be managed by the distracting forces between a halo and pelvic hoop (Fig. 24-10). Like the halo, the pelvic hoop is a metal ring secured to bone. Fixation is provided by two heavy pins driven across the pelvis between the tables of the ilium. Thus, each pin is supported by four cortices of bone. The iliacus muscle, which lines each ilium, protects the major pelvic blood vessels and abdominal contents.

Halo-hoop traction maintains fairly rigid spinal immobilization and traction yet allows the wearer to ambulate and shower. Four metal uprights distract the halo and pelvic hoop so that respiratory function and skin integrity are not disturbed by restrictive casts (Fig. 24-11).

Application of pelvic hoop. Application of the pelvic hoop is best done with the patient under general anesthesia. The patient is turned to one side to allow the abdominal contents to fall away from the iliac fossa. The hemipelvis is then prepped and draped in the usual manner. A trans-

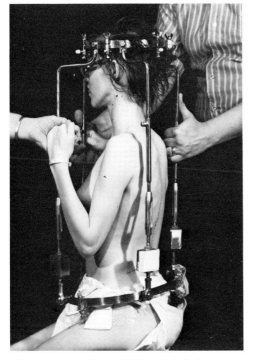

Fig. 24-11. Patient in experimental halo-hoop apparatus used for force measurement studies. (From Ahstrom, J. P., Jr.: Current concepts in orthopaedic surgery, vol. 5, St. Louis, 1973, The C. V. Mosby Co.)

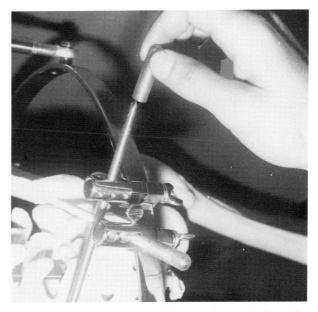

Fig. 24-12. Illustration of holders used posteriorly with multiple hole selections so that variations in rod position will not be hampered when applying the hoop. Also notice distance between rod and vertebral canal.

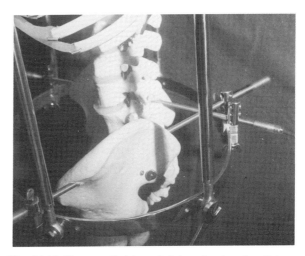

Fig. 24-13. Hoop applied to a skeleton showing the distance of the hoop from the patient as well as the fact that many times, depending on the slant of the iliac crest, the rods may cross posteriorly.

verse incision is placed slightly lateral and inferior to the anterosuperior iliac spine. One inch lateral to the spine and directed toward the posterosuperior iliac spine, a drill hole is made and then enlarged with a curette. Next the ¼-inch iliac pin of appropriate length is driven across the pelvis toward the posterior spine, while the pin is kept approximately perpendicular to the longitudinal axis of the vertebral column. On occasion, the pelvis may be tilted anteriorly, such as in a severe lumbar lordosis, and one must plan accordingly when introducing the pins (Fig. 24-12). Equal portions of the iliac pins are left protruding anteriorly and posteriorly (Fig. 24-13). Incisions are then closed.

The patient then is turned to the opposite side, and the procedure is repeated. While the patient is still lying on his side, the hoop is brought up around the patient's legs and attached to the iliac pins. This is best performed by completely disassembling the pin holders, threading them over the iliac rods, and then clamping them onto the hoop. After pelvic-hoop attachments are made, all portions of the system are left loose and the patient is returned to the supine position with a pil-

low support under the lumbar spine. The hoop is then adjusted around the pelvis and iliac pins until there is an equal amount of room between the patient's skin and the hoop in all directions. This is a critically important adjustment that equalizes forces supported by each pin.

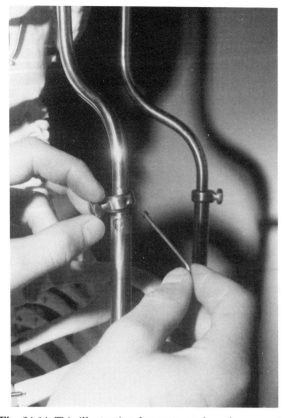

Fig. 24-14. This illustration demonstrates how the apparatus can easily be made shorter by simple reduction of length of slide mechanism.

Halo-hoop uprights. When attaching the halo to the hoop, four turnbuckle uprights with universal joints at the lower end are secured first to the hoop and then to the halo. One would be wise, before applying the halo-hoop system, to assemble the apparatus and prefit it to the patient to be sure that the apparatus allows the halo and hoop to be in the correct position. It is best to have the uprights in the shortest position when first connecting the halo to the hoop, since it is very difficult and also dangerous to distract the patient's spine while he is under anesthesia. Uprights allow approximately 7 inches of distraction from the shortest position, and this should provide enough corrective force for gradual correction of any type of scoliotic condition except a severe collapsing type of curve (Fig. 24-14). Once the uprights are attached to the halo and the hoop, the set nut for the sliding mechanism is loosened and the pelvis is placed in the correct position. Slight traction is placed on the head and halo so that the spine is under some distraction before tightening of the set screws on the sliding mechanism. This procedure assures head position directly over the pelvis and corrects pelvic obliquity, or forward tilt if present. Any rib hump will also be directed away from the posterior upright.

General considerations. Patients with the halo-

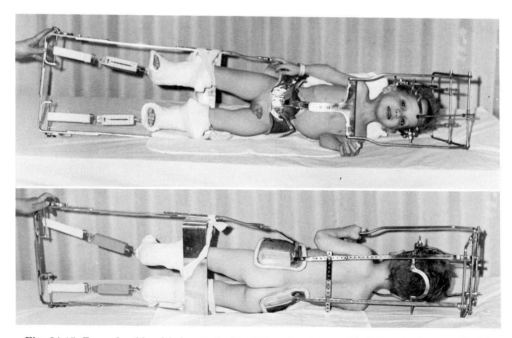

Fig. 24-15. Example of head halo attached to Milwaukee brace with Hoke attachment. Useful for correcting pelvic obliquity. (From Blount, W. P., and Moe, J. H.: The Milwaukee brace, Baltimore, 1973, The Williams & Wilkins Co.)

hoop apparatus need to be continually monitored so that the device is kept rigid. Should the iliac pins loosen, more distraction is needed so that the pins will settle into the pelvis if bone resorption takes place around them.

All pin skin surfaces should be cleaned daily with an antiseptic solution such as povidone-iodine complex (Betadine) and a topical antibiotic should be applied twice daily. Should more than the usual amount of skin drainage occur, it may be necessary to remove a head pin and place a fresh one in a new area of skin. Iliac pins that are grossly infected need to be removed and some other means of countertraction such as a halo-cast will be necessary. With more rigid halo-hoop fixation, there is less possibility of pin traction drainage and problems. It is important to check each nut and increment of distraction on the halo-hoop daily to be sure that the device has not loosened. As patients lie in bed, the apparatus may tend to shift about, depending on the body weight.

Combination halo-Hoke device

The halo can be combined with Hoke traction as a halo-Hoke system, which uses tibial traction, halo traction, a Milwaukee type of pelvic girdle, and a fitted Milwaukee brace. Pins placed through each tibia are incorporated into short-leg casts and suspended from a sturdy metal frame (Fig. 24-15).

Since tension for each leg can be individually adjusted, the halo-Hoke device can control pelvic obliquity as well as distal spine deformity. The pelvis is gradually leveled by the application of greater tension to the higher pelvic side.

As with other form of skeletal traction, nerve injuries are a possible complication during the treatment period. Patients in this device are restricted to complete bed rest. Halo-Hoke traction also requires an extralong bed to adequately support its framed components.

PART SIX

Mobility aids

CHAPTER 25

Canes, crutches, and walkers*

ERNEST M. BURGESS, M.D.
ANNE G. ALEXANDER, R.P.T.

The upper limbs must frequently be used to assist the disabled lower limbs in providing locomotion. Canes, crutches, and walkers in ascending degree serve as extensions that permit the upper limbs to transmit force to the floor, providing support and protection for the lower limbs and improving balance.

Almost all patients who can use a simple cane can walk without it. Although a cane is an important mobility aid, it provides little in the way of support and should not be used if more than 20% to 25% of the body weight is to be borne on it. This is true because a cane has only a single point of contact with the body, namely, the handgrip. Crutches have at least two points of contact to provide much better stability. A walker provides even greater stability for the patient who has poor balance.

The first use of canes and crutches to assist the disabled is not known. Surely external aids have been used since man has walked. The first recorded evidence of their use was found in the Egyptian tombs of Herkhuf in 2830 B.C. and of Runi, where there is pictorial evidence of what we have come to know as poliomyelitis, showing the use of a staff as support. Ancient Greek vases

and other pieces of art as well as manuscripts, such as the *Codex of Echternach* and the *Luttress Psalter* of about the year 1000, have been found documenting the early use of crutches. In 1412 a book by John of Adrene depicts a man with atrophied limbs using crutches. Much documentation on the history of ambulation aids can be found in the Division of History and Medicine at the Smithsonian Institution in Washington, D.C. The staff, constructed of endless variations of animal, plant, and mineral structures, has a significant place in the middle ages for its use by pilgrims and shepherds to assist in hill climbing. It became an item of dress about the eleventh century and later came to depict one's station in life. Generations of schoolboys have known the force of the cane for discipline.

The development of crutches since the eighteenth century following the needs of the time. From the original single upright, with top piece, have come many types and adaptations. These early crutches were made of a variety of woods, usually hickory, maple, or birch. Custom-made crutches were constructed of Brazilian rosewood, the hard or rock maple, and lemonwood, since they provide a finer finish and resisted splintering. Early use of metal was unsuccessful because of its excessive weight. With the advent of tubular aluminum and other light alloys, metal-resistive

*Prepared under Veterans Administration Contract No. V663P-718.

421

aids came into vogue. Aluminum crutch design followed the development of wood crutches, with the single upright type first being used (Fig. 25-6).

A wide variety of both wooden and aluminum crutches with the axillary, platform, and forearm design have been developed and are available today (Figs. 25-7 and 25-8). Ingenuity and function requirements have resulted in a large armamentarium of accessories designed over the years to fit specific needs.

Various types of walkers, the last to be introduced into the family of assistive aids, also appeared in simple form for rehabilitation several hundred years ago. The walker affords the most stability of all of the ambulation aids. Transition ordinarily progresses from walker to crutch to cane as the need for support decreases.

TYPES OF GAIT PATTERN

One needs to understand the basic gait patterns using supportive aids in order to prescribe properly. Prescription of the proper assistive aid or aids and training in the appropriate gait pattern for energy conservation and function will maximize progressive rehabilitation. Gait patterns using assistive upper-limb aids are as follows:

1. *Drag-to:* Slow and laborious. Alternate weight shifting side to side as first one crutch and then the other is brought forward. Feet are then dragged to crutches.
2. *Swing-to:* Crutches are simultaneously brought forward. Lift body so that both feet move forward simultaneously between crutches.
3. *Swing-through:* Progress of swing to. Instead of the feet only moving to the crutches, they progress through before making contact with the floor.
4. *Four point:* Always three points of contact with the floor. Move one crutch forward; shift weight and advance the opposite foot; shift weight and advance the ipsilateral crutch; shift weight and advance the contralateral foot.
5. *Alternating two point:* A progression of the four point. Advance contralateral foot and crutch simultaneously; shift weight and advance the other foot and crutch.
6. *Non–weight bearing swing-through:* Most commonly used gait. Advance both crutches, shift weight, and advance sound leg.

PREFITTING EXERCISE PROGRAM

Any patient requiring canes, crutches, or walkers needs to participate, if possible, in a prefitting physical therapeutic exercise program. Maximal functional proficiency will be achieved only when maximal muscle strength in the upper limb and trunk is obtained before assistive devices are prescribed and during their use. Exercises should be designed to strengthen especially the muscle groups that enhance crutch, cane, or walker use. Physical therapy should include programs to improve range of motion, balance, coordination, general endurance, and strength. The most important muscles for assisted walking using aids are those of the upper limb and trunk. These are specifically the abdominal and paraspinal muscles in the trunk; the shoulder abductors, depressors, adductors, and extensors; the elbow extensors; and the forearm rotators, wrist extensors, and finger flexors in the upper limb. Accessory devices that are available to supplement upper-limb muscle weakness include triceps bars, wrist-extensor straps, finger-flexor gloves, and forearm-platform supports.

BODY POSITION WHEN CANES, CRUTCHES, OR WALKERS ARE USED

The following body positions appear with aids:
1. Maintenance of erect posture.
2. Upper arm(s) (depending on unilateral or bilateral use of appliance or appliances) adducted against chest wall for lateral control of body and added weight transfer.
3. Wrist(s) held firmly in extension.
4. Placement of shaft of cane(s) or crutch(es) opposite the midfoot of side being assisted.
5. Step lengths initially short then increasing as balance allows.
6. Hips in neutral position or slightly hyperextended, if possible. Hip joints should be opposite the wrist(s) of hand(s) holding the appliance(s). The appliance or appliances are perpendicular to floor.

The body can be advanced without concern of falling either forward or backward if the preceding rules are followed. For a patient who has very poor balance, even two axillary crutches may not be sufficient and such a patient may require a walker. The walker has the advantage of stability, but it is difficult on stairs and tends to greatly slow the gait. The walker is helpful for the early training of patients who eventually will progress to lesser ambulation aids, and as a permanent aid for the more severely disabled.

Gait patterns applicable for use with a walker include the drag-to, swing-to, and, with the reciprocal walker, alternating two point.

Maximum stability will be afforded if all four legs of the walker are in secure contact with the floor before forward motion of the body is initiated. Walkers with wheels can be unsafe.

MEASURING FOR CANES, CRUTCHES, AND WALKERS

The correct length for canes, crutches, and walkers can be determined in several ways:

Canes	With the cane tip approximately 6 inches lateral to the base of the fifth toe, there should be a 20-degree flexion angle at the elbow.
Crutches	
Axillary	Use 77% of the patient's overall height. Subtract 16 inches from the patient's height. Find the distance from the anterior axillary fold to the heel and add 2 inches measured with the patient in the supine position. With the patient standing, the crutch should be two finger breadths below the axilla, while the crutches are placed with tips 6 inches lateral from the base of the fifth toe.
Forearm	With the crutch tip 6 inches lateral to the base of the fifth toe, the handgrips should be at a sufficient height to give 20 degrees of flexion at the elbow.
Walkers	Handgrips should be at a sufficient height to allow a 20-degree flexion angle at the elbow.

Particular mention should be made as to the specifications for canes. The customary length supplied is 36 inches, which is too long for most people. Too long a cane causes undue elbow flexion, placing excessive demands on the triceps muscles and leading to inadequate support. Also, too long a cane causes excess load on the wrist because of ulnar deviation unless the hand is slipped around the handle of the cane. This sacrifices grip strength and is unsatisfactory. Also, a long cane can cause elevation of the shoulder with poor cosmesis and trunk deviation.

A short cane, too often used, demands complete elbow extension. This produces inadequate support after heel contact and insufficient assistance at toe-off. Also, a short cane causes difficulty in lifting the body weight during stair climbing and thus requires excessive hip flexion and forward tilting of the torso.

The orthopaedic cane handle is curved slightly more than 180 degrees so that it will sit comfort-ably over the forearm even when the patient wears an overcoat. The cane handle is often too small, particularly a decorative cane that is being used for orthopaedic needs, but it may be too large when supplied for a child. The index finger should extend down the shaft to guide the cane. The cane should have sufficient strength to support up to one half of the body weight, and the cane tip should have a nonskid design with a gently flaring tip, flexible with concentric rings for stability.

AVAILABLE TYPES OF CANES, CRUTCHES, AND WALKERS

Single canes can be purchased in either tubular aluminum or a variety of wood grains with various styles of handgrips (Figs. 25-1 to 25-4). The length is adjustable or nonadjustable, even for the folding variety.

Four-legged or quad canes provide increased support and balance for the patient (Fig. 25-5). Available styles vary in both width and design of base. All quad canes are constructed of tu-

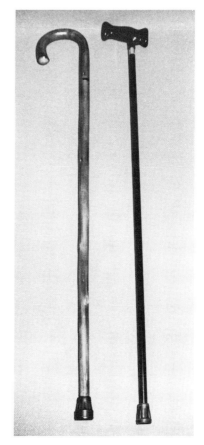

Fig. 25-1. Standard wood canes.

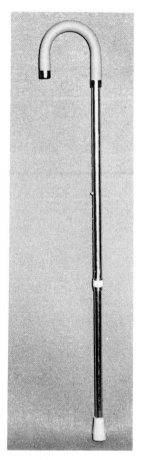

Fig. 25-2. Adjustable-length metal cane.

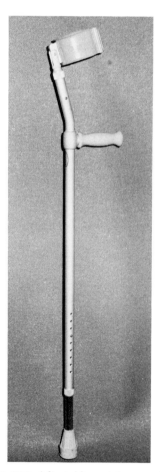

Fig. 25-3. Adjustable metal cane with forearm support.

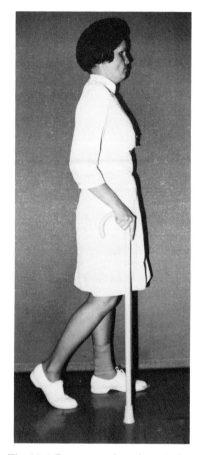

Fig. 25-4. Proper cane length carried on opposite side from injury.

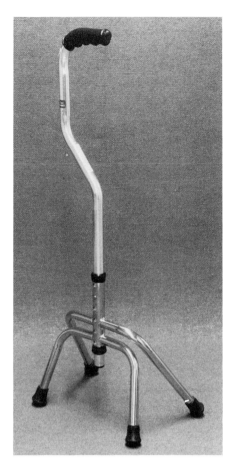

Fig. 25-5. Quad cane. A wide variety of base modifications are available.

bular aluminum, are adjustable in height, and come in a variety of handgrip styles.

These are useful only in a slow gait. With a more rapid gait, a rocking action from the rear legs to the front legs develops, nullifying the stability of the four-legged base. This cane is particularly useful for hemiplegics who have a very slow gait.

Gait patterns applicable to cane use are four point, three point, and alternating two point. Canes primarily provide balance support but can provide up to 40 pounds of weight reduction of the involved side, thereby reducing a Trendelenburg gait. Compressive forces greater than body weight alone are active on a hip in unassisted weight bearing because of the pull of hip-abductor muscles. A cane used on the opposite side provides a counterforce to keep the pelvis level and reduce excursion of the center of gravity. The cane in the opposite hand may decrease the total force by more than the actual weight taken on the aid since any

weight taken by the cane unloads the hip abductors. Even a slight touch of the cane can prevent a grossly visible limp in a patient with weakened hip abductors. The use of a cane should be one of the first measures of treatment in degenerative arthritis and other disabilities of the hip or knee. When using one cane, the patient should use the cane in the hand opposite the involved side (Fig. 25-4). There are several reasons: (1) It is physiologic because in normal walking the opposite arm and leg move together; (2) a wide base provides better balance; (3) probably most important, the center of gravity does not need to shift considerably from side to side with each step, as it does with a cane in the ipsilateral hand.

Canes are often used by amputees. The above-knee amputee must tense his abductor muscles in the socket for stability. A cane on the opposite side acting in a long lever arm from the ischial support can sustain a much larger force than that exerted on the cane, thereby reducing the horizontal counterforces to be developed between stump and socket.

The value of a cane in checking forward motion of the body directly after heel contact and transmission of force at pushoff is not usually recognized. Thus the arm and shoulder muscles transmitting forces through the cane can reduce demands on the hip extensors, quadriceps, calf, and other muscles. Lessened muscle effort in turn may reduce demands on impaired circulation in the leg and may be of advantage to patients with peripheral vascular disease. The cane can also provide valuable sensory feedback. It can detect body sway during standing at a considerable distance from the ankle, and small corrective forces can then be applied at a substantial lever arm. Crutches offer more support, but canes are lighter, more easily stored, and cause less clothing damage. When medically feasible, canes are preferable to crutches.

CRUTCHES

Body weight is to be borne on the hand pieces not the axillary pieces (Figs. 25-6 to 25-7). Long-term pressure in the axilla can cause nerve damage and loss of function in the upper limb. This condition is the so called crutch paralysis. Patients who are debilitated or who have pain or weakness in the upper limb are particularly prone to use the axillary bar for weight bearing. It is important to check the extensor muscle strength

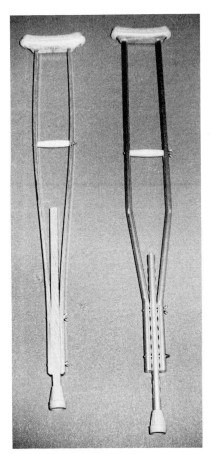

Fig. 25-6. Adjustable standard crutches, wood and aluminum types.

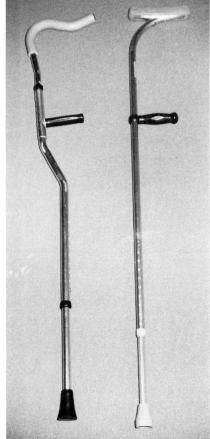

Fig. 25-7. Adjustable aluminum crutch with axillary support modifications.

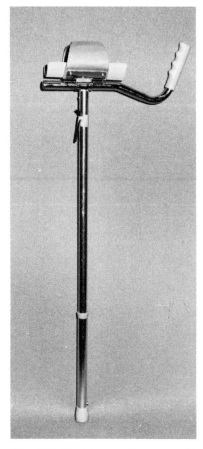

Fig. 25-8. Crutch type of support with forearm assist, no axillary platform.

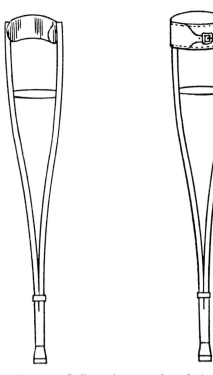

Fig. 25-9. Cuff crutches; two short designs.

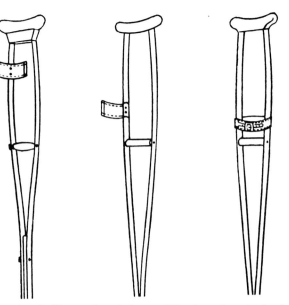

Fig. 25-10. Types of assistive modifications for standard crutches.

frequently, to be sure that the muscles are not developing crutch paralysis. The top one third of the axillary crutches improve balance when pressed against the rib cage by the upper arm.

The forearm style of crutches require the patient to have better balance control and more upper-limb strength than do the axillary styles (Figs. 25-8 to 25-9). The forearm style of crutches usually produce a gait pattern better than the axillary style, since the patient may stand more erect with no axillary pad to tend to lean on.

ACCESSORIES FOR CANES, CRUTCHES, AND WALKERS

There are numerous accessories for ambulation aids (Fig. 25-10). Many styles of handgrips and pads are available for canes and crutches (Fig. 25-11). The same applies to axillary pieces and pads. These are not for axillary support, rather they are for rib and chest wall cushioning. The forearm crutch has a variety of cuff designs and handgrip styles.

Also, many tips are available for all ambulatory aids. As noted previously, the flexible, concentric ring, moderately large at its base, is most

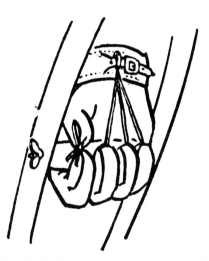

Fig. 25-11. Crutch hand-grasp assistive aid.

uniformly acceptable. Nonskid construction is imperative regardless of tip design.

WALKERS

Walkers are constructed of tubular aluminum, most are adjustable in height, and some fold for easy transportation (Figs. 25-12 to 25-13). There are various types of wheel tips available as well as sled type of tips that could be used on soft surfaces. Some come in child sizes as well as tall types for those patients over 5 feet, 10 inches.

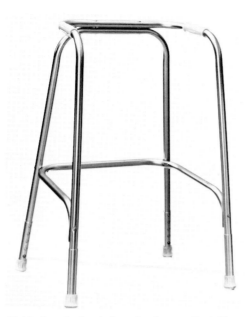

Fig. 25-12. Standard tubular aluminum adjustable walker.

Walkers with wheels must be considered to some degree hazardous. Specific instructions should be given in their use (Fig. 25-14).

The parapodium and parallel bar walkers have been developed at Ontario Crippled Children's Centre* for the severely involved such as the child with spina bifida and cerebral palsy. The parapodium provides rigid stability yet has knee and hip joints that allow for ease of sitting.

AMBULATION AIDS FOR THE BLIND

The ability to navigate within the environment is directly related to the training received by the blind in assimilating the feedback from the hardware of our society.

The most prominent aid to navigation, the long white cane, has been in existence for a considerable amount of time. The sophisticated level of training in assimilating the information obtained from the aid is responsible for its wide acceptance.

*350 Rumsey Road, Toronto 350, Ontario, Canada.

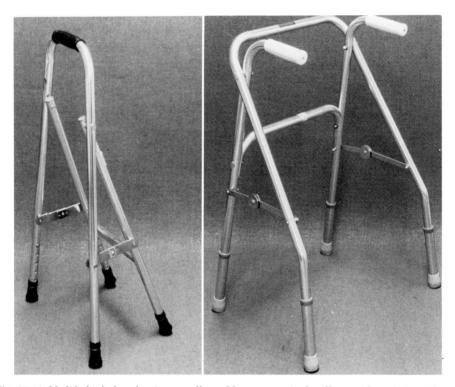

Fig. 25-13. Modified tubular aluminum walkers. Many customized walkers with assistive aids are available.

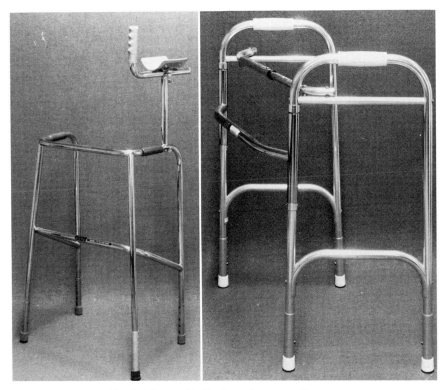

Fig. 25-13, cont'd. For legend see opposite page.

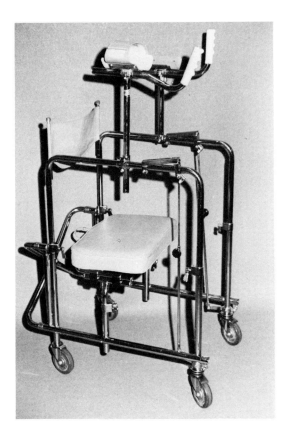

Fig. 25-14. Wheel walker with seat. Note several assistive attachments.

Seeing-eye dogs are used by 1% or 2% of the blind. Reasons for such limited use include the size of the dog, for it may require a fairly strong person to handle it. Many people are allergic to dogs, and the expense and time invested in acquisition, training, exercise, care, and food is considerable. Also to be considered is the fact that the master must be completely aware of his surroundings in order to command the dog. A dog can prevent his master from walking into traffic or like situations of danger, but it cannot tell his master where an object is located, what it is, or whether a traffic light is red or green.

Electronic aids, be they sonar, laser, or whatever, are used on a limited basis and are only as useful as the training program administered. It has been the experience of some that too much useless information is provided, but this may be attributable to inadequate training in assimilating the information provided by the device.

Research continues in many areas to provide the blind with an improved information-gathering system that is simple, practical, inexpensive, and lightweight.

SUMMARY

It is important to remember that in order of increased assistance, one goes from a single cane to the aluminum forearm crutch, to two forearm crutches, to two axillary crutches, to the walker. The correct length of the appliance is of extreme importance. The cane should be used in the contralateral hand. Forearm crutches are preferable to axillary crutches if feasible. Assistive aids added to the basic appliance may be used if necessary. It is important to watch for axillary pressure, particularly in the weakened patient and to understand each patient's functional deficit to the end that the appropriate assistive aid or aids is prescribed and properly used.

REFERENCES

1. Bachynski, B.: Mechanical aid to walking; crab crutch with universal joint, J. Bone Joint Surg. **35A:**1013, 1953.
2. Blodgett, M. L.: The art of crutch walking, Occup. Ther. Rehab. **25:**27, 1946.
3. Jebsen, R. H.: Use and abuse of ambulation aids, J.A.M.A. **199:**5, 1967.
4. Harris, D. M.: Crutch balancing, Phys. Ther. Rev. **30:**424, 1950.
5. Holliday, R. C.: Walking-stick papers, New York, 1918, George H. Doran Co.
6. Licht, S.: Therapeutic exercise, New Haven, Conn., 1965, Elizabeth Licht, Publisher.
7. Park, H. W., Malone, E. W., and Steglich, R.: Tilted crutch hand piece, Arch. Phys. Med. **33:**731, 1952.
8. Rial, A., and Michael, F.: The story of the stick, (Smithsonian Institute), 1875, J. W. Bouton.

Special appreciation to Abbey Rents and Rainbow Ambulance Company for use of appliances in pictures.

CHAPTER 26

Wheelchairs

EDWARD PEIZER, Ph.D.
DONALD W. WRIGHT, M.Ed.

Until recently relegation to a wheelchair was an admission of medical failure and so only the most general features of the chair were of concern. Now the wheelchair is looked upon as a rehabilitation tool to replace functional loss. As such, there must be judicious prescription of the most appropriate components from a vast number of options.

The idea of placing wheels on chairs to which the infirm were confined goes back several hundred years.[9,10] In 1918 Herbert A. Everest designed a patient-propelled folding wheelchair, a radical departure from previous models. It was later redesigned with Harry C. Jennings, Sr., and became the prototype of the modern wheelchair.[4,5] About 30 years ago, electric motors were introduced to provide mobility to persons too weak to push their chairs manually. The present-day descendants of the early models now manufactured by a number of companies are deceptively complex. They offer a staggering number of special functions to meet the needs of a large variety of wheelchair users. As perhaps nowhere else in the field of orthopaedic aids, the modern wheelchair expresses the now current trend toward modularity. The art and science of prescribing a wheelchair is the matching of specific wheelchair features and functions to clearly identified needs of a particular patient.

Wheelchair usage is dependent on the degree of disability, the parameters of wheelchair use, indoors, outdoors, patient transfer capability,

seating posture, the need for external power, and model of control of external power. Prescription recommendations should include functional disability, general physical condition, prognosis, and the environment within which the chair will be used.[4,6,7] A patient is to be considered as a functional rather than a medical entity. The completed prescription must then be checked out functionally with the patient so that it may be modified if necessary to provide maximum patient benefit.

From experience in satisfying the needs of their clientele, wheelchair manufacturers produce specific "lines" or models. Each type is basically designed to meet a particular set of patient needs. Many are highly modifiable through a wide choice of optional or interchangeable features. Each year thousands of wheelchairs are purchased by patients with merely the guidance of rental and direct-sales agencies. If the need is for temporary or casual transportation, this is often an adequate answer. However, patients who have the potential to be active and yet must look to a wheelchair as their only mode of mobility, require one that best complements their physical disability, their functional potential, and the environment in which it is to be used. Such matching of patient with device requires the composite knowledge of a medical prescription. Also advised is a "checkout" procedure using a formal checklist to determine that every significant feature is included as specified in the prescription. This procedure also functions as a check on the validity of the original prescrip-

431

tion, since the patient's ability to use the device is also examined.

TYPES OF WHEELCHAIRS
Manually propelled wheelchairs (Fig. 26-1)

A wheelchair is generally viewed as equipment that provides a person with support and mobility in the sitting position. Through largely empirical knowledge of the purposes for which wheelchairs are used, the concept of a basic, or conventional, wheelchair has evolved. It consists essentially of a supporting structure and a propulsion system. The supporting structure includes a backrest, seat, armrests, and footplates. The propulsion system consists of wheels, drive mechanism, and brakes. The preferences of patients and professional staff for particular features that enhance safety, comfort, and independent function complete the wheelchair design. The most common types of components are flexible backrest, hammock seat, padded armrests with skirtguards, leg rests of adjustable length with folding footplates, 24-inch wheels attached to the rear axle, handrims, hand-operated brakes, and a folding mechanism. There are several general classes of wheelchairs specified by the manufacturers. Unfortunately, the terminology is not standardized although it is in most cases well understood.

Standard wheelchairs are generally constructed of cold-rolled steel and are suitable for most individuals (adults weighing less than 200

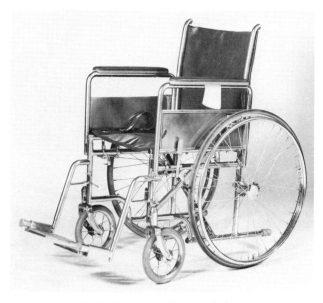

Fig. 26-1. Typical manually propelled wheelchair.

pounds). The average weight of this type of chair is approximately 45 pounds. Most of the wheelchair components available as options are adaptable to the standard models. Metal is preferred material, since it can easily be worked to provide variations in design combined with strength.

Heavy-duty wheelchairs (Fig. 26-2) are especially designed for individuals that are very active, operate on rough terrain or weigh over 200 pounds. Seats up to 24 inches wide are available in these chairs, which remain both foldable and portable. These chairs weigh approximately 55 pounds primarily because of the added reinforcement of the axles and cross members. These heavy-duty features are also available on models with seats less than 18 inches wide, if specified on a prescription. These models are all cold-rolled steel.

Lightweight models (Fig. 26-3) are constructed of special chrome-alloy thin-wall steel tubing, which effectively reduces the overall weight but also sacrifices some strength. In general, the lighter the wheelchair, the more strength is sacrificed. Several companies market lightweight chairs ranging from 30 to 42 pounds. Where the patient is light, relatively inactive and has a need for lifting and moving the chair in and out of his car, for example, the lighter models in the lightweight class will suffice.

In the *amputee chair* (Fig. 26-4, *A*), the center of gravity has been shifted forward to accommodate the difference in body balance of patients who have had both legs amputated. Such a loss of anterior mass reduces stability, making it easier to tip over backwards. The risk is more acute when an incline is climbed, when the amputee shifts his trunk backwards, or when he propels the chair very forcibly. The rear wheels and axles of a so-called amputee chair are set back 2 to 2½ inches, creating a longer wheelbase. As a result, the drive wheels of an amputee chair are somewhat more difficult to operate. One does not automatically order an "amputee" chair. It should be considered only if the amputation is at a sufficiently high level (and perhaps bilateral) to significantly shift the center of gravity of the total man-chair system.

Of the *indoor chair* (Fig. 26-4, *B*), the distinguishing feature is the location of the large drive wheels. They are aligned with the front edge of the seat rather than the rear axle. This makes the chair 1 to 3 inches shorter than a conventional model because the same area accommodates the wheel radius and foot plates. As a

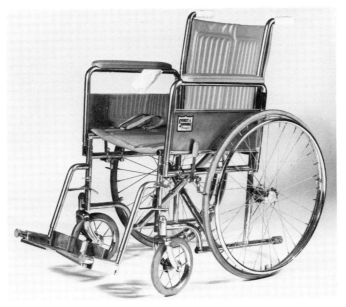

Fig. 26-2. Heavy-duty wheelchair with posteriorly placed, large-diameter axle and spokes.

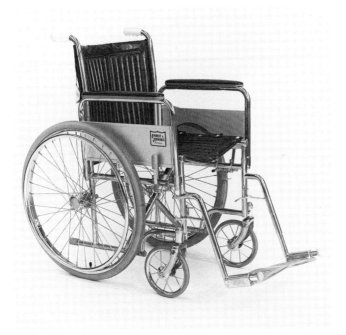

Fig. 26-3. Typical lightweight wheelchair.

result, less space is needed for turning space. It is especially useful in cramped spaces or small rooms, but propulsion requires the user to lean forward slightly. To do so, he must have strong trunk extensors or the 24-inch wheels should be replaced with 26-inch wheels. Having the large wheels anterior makes it difficult for many pa-tients to transfer in and out of the chair and for attendants to manage curbs and stairs. Hence, the indications are very limited.

Other chairs are often classed by their special mode of propulsion, such as one-arm drive or electric. This will be discussed in the section on propulsion.

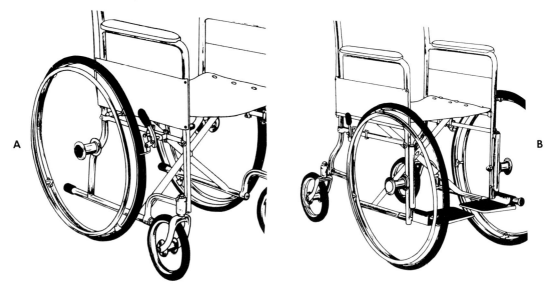

Fig. 26-4. A, Wheelchair with rear-drive wheels set back for amputee use. **B,** Wheelchair with drive wheels in front, designated "indoor" chair.

WHEELCHAIR COMPONENTS
Supporting structure

The supporting structure consists of two side frames and a crossbrace of chrome- or nickel-plated tubular steel and upholstery that is flexible, nonabsorbent, stain resistant, and flame resistant. Vinyl-coated fabric seems to meet these requirements best, although it stiffens and cracks at freezing temperatures (a consideration in colder climates). Nylon and Dacron fabrics tend to stretch, are warmer, but are harder to clean.

Frames. The wheelchair frame is generally designated as standard (Fig. 26-1), heavy-duty (Fig. 26-2), or lightweight (Fig. 26-3).

Size. A wheelchair must fit a patient in the same sense as an artificial limb; it must be comfortable to be functional and to avoid exacerbating the condition for which it was prescribed.[4] An ill-fitted chair may not only be uncomfortable but also restrict function and lead to pressure sores. There are five sizes of wheelchairs produced in the United States: small child, large child, junior, adult, and oversize. Actually, manufacturers vary the basic types they market as increasing numbers of patients become capable of operating wheelchairs. The size of the chair determines the width and height of the seat. Seats range in width from 12 to 24 inches and in height from 16 to 20 inches.

Selecting the best chair for a child is often

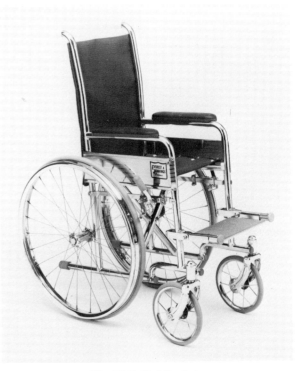

Fig. 26-5. Child's chair.

difficult because they grow quickly, occasioning the need for concomitant changes in the dimensions of the chair or its accessories. A partial solution to these problems is the use of units that allow adjustment of foot-rest height, chair width, and sometimes chair depth. Cushions can be used to change the size in many cases.

There are usually two seat heights available for the small child's chair, 16 and 20 inches (Fig. 26-5). The higher seat is better for the child who will be pushed by an adult since the handgrips are higher and a seat at this height places the child at table level. The lower seat height (16 inches) permits the child to get off and on the chair independently. This chair is approximately 12 inches wide.

A larger child's chair is for children from 6 to 12 years old. This is called a "growing chair" but is actually a junior chair that permits the components to be replaced as the child grows. The seat is 14 by 11 inches, but it can be converted to 16 by 13 inches by new upholstery.

The junior, or youth, chair is for large children or small adults. The chair is 16 inches wide and the seat is 18 inches high. This chair is often appropriate for small older people.

The adult chair is 18 inches wide and the seat is 20 inches high. It is designed for an adult of normal size. It will fit through a passage 25 inches in width. A "narrow" adult chair with a seat 16 inches wide is also available.

An oversize chair is designed for especially large, heavy people. It is both larger and made of heavier and more durable materials.

Seat. The wheelchair seat is designed to distribute the patient's weight over the greatest possible area. Good seat design provides sufficient clearance to prevent the patient from rubbing against the sides of the chair while keeping the overall width of the wheelchair as narrow as possible. It should relieve the buttocks of some body weight by distributing it on the thighs to minimize the threat of pressure sores. The objective is to assure that the patient is provided with the smallest total seat area consistent with his size, disability, and clothing.

If the seat is too wide, the patient will have more difficulty in maintaining trunk alignment and in reaching the handrims. Too wide a seat will also increase the overall width of the chair, making it difficult to pass through doorways, particularly interior doorways such as bathrooms. If the chair seat is too narrow, it may create skin abrasions or pressure sores on hips or thighs. If it is too shallow from front to back, it will reduce the weight-bearing area and raise unit pressure on the buttocks; too deep a seat will apply undue pressure in the popliteal area.

It is a common misconception that manufacturers make only a standard seat dimension. The "standard" dimensions are simply based upon common or average needs. One can and should specify the exact seat dimension for his patients' needs. Because precise calibration is extremely difficult, it is acceptable to specify both width and depth in whole-inch increments. The seat or weight-bearing surface is critical and should be carefully measured for the patient.

Seat width. To assure the correct relationship between the patient's size and the wheelchair width, measure straight across the hips or thighs, whichever is the widest point, and then add 2 inches to this measurement (Fig. 26-6, *A*). This relationship will usually result in a seat with minimally sufficient width since it allows for clothing and some relative movement within the seat. For patients who are above-knee amputees and wear prostheses, it will be necessary to increase this dimension approximately 2 inches more (a total of 4 inches in order to accommodate the thigh section of the prostheses. Certain patients may require an exceptionally wide seat, making it difficult to pass through doorways.

Seat depth. To distribute the patient's weight over the maximum surface and reduce the concentration of weight on the bony prominences, the deepest seat possible should be prescribed. At the same time, the front edge of the seat upholstery must not be allowed to press against the popliteal area behind the knee. To meet these two requirements, the patient is measured from the rear of the buttocks to the rear of the bent knee while he is seated. Then 2 or 3 inches are subtracted depending on the patient's overall size (Fig. 26-6, *B*). Empirically, this provides the optimum weight-bearing platform for an individual and at the same time makes it virtually impossible for him to assume any sitting position that applies pressure behind the knee. Also to be considered are other devices worn by the patient. Back cushions, inserts or Ortho-Backs, in addition to certain types of body orthoses, will make the patient sit further forward in the seat. Incidentally, the use of a 1- or 2-inch back cushion is a useful method of

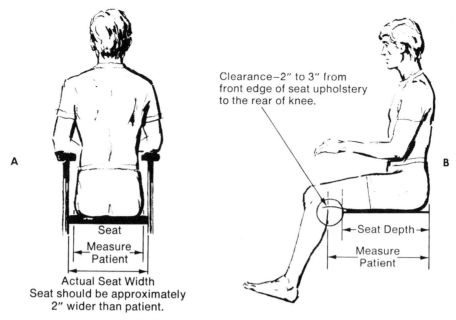

A

B

Clearance–2″ to 3″ from front edge of seat upholstery to the rear of knee.

Seat
Measure Patient
Actual Seat Width
Seat should be approximately 2″ wider than patient.

←Seat Depth→
Measure Patient

Fig. 26-6. A, Seat width. **B,** Seat depth.

fitting the chair to the patient when a "standard" seat depth is too deep. Relatively minor but expensive modifications may thus be avoided. Although it is essential to avoid pressure directly behind the knee, it is also imperative to prevent excessive pressure on the underside of the thigh that may be caused by the sudden dropoff at the front edge of the seat upholstery.

Seat height. Whether or not the patient will use one or both feet in propelling the chair is the first determinate of seat height. If not, the second objective is to have the supporting footrests be sufficiently high to clear average threstholds and rough terrain.

To determine proper seat height for foot propulsion, measure the dimension from the rear of the patient's knee (popliteal area) to the bottom of his heel while his foot is flat on the floor. One inch is subtracted to avoid the anterior seat edge cutting into the thighs. Caution must be exercised to prevent elevating the thighs too high and losing a significant portion of the weight-bearing surface by forcing the weight back onto the buttocks. A "wedge-shaped area of clearance," approximately 1 inch high and 1½ inches deep is optional. For patients who will be depending on a footrest, at least 3 inches should be added to the measured height. With the footrests at their proper level, the lowest point of the foot-support unit should be at least 2 inches above the floor, the minimum

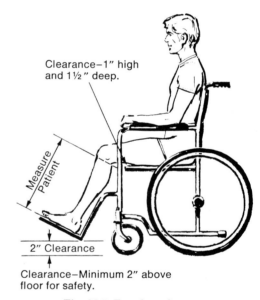

Clearance–1″ high and 1½″ deep.

Measure Patient

2″ Clearance

Clearance–Minimum 2″ above floor for safety.

Fig. 26-7. Footplate clearance.

safe distance to allow the foot plates to clear the floor after descending a 14-degree (or 25%) incline (Fig. 26-7). A 1-inch increase in seat height allows approximately 1⅓-inch additional foot-plate clearance. Seat cushions are a convenient and relatively inexpensive way to revise seat height. A foam-rubber seat cushion will compress to approximately half of its original thickness. A potential disadvantage of this procedure is that even

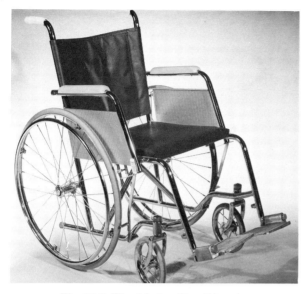

Fig. 26-8. Wheelchair with solid seat.

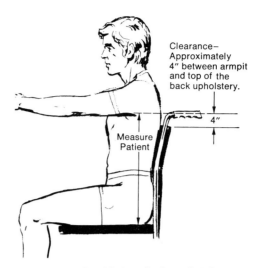

Fig. 26-9. Establishing backrest height.

though the arm and back heights have not been changed, they will appear to have been lowered.

Specific needs such as to accommodate a work-bench level or to raise an unusually small adult may dictate a higher seat.

Type of seat. For persons with a tendency toward internal rotation at the hip or spasticity of the high adductors, the hammock type of seat may contribute to improper alignment of the legs. In such instances and where prolonged use leads to increasing sag of a fabric seat, a solid seat is recommended (Fig. 26-8). Seat boards can be handmade from materials such as upholstered plywood and should be used with a seat cushion. A solid seat and seat cushion will increase the height of the occupant in the chair by several inches. This should be remembered at the time measurements for a wheelchair are made. For those patients with anesthetic skin, special cushions will be required.[3] This subject is fully discussed in the following chapter. The underside of the thigh must be raised above the leading edge of the seat upholstery in order to relieve pressure. One should assure a clearance space 1 inch high and 1½ inch deep by specifying the most functional seat height while still permitting footrest adjustment to provide 2 inches of floor clearance.

Commode seats, which consist of a contoured or padded toilet seat, a seat-board cover and a removable pain or bedpan below, are desirable for use in homes where size and arrangement of the bathroom prohibits entry and maneuvering by a person in a wheelchair. Incontinent persons may be toileted in a commode chair, although prolonged sitting on the toilet seat is not recommended. Since access to the toilet seat is gained by removing or folding up the seat-board cover, the wheelchair occupant must be capable of raising up from the seat or he must be lifted to effect this procedure.

Backrests. The specific type and height of the back will depend on the patient's size and his needs for passive trunk support and his activity capability.

Back height. The individual with good to normal trunk musculature and the capability of propelling his chair independently requires minimal back support. The height of his chair back should be 2 to 4 inches below the axilla to afford maximum freedom of arm movement and reduce skin irritation (Fig. 26-9).

For those who require full or maximum trunk support, the distance from the seat level to the required level of support is measured. This may be midscapular, midcervical or midhead level depending on the functional residuals. This patient also may be a candidate for one of the two reclining-back chair styles. Headrests attached to extensions of the back uprights are also available. The backrest is inclined backwards not less than 10 degrees from the vertical for support and comfort.

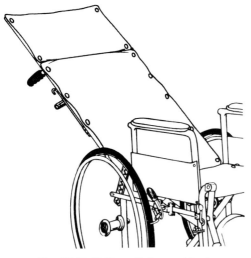

Fig. 26-10. Fully reclining seat back.

Reclining backs. Two models are available: semireclining, which can be inclined 30 degrees from the vertical, and fully reclining (Fig. 26-10), which goes almost horizontal. The reclining backs may be adjusted to a selected angle of rearward inclination and stabilized in that position. However, unless a special powered aid is added, the control is behind the wheelchair, precluding independent operation by the occupant. As the angle of reclination increases, contact with the armrests is lost.

Both types have seat-back heights approximately 8 inches higher than the standard upright back models, and they are equipped with a telescoping headrest extension to support the head while reclined. To provide stability in the presence of this backward displacement of the center of gravity, the wheelbase is lengthened. These chairs are larger and heavier than the standard wheelchair. They are more cumbersome to fold, transport, and store.

The semireclining chair is indicated for persons who cannot sit erect. Hip-extension contractures, spine deformity, or severe paralysis of trunk musculature or dependence on a chest respirator are typical examples. Seldom is this chair adequate to provide relief from the erect position.

Propulsion of the rear-drive wheels is facilitated when the chair back is semireclined, not only for those persons who have difficulty reaching backward, but also for persons with weak elbow extensor muscles. The latter can place their hands in a more posterior position on the handrims and turn the wheels by flexing their elbows. Patients who need to rest periodically because of fatigue or to protect sensitive skin should have fully reclining chairs. These chairs allow the more severely handicapped individuals to remain out of bed and potentially mobile most of the day. With proper placement of pillows under the abdomen and hips they even can be made prone.

Reclining backs for otherwise conventional chairs should be distinguished from those special chairs in which the entire supporting unit (back and seat) tilts back, maintaining a fixed angle of approximately 90 degrees between the seat and back; this action is accomplished either independently of the driving parts or through utilization of reclining or antitipping bars, which enable the entire chair to be tilted backwards.

Detachable back. For some persons, the safest and most easily accomplished method of transfer to and from wheelchair, bed, stationary furniture, car seat, or toilet is through the back of the chair rather than the front. To permit this, back openings, which fasten with zippers, snaps, screw studs, turn buttons, or Velcro, can be obtained. A sufficient degree of manual dexterity on the part of the wheelchair occupant is necessary for independent manipulation of such a back opening.

Armrests. Armrests provide support for the arms and hands and also serve as a base for change of position, pushups, and transfers. A basic wheelchair has fixed arms that include skirtguards and padded armrests. Skirtguards protect the person and clothing of the wheelchair occupant from entanglement in or injuries from the drive wheels and spokes as well as from soilage. This is particularly helpful to the person with flaccidity of the upper limbs.

Arm height. Correct arm height is important for several reasons. If the arms are too low, the patient will have a tendency to slump forward and lose trunk stability. This may have serious consequence for those with respiratory restrictions since leaning forward reduces thoracic expansion capacity. If the arms are too high, the shoulders will be forced up, making it difficult to sit upright for extended periods. Occasionally, patients will require a special arm height because of a specific disability.

Arm height for the average patient is determined by measuring the distance from the seat level to the lateral epicondyle. Add 1 inch to compensate for the fact that the normal location of the

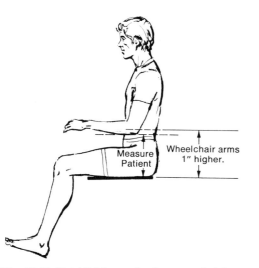

Fig. 26-11. Establishing optimal armrest height.

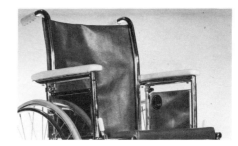

Fig. 26-12. Height-adjustable armrests compensate for cushions or body dimensions.

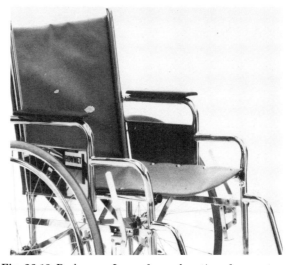

Fig. 26-13. Desk arms. Lower forward portion of armrest permits chair to be positioned under a table or desk.

elbow, while the patient is seated, is slightly forward of the trunk midline, rather than straight down as measured (Fig. 26-11). Proper armrest height will not only provide assistance in maintaining good posture, it will also allow the patient to shift his sitting position slightly and relieve seat-pressure points. By sliding the elbows further to the rear of the armrest and depressing the shoulders, he will be able to elevate himself in the seat. The use of a seat cushion, which is quite common, will alter these relationships by raising the patient's sitting level and effectively lowering arm height.

Types of armrests. There are two types of arms, detachable and nondetachable. Both are available with either a full-length or desk type (two-level) of top sections. Also available is a wrap-around design. A wheelchair with removable arms is heavier and up to 2 inches wider than a chair with fixed arms. It also is harder to lift, as the arms tend to pull out.

Some armrests, in both standard and desk types, are adjustable in height, with the range of height varying with the manufacturer (Fig. 26-12). The adjustable arm would have obvious advantages when asymmetries occur as in the addition and removal of seat cushions or lap trays.

Wheelchair arms may be offset, that is, attached to the outer side of the chair's frame, to allow more room for the user without further increasing the width of the wheelchair. Persons who wear bulky braces or who have a wide beam may be better accommodated with offset arms.

Full arms are usually as long as the depth of the seat and have a flat, widened surface on the superior dimension, which serves as a supportive rest for the forearms and hands. Padded, upholstered armrests are recommended for general use, whereas hard plastic or wood are useful with tray attachments. Padding protects against pressure sores in the presence of diminished sensation.

Desk arms (Fig. 26-13), have the forward height lowered more than 4 inches so that the wheelchair occupant can effectively sit at most desks and tables. Desk arms are usually removable and reversible. In the reversed position, access to the drive wheel is improved and a higher hand grip is created for use in position changes and transfers. Arm locks are positioned so that armrests can be locked in the forward or reversed position.

Detachable armrests should be specified for those users who prefer a side-sitting transfer or who require manual lifting. Removable arms

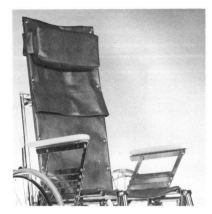

Fig. 26-14. Retractable armrests allow chair to be positioned under desks and tables.

should be equipped with some type of lock, usually pushbutton or pin, to improve their stability and prevent their unexpected detachment. Choice of arm lock should involve consideration of the user's manual abilities: pushbutton locks require finger power; pinlocks require steady precision; lever locks (which flip on) require minimal dexterity. Reversing removable arms, where the armrest is offset to the outside of the frame, narrows the internal distance between the arms but makes access to the drive wheels easier.

Retractable armrests (Fig. 26-14), similar in function, are also available. They provide maximum support in the forward position but permit close approach to table-like furniture when retracted. The front is usually angled toward the back of the chair in the retracted position; thus the obstruction to side transfer is minimized. Retractable arms are fixed and not reversible, offering most advantages of removable arms without the necessity to detach and store them.

Foot and leg rests. This assembly is designed to provide support for the lower limbs, support them above the floor, and aid in reducing the concentration of pressure under the thighs. The leg rests may be stationary (standard), swing-away, detachable, or elevating. The choice between stationary and removable units depends on the patient's method of transfering in and out of the chair.

Leg rests extend from the front of the chair and angle downward and forward (about 20 degrees) so that they do not obstruct the front casters. They have a sliding tubular midshaft connection to allow length adjustment to fit the individual

needs. This junction must fasten securely to prevent slipping if the patient steps on it.

Swing-away, detachable leg rests have a cam type of automatic lock. The lock release is within easy reach of the person sitting in the chair. These leg rests are indicated whenever the patient cannot stand up and walk out of the chair. It permits a closer forward approach to objects such as tubs, beds, and automobiles.

Elevating leg rests provide a means of positioning the limb horizontally. Indications are edema or a knee that lack sufficient flexion to rest on the usual support.

The distal end of each leg-rest bar is bent at right angles to form a pivot about which the footplates rotate 90 degrees. This allows the footplates to either provide a central support surface or to fold up against the leg rest leaving the area clear so that the feet can be placed on the floor for wheelchair propulsion or standing transfer.

Standard footplates must be manually placed in the up position, or nudged up with the foot, which requires motor function in the legs or bending forward and motor function of the upper limb. Lowering the footplates is easier, but the same abilities are necessary. The possibility of soiling a hand or foot, or of injury to limbs is always present.

The "standard" footplate is 6 inches deep from front to rear. However, oversize plates are available for patients with large shoe sizes (10 or larger) or to protect the toes of patients who do not normally wear a hard-sole shoe. These oversized footplates will extend 2½ inches to either the front or rear as specified.

Steering systems. The swivel casters are the steering device for wheelchairs. Their ability to rotate with minimum effort is determined by the amount of friction that has been introduced to the stem bearings. In most instances, the original (manufacturer's) settings will be acceptable, but for the very active wheelchair user, it may be desirable to apply greater friction to reduce or eliminate the flutter that occurs at high rates of speed. There are two basic casters available, one 8 inches in diameter and the other 5 inches. The 8-inch caster is the more effective for all-around application, since its greater diameter makes it possible to go over small obstacles and avoid getting stuck in sidewalk or elevator cracks (Fig. 26-15). The 5-inch caster is capable of turning in a smaller radius, but the effective radius will usually be

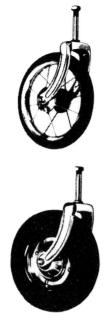

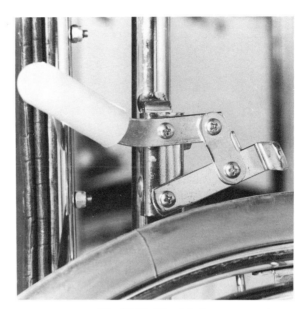

Fig. 26-15. Eight-inch casters with solid and balloon tires.

Fig. 26-16. Wheel lock.

determined by the large wheel size and the position of the leg and footrests; hence, the indications for this caster are obscure. The tires used on an 8-inch caster may be either solid rubber or semipneumatic (zero pressure). The decision in this regard will depend on the general environment of use or the patient's ability to withstand bumps. A swivel lock is available for use on 8-inch caster forks, which can be locked on by the user to stabilize the front of the wheelchair during side-transfer activities.

Wheel safety locks. Wheel safety locks, though once considered accessories to be specified on the prescription, are now standard equipment. The decision is merely one of choice. There are two basic types: (1) the lever and latch and (2) the over-center locking toggle type (Fig. 26-16). Lever and latch locks require the individual to perform two functions each time they are operated: unlatch and move the lever to the off position or the reverse. This combined movement may not be possible for some patients. The over-center toggle locks require only a single movement to lock or release. In addition, the prescriber has the added option of selecting either a forward or rearward locking action in order to provide the desired capability of the patient. Extended handles are needed by patients with limited arm reach.

A "hill holder" (Fig. 26-17) is of significant

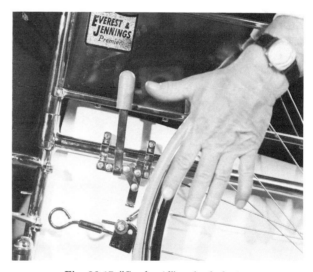

Fig. 26-17. "Grade-aid" no-back device.

advantage to those who operate their chairs on hills or ramps, preventing the chair from backing down the hill.

Propulsion systems. Selection of a specific method of propelling the chair should be based upon the individual's limb capabilities and his source of energy. Wheelchairs may be patient propelled, pushed by an attendant, or powered with an electric motor. The conventional wheelchair is propelled by force manually applied to the

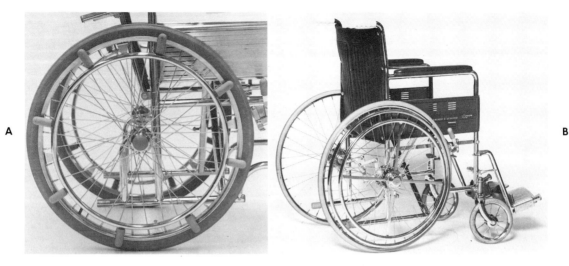

Fig. 26-18. A, Handrims with knobs to aid propulsion. **B,** One-arm drive wheelchair in which force applied to one wheel is transferred to the other.

handrims connected to the large rear wheels. If the patient's hand is weak and he cannot grasp the handrim, projections or knob projections can be placed on the handrims (Fig. 26-18, *A*). The projections are available in three different positions: vertical, oblique, and horizontal. This enables the wheelchair user to turn the wheels with his wrist, heel of his hand, or forearm.

The standard wheelchair also has a pair of handles attached to continuations of the rear uprights, which permit a person other than the occupant to push the chair. The handles are usually placed 35 to 40 inches above the floor.

One-arm drive (Fig. 26-18, *B*). To permit a person to propel a chair with just one hand, two handrims are mounted on one side. One turns the wheel to which it is attached; the other turns the wheel on the opposite side. If both handrims are turned together, the chair will go straight forward. Either rim can be turned separately. The one-arm drive usually makes the chair about 2 inches wider than a conventional chair and also more expensive. Indications for this chair are quite precise because its operation is very demanding of the controlling hand. It is appropriate only when the patient cannot employ his foot (or feet) to assist his one good arm in propelling the chair. For example, hemiplegia, per se, is not an indication. These patients have no difficulty with a conventional chair. Also this drive system is too complex for confused patients.

Electrical power (Fig. 26-19). In the past, medi-

cal opinion discouraged the use of electrically powered chairs on the premise that residual function should be exercised. As long-term function became the focus rather than immediate physical development, this attitude changed. It became apparent that severely disabled persons should save their limited energy for job performance once they arrive at their destination.

Although there are standards for conventional wheelchairs, there are none for electrically propelled systems. Certain basic requirements however have been proposed:

1. Speed, adjustable to a low of 1 mile per hour
2. Capable of negotiating a 1-inch obstacle
3. Ascend a 10% (6-degree) ramp and come down at a safe speed
4. Turning radius not to exceed 30 inches
5. Adequate maneuverability
6. Removable motor and battery; that is, they must not be riveted or welded to the chair frame
7. A power supply that will operate under normal conditions for one full day without recharging and that can be fully recharged overnight

Options. Among chairs options relate to the type of battery, mode of control, and method attaching the power to the chair. The basic chair is also being redesigned by some manufacturers. In regard to control, a joystick unit mounted on the armrest of the chair is the standard control mechanism. When hand function is lacking, this same

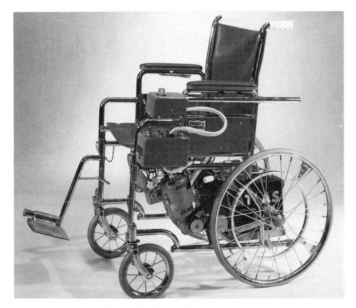

Fig. 26-19. Typical electrically powered wheelchair.

unit can be mounted opposite the patient's head so that he can move the joystick with his cheek. A modification of this is to replace the joystick with a chincup. The most serious disabled, with very limited head motion, require a pneumatic system or electric tongue switch.

The *VAPC chin control* (Fig. 26-20) is a power pack designed for relatively easy installation on any conventional wheelchair to convert it to a power-driven chair. Essentially the chin control is a modified joystick mounted for operation by movement of the chin. The bracket provides several adjustments and a relatively large clamping surface for a rigid chin-control suspension. The horizontal bar swivels 180 degrees away from the patient to permit entry and exit. The bracket is mounted on the frame of the wheelchair.

The *Rancho tongue switch* (Fig. 26-21) is operated by the tongue, lips, or teeth of the patient. Three switches activated by three levers control the direction in which the chair is driven and the power input. A separate switch mounted near the occupant's head allows him to move the tongue switch unit (Fig. 26-22) into a driving position or out of the way for reading, eating, and so forth.

The *VAPC pneumatic control* is designed for quadriplegic patients with relatively high-level lesions who are not capable of employing a chin control. A number of such systems have been developed. One example, developed by the Veterans Administration is operated by four sensitive air

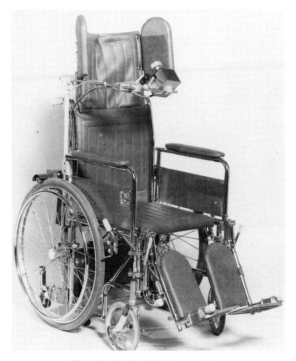

Fig. 26-20. VAPC chin control.

pressure switches and four relays that can be made responsive to positive or negative air pressure (Fig. 26-23). They control the operation of each of the power relays, which transmit battery power directly to the motors. Two air switches respond to positive breath pressure and activate two relays

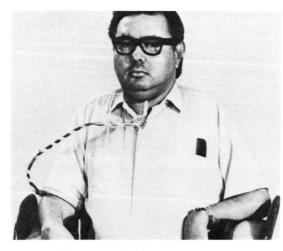

Fig. 26-21. Rancho tongue switch.

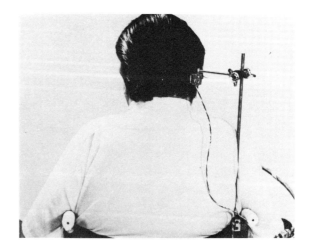

Fig. 26-22. Rancho occipital switch to position tongue-switch assembly.

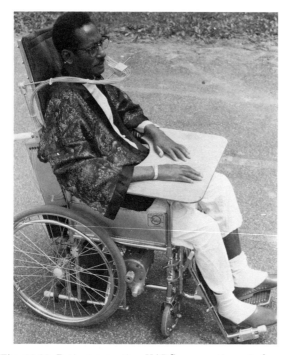

Fig. 26-23. Patient operating VAPC pneumatic control, permitting variable speed and improved maneuverability.

so that both motors propel the chair forward. The other two air switches respond to negative breath pressure and activate the other two relays so that both motors propel the chair backward. Control of the wheelchair is achieved by means of two air tubes in the patient's mouth. An improved model provides a variable speed control. However, light breath pressure must be maintained.

This version is commercially available and is in use at several Veterans Administration spinal cord injury centers. A recent modification permits operation with intermittent rather than continuous blowing into a tube.

Power systems. The basic powered wheelchair is a simple system employing microswitches and circuit breakers powered by a 2- to 6-volt battery (Fig. 26-19). A more advanced model employs a proportional speed control and is powered by a single 12-volt battery. The modular design approach employs the use of special male and female connectors. This is a useful technique for maintaining and repairing motorized wheelchairs in an environment that usually lacks engineering and other technical support. By maintaining spare modular parts and plug-in subassemblies, patient "downtime" is minimized and actual repair is effected by returning the malfunctioning units to the manufacturers.

An attachable power pack enables one to convert almost any conventional wheelchair to a powered chair (Fig. 26-24, *A*). Coupled with a modern solid-state proportional control system, such a unit provides a high-performance powered wheelchair. Being an attachable unit makes it also removable to permit temporary use, loans, trials, and exchanges without excessive expense or inconvenience. It provides proportional speed control to a maximum of 5 miles per hour. Although considerable evidence exists that proportional speed and maneuverability are highly desirable, the relatively high maximum speed of 5 miles per hour that the system provides may be

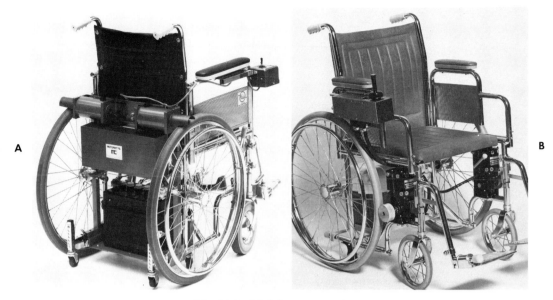

Fig. 26-24. Modular power systems.

the determining factor for its preference among patients.

Another system (Fig. 26-24, *B*) follows the modular design with both motors, control box, and battery joined by special connectors. Only manual control is available.

Printed circuit motors. The development of an electric wheelchair with performance characteristics higher than those of commercially available models has long been sought.

Many patients need to negotiate ramps with inclines of up to 8 degrees. Greater speed capability is not only desirable but may be a necessity. Outpatients who wish to pursue a college career require sufficient wheelchair speed to attend classes in different campus buildings. Patients who take their chairs into traffic must be able to cross at intersections with traffic-light changes. Conventional electric wheelchairs do not have these capabilities.

Efforts in this field have led to a 24-volt power package that makes use of printed-circuit motors (Fig. 26-25). This wheelchair has a speed of 5.5 miles per hour on level ground, which is considered maximum velocity for conventional wheelchair structures to maintain stability.

OTHER MOBILITY AIDS
Stair-climbing wheelchairs

Stairs are a problem for wheelchair users. Without ramps or lifts, an otherwise independent

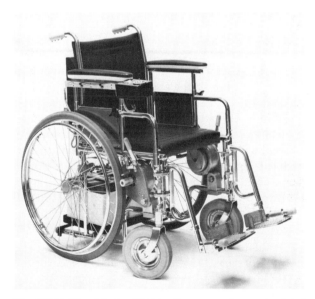

Fig. 26-25. Wheelchair with 24-volt power system and printed circuit motors.

person requires assistance in ascending and descending stairs. This problem has generated an inadequate solution to date: the stair-climbing wheelchair. Stair-climbing wheelchairs, generally speaking, tend to evolve into stair-climbing vehicles, losing in the process most of the features required for a foldable, hand-propelled wheelchair. One example (Fig. 26-26, *A*) has two main sections: (1) a conventional heavy-duty wheel-

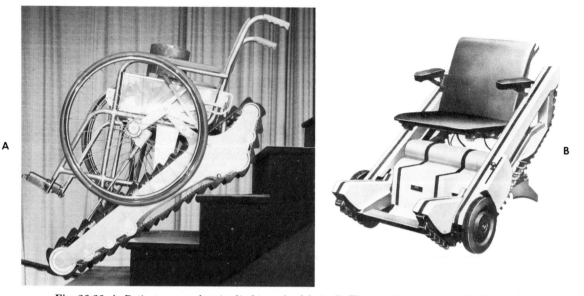

Fig. 26-26. A, Patient-powered stair-climbing wheelchair. **B,** Electrically powered stair-climbing wheelchair.

chair, with (2) a stair-climbing assembly consisting of two cleated rubber tracks mounted on idler and drive wheels. It was designed to operate on level ground as a conventional wheelchair carrying the stair-climbing assembly beneath the frame. To climb stairs, the patient backs the chair against the first step until a rubber cleat catches the top of the step. He rotates the drive wheel, which causes the track to climb the step, slipping to readjust itself every time the one cleat that is supporting the load reaches the end of its travel and another load-bearing cleat becomes engaged. At the top of the flight of stairs, the chair tilts backward and the track slips until a second cleat engages the top step. The chair pivots about the top step until the track is flat on the landing. The patient drives the chair clear of the stairs and retracts the climbing gear and repositions the seat to a level attitude. Operations of this chair needs an extraordinary amount of upper-limb power.

Concomitant with the enormous power demand and the "tank-like" tracks is its great weight. This makes such a vehicle incompatible with the standards for conventional wheelchairs. Another device (Fig. 26-26, *B*) is electrically powered and streamlined.

Further, it is not clear who would use stair-climbing wheelchairs. In the home, other means of negotiating stairs are available, such as lifts, ramps, and the assistance of others. However, for ordinary outdoor use, climbing both curbs and stairs must be considered.

Curb-climbing wheelchairs

As a result of the impasse in designing stair climbers, designers have sought an intermediate goal; the design of a vehicle to ascend and descend one step, that is, a curb climber. The problem of climbing one step versus a flight of stairs is simpler and also the frequency of having to climb one step is probably greater than a flight of steps. Power requirements will be lower and probably the climbing gear would be lighter.

An available curb climbing (Fig. 26-27) system employs a dropback dolly. This facilitates the ascent of obstacles up to 4 inches high and, in addition, permits the patient to alter his sitting position by tilting backward. Once attached, the device adds 15 pounds to the overall weight of the chair. If curb-climbing represents an essential requirement for a patient and he is physically capable of generating the force needed to operate the unit, this device will be useful to him.

Other methods of negotiating stairs and curbs

Ramps. The easiest and least expensive method of overcoming stairs and curbs is by means of ramps. A ramp is a gradual change in

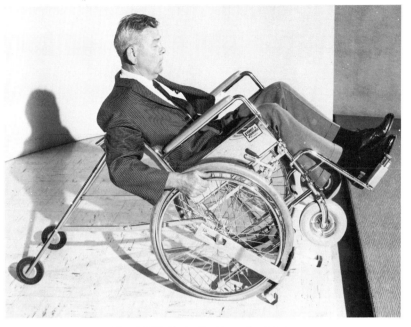

Fig. 26-27. Curb-climbing wheelchair.

elevation. It is recommended that ramps not exceed an 8% (or 4.8-degree) incline. Thus for every foot of vertical rise, there is a horizontal expanse of 10 feet.

Elevators and lifts. When assistance in climbing stairs is inconvenient or unavailable or if the wheelchair user prefers independence, there are other means of climbing flights of stairs. An elevator can be installed either inside of outside a house, though this may be expensive. There are three types of elevators: enclosed, open, and platform. An enclosed elevator has walls on all four sides and perhaps a ceiling and travels vertically. An open, or platform, elevator can move either vertically or obliquely, perhaps along a staircase. A platform elevator is merely a platform onto which a person wheels his chair. Either siderails or strips on the platform prevent the chair from rolling. Many of these elevators fold up against the wall in order not to obstruct the stairs.

At least one system employs an overhead trolley running through several rooms of a home. Suspended from the trolley is an electric hoist that lifts a sling type of seat. The lift controls enable the patient to lift himself out of bed and transport himself anywhere in the house into which the overhead rail and trolley have been installed.

Systems of this type require extensive installation procedures, extensive home modifications, or the design of a special house.

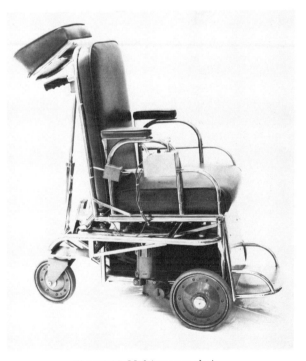

Fig. 26-28. Multipurpose chair.

Multipurpose chairs

Included in this category are devices designed principally as wheelchairs but with several auxiliary functions. They are intended to fulfill a number of functions that certain patients require in

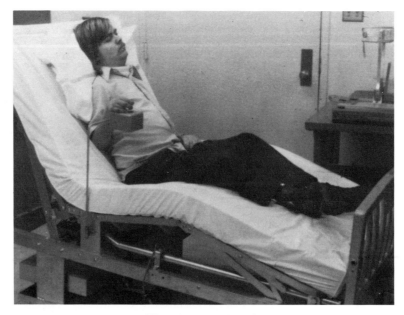

Fig. 26-29. Mobile bed.

addition to wheelchair use, such as transfer assistance, commode service, treatment accessories, standing assistance, and exercise aids (Fig. 26-28).

As a class, all these devices suffer from the same malady. None of the multiple functions they furnish is performed as efficiently as the individual devices they are intended to replace. Few patients require this combination of assistance. The individual must generally utilize a cumbersome nonfolding heavy wheelchair all day in order that he might conceivably use one of the secondary functions once or twice daily.

Mobile beds (Fig. 26-29)

The mobile bed is capable of being adjusted into a "chair" attitude and then driven like a powered wheelchair. In the model illustrated, the sides fold up to provide a railing for safety purposes. This type of bed is designed for patients who cannot independently transfer to a wheelchair. It enables such a person to visit other rooms in the hospital, the cafeteria, or the recreation areas. In appropriate climates, it permits patients to leave the building and to move about the grounds. Similar uses can be found for certain individuals who live at home.

Mobile standers

The concept is to provide wheelchair-like mobility while the patient has the therapeutic benefits of standing. These devices enable the patient

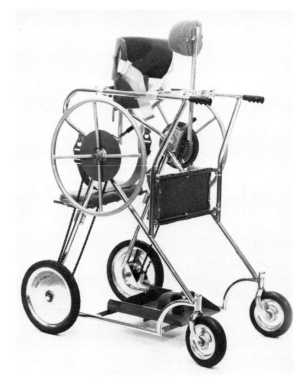

Fig. 26-30. Mobile stander.

to stand erect and move himself about by hand propulsion[12] (Fig. 26-30). Another device has spring-loaded lifters to assist patients who are capable of tilting themselves forward in the wheelchair and releasing the spring catchers, allowing them to stand in a reasonably erect position. Three-point support is provided by bolsters to stabilize the knee. In this position, the patient has access to higher space levels, but he remains immobile.

Wheelchair transporters

There is a rather large gap between the performance levels of wheelchairs and an automobile or a van, particularly if distances between 2 to 10 miles are to be traversed cross-country, or by peo-

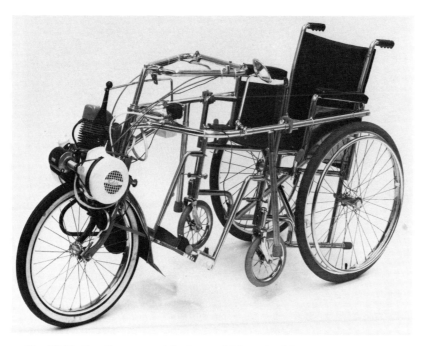

Fig. 26-31. Gasoline-powered device to which a wheelchair may be attached.

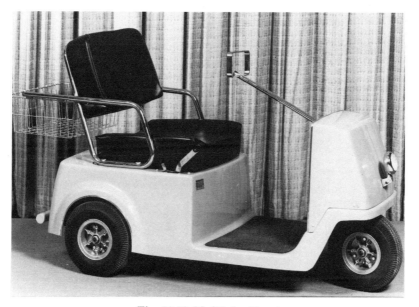

Fig. 26-32. Modified golf cart.

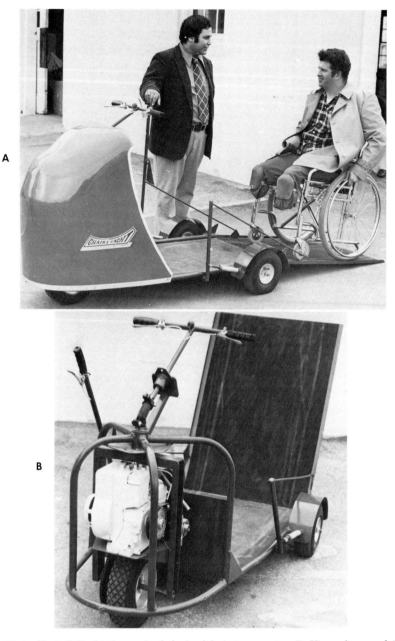

Fig. 26-33. A, Chair-E-Yacht three-wheeled wheelchair transporter. **B,** View of power-drive system with cowling removed.

ple who are not licensed or do not have an automobile. This area of transportation is being filled by the designers of wheelchair transporters, vehicles that permit a person to drive his wheelchair into them and then drive away from the power provided by the wheelchair transporter.

A gasoline-powered vehicle to which a wheelchair may be attached is one design (Fig. 26-31). This provides a three-wheeled vehicle powered by a gasoline engine with speeds of 10 miles an hour and relatively long driving ranges. There is some question about the safety of such a device and the stability of a three-wheeled system at speeds in excess of 6 miles per hour.

Another vehicle, similar to a golf cart, requires a patient to transfer to it from his chair (Fig. 26-32). This unit travels at approximately 8 to 10 miles per hour and has a range exceeding 10 miles. The idea of transferring to another vehicle, of course, implies a patient with sufficient strength and residual function and circumstances to be able to leave a wheelchair in one place and to drive a cart for significant periods of time.

Another three-wheeled gas-powered device has a folding tail gate that functions as a ramp, enabling a patient to enter the vehicle (Fig. 26-33). It is capable of speeds of 10 to 15 miles per hour, provided that the user has sufficient arm function to handle the throttle, brakes, and steering controls. As currently designed, there is no provision for locking the wheelchair securely in place. At speeds of 10 to 15 miles per hour, the chair is likely to be unstable, particularly on turns. The whole question of maximum safe speed for three-wheeled vehicles of this type needs further investigation.

WHEELCHAIR CHECKOUT

When a new wheelchair is delivered, it should be evaluated carefully by the prescribing physician or his delegate (therapist). An item-by-item check should be made against a copy of the original prescription,[7,11,13] The chair should be inspected for general construction features and correct measurements, as well as be evaluated for patient fit and for functional operation by the patient, family, or attendant. The manufacturer or a reliable distributor will usually rectify defects or mistakes made in ordering a new chair. Reliable sources also provide repair or replacement of defective parts within the first year after purchase.

Check against prescription

An overall inspection of the chair should answer the following questions: Is the chair firmly and properly assembled? Are removable parts easily removable? Is the quality of workmanship and materials satisfactory? Do attachments, such as overhead slings, headrests, or trays fit properly? Are handgrips and rubber tips firmly attached?

Do all wheels move freely and easily? Are the brakes and caster locks easy to apply? Do they hold? If the back reclines, is it easy to adjust? Is it stable? Are the armrests easily removable? Are they adequately padded? Do telescoping parts show a tendency to bend? Do the foot rests swing aside and detach easily? Is it in proper alignment? Is it stable when transferring in and out? Does it fold and unfold without difficulty?

The small swivel-caster assemblies should rotate easily but without excessive looseness. Test the chair to determine if excessive wheel flutter or shimmy occurs during normal operation speeds.

Check the large wheels by lifting one side of the chair and spinning the wheel slowly. It should not come to an abrupt stop but simply run down to a stop. The following defects are commonly found:

    Tires
        Faulty joints and loose fit of solid tires
        Faulty mounting and leaks of balloon tires
    Wheels
        Malalignment
        Loose of faulty bearings
        Loose or bent spokes
    Brakes
        Improper placement making them either too tight to apply easily or too loose to restrain the chair.
    Casters
        Malalignment leading to wobble
        Loose stems
        Bent forks
        Loose tires
    Frame
        Loose sections during manufacture or shipment
    Upholstery
        Loose screw fasteners

If the chair seems to be soundly constructed and fulfills the prescription specifications, the quality of its fit to the patient should be checked with the patient seated in the chair with the seat cushion he will use and his braces, if he wears them.

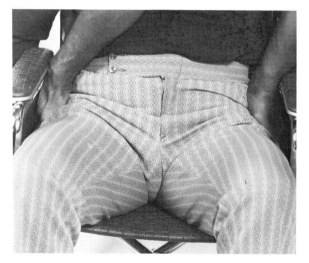

Fig. 26-34. Actual seat width should be 2 inches wider than patient.

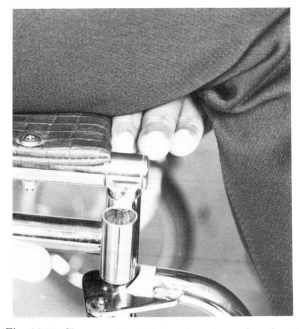

Fig. 26-35. Clearance 2 to 3 inches from front edge of seat upholstery to rear of knee.

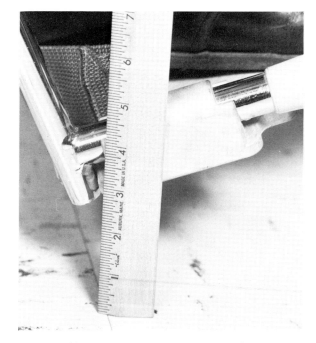

Fig. 26-36. Clearance minimum 2 inches above floor for safety.

Chair size. The evaluator should be able to put his hand between the patient's hips and the chair skirtguards touching both without pressure, if the seat width is correct for the patient (Fig. 26-34). The length of the seat should permit the breadth of a hand (at least 2 to 3 inches) between the end of the seat and the posterior knee (Fig. 26-35).

Seat. Seat height should permit the patient's posterior thigh to rest firmly on the seat cushion and still allow at least a 2-inch minimum clearance of the foot pedals from the ground (Fig. 26-36). If the foot rests are of proper length, the evaluator can slip his fingers under the patient's thigh at the front of the seat upholstery, without effort. Solid seats should not interfere with the foldability of a chair.

Armrests. When the patient is seated, with the arms supported on the armrests and the seat cushion in place, his shoulders should not be forced up nor allowed to drop.

Legrests and footplates. The length of the legrests should permit firm contact between the upper thighs and the wheelchair seat. The position of feet on the footplates and of the lower leg should leave a clearance of at least 2 inches between the popliteal area and the front edge of the wheelchair seat; at the same time, the distal, posterior thigh should be raised 1 inch above the front 2 inches of the seat.

Backrest. For the patient requiring minimal trunk support, the evaluator should be able to insert four or five fingers between the patient's axilla and the top of the back upholstery. There should be unhindered arm movement for propelling the chair without friction or irritation from the backrest. The backrest should be as wide between the uprights as the seat. When full trunk support is required, the scapulae should be fully covered by the backrest. If the patient with trunk instability is accustomed to stabilizing himself by hooking his arms over the push handles, one should note whether he can accomplish this.

Operational check

A brief trial period of operation of the wheelchair should be carried out by the person (patient, family member, or attendant) who will be operating the chair. The following should be determined:

1. Can the patient wheel or attendant push the chair without undue exertion?
2. Can he apply the brakes quickly and effectively?
3. Can he detach, remove, store, and replace armrests and footrests without much difficulty?
4. Can he maneuver the chair with adequate facility in conditions simulating the space

and surfaces of the patient's environment (home, office, school)?

5. Can patient transfer (independent, assisted, or dependent) be effected safely?

6. Can folding, placement, and removal of the wheelchair from a transportation vehicle be accomplished by those who will be doing it?

7. Is routine wheelchair maintenance understood by those responsible?

8. Do they have the name, address, and phone number of the distributor or manufacturer whom they could contact for servicing or repairs?

REFERENCES

1. Beaumont, E.: Wheelers, Nursing, pp. 48-57, Nov. 1973.
2. Bergstrom, D. W., editor: Report on a conference for wheelchair manufacturers, Bull. Prosthet. Res. BPR 10-3, Spring 1965.
3. Cochran, G. V. B., and Slater, G.: Experimental evaluation of wheelchair cushions, Bull. Prosthet. Res. BPR 10-20, Fall 1973.
4. Everest and Jennings, Inc.: Wheelchair prescription: Measuring the patient, Los Angeles, 1968.
5. Everest and Jennings, Inc.: Wheelchair features and benefits, Los Angeles, 1969.
6. Fahland, B., and Grendahl, B. C.: Wheelchair selection: More than choosing a chair with wheels, Minneapolis, 1967.
7. Fowles, B. H.: Evaluation and selection of wheelchair, Phys. Ther. Rev. 39:525-529, Aug. 1959.
8. Gutman, E. M., and Gutman, C. R.: Wheelchair to independence: Architectural barriers eliminated, Springfield, 1968, Charles C Thomas, Publisher.
9. Kamenetz, H. L.: Wheelchairs. In Licht, S.: Orthotics etcetera, New Haven, Conn., 1966, Elizabeth Licht, Publisher.
10. Kamenetz, H. L.: The wheelchair book, Springfield, Ill., 1969, Charles C Thomas, Publisher.
11. Peizer, E., Wright, D., and Freiberger, H.: Bioengineering methods of wheelchair evaluation, Bull. Prosthet. Res. BPR 10-1, Spring 1964.
12. Peizer, E., and Bernstock, W.: Bioengineering evaluation and field test of the stand-alone therapeutic aid, Bull. Prosthet. Res. BPR 10-2, Fall 1964.
13. Peizer, E., and Wright, D.: Five years of wheelchair evaluation, Bull. Prosthet. Res. BPR 10-11, Spring 1969.
14. Spiegler, J. H., and Goldberg, M. J.: The wheelchair as a permanent mode of mobility, Parts I and II, Am. J. Phys. Med. 47(6):315, 1968; 48(1): 1969.

CHAPTER 27

Wheelchair cushions and related protective devices

JOHN ROGERS, M.S.

Patients who require wheelchairs have the potential for developing a significant problem of "pressure sores," "ischemic ulcers," or "decubitus ulcers." Decubitus ulcers are literally caused by prolonged pressure, or shear, therefore, the term "pressure sore" is more appropriate. Their prevention has a direct bearing on equipment ordered for the wheelchair as well as the fit of the wheelchair.

Pressure is weight or force divided by area of support. Mooney et al.,[10] Fellars,[3] Houle,[6] Kosiak,[7] Lindan,[8] and others indicate that the highest pressures encountered while sitting are under the ischial tuberosities. Lowering this pressure below 25 millimeters of mercury would be ideal for long-term sitting. However equal distribution of pressure over the entire buttocks area will mathematically result in pressures greater than 25 mm. Hg over the ischium and result in tissue breakdown in most instances. This is why nurses "bridge" patients, and prosthetists and orthotist "relieve" high pressure areas. I must emphasize that pressure found in testing normal individuals is considerably less than in patients,[10] with atrophy of muscles as well as loss of tissue over bony prominences. Fellars[3] reports that clinical experience indicates that greater trochanters and thighs withstand higher pressure or shear than do the ischial tuberosities. This is the key to fitting special cushions for long-term sitting (Figs. 27-1 and 27-2).

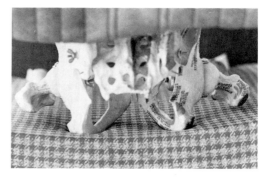

Fig. 27-1. Demonstration of ischial tuberosity loading.

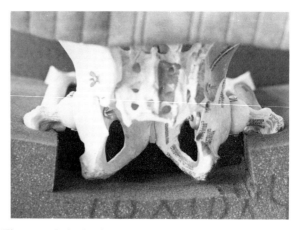

Fig. 27-2. Ischial tuberosity relief by loading of trochanters.

454

CLINICAL PROBLEMS

In evaluating patients for wheelchair padding, they must first be separated into two categories: (1) those with sensation but anatomic variations or muscle weakness, and (2) those with limited or no sensation.

Patients with sensation, such as those with arthritis or muscular dystrophy, or those who have had poliomyelitis, often have skin and muscle atrophy that accentuate bony prominences. Special fittings may be required, however, to lower pressure in certain areas where the concentration of forces cause pain or skin breakdown.

Patients with limited or no sensation, such as with multiple sclerosis or spinal cord injury, require controlled pressure distribution rather than equalized pressure over the entire buttocks. This may require specially configured padding judiciously modified over bony prominences or sites of previous breakdowns or scars with less tolerance than healthy tissue would have (Fig. 27-3).

BREAKDOWN SITES

In many cases, patients to be fitted for wheelchairs have had previous tissue breakdown while lying in bed. Although there are special beds,[4,13] pads,[1,5,15] mattresses,[14] and techniques to relieve pressures, breakdowns do occur in uncontrolled circumstances. The usual sites affected are the heels, sacrum (or coccyx), scapulae, trochanters, anterior tibia, patellas, iliac crest, elbows, or wrists (Fig. 27-4 to 27-6). Of these areas, the heels, sacrum, coccyx, and scapula affect sitting tolerance. Trochanter breakdown from bed rest is usu-

ally above the location of the support site used while the patient sits, except where air or ballooning types of seat cushions or pads are used. Heels may be adequately protected without excess pressure on the posterior aspects, if calf supports are provided on the legrest part of the wheelchair. Legs should be placed in a near-vertical position to relieve minimize pressure on the posterior aspect of the heels.

The sacrococcygeal areas are relieved by sacral cutout pads[14] with care taken to ensure that the coccyx is clear of the lower seat cushion (Fig. 27-7). Air or ballooning types of seat cushions should not be used in these instances, since excessive pressure on the coccyx can result. Relief of sacral pressure may be obtained in some cases by the placing of two pieces of 1 by 3 by 16 inch firm polyfoam on either side of the vertebral spine, spaced so that the pressure on the sacral site is relieved.

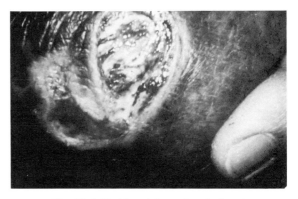

Fig. 27-4. Heel breakdown from bed rest.

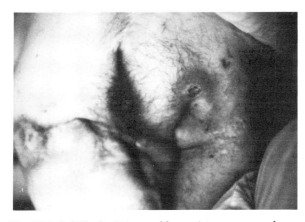

Fig. 27-3. A difficult sitting problem exists over scarred areas allowed to "granulate in."

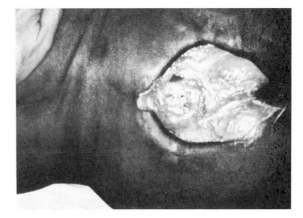

Fig. 27-5. Sacral breakdown from bed rest.

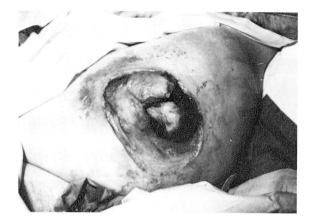

Fig. 27-6. Trochanter breakdown from bed rest.

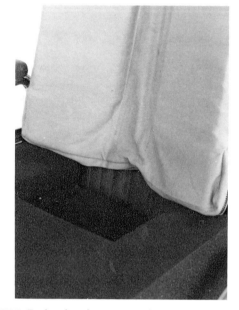

Fig. 27-7. Backpad and cut-out cushion to relieve vertebral spine, sacrum, coccyx, and ischia.

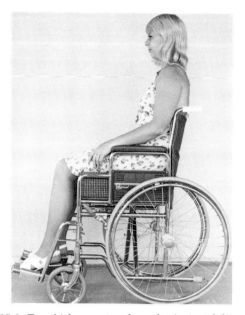

Fig. 27-8. Too thick a seat pad results in instability, overloading of ischial tuberosity, and excessive popliteal pressure. (Compare Fig. 27-14.)

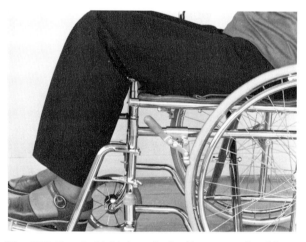

Fig. 27-9. Poor ischial tuberosity loading—no pad and knees elevated.

INFLUENCE OF WHEELCHAIR PRESCRIPTION

In determining wheelchair size, one factor that must be taken into account is the size of pressure-relief padding that will be required for a patient with obvious or suspected breakdown sites (Fig. 27-8). Too thick a pad will raise the patient above the footrest and armrest and may lead to trunk instability and increased pressure on the thighs. Sitting without proper protective padding, or improper positioning in a wheelchair (Fig. 27-9) with knees raised and ischiium overloaded, may cause skin breakdown. To minimize this possibility, a clinical pressure-transducer system has been developed and used in a clinical setting for over 4 years.[3] This technique uses pneumatic pressure grids that allow pressure over suspected sites. The padding is then applied or modified, and the pressure is rechecked to assure effectiveness. This requires custom fitting. Some companies[14] circumvent this by supplying a series of pads with varying relief capabilities for trial purposes.

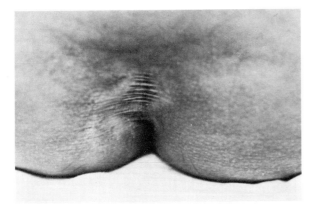

Fig. 27-10. Coccygeal area healed under extreme tension when patient was sitting on normal pad.

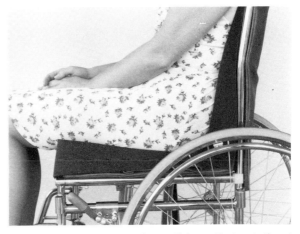

Fig. 27-12. Wheelchair wedges aid in patient rotation to transfer some loading to back.

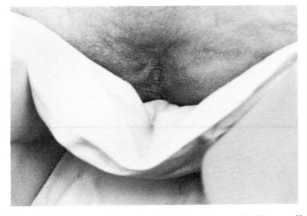

Fig. 27-11. Coccygeal area healed when given relief by small lateral pressure pads on top of normal cushion.

Prior to specification of a particular wheelchair, the following checklist should be used:

Previous tissue damage. If a patient has had tissue damage from previous surgery, pressure, impact, or shear, the site should be relieved of excessive pressure or shear. Care should be taken to ensure that tissue is not stretched excessively, thereby creating high internal pressure that reduces blood flow to the affected area. A specially configured pad may, for example, be required for a patient with a healed pressure sore directly over the coccyx, because as the patient sits, the buttocks spread and tend to tear the previous pressure site (Fig. 27-10). This tendency is removed by padding that pushes the buttocks together (Fig. 27-11).

Positioning. Most patients prefer to sit as upright as possible. A patient with bilateral hip disarticulations, however, has too little an area available for sitting, and thus vertical positioning may be unrealistic unless support can be obtained by special devices under the axillae.

This solution, however, causes many additional problems and is not realistic. Therefore the best expedient is to recline the wheelchair back as far as necessary to provide partial vertical trunk support. Some companies[14] provide total wheelchair inserts to support both the ischial tuberosities and the back and to maintain adequate pressure distribution. The reclining back is necessary in all cases where proper distribution of sitting pressure is compromised by the patient's lack of skeletal support area.

Seat size, leg length, and back height. If the wheelchair back is reclined, it is desirable to raise the anterior portion of the seat to relieve shearing tendencies. In some instances, suppliers[14] have available either pads that automatically convert some of this sliding shearing force into perpendicular pressure force or wheelchair inserts that tilt the seat angle to minimize shear (Figs. 27-12 and 27-13).

Seats are variable in size and may be located at different heights above wheels. If padding for the buttocks is too thick, the patient may be too high above the wheels and may easily tip over (Fig. 27-8). Thus, if buttock pressure is to be relieved by padding, the expected final seated height should be known prior to completing the wheelchair prescription. The seated height also dictates the length of footrests and back height. If the seat height is raised, the footrests may be too low and the patient's feet will dangle without adequate

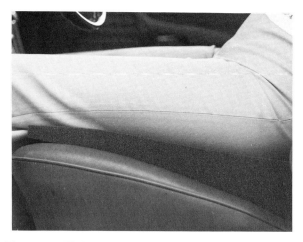

Fig. 27-13. Wedge in car seat provides control of pressure over ischia with suitable cut-out.

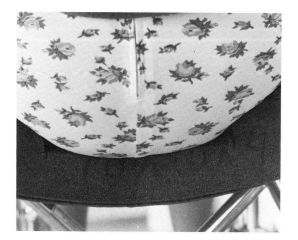

Fig. 27-15. Ischial tuberosity pressure is readily controlled by transferal of load to trochanters and thighs.

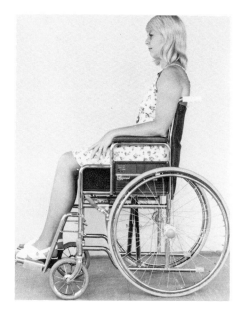

Fig. 27-14. Correct padding allows arms, feet, and back to be properly positioned. (Compare Fig. 27-8.)

support. Wheelchair footrest length should be such as to allow feet and legs to act as counterbalances to raise the ischium and reduce ischial tuberosity loading (Fig. 27-14). Shoe thickness and shoe-heel height will also affect these considerations.

SOURCES AND CONTROL OF EXCESSIVE PRESSURE

There are many ways in which the seated patient generates excessive internal pressure over the ischial tuberosities, trochanters, coccyx, and sacrum.

Direct loading

Direct loading has the most obvious effect on internal pressure and as previously mentioned[3] can be tolerated by the body more adequately over fleshy portions of the buttocks or thighs than over the bony prominences. Direct loading is determined by patient position, weight, bony prominence, skin and muscle atrophy, weight of objects being carried, and the available area of support. If loading is applied to a rounded or pointed support, then shear forces operate at that site. This is a factor in breakdown over ischial tuberosities when ballooning occurs or very pliable padding is used, because upward forces around the tuberosities create excessive internal shear and pressure. High direct loading is better tolerated over thighs than the ischium. The loading should be gradually increased from the ischium to the thighs (Fig. 27-15). Too abrupt an increase may result in tissue breakdown at the transition points. A patient who has no femoral head may require unloading of that thigh or femur and increased loading of opposite side. Trunk supports (Figs. 27-16 and 27-17) in a wheelchair and in a car may be used to support some lateral tilting of the trunk and in turn reduce ischial pressures by tending to level the pelvis.

Shear loading

Shear loads cannot exist without vertical loading also being applied. Many researchers believe

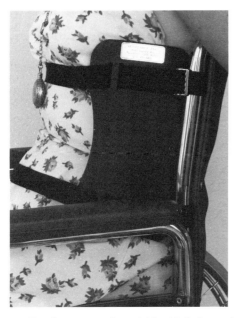

Fig. 27-16. Trunk supports that yield with body motion and padded with Sifoam provide trunk stability and negate excessive rib-cage pressure.

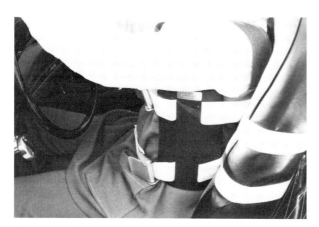

Fig. 27-17. Car trunk supports aid in lateral and forward stability.

that shear is more devastating than direct loading. It is mandatory that all loading aspects be kept to a minimum, since two adjacent areas loaded differently cause high shear forces at the interface. Also shear exists beneath the skin even though the external shear may be reduced. This situation is encountered where hammocking of the wheelchair is present and ischial tuberosities are manifested directly when tissue is pulled tight over the bony prominences. If the patient is fair skinned, tissue may be more susceptible to pressure.

Hammock effect

This describes an effect whereby a material or membrane is supported by its edges while the load rests in the center of the material or membrane. In a folding wheelchair the fabric seat between its two side supports creates this sling-effect situation. This hammock effect is also encountered with clothing stretched tightly over the ischial tuberosities when the patient sits (Fig. 27-15). If clothing is tight or inflexible when patients push themselves up to relieve pressure, little relief is actually obtained. Thus loose, double-knit, open-weave, and silk clothing minimize friction and hammock effects.

A hammock effect also occurs when envelope seat pads are used to contain fluids, gels, water, and so forth and must be carefully evaluated when a cushion or pad selection is made, as it has the same effect as tight clothing. If an envelope is only semipliable, it inhibits performance.

OTHER CONSIDERATIONS
Rehabilitation goals

Rehabilitation is directly related to mental attitude and ability. Where long-term sitting is anticipated, special padding may be required. It is very hard for some people to diligently do "push-ups" where they are likely to be more conspicuous than usual, such as in school or at a theatre or sports event. Many institutions emphasize and reemphasize pressure-relief methods for people with poor sensation. With these patients, who may work or be sitting for extended periods of time, some type of padding should be used to alleviate possible tissue breakdown if their relief regimen is interrupted. It is also of prime importance to realize that some active patients will become preoccupied with their endeavors and neglect to relieve their pressure areas.

Assistive equipment

Where some additional type of assistive equipment is anticipated, such as upper-limb mobile arm supports for spinal cord patients, additional care should be exercised in selecting the correct padding for lowering pressure below the 50 mm Hg encountered with equal distribution of pressure claimed by most manufacturers.[10] This is where breakdowns occurs. Because considerable time is spent in setting up upper-limb equipment, patients are hesitant to relieve pressures as much as may be required. Pressure-relief padding to fit these patient requirements is of prime importance.

Padding requirements

Some manufacturers claim equal pressure distribution is achieved with the same pad under eighter lying or sitting conditions. This is probably not valid because the pressures encountered while the patient is lying are considerably less than while sitting, such as 40 mm Hg versus 100 mm Hg. This is the reason why some pads may be reasonable for lying upon but will cause skin breakdown when used as seat cushions. Sitting and lying are two separate problems and should be handled as such.

Generally the manufacturer is faced with problems of fabricating a low-cost functional long-life pad to satisfy all problems. This is a goal seldom attained. The following may be used as guidelines in selecting proper padding:

1. *Breathing.* Air should circulate freely to minimize maceration.
2. *Incontinence protection.* The padding interior should be adequately protected for incontinent patients. Some manufacturers supply washable or dry-cleanable covers to alleviate this problem.
3. *Handling.* Where poor function of the upper limbs or trunk may be anticipated, the padding should be lightweight (less than 5 pounds) for ease of transfer from a wheelchair to a car. Major problems occur if the cushion interior is too soft because the cen-

Table 4. Wheelchair cushions and related protective devices

Cushion	Thickness (inches)	Weight (pounds)	Characteristics
Bioclinic P.O. Box 1505 Saugus, California 91350	2	10	Water- and foam-filled vinyl envelope; gel filled also available
Decubitex (In Sweden)	2	1	Tiny plastic balls are displaced by concentrated weight
De Puy Warsaw, Indiana 46580	2	10	Water and squared foam; nylon covers
Jobst 6360 Wilshire Blvd., Suite 305 Los Angeles, California 653-3127	2	22	Open-pored synthetic foam filled with water and contained in a nylon cover
Ken McWright Supplies, Inc. 7456 South Oswego Tulsa, Oklahoma 74135	4	2	Compartmentalized rubber envelope for air inflating; depressions or buttons near ischial tuberosities
Ortho Industries 49 Lawton Street Rochelle, New York 14603	2	16	Special gel
Orthopedic Equipment Burbin, Indiana 46504	2	15	Silicon fluid and foam are contained in a rubber envelope
Scimedics, Inc. 700 North Valley St., Suite B Anaheim, California 92801			
Solid Adaptaire	3	3½	Nonflammable resin-filled polyurethane; Sifoam liners
Standard Adaptaire	3	3½	As in Solid Adaptaire with 8 by 10 by 1 inch cut-out
Double Cut-out Adaptaire	3	3	As in Solid Adaptaire with 8 by 10 by 2 inch cut-out
Stryker 490 East Walnut, Suite 6 Pasadena, California 91101	2	14	Special gel contained in a latex cover

ter of gravity moves when the padding is moved and patients with weakness are unable to handle it adequately. If the pad cover is broken, the pad must still function and not exude its contents over the clothing or on the wheelchair or floor. This aspect is important where poor sensation is exhibited by the patient as he may be unaware that his padding is no longer protecting his body adequately against pressure sores.

4. *Car use.* The pad used in the wheelchair may be suitable for car use if the angle of the car seat is accommodated (Fig. 27-13). Ischial tuberosities are relieved by cutouts in the ischial area (Fig. 27-7). Usually any padding is better than none as most cars or vans are not suitably upholstered for the handicapped.

5. *Cost.* Pads range from $5 to $350. Their cost is not necessarily related to performance.

6. Specifications and sources of supply for wheelchair pads or cushions are found in Table 4.

REFERENCES

1. BioClinic Company, P.O. Box 1505, Saugus, California 91350.
2. Everest & Jennings, Inc., 1803 Pontius Avenue, Los Angeles, California.
3. Fellars, P. H.: Preliminary evaluation of the Adaptaire cushion. Paper presented June 10, 1972, Orthopedic Conference, Rancho Los Amigos Hospital, Resident Research Papers, Vol. V, Rancho Los Amigos Hospital.
4. High density fluid system bed (H.D.S. bed) by Gaymar, Inc., Representative: Gene Daniels Sales Company, 128 Bielec Lane, City of Industry, California 91746.
5. Hot Springs, Rehabilitation Center, Arkansas.
6. Houle, R. J.: Evaluation of seat devices designed to prevent ischemic ulcers in paraplegic patients, Arch. Phys. Med., Oct. 1969.
7. Kosiak, M.: Etiology of decubitus ulcers, Arch. Phys. Med. **42**:19-28, Jan. 1961.
8. Lindan, O., Greenway, R. M., and Piazza, J. M.: Pressure distribution on surface of the human body: I. Evaluation in lying and sitting positions using a bed of spring nails, Arch. Phys. Med. **46**:378-385, May 1965.
9. Mooney, V.: Progress in improved prosthetic design, Paper presented in Bermuda, 1972.
10. Mooney, V., Einbund, M. J., Rogers, J. E., and Stauffer, E. S.: Comparison of pressure distribution qualities in seat cushions, Bull. Prosthet. Res., Spring 1971.
11. Rancho Los Amigos Hospital, Rehabilitation Engineering Center, Control, Power, and Communication Engineering, 7425 Leeds Street, Downey, California 90242.
12. Rancho Los Amigos Hospital, 7601 East Imperial Highway, Downey, California 90242.
13. Royalaire by Milton Roy Company, 717 South Garfield, Alhambra, California 91801.
14. Scimedics, Inc., 700 North Valley St., Suite B, Anaheim, California 92801.
15. Stryker Company, Kalamazoo, Michigan. (Main office; for branch office, see Table 4.)

CHAPTER 28

Adaptive devices for automobiles

ANTON J. REICHENBERGER
PAUL H. NEWELL, Jr., P.E., Ph.D.

A variety of assistive automotive control systems is commercially available for use by handicapped drivers in operating standard types of automobiles. The vehicle in question must be equipped with an automatic transmission, power steering, and power brakes. All commercial hand-control systems are designed so that both the throttle and the brakes can be operated with one hand, leaving the other hand exclusively for steering. Left-hand operation of a control system offers maximum driving comfort and is therefore the preferred mode, although most adaptive equipment manufacturers can provide a right-hand operated control system on request. In some cases either a dimmer switch or horn button or both are mounted on the control handle, however, none of the adaptive automotive equipment manufacturers offers a system with the directional signal switch mounted on the control handle. Consequently, activating the directional signal requires one to release the control handle momentarily to accomplish this task.

With the exception of custom-designed foot-control steering systems and several design configurations of an adaptive left-foot accelerator, controls listed in Table 5 should be used by disabled drivers with little or no use of the lower limbs and nearly normal upper-limb strength and mobility.

ADAPTIVE HAND-CONTROL SYSTEMS

The class of commercially available hand-control systems consist of mechanical linkages, a

Table 5. Driving aid for loss or paralysis of limb

Special controls required	Right leg	Left leg	Both legs	Right arm	Left arm	Both arms
Brake and accelerator			*			
Dimmer switch		*	*			
Left foot accelerator	*					
Parking brake		*	*			
Steering assists				*	*	
Turn lever, right-hand operated					*	
Shift lever, left-hand operated				*		
Foot steering						*

control handle, and associated hardware. With the exception of mechanical advantage, no form of power augmentation is provided for any of these devices, thus there is a suggestion that the usefulness of a particular hand-control system must be determined by the individual handicapped driver. We classify all known adaptive hand-control systems into four types, push-pull, push-right angle pull, push-twist, and the crank type.

1. *Push-pull control system* (Figs. 28-1 to 28-3). Activation of the brakes requires a force applied to the control handle in the direction away from the driver and parallel to the steering column, whereas the accelerator pedal is operated by pulling the control handle in the opposite direction.

2. *Push–right angle pull control system* (Figs. 28-4 to 28-6). The brakes are actuated in a manner similar to type 1, whereas the accelerator pedal is operated by pulling the control handle toward the driver's lap.

3. *Push-twist control system* (Figs. 28-7 and 28-8). Again the brakes are activated in a manner similar to type 1, and operation of the accelerator is achieved by a twisting motion of the control handle.

4. *Crank control system* (Figs. 28-9 and 28-10). Finally, this system requires cranking of the handle in a clockwise direction away from the driver for brake actuation, whereas actuation of the accelerator is achieved by cranking the handle in the opposite direction toward the driver.

Text continued on p. 468.

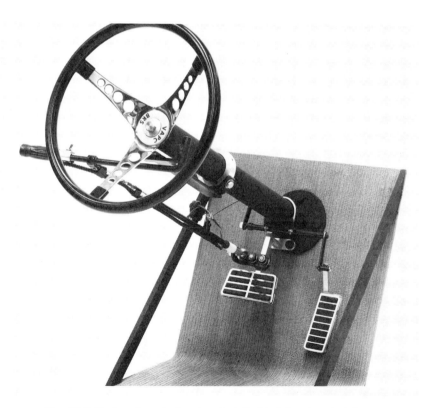
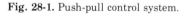

Fig. 28-1. Push-pull control system.

Fig. 28-2. Push-pull control system installed to laboratory test jig.

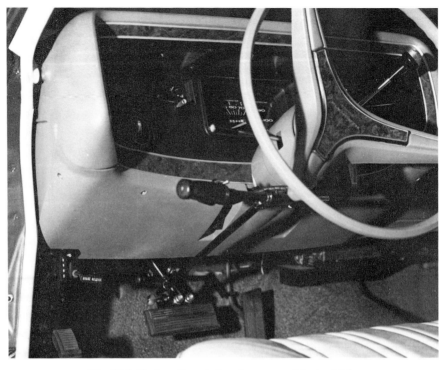

Fig. 28-3. Push-pull control system on road-test vehicle.

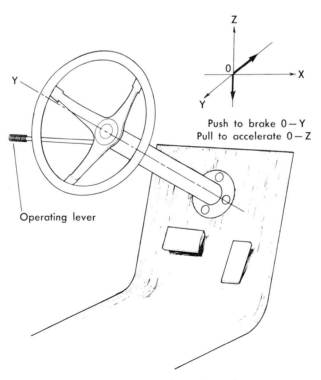

Fig. 28-4. Push–right angle pull control system.

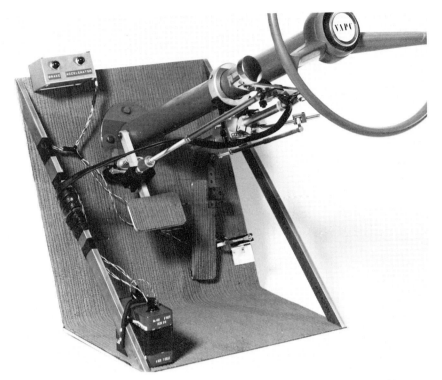

Fig. 28-5. Push–right angle pull control system installed to laboratory test jig.

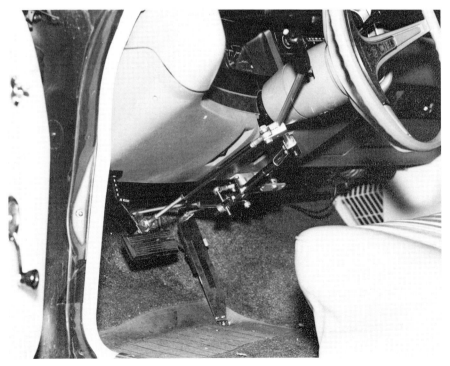

Fig. 28-6. Push–right angle pull control system on road-test vehicle.

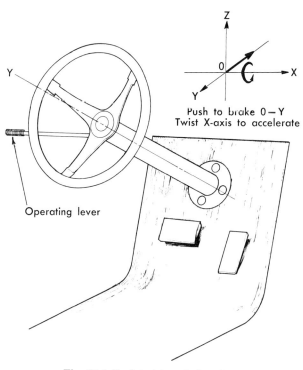

Fig. 28-7. Push-twist control system.

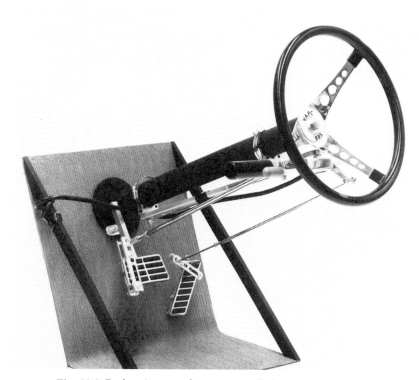

Fig. 28-8. Push-twist control system installed to laboratory test jig.

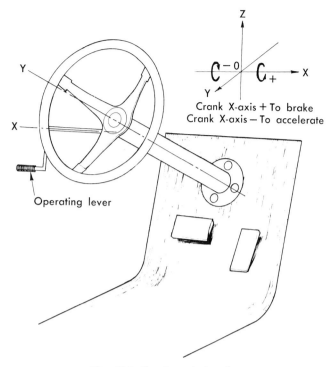

Crank X-axis + To brake
Crank X-axis − To accelerate

Fig. 28-9. Crank control system.

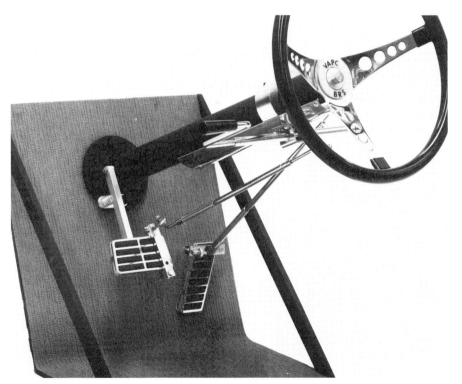

Fig. 28-10. Crank control system installed to laboratory test jig.

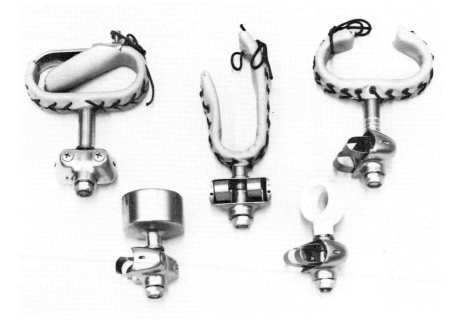

Fig. 28-11. Assortment of steering assists.

For handicapped drivers with nearly normal upper-limb strength and mobility but requiring some assistance in steering the motor vehicle, there are a number of devices that can be simply adapted to any standard-sized steering wheel. Fig. 28-11 shows a typical assortment of steering assists, with their usefulness much depending on available physical strength and mobility of upper body and limbs of the individual handicapped driver. Experimentation with the potential driver should ascertain whether a particular steering assist is useful in operating the automobile safely.

Provided that the particular hand-control system selected can be easily operated by the handicapped driver, the principal design features to look for are the methods of attaching the device to the vehicle and the pedals. Bolted connectors are preferred in all cases, as opposed to clamping types. The internal hardware is also important, and the use of ball joints at all pivot points and locking fasteners indicate good design. All adaptive automotive hardware should be accompanied by installation instructions, but installation of any device should only be attempted by an experienced mechanic to assure maximum safety in operating the automobile. Because of the difficulty in locating this type of equipment and service, the present available sources are listed in Table 6.

VAN MODIFICATIONS AND SPECIAL SYSTEMS

For those patients who do not have sufficient strength in their arms and upper body to make the wheelchair-car-wheelchair transfer and for those who, for any reason use an electric wheelchair, the needs of these individuals are best met by the use of a van with some type of power lift to allow them to remain in the wheelchair. Table 7 lists companies that are presently available to modify vans, install power lifts, and manufacture special equipment specifically for use by disabled drivers. The lifts operate at either the right side or the rear doors of the van, and most use an electric motor as either a direct source of power for the lift or as a source of power for a hydraulic pump, which is in turn used to power the lift. There are also some lifts designed for operation by an attendant, simply providing a device for transferring wheelchair-bound individuals in and out of the van. Naturally, when the van is to be operated independently by the handicapped driver, additional equipment is required for opening and closing doors, controlling the operation of the lift, positioning and securing the wheelchair in the van, and driving the van from a wheelchair.

The interior of these motor vehicles can be supplied to resemble a panel truck, or perhaps

Table 6. Present manufacturers of adaptive automotive equipment

Manufacturer	Type of hand control	Notes	Manufacturer	Type of hand control	Notes
Blatnik Precision Controls 1523 Cota Avenue Long Beach, California 90813 (213) 436-3275	2		**Mechtronic Industries** 15315 S. Broadway Gardena, California 90247	2	
Cameron Ens 13637 South Madsen Avenue Kingsburg, California 93631 (209) 897-2749		Left-foot steering manufacturer	**Manufacturing and Production Service Corp.** 4666 Mercury Street San Diego, California 92111 (714) 292-1423	2	
Card Hand Controls P.O. Box 907 Garland, Texas 75040 (214) 278-2676	2		**National Institute for Rehabilitation Engineering** 238 Poplar Avenue Pompton Lakes, New Jersey 07442 (201) 694-9100		Custom fabricator, special systems
Drive Master Corporation 61 North Mountain Avenue Montclair, New Jersey 07042 (201) 744-1998	1		**Nelson Products** 3112 Wilder Avenue Sarasota, Florida 33580	3	Also complete line of steering assists
Paul A. Dunn, Jr. 1582 Kenmore Avenue Buffalo, New York 14216 (716) 875-3351	1		**O.K. Brakes, Inc.** 416 3rd Avenue Brooklyn, New York 11215 (212) 624-4790	1	
Gresham Driving Aids 30800 Wixom Road Wixom, Michigan 48096 (313) 624-1533	2	Also complete line of steering assists	**Royce International** 4345 South Santa Fe Drive Englewood, Colorado 80110 (303) 789-1032	2	Also quadriplegic control steering assists
Hughes Hand Driving Controls Tevis Bridge Road, Box 275 Lexington, Missouri 64067	2				
Kope Engineering and Manufacturing 8674 South Reed Avenue Reedley, California 93654 (209) 638-3429		Custom fabricator, left-foot steering, special systems	**Safety Magic Sales Co.** Box 602 Janesville, Wisconsin 53546 (608) 752-4801	4	
Kroepke Kontrols, Inc. 104 Hawkins Street Bronx, New York 10464 (212) 885-1547	1		**Smith's Hand Control Service** 1472 Brookhaven Drive Southaven, Mississippi 38671 (601) 393-0540	2	
Leverage Hand-Brake Co. P.O. Box 853 Fargo, North Dakota 58102 (701) 232-2133	2		**Trujillo Industries** 815 Nash Street El Segundo, Calif. 90245 (714) 492-6207		Complete line of steering assists
Alfred F. Morris 2512 Banner Street Durham, North Carolina 27704		Left-foot steering manufacturer	**Wells Engberg Co.** 2505 Rural Street Rockford, Illinois 61107 (815) 399-2314	3	

Table 7. Van modifiers and manufacturers of wheelchair-access systems and special equipment

Braun Corporation
(formerly Save-A-Step
  Corporation)
1014 South Monticello
Winamac, Indiana 46996
(219) 946-3647

Cheney Company
7611 North 73rd Street
Milwaukee, Wisconsin 53223
(414) 354-8510

Compass Industries
715 Fifteenth Street
Hermosa Beach,
  California 90254
(213) 379-7080

Drive-Master Corporation
61 North Mountain Avenue
Montclair, New Jersey 07042
(201) 744-1998

Handi-Ramp, Incorporated
1414 Armour Blvd.
Mundelein, Illinois 60060
(312) 566-5861

Helper Industries, Inc.
832 N.W. 1st Street
Ft. Lauderdale,
  Florida 33311
(305) 524-7231

David G. Kope
1378 N. Reed
Reedley, California 93654
(209) 638-3429

Motorette Corporation
6014 Reseda Boulevard
Tarzana, California 91356
(213) 345-6490

Robin-Aids, Inc.
3353 Broadway
Vallejo, California 94590
(707) 643-1785

Royce International
4345 S. Santa Fe Drive
Englewood, Colorado 80110
(303) 789-1032

Safety Van Lift
1627 Linnea Avenue
Eugene, Oregon 97401
(503) 686-9706

Charles M. Scott
U.C.L.A. Rehabilitation
  Center
1000 Veteran Avenue
Los Angeles,
  California 90024

Fred Scott & Sons
70 Scott Street
Elk Grove, Illinois 60007
(312) 437-7666

Speedy Wagon Sales Corp.
2237 Harvester Road
St. Charles, Missouri 63301
(314) 723-1119

Strong Engineering Mfg.
630 Venice Way
Ingelwood, California 90302

**Warren Equipment
  Company**
1120 Dartmoor Avenue
Parma, Ohio 44134

stylishly finished for maximum comfort and utility, depending on preference and of course on how much one is willing to pay.

In Figs. 28-12 to 28-14, typical modifications of a van for use by handicapped drivers is shown. Side-loading wheelchair entry-exit system, automatic opening and closing of sliding right-side door, hand controls, and so forth make this motor vehicle useful for many disabled drivers. Although a Chevrolet Sportsvan was used for this particular adaptation, most van modifiers are able to supply customers with their choice of a standard-sized van. This particular motor vehicle requires that the driver has enough upper-limb strength

and mobility to operate conventional hand-control systems similar to those listed for sedans. Of course, the steering wheel can be equipped with steering assists as needed.

The vehicle shown in Figs. 28-15 to 28-17 is modified so that the reinforced automotive right-side door provides a ramp for wheelchair entry and exit. Once the driver has entered the van, transfer is made to a specially designed driver chair that provides some adjustments to bring the driver into the desired driving position. The driver chair fastens to the automotive structure, protecting the driver against problems arising through sudden inertial changes of the motor vehicle. Again, to operate this van, the handicapped driver must have enough upper-limb strength and mobility to work with hand-control systems used in sedans.

The Veterans Administration is currently evaluating an experimental van for handicapped drivers unable to control a motor vehicle by the variety of available hand-control systems. This Ford Econoline 100 van is specially equipped with a control system that requires a minimum of physical effort to operate (Figs. 28-18 to 28-21). The standard automotive steering mechanism and brake-accelerator control systems were removed from the vehicle and replaced by a hydraulic servo-system to permit operation in a joystick-like manner. The magnitude of forces required to actuate brakes or accelerator is in the order of a few ounces, whereas steering can be controlled with limited wrist motion of either the right or left hand. A touch type of pushbutton control module places all required functions of automobile driving within easy reach of the handicapped driver, such as starting and stopping the engine, gear selection, signal lights, opening and closing rear doors, operation of wheelchair lift, and opening and closing windows. In Fig. 28-22 a specially designed wheelchair is shown. This chair is for use with or without the van, equipped with the necessary safety features of standard automotive seating, eliminating the problem of transfer for seriously handicapped drivers. The complexity of this *experimental* motor vehicle requires that development continue, so that a van type of vehicle can soon become *commercially* available for safe and dependable use by severely handicapped drivers.

Future expectations

Areas where further improvements are most needed are positioning and securing the driver

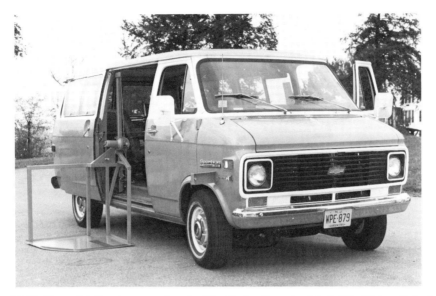

Fig. 28-12. Chevrolet Sportsvan equipped with side-loading wheelchair lift. (Helper Industries, Inc., Fort Lauderdale, Florida.)

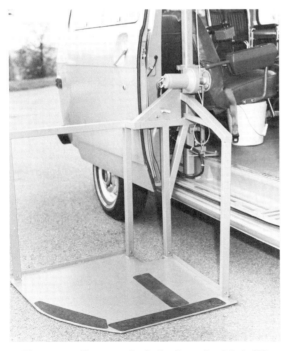

Fig. 28-13. Close-up of side-loading wheelchair lift.

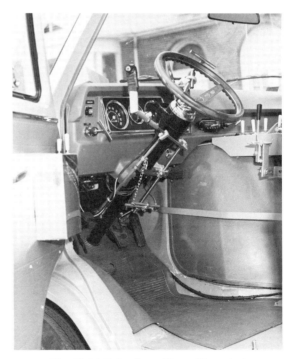

Fig. 28-14. Driver's position with controls.

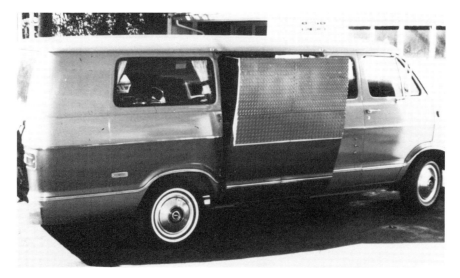

Fig. 28-15. Dodge Sportman Van including integral wheelchair entry-exit system. (Royce International, Englewood, Colorado.)

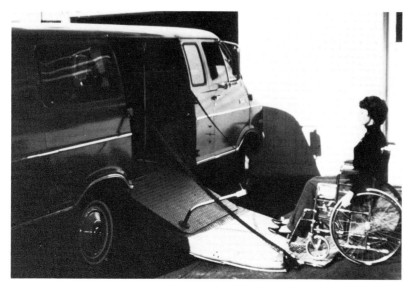

Fig. 28-16. Wheelchair-bound driver entering vehicle.

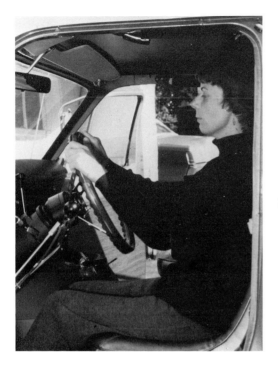

Fig. 28-17. Driver in operating position.

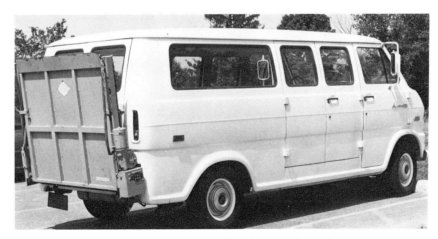

Fig. 28-18. Scott Van-Ford Econoline 100 Super Van.

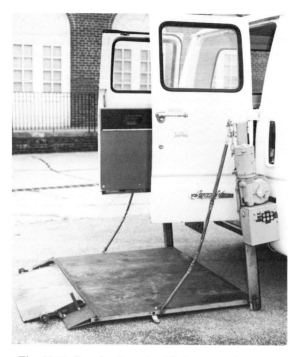

Fig. 28-19. Rear-loading wheelchair entry-exit system.

and wheelchair in a good driving position, providing adequate man-machine interfaces to allow safe driving and ensuring reliability of the assistive systems, particularly the lifts. Being constructed is a prototype van that uses a two-axis joystick similar to that on an electric wheelchair to control the primary functions of steering, acceleration, and braking (Fig. 28-23) and provides automatic or electronically controlled actuation of the secondary functions necessary for driving (Fig. 28-24).

Since handicapped drivers should be protected from unsafe adaptive automotive equipment in the same manner nonhandicapped drivers are protected by Federal Motor Vehicle Safety Standards (FMVSS), it is crucial to develop standards and specifications applicable to equipment provided for handicapped drivers.

Federal Motor Vehicle Safety Standards do not presently apply to vehicle modifications that occur after the original sale.

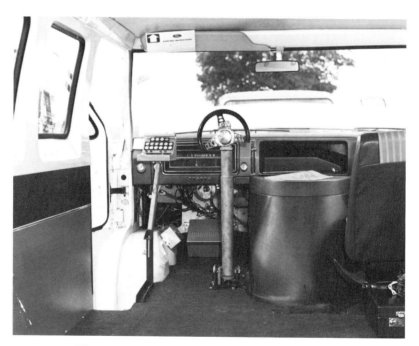

Fig. 28-20. View of specially designed control system.

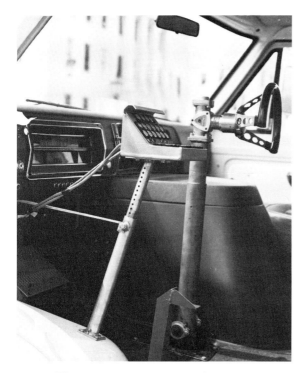

Fig. 28-21. Side-view of control system.

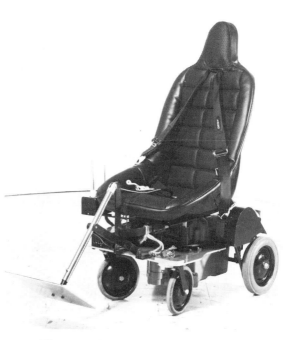

Fig. 28-22. Special automotive wheelchair.

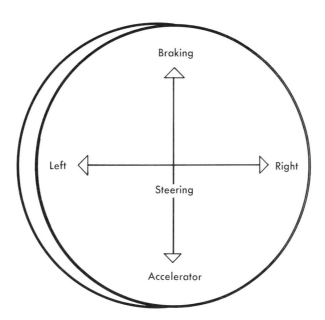

Fig. 28-23. Joystick operation for primary control.

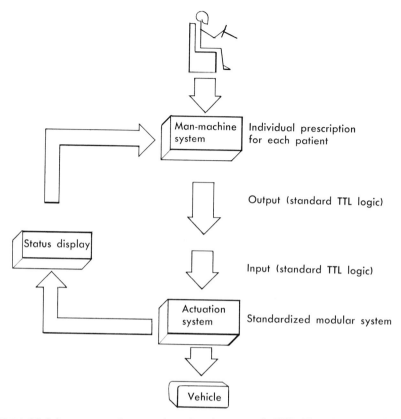

Fig. 28-24. Modular systems for secondary function control. *TTL,* Transistor-transistor logic.

SUGGESTED READINGS AND REFERENCES

1. Aimers McLean Co.: "The Amnel Wildcat," a cross-country vehicle designed for paraplegics, Galashiels, Scotland (Undated).
2. American Automobile Association, Traffic Engineering and Safety Department: Vehicle controls for disabled persons, Washington, D.C., 1972.
3. American Medical Association, National Conference on Medical Aspects of Driver Safety and Driver Licensing, 1964:
   Erickson, H. M., and Waller, J. A.: Medical deficiencies, detection, evaluation, reporting.
   Kerrick, J. C.: Medical advisory committees.
   McFarland, R. A.: Research–driver capability.
   Mirkin, A. J.: Medical factors related to driving ability.
   Scheidt, E.: Administrative procedures.
   Terry, L. L.: Public health and driver licensing.
4. American Medical Association, Committee on Medical Aspects of Automobile Safety, 1968, Physicians guide for determining driver limitations.
5. Bardach, J. L.: Psychological factors affecting driving behavior in the disabled, Med. Clin. N. Am. 53:692, 1969.
6. Bardach, J. C.: Psychological factors in the handicapped driver, Arch. Phys. Med. Rehab. 53:328, July 1971.
7. Bell, E., Elliott, R. M., and Von Werssowetz, O. F.: Muscle strength and resultant function in cervical cord lesions, Am. J. Occup. Ther. 15:106, 1961.
8. Berner, L.: Driver training for the severely handicapped, Am. Correct. Ther. J. 22:18, 1968.
9. Brandaleone, H., Blaney, L., Irwin, G. H., et al.: Physical standards for vehicle operators, Industrial Med. Surg. 25:17, 1956.
10. Brandaleone, H., and Friedman, G. J.: Recommendations for medical standards for motor vehicle drivers, Industrial Med. Surg. 26:25, 1957.
11. Brandaleone, H.: Medical aspects of motor vehicle accident prevention. Study of the driver, Clin. Orthop. 9:291, 1957.
12. Bray, P., and Cunningham, D. M.: Vehicles for the severely disabled, Rehabil. Lit. 28:98, 1967.
13. Connecticut State Motor Vehicle Department: Some of our best drivers, Hartford, 1970.
14. Consumers' Association: "Which?" London, No. 8, p. 248, August 1969.
15. Crancer, A., and McMurray L.: Accident and violation rates of Washington drivers with medical licensing and driving restrictions, Division of Research, State of Washington Department of Motor Vehicles, 1967, Seattle, Wash.
16. Darlington, J. O.: Road accidents–human causes and general remedies, J. Institution of Highway Engineers, vol. 19, August 1967.
17. Department of Transportation, Traffic Laws Commentary, Medical advisory boards, Vol. 1, No. 1, 1972.
18. DePian, L., and Wiggins, T. B.: One handed automobile

control, Final report to VRA, RD-1450-G, September 1964, Washington, D.C.

19. Domey, R. G., and Duckworth, J. E.: Comparative study of highway accidents among 625 physically impaired licensees matched with 625 nonimpaired licensees, Cambridge, Mass., 1963, Harvard School of Public Health, Boston.

20. Finesilver, S. G.: A survey of physically impaired drivers —their answers and observations, University of Denver College of Law, 1969, Denver.

21. Finesilver, S. G.: The accident involvement and driving capabilities of physically impaired drivers, University of Denver College of Law, 1969, Denver.

22. Gart, W. R.: A comparison of severely handicapped and able bodied drivers, Master's thesis, University of Illinois, Urbana, Ill., 1957.

23. General Motors Corporation, Public Relations Office: Personal communication, 1972.

24. Goldstein, L. G.: Human variables in traffic accidents, a digest of research and selected bibliography, U.S. Public Health Service, 1961, Washington, D.C.

25. Gutshall, R. W.: The handicapped driver, Safety Education, p. 6, Dec. 1961.

26. Harvard School of Public Health, Harvard University, Cambridge, Massachusetts.

27. Henderson, H. L., and Kole, T.: The automobile as a prosthetic device in physical rehabilitation, J. Rehabil. **31:** 30, 1965.

28. Highway Research Board: Publications, Washington, D.C., 1972.

29. Highway Safety Research Institute, University of Michigan, Ann Arbor, Michigan. (A bibliography is available.)

30. Hofkosh, J. M., Sipajlo, J., and Brody, L.: Driver education for the physically disabled, Med. Clin. N. Am. **53:** 685, 1969.

31. Hyman, W. A.: Suggested standards for adaptive control devices for vehicular driving, Bioengineering Program, Texas A. & M. University, College Station, Texas, Oct. 1972.

32. Hyman, W. A.: Survey of domestic automobile manufacturers with respect to approval of existing adaptive aids, Bioengineering Program, Texas A. & M. University, College Station, Texas, Nov. 1972.

33. ICTA Information Centre, Bromma, Sweden: Conversion of cars for disabled drivers, Report 1971, Stockholm.

34. Imrie, J. A.: Medical standards of fitness for driving, The Practitioner **188:**508, 1962.

35. Insurance Services Office, New York, and American Mutual Insurance Alliance, Chicago, Personal communications, 1972.

36. J.A.M.A. special addition, Committee on Medical Rating of Physical Impairment. A guide to the evaluation of permanent impairment of the extremities and back, Feb. 15, 1958.

37. J.A.M.A. **203:**879, 1968. Determination of need for medical evaluation in driver licensing.

38. J.A.M.A. **169:**1195, 1959. Medical guide for physicians in determining fitness to drive a motor vehicle.

39. Kaplan, L., Rowell, B. R., Grynbaum, B. B., and Rusk, H. A.: Comprehensive follow-up study of spinal cord dysfunction and its resulting disabilities, Institute of Rehabil-

itation Medicine, New York University Medical Center, 1969.

40. Lehneis, H. R., Hofkosh, J. M., Sipajlo, J., and Wilson, R. G.: Driving aids: Design and development, Med. Clin. N. Am. **53:**689, 1969.

41. Leonard, E. J.: Personal communication, President's Committee on Employment of the Handicapped, 1972.

42. Little, Arthur D., Inc.: The state of the art of traffic safety, New York, 1970, Frederick A. Praeger, Inc.

43. Long, C.: Congenital and traumatic lesions of the spinal cord. In Krusen, F. H., Kottke, F. J., and Ellwood, P. M., editors: Physical medicine and rehabilitation, Philadelphia, 1971, W. B. Saunders Co.

44. Long, C., II, and Lawton, E. B.: Functional significance of spinal cord lesion level, Arch. Phys. Med. Rehabil. **36:**249, April 1955.

45. Lowman, E., and Klinger, J. L.: Aids to independent living, Chapter 63, "Automobile controls and adapted vehicles," New York, 1969, McGraw-Hill Book Co.

46. Malfetti, J. L.: The impaired driver, New York State J. Med. **63:**1778, June 15, 1963.

47. Mayyasi, A. M., Pulley, P. E., and Swarts, A. E.: (a) A complete one-handed pistol-grip automobile controller, (b) Complete single-footed automobile controller, (c) Adaptability of the PGC/SFC for special applications, Bioengineering Program, Texas A. & M. University, College Station, Texas, Nov. 1972.

48. Mayyasi, A. M., Pulley, P. E., Hyman, W. A., and Swarts, A. E.: Categorization of disabilities and functional limitations imposed in the driving task, Bioengineering Program, Texas A. & M. University, College Station, Texas, Nov. 1972.

49. McFarland, R. A., Domey, R. G., Duggar, B. C., Crowley, T. J., and Strudt, H. W.: An evaluation of the ability of amputees to operate highway transport equipment, Cambridge, Mass., 1968, Harvard School of Public Health.

50. McKenzie, M. W.: The role of occupational therapy in rehabilitating spinal cord injured patients, Am. J. Occup. Ther. **24:**257, 1970.

51. Millichamp, D.: Who cares about the disabled driver? Engineering, p. 192, Aug. 1970.

52. Mitchell, H. H.: Medical problems and physical fitness as related to occurrence of traffic accidents, Rand Publications RM-5363-DOT, 1968.

53. National Highway Traffic Safety Administration: Highway safety literature, Washington, D.C.

54. National Highway Traffic Safety Administration: Personal communication, 1972.

55. National Safety Council: Accidents facts, 1972, Chicago.

56. PVA Conference: Presentation by Veterans Administration, Miami, Florida, July 1972.

57. Rees, W. D.: Physical and mental disabilities of 1,190 ordinary motorists, Br. Med. J. **1:**593, 1967.

58. Reynolds, J.: A study to demonstrate the practicability and methodology of teaching driving to the physically disabled high school student, Final report to SRS, Report No. RD-1852-G, June 1968, Washington, D.C.

59. Rhoads, M. D., and Matthews, P. W.: New resources and new techniques in teaching the handicapped to drive are proving out in Oklahoma, Highway User, p. 21, Nov. 1971.

60. Rozin, R., and Tolani, D.: Car independence for patients with triplegia, Arch. Phys. Med. Rehabil. **52:**80, 1971.

61. Schwerhert, H. A.: Transportation for disabled, Paraplegia News, 1970.
62. Science News Letter, **88:**1965: Limbless youth drives specially engineered car.
63. Stock, M. S., Light, W. O., Douglass, J. M., and Burg, F. D.: Licensing the driver with musculoskeletal difficulty, J. Bone Joint Surg. **52A:**343, 1970. (Musculoskeletal section of reference 30.)
64. Street, R. L., Mayyasi, A. M., and Berngen, F. E.: Diagnostic studies of highway visual communications systems, Texas Transportation Institute, Texas A. & M. University, Project RE 606, 1969.
65. Talbot, B.: Automobile modifications for the disabled, In Licht, S., editor: Orthotics, Baltimore, 1968, Waverly Press.
66. Texas Transportation Institute, Texas A. & M. University, College Station, Texas.
67. U.S. Dept. of Transportation, National Highway Traffic Safety Administration, Standards, June 1972.
68. U.S. Public Health Service: Driver licensing guidelines for medical advisory boards, 1969.
69. VA tentative standards and specifications for automotive driving aids (adaptive equipment) for standard passenger automobiles, VAPC-A-7404-T5, 1974, U.S. Veterans Administration.
70. Vernon, R. J., and Phillips, M. B.: A study of public school driver education in Texas, Texas Transportation Institute, Texas A. & M. University, College Station, Texas, April 1972.
71. Vodovnik, L.: An electromagnetic brake activated by eyebrow muscles, Electronic Engineering, Oct. 1964.
72. Waller, J. A.: Guide for the identification, evaluation, and regulation of persons with medical handicaps to driving, Washington, D.C., 1967, American Association of Motor Vehicle Administrators.
73. Waller, J. A., and Thunen, R. V.: Medical handicaps to driving, Calif. Med. **98:**275-278, 1963.
74. Ward, H. L., and Gingras, G.: Medical aspects of traffic accidents in paraplegics, Can. Serv. Med. J. **12:**459, 1956.
75. West, I.: The impaired driver, Calif. Med. **98:**271, 1963.
76. Wheatley, G. M.: The health of the driver, J. Traffic Safety Educ. p. 16, Jan. 1966.
77. Ysander, L.: The safety of the physically disabled driver, Br. J. Indust. Med. **23:**173, 1966.
78. Zino, R. L.: Selecting a car for the instruction of physically handicapped students, J. Traffic Safety Educ. p. 34, April 1972.

CHAPTER 29

Architectural barriers

TIMOTHY J. NUGENT, Ph.D.

THE PROBLEM

The most frustrating of all problems to physically disabled individuals are buildings and facilities, supposedly created for the public, that are designed and constructed in such a manner that they prohibit the full participation of the physically disabled.

Standards that are recommended to facilitate the permanently physically disabled will be of benefit to everyone.

The standards herein referred can be incorporated in any type of building regardless of the basic architectural concept.

Approximately one out of every seven people in our nation has a permanent physical disability. Among these are many different causes and manifestations of physical disability and each has its own particular associated problems.

We are basically concerned with making it possible for the physically disabled individuals to be put to increased use by the elimination of architectural barriers.

It has been our purpose to develop standards and specifications for all buildings and facilities used by the public so that they will be accessible and functional to the physically handicapped to, through, and within their doors.

It is quickly recognized that the majority of buildings to be used in the next decade or two are already built. Therefore, the first problem is to determine what might be done to make accessible and functional existing buildings that are now

nonaccessible. The second task, the simpler of the two, is the development of the standards for proper design and construction of new buildings and facilities.

TYPES OF HANDICAPS

We are concerned with the following functional groups:

Nonambulatory, those individuals who for all practical purposes are bound to wheelchairs

Semiambulatory, those individuals who walk with difficulty or insecurity such as persons using orthoses or crutches, or both

Sight handicapped, those who are totally blind and whose sight is impaired to the extent that ambulation in public areas is insecure and hazardous

Disabilities of incoordination, faulty coordination or palsy from brain, spinal cord, or peripheral nerve injury

Hearing handicapped, persons who are deaf or have a hearing handicap to the extent that they might be insecure in major public areas or in industrial situations because they are unable to communicate or hear warning signals

Aging, those manifestations of the aging processes that significantly reduce mobility, agility, and perceptiveness

EXISTING BUILDING STANDARDS

The American National Standards Institute approved and published their specifications in

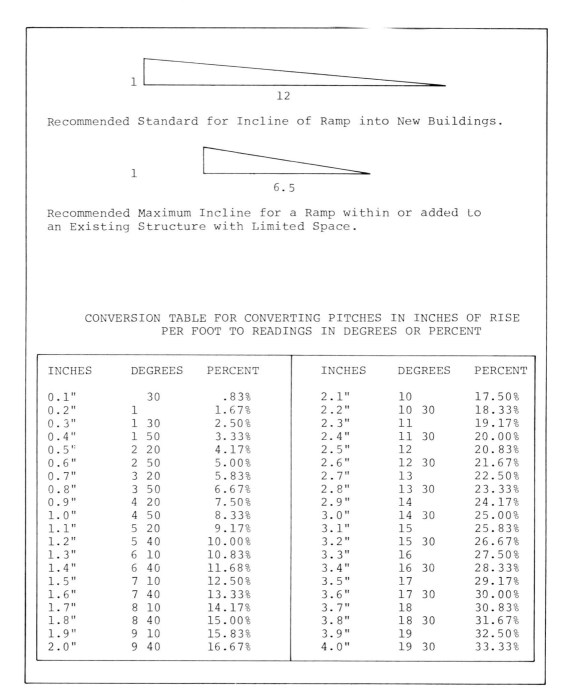

Fig. 29-1. Ramp gradients.

October 1961 for making buildings and facilities accessible to and useable by the physically handicapped.

The specifications are referred to in all national and state laws dealing with construction of facilities for the handicapped. They are in the process of being reviewed and revised, but the 1961 edition is currently in use. These specifications were made with the following wheelchair dimensions in mind.

The fixed turning radius of a standard wheelchair is 18 inches. The turning space required is 60 by 60 inches. A minimum of 60 inches is required for two wheelchairs to pass. The following are a few specifications taken from the 1961 information:

Walks

Public walks should be at least 48 inches wide and should have a gradient not greater than 5%.

Wherever walks cross other walks, driveways, or parking lots, they should blend to a common level.

A walk shall have a level platform at the top which is at least 5 feet by 5 feet, if a door swings out onto the platform or toward the walk.

Parking lots

Parking spaces for individuals with physical disabilities when placed between two conventional diagonal or head-on parking spaces should be 12 feet wide.

Ramps with gradients (Fig. 29-1)

A ramp shall not have a slope greater than one foot rise in 12 feet. This is a grade of 8.33% or a 4-degree, 50-minute angle.

It shall have handrails on at least one side, and preferably two sides, that are 32 inches in height . . . there shall be a nonslip surface.

Each ramp shall have at least 6 feet of straight clearance at the bottom and level platforms at 30-foot intervals. . . .

Doors and doorways

Doors shall have a clear opening of no less than 32 inches and shall be operable by a single effort.

Stairs

Stairs shall have handrails 32 inches high. . . . risers no higher than 7 inches.

Toilet rooms

Toilet rooms shall have at least one toilet stall that:

is 3 feet wide

is at least 5 feet deep

has a door that is 32 inches wide and swings out

has handrails on each side, 33 inches high and parallel to the floor, 1½ inches in outside diameter, 1½ inches from wall

Public telephones

Such telephones should be placed so that the dial, coin slots, and handset can be reached by individuals in wheelchairs. . . .

Controls

Switches and controls for light, heat, ventilation windows, draperies, fire alarms, water fountains, and all similar controls of frequent or essential use shall be placed within the reach of individuals in wheelchairs.

MATERIAL AVAILABLE ON ARCHITECTURAL BARRIERS

Guidebooks for motels, parks, public buildings, and so forth in each state that are accessible to the handicapped in wheelchairs or using ambulatory aids are available through the National Easter Seal Society, 2023 West Ogden Avenue, Chicago, Illinois 60612.

SUGGESTED READINGS

American Standards Association (now American National Standards Institute): American standard specifications for making buildings and facilities accessible to, and usable by, the physically handicapped, 1961. Single copies free from National Easter Seal Society for Crippled Children and Adults, 2023 W. Ogden Ave., Chicago, Illinois 60612. Additional copies may be purchased from American National Standards Institute, 10 E. 40th St., New York, New York 10016. $2 a copy.

Gives details of specifications for building approaches, ramps, doorways, floor surfaces, drinking fountains, telephone, and warning signals.

Callender, M. C., Corcoran, S. P., and Minden, M. B.: Bibliography on home management, with emphasis on work simplification for handicapped homemakers, 1960. Handicapped Homemaker Research Center, School of Home Economics, University of Connecticut, Storrs, Connecticut 06268.

Dantona, R., and Tessler, B.: Architectural barriers for the handicapped: A survey of the law in the United States, Reprinted from Rehabil. Lit. 28(2):34-43, Feb. 1967.

Hilleary, J. F.: Buildings for all to use: The goal of barrier-free architecture, AIA J. March 1969.

Kira, A.: Housing needs of the aged, with a guide to functional planning for the elderly and handicapped, Rehabil. Lit. 21(2):370-377, Dec. 1960. Reprint from National Easter Seal Society for Crippled Children and Adults, 2023 W.

Ogden Ave., Chicago, Illinois 60612. Free on request; ask for L-20.

Discusses types of housing needed and includes design and planning criteria for housing for the aged.

Laging, B.: Furniture design for the elderly, Rehabil. Lit. May 1966. Reprint from National Easter Seal Society for Crippled Children and Adults, 2023 W. Ogden Ave., Chicago, Illinois 60612. 25¢ Reprint DR-36.

Identifies the needs of the elderly and relates these to the design and construction of furniture that is scaled to the older person's living space requirements. Included are suggestions on well-planned storage units.

Mathiason, G., and Noakes, E. H.: Planning homes for the aged, 1959. Published by F. W. Dodge Corp. and available from McGraw-Hill Book Co., 330 W. 42nd St., New York, New York 10036, or from National Council on Aging, 1828 L. St., N.W., Washington, D.C. 20036. $12.75.

May, E. E., Waggoner, N. R., and Boettke, E. M.: Homemaking for the handicapped: A resource book in home management for the physically handicapped and their families and for professional personnel concerned with rehabilitation, 1966, Dodd, Mead & Co., 79 Madison Ave., New York, New York 10016. $7.50.

Sections on management and work simplification and on housing and kitchen planning for the handicapped contain suggestions useful for the architectural planning of homes for the disabled. Commercial sources of equipment and devices and information on adaptations incorporated in such homes are included.

McCullough, H. E.: Space and design requirements for wheelchair kitchens, 1960, Bull. 661. Available on request to Information Office, College of Agriculture, Mumford Hall, University of Illinois, Urbana, Illinois 61803.

McCullough, H. E., and Farnham, M. B.: Kitchens for women in wheelchairs, 1961. Extension Service in Agriculture and Home Economics, circ. no. 841. Available on request to Information Office, College of Agriculture, Mumford Hall, University of Illinois, Urbana, Illinois 61803.

Construction details for three major work centers (sink, range, and food preparation areas), for storage units, and for adaptations of commercial cabinets. Includes basic arrangements for U- or L-shaped and corridor type of kitchens.

Musson, N., and Heusinkveld, H.: Buildings for the elderly, 1963, Reinhold Publishing Corp., 430 Park Ave., New York, New York 10022. $17.50.

Authored by an architect and a member of the National Council on the Aging, this book is written mainly for architects and builders, laymen and community leaders interested in providing adequate satisfying housing for older people, and the elderly planning to build or resettle. About half the book is devoted to photographs, architectural plans, and drawings of existing or planned homes in many areas of the U.S.

National Easter Seal Society for Crippled Children and Adults: Easter seal guide to special camping programs, 1968, E-45, National Easter Society for Crippled Children and Adults, 2023 W. Ogden Ave., Chicago, Illinois 60612. $1.50.

Includes sections on camp site selection, buildings, and facilities, and health and safety.

New York State Department of Conservation. State Council of Parks and Outdoor Recreation: Outdoor recreation for the physically handicapped: A handbook of design standards, 1967, Albany, New York 12226.

Standards approved and adopted by the state council cover adaptations that are recommended for existing parks and for all future construction of public outdoor recreation areas in New York state.

Salmon, F. and Salmon, C. F.: Sheltered workshops: An architectural guide, 1966, Office of Engineering Research, Oklahoma State University, Stillwater, Oklahoma 74075. 90¢.

Describes the role of the sheltered workshop in the community and provides programming and planning information specific to this type of building. Applications of architectural planning principles are illustrated; since no two workshops are alike, there is no attempt to establish standards.

Schoenbohm, W. B.: Planning and operating facilities for crippled children, 1962, Charles C Thomas, Publisher, 301-327 E. Lawrence Av., Springfield, Illinois 62703. $11.50.

Part III of this book, "Planning a camp for crippled children" (p. 239-291), is mainly a discussion of preliminary planning for the residential camp, the various buildings to be included, and the planning of special facilities for swimming and recreational activities.

U.S. Bureau of Outdoor Recreation: Outdoor recreation planning for the handicapped. Prepared in cooperation with the National Recreation and Park Association, 1967, Technical Assistance Bull., April 1967. Available from Superintendent of Documents, U.S. Government Printing Office, Washington, D.C. 20402. 40¢.

Suggests methods for adapting and modifying playgrounds, swimming, and camping facilities, and other areas of recreation; specifications for adaptations of facilities are given.

U.S. Department of Transportation: Travel barriers, 1970. Available from Office of the Secretary, Department of Transportation, Washington, D.C. 20590.

This report summarizes the findings of a research program on the accessibility of public transportation to all Americans. The complete report entitled *Travel barriers* is available from the Clearinghouse for Federal Scientific and Technical Information, Springfield, Virginia 22151. PB #187 327, $3 a copy.

Washington State Department of Health: Guide to planning and equipping a handicraft facility for a nursing home activity program, prepared by Evelyn H. Bengson, 1964, Washington State Department of Health, Public Health Building, Olympia, Washington 98501. $2, plus 24¢ postage. (Address orders to: Mrs. Vera H. McCord, Coordinator, Rehabilitation Education Service Unit, Washington State Department of Health. Checks should be made payable to Treasurer, State of Washington.)

An aid for the nursing home administrator planning to install an extensive (or limited) craft area. The guide is quite specific in regard to location, space requirements, and special features of equipment. Suggested floor plans for a single-room and multiple-room activity area are included.

Wheeler, V. H.: Planning kitchens for handicapped homemakers, 1965, Rehabil. Lit. monograph XXVII, Publications Unit, Institute of Rehabilitation Medicine, 400 E. 34th St., New York, NY 10016. $2.00.

A monograph specifically concerned with the needs of severely disabled homemakers; emphasis is on the disabled person working in a wheelchair and on solutions that can be adapted for low-income families. It is equally useful in any kitchen planning service for the less severely disabled and in "long-distance" planning, when the rehabilitation center is not located near the patient's home. A suggested list of equipment and appliances is included.

Yuker, H. E., Cohn, A., and Feldman, M. A.: The development and effects of an inexpensive elevator for eliminating architectural barriers in public buildings, 1966, Hofstra University, Program for Higher Education of the Disabled, Hempstead, Long Island, New York 11550.

Describes the project to design, develop, install, and evaluate an inexpensive prototype wheelchair lift for use in public buildings; architectural specifications are included in the appendix.

Trends in research

COLIN A. McLAURIN, Sc.D.

Even a cursory examination of the needs for research in orthotics indicates the enormity of the work yet to be done. One may state with considerable validity that problems in orthotics, both in numbers and complexity, exceed those in prosthetics. Yet the number of practicing orthotists is about the same as the number of prosthetists. One may conclude that most of the patients requiring orthoses are either going without, or using some appliance that is less than satisfactory. If we are going to approach this problem intelligently, we must not only try to assess the requirements but build up as quickly as we can technical competence to a high level. The future of orthotics depends not so much on extending our present knowledge as on the ability of those we are now preparing for the future. It is, however, important that we do look at the present state of the art and especially the indicators that point the way to the future. To this must be added an open mind—readiness to accept new concepts, evaluation of them in a practical way, and a willingness to view the problems comprehensively as part of a total program. This is true whether they are problems of individual patient care or problems in the provision of service on a national basis.

From the standpoint of patient care, the development and adoption of standard patient assessment methods and standard prescription forms can do much toward adding logic to the design of the orthotic system. Although basing such design on biomechanical principles is a significant step, one must look further to include values that affect other physiologic factors and indeed the life style of the patient. For example, if we are considering orthoses for a paraplegic patient, are we trying to prevent contractures or provide joint stability for standing? Why do we want standing—for function and mobility, for physiologic reasons such as the prevention of osteoporosis and improved bladder function, or to provide self-esteem? It may be one or all of these reasons, but several questions must be asked. In what other ways can these be provided, either with one or several devices? What are the shortcomings? What are the costs in terms of appearance, difficulty in dressing, or difficulty in rising from a chair? We must also ask how much of the patients' time and effort will be absorbed in learning to use the appliance(s) and how much money it will cost.

Let us examine some of the newer concepts pointing the way to what we might expect in the future—areas where we might well invest some of our energy. These can be listed as follows:

1. Increased biomechanical information
2. New materials and techniques
3. Functional electrical stimulation
4. Biofeedback
5. Internal orthotics
6. Establishment of centers of competence
7. Education and training
8. The development of national programs

BIOMECHANICAL ANALYSIS

For anyone trained in engineering, the analysis of a problem situation in terms of the forces involved is a logical and necessary step toward the solution. In most orthotic problems the purpose of the orthosis is to impose or control sets of forces on the body to provide stability, mobility, and deformity prevention. The three-point principle has long been accepted and most orthotists can estimate the gross magnitude of the forces involved in simple applications such as long-leg orthoses. We are less aware of the dynamic requirements of an orthosis and less able to estimate the resisting forces on the internal structures of the body—bone, ligaments and tendons. We also have little information regarding what force patterns are necessary and safe in both magnitude and time cycle.

This rather gloomy picture does leave some measure for hope. The main reason why biomechanics has failed to make a significant impression in orthotics has been the lack of basic knowledge of the science among those actually working in the field. Most professionals who have made contributions in mechanics, either in prosthetics or orthotics, are academicians who have worked out force diagrams for various existing appliances and used this information in teaching orthotists, physicians, and therapists the rudiments of the analytical system. There are now a number of engineers who have graduated from bioengineering schools who are employed full time in clinical situations. Therefore we have, for the first time, technical competence at the working level. This alone does not ensure dramatic results in the near future, but it does provide a basis whereby the analytic process can develop as a useful tool in the clinic and the research labs. This technique is a way of determining patient requirements and establishing orthotic design goals.

Biomechanics can play a major role in such areas as the spine and the foot. Anyone who has witnessed a Harrington or Dwyer procedure for correcting scoliosis might wonder if there is not a better way of achieving spinal correction without sacrificing mobility of the spinal segments. The fact that a Milwaukee brace works at all, indicates that spinal correction can be achieved by force patterns induced either externally from the orthosis itself or internally from the muscle activity used in pulling away from throat mold and pads.

Galente in Chicago is recording data on the forces that occur between the orthosis and the patient. Frankel in Cleveland is developing a three-dimensional x-ray technique for accurately determining spinal curvature. Morris, Lucas, and Bressler in San Francisco have shown that the normal spinal column can barely support itself and therefore must rely on muscle activity and other force producing elements to maintain structural integrity. The work of these researchers and others, however, does not yet add up to sufficient knowledge to allow one to estimate what force pattern, internally or externally, might prevent spinal deformity. The evidence, however, is clear, that a thorough understanding of the structure and function of the back, the spinal column, with its ligaments and intrinsic muscles, and the abdominal and trunk musculature could open the possibility of providing more subtle ways of preventing deformities. The actual solutions to the problem might be in the form of new surgical procedures, stimulation of existing muscles, interference with bone formation, external application of forces on a consistent or intermittent schedule, or even a system of exercises. Whatever the solution, a more searching examination of the complex structural system of the spine and its supporting members might yield information leading to a variety of possibilities in managing spinal problems. Essential to such progress is a more thorough understanding of the biomechanics of the spine. It is important that we strongly encourage research in this area.

Similar arguments can be set forth supporting the biomechanical studies of the foot. Inman has shown the importance of the skeletal configuration in maintaining structural stability of the arch, but far too little is known about the role of the ligaments, fascia, and the intrinsic muscles. Furthermore most of the knowledge is related to feet that once were normal, but now present problems because of neurologic or physical impairment. It has been stated that most of the foot problems in the Western world are caused by improper footwear. The question arises as to what magnitude those forces are and where they should be applied. To this end a careful analysis of foot structure, both normal and pathologic, is indicated, even though the problem is complex in engineering terms. The solution lies in supporting the work of competent persons in continuing intensive investigation. As a nation we support tens of thousands of engineers doing mechanical analyses of man-made structures such as bridges, aircraft, and space vehicles that become obsolete in a matter of years. It is a pity that some of this effort cannot be directed to the human body, which we hope will remain with us for a long time with only slight modifications.

The affect of external pressure on tissue was the subject of a conference at Charlottesville, North Carolina, sponsored by the National Academy of Sciences, Committee on Prosthetics Research and Development. This included the soft tissues of the body, namely skin, subcutaneous tissue, and muscle. This work is important in the control and prevention of pressure sores in paralysis and myopathy. It has application in determining allowable skin pressures in orthotic applications and assessing allowable force requirements for preventing or correcting deformities.

In summary, increased knowledge of the properties of human tissue, an increased understanding of the mechanics involved in functional or correctional orthotics, and the use of engineering principles can lead to a more effective approach to problem solving. The foundations are being laid. Most professionals in orthotics and orthopaedics have some appreciation for the method. It remains to encourage growth in related studies and application before significant results can be expected in the years to come.

There are meanwhile some encouraging examples where biomechanical instrumentation and methods are being applied on a routine clinical basis. One such example is at Rancho Los Amigos, Downey, California, where Dr. Jacquelin Perry's kinesiology lab is used to assess patients as part of a diagnostic process before surgery and to assess the results of surgical and orthotic treatment. Another example can be found at Moss Rehabilitation Center, Philadelphia, Pennsylvania, where the locomotion laboratory is used to assess neurologic dysfunction prior to the precription of treatment and as a means for assessing results. From these and other laboratories we should expect a series of simple devices and procedures that can be used in less sophisticated clinics for routine diagnostic and evaluation purposes. The devices and method for recording the stance time in locomotion, as developed at the Rancho Los Amigos laboratory is one such example. Practical science in the clinic is an indication that we are at last coming of age in the routine application of mechanical principles.

MATERIALS AND TECHNIQUES

Almost every day some new material or some variation on an old material, with advantages in physical properties, lower cost, or formability, is introduced into the industrial market. Usually the advantages are slight and can have significance only in a large-scale production facility. Some of these newer materials can have direct application in orthotics often without any design change. For example, many of the metals used nowadays are aircraft-quality aluminum and steel. Even if there were minor changes in the composition of these materials, the result would be scarcely noticeable. In order for any dramatic changes to occur, we have to look beyond simple substitution of materials, into new concepts and fabrication methods. The most notable example of this can be found in the vacuum-formed plastic (AFO), ankle-foot orthoses, which are gradually replacing the conventional metal upright type. They are lighter, look better, may support the foot better, can be worn with a variety of footwear, and are easily fabricated. However, this is not a simple case of material substitution. It requires different thinking on the part of the orthotist and physician, different skills in fitting and fabrication, and different facilities, in particular a vacuum-forming machine. The introduction of this new thinking, new skill, and new equipment into the orthotic industry is opening up and will continue to open up, new applications for lower- and upper-limb orthoses at all levels. This might include spinal and cervical orthoses, custom-fitted seats and footwear, and even protective headwear. Some of these appliances can be preformed and adjusted individually. Some must be completely custom made. Materials can vary from rigid to flexible, and brightly colored to transparent; they can be made with a hard surface or a foam liner, or can be made with various combinations of these properties. New thermoforming plastics are being introduced rapidly. Some materials are now available that contain reinforcing glass fibers to give increased stiffness and strength and still be suitable for the same forming process. Fiber glass strips can be sandwiched between two layers of plastic to produce increased strength and rigidity in specific areas of the orthosis. Problems in ventilation or breathing seem to be the most serious difficulty in the use of plastic orthoses. Even here possibilities exist for forming porous sheets, requiring, in fabrication, a removable skin to seal the vacuum.

Perhaps the most suitable application of vacuum forming is in the construction of orthopaedic shoes. The traditional shoemaker is rapidly disappearing, and leather, although it has many desirable properties, tends to lose its shape and support characteristics. The shoes introduced by Tuck made from vinyl-covered Plastazote offer an inexpensive and comfortable substitute. They can be formed over a plaster cast of the foot to give more accurate fit than was ever possible with leather. With rubber soles and vinyl covers, durability is reasonable. This type of shoe is already finding favour with geriatric, arthritic, and leprosy patients and there is little doubt that the application will be expanded to include nearly all those for whom standard footwear is unsuitable.

In recent years, as more prosthetists have become involved in orthotics, the use of plastic laminates has crept into orthotic use. Often vacuum forming can replace the laminating procedure with saving in time and labor. There are still some applications where extra strength is required such as in joints or the springs used in some AFOs. Experience at the Veterans Administration Orthotic Center has shown that glass epoxy springs last very much longer than do steel springs. They are lighter and are also available in preimpregnated strips or rods that can be readily formed to almost any shape. The use of this technique to provide either a simple structural member or a reinforcing element has yet to be exploited. Its use in forming a framework for spinal orthoses is one obvious example.

The more exotic composite materials using fibers such as carbon and boron filaments are now approaching a cost low enough to be seriously considered. If properly used, they can provide a strength and stiffness equivalent to the finest steel at about one third the weight. However, when they break, they do so suddenly, like wood, leaving jagged splinters. It is possible that they can be used where stiffness and lightness are mandatory, but general application can be expected to be limited. Some possibility exists that they can be used for side bars and joints, obtained in the prefabricated condition and placed over a cast for curing in the desired contours.

Long neglected in orthotic practice is the use of pressure-distribution pads. In the past these have been combinations of leather, felt, and foam rubber with pneumatic pads in rare exceptions. Plastozote or foam polyethylene, when heat softened and molded to the proper contours, is finding its way into use, particularly for shoe insoles. Recent years have seen a variety of gel type of seat cushion introduced for paraplegic and quadriplegic patients. These provide both good and bad features. Gel or fluid, or even powder-lined cushions, seem to have an ability to distribute pressure more evenly. The same principle may be useful in pads over the knees, or malleoli, or other bone prominences where forces must be applied for stability or prevention of deformity. The advantages include adjustment by increasing or decreasing the amount of fluid in the pad. At the present time there is no easy method for the custom fabrication of the sacs or containers for the fluid, but the technical difficulties do not appear great and should be easily solved. The ability to fabricate custom-shaped, flexible, liquid-proof bags leads also to a whole new area in orthotics—the pneumatic orthosis. Introduced by the French and appearing very much like a pilot's g suit, these tightly laced garments contain tubes that when inflated produce sufficient rigidity at the knee, hips, and waist for a paraplegic to stand. The orthosis is light in weight and almost unnoticeable under male clothing but still presents some major problems. A major deterrant is the difficulty in obtaining a source of compressed air or gas. A portable bottle of CO_2 provides only enough for a few inflations. Pumps are even less portable. The principle, however, warrants further development and many possibilities exist, such as using the tubes only on joints and substituting plastic strips in other areas, or the use of incompressible fluids instead of gasses.

One possibly less critical use for the pneumatic principle is in spinal orthotics, where the ability to flex or extend is not a major concern. In the spinal brace, inflation after donning with the aid of a pump in the home is all that would be necessary. The ability to work with such materials is all that is needed in the orthotic industry to exploit the possibilities.

Plaster substitution is one other area where materials and techniques can play a major role. Vacuum forming for splints, shoes, and seats has generated the need for plaster casts and plaster models with the time, labor, and mess that it entails. At the present time there seems to be no direct substitute, but for some applications, the use of penumatic bags filled with pellets or powder can be used for taking impressions. When a vacuum is applied to the bag, it is pulled tightly over the pellets or powder causing them to become rigid or firm. A plaster positive can then be made of the impression and the seat vacuum can be formed in the usual manner. This technique is being effectively used in Little Rock, Arkansas. A similar procedure is used for casting below-knee stumps in the fabrication of prosthetic sockets in Holland. It remains to extend the technique so that the plastic seat can be formed directly over the pellet bag; thus the plaster can be eliminated completely. One of the difficulties is in eliminating the wrinkles and crevices in the pneumatic bag and in providing a smooth and acceptable contour. If this or other methods could be developed for general use in orthotics, great savings in time and money could be realized.

No review of orthosis would be complete without consideration of internal orthotic devices. These are highly specialized, but some developments may eliminate, assist, or replace external prosthesis. Possibilities that may have future application include artificial muscles in the form of rubber compounds that can serve as elastic internal structures. Possible examples also include pretibial or toe-lift devices for hemiplegia and hip extensors for the paraplegic. In some ways the springs used by Weiss to stabilize the spine can be considered as dynamic internal orthotic devices. The development of reliable, nonallergenic, inert materials is an essential first step. End fixation of such devices presents problems similar to those in joint replacement. The current work in finding substitutes for methylmethacrylate might well apply in future orthotic practice.

FUNCTIONAL ELECTRICAL STIMULATION

The electrical stimulation of paralyzed muscles into functional activity is at last approaching practical application, and the pioneering work of Leiberson and the remarkable vision of Reswick some 15 years ago are no longer distant possibilities.

It is true that the peroneal stimulator using surface electrodes (functional electrical stimulator) at present offers little or no functional advantage over a drop-foot orthosis. The wires and other paraphernalia are a nuisance to the wearer. Implanted devices require considerable surgery with associated expense and risks. From the evaluation program conducted by the Committee for Prosthetic Research and Development, however, some rather conclusive results are emerging. Patient acceptance is encouraging in selected cases, in particular with implanted devices. The stimulators and the muscles continue to perform after continued use. Wearers report less fatigue when using the stimulator as compared with a mechanical orthosis. Although this has yet to be proved, it is a good indication of patient acceptance. Other encouraging aspects include the possibilities for use in hip extension and other important muscle functions that are difficult, if not impossible, to achieve by use of external mechanical orthoses. In simple form the stimulated muscle could be used to effect a standing posture. It might be, we hope, programmed to selectively provide contraction during the stance phase. The variable control of muscle has been demonstrated by Mortimer and Marselais in Cleveland in producing hand function in quadriplegia. Their work has also indicated success in overcoming fatigue by cycling the stimulation sequentially through a pattern of electrodes. The recent introduction by Medronics Corporation of long-life batteries, avoiding the need for external power sources, and precutaneous transmission by induction also may enhance future possibilities. It remains only to develop an internal control system to render the systems capable of implantation.

The work at Rancho Los Amigos and elsewhere in using electrical stimulation for inducing therapeutic exercise to strength muscle and overcome contractures will stimulate its use in rehabilitation. Continued development in hardware, basic physiologic studies, and clinical experience can lead to a much wider application in the future. Note should be taken of the work of Clippinger at Duke University in implanting a stimulator in the peripheral nerve of a below-elbow amputee to provide some feedback of information on prehensile force. The same principle, if developed further, might well be an integral part of a stimulation system, providing position and force information from the activated muscles and limbs. The advent of microcircuitry makes possible intricate control systems—logical patterns of muscle activity to suit a variety of physical performances, triggered by sensors on the intact nervous system—heel switches, or joint- or posture-sensing devices. Many of the problems are complex and are still a long way from solution, but the way is clear however to the era when artificial neurosystems may become a routine practice.

Artificial neurosystems can also be considered as afferent, or feedback systems, to provide sensory information on a routine functional basis or as part of a therapy or training program. Biofeedback therapy for the physically handicapped may open a whole new field in orthotics, particularly for those patients with a sensory or proprioceptive neurologic deficit, but with intact motor power. Stroke and cerebral palsy are two examples of patients with such deficiency. The principle implied is that learning requires immediate and accurate feedback of information so that errors can be corrected and performance improved by repetition. Information that can be sensed and imparted to the patient can be derived from pressure transducers, joint-motion sensors or electrogoniometers, gravity-position sensors such as mercury switches, or muscle-action sensors as in electromyography. Information can be imparted to the patient by tactile devices, visual displays, or auditory signals. The validity of the principle is easily demonstrated. Patients, provided that they have the physical motor ability to perform the functional task, can quickly learn to control muscle activity, posture, joint position and weight bearing, when given the appropriate cues. Devices that provide this information can properly be called orthoses for the neurologic system and may play an important role in future therapy programs.

SCOPE

A few years ago orthopaedic appliances could be described in terms of special footwear, long and short leg braces, spinal and cervical braces, wheelchairs, crutches, and some rather complicated upper-limb orthoses. This group has already been expanded to include the vacuum-formed and pneumatic appliances, electrical stimulation and feedback, and consideration of internal devices of either electric or mechanical nature. The scope is further broadened into the area of special seats for improved support, function and pressure tolerance, mobility devices to allow various postures

and positions from lying, sitting, and standing. There is an increasing demand for improved powered mobility, particularly for the high-level spinal cord–injured patient. The conventional electric wheelchair, practically unaltered for a quarter of a century, is too cumbersome, heavy, costly, and unreliable and is limited to a smooth level environment. Smaller, neater electric wheelchairs are being developed, especially in Europe, for home or office use. Outdoor chairs are also becoming available. As yet the price in either category exceeds that which would permit a larger market, not just for the paralyzed patients but for the hundreds of thousands of geriatric and arthritic patients whose life style could benefit from some means of self-mobility. Vans, modified for wheelchair use, are becoming popular. Scott of Denver has shown that even a quadriplegic patient can operate one from an electric wheelchair. The need and technical feasibility have been established; it remains to work out the design criteria, technical details, and production models. The area of mobility is certainly the main area where external power can be used in rehabilitation appliances. Although some elaborate work has been done in powering both upper- and lower-limb orthoses, the technical and labor cost in fabricating, fitting, and maintaining such devices seems to far outweight the possible dividends. The experience at Rancho Los Amigos with a total electric arm clearly illustrates the limitations of powered devices that do not have control systems with a feedback loop. Even with a good feedback control system, the complexity and expense might well be excessive.

Another type of appliance is proving to be very useful to the severely handicapped. The environment control devices were introduced many years ago. In simple form they consist of a switching system, using breath or other available body motion to turn on lights, answer telephones, operate typewriters or computers, or any similar household or office task. Many centers throughout the Western world have reinvented their own models and from this first generation of design some new concepts utilizing computer logic offer vastly increased possibilities for the physically and neurologically impaired. Homebound vocational opportunities exist in computer-based industries such as hotel and travel reservation systems.

The list of environmental aids should include robot technology, particularly wheelchair-mounted manipulators. Present manipulators are grossly inefficient compared to normal hand operation. The need however for reaching and handling books and appliances, opening doors, pushing elevator buttons, eating, drinking, and other personal tasks is very great. It is interesting that so far no one has yet exploited the possibilities offered by more sophisticated manipulators and robots for these routine tasks.

CENTERS OF EXCELLENCE

The variety and complexity of existing appliance systems and the medical engineering knowledge required in their prescription and fitting challenges the competence of rehabilitation centers and their professional expertise in the original development of such appliances and their application. In addition to the customary medical specialties, experts in both mechanical and electrical engineering with a complement of trained technicians is required. Experience has shown that these technical experts must be well versed and involved in clinical problems and must be able to communicate easily with the medical and paramedical specialists. With this in mind the concept of rehabilitation engineering was formed. Well-established rehabilitation centers with large case loads would be reinforced with engineering and technical personnel on a full-time, essentially permanent, basis, with definitive and practical clinical goals to achieve. Ideally the center should be associated with medical and engineering schools so that students could be an integral part of the program and a new generation of rehabilitation engineers and medical students with an appreciation of practical engineering could develop.

These rehabilitation engineering centers could become centers for applied research, evaluation, clinical application, and staff education—centers where the more sophisticated yet practical possibilities that exist in technology for the handicapped can grow and flourish. The concept also includes cooperation with other centers so that a national program can emerge. Each center might have a specialty—a core program that could serve as a focus for other centers and projects. Each center could, if the case load and professional experience is suitable, also serve as a proving ground or evaluation unit for devices and techniques developed elsewhere.

Research should never be dissociated from the total program. This should include evaluation, education, production, distribution, and patient services. Evaluation and testing are an integral part of the development process and serve to introduce new techniques and devices into clinical practice in a controlled manner. Wider dissemination usually includes an education or training program, but the effect of education on research capability is a much larger story. It has already been stated that the potential need for orthotists is perhaps five or ten times the present number. Many of those will find their way into research programs, and the training they receive will determine to a considerable extent their ability and aptitude for research. This is of paramount importance in a program that must, through its own efforts, increase in scope and size in the next decade or so. The future depends not so much on the achievement of today as on the quality and competence of the people we are training for tomorrow. Many kinds of experts such as specialists in plastics, metals, and electronics, are required, but the people that are most needed are those who can combine their technical knowledge with the ability to relate to patients and to their colleagues in medicine. More and more the requirements are for the orthotist to be a true professional in his own right. Degree-level education, with possibilities for further advancement, is becoming almost mandatory.

With the current trend toward technical complexity, the orthotist might well benefit from an education in engineering instead of traditional brace making. If such a person is well schooled in clinical problems and has an appreciation for practical solutions, we can feel confident in the continued development in orthopaedic appliances and their application.

A NATIONAL PROGRAM

There are many facets to the provision of a national program that includes research, education, manufacturing and delivery of services. Perhaps one of the more important facets is acceptance by society of the handicapped person and of his right to participate in our way of life. This not only helps the handicapped psychologically by opening doors to a broader social and vocational life but renders possible political action leading to public transportation and building codes that do not exclude the disabled. If we openly accept the disabled person as a public responsibility, we are more likely to expect a dollar's worth of benefit for every dollar spent on his behalf. This can only lead to better rehabilitation and better assessment of the value of the various aspects of rehabilitation. This includes orthopaedic appliances and technical aids that are becoming possible. Hospital and institutional costs are presently enormous, so that an independent life for as many as possible of the 15 to 20 million handicapped persons in America is fast becoming an economic necessity.

The basis for such a program must include the ability to allocate funds, be they federal, state or private, in the most appropriate manner. Complete management programs for the handicapped are needed so that each professional person involved, from the physician to the vocational officer, can carry out the program in a coordinated manner.

The national program must also include means whereby evaluation can indicate which of the many possibilities is to be encouraged so that large production runs can be used to reduce costs and gain reliability. Above all, it must provide an information system so that all may share in newfound knowledge and so that no funds are misspent on duplicating research that has already been carried out.

Index